OPHTHALMOLOGY CLINICS-2
for Postgraduates
Basic Sciences, Instruments, Investigations, Imaging, Interpretation & Viva Voice

OPHTHALMOLOGY CLINICS-2
for Postgraduates
Basic Sciences, Instruments, Investigations, Imaging, Interpretation & Viva Voice

Second Edition

Editors

Prafulla Kumar Maharana MD DNB
Additional Professor
Dr Rajendra Prasad Centre for Ophthalmic Sciences
All India Institute of Medical Sciences
New Delhi, India

Namrata Sharma MD
Professor
Dr Rajendra Prasad Centre for Ophthalmic Sciences
All India Institute of Medical Sciences
New Delhi, India

Atul Kumar MD FAMS FRCS (Ed)
Medical Director
Department of Ophthalmology
AK Institute of Ophthalmology
New Delhi, India

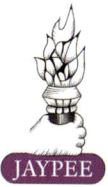

JAYPEE BROTHERS MEDICAL PUBLISHERS
The Health Sciences Publisher
New Delhi | London

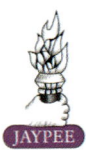 **Jaypee Brothers Medical Publishers (P) Ltd**

Headquarters
Jaypee Brothers Medical Publishers (P) Ltd
EMCA House, 23/23-B
Ansari Road, Daryaganj
New Delhi 110 002, India
Landline: +91-11-23272143, +91-11-23272703
+91-11-23282021, +91-11-23245672
Email: jaypee@jaypeebrothers.com

Corporate Office
Jaypee Brothers Medical Publishers (P) Ltd
4838/24, Ansari Road, Daryaganj
New Delhi 110 002, India
Phone: +91-11-43574357
Fax: +91-11-43574314
Email: jaypee@jaypeebrothers.com

Overseas Office
JP Medical Ltd.
83, Victoria Street, London
SW1H 0HW (UK)
Phone: +44 20 3170 8910
Fax: +44 (0)20 3008 6180
Email: info@jpmedpub.com

Website: www.jaypeebrothers.com
Website: www.jaypeedigital.com

© 2025, Jaypee Brothers Medical Publishers

The views and opinions expressed in this book are solely those of the original contributor(s)/author(s) and do not necessarily represent those of editor(s) or publisher of the book.

All rights reserved. No part of this publication may be reproduced, stored or transmitted in any form or by any means, electronic, mechanical, photocopying, recording or otherwise, without the prior permission in writing of the publishers.

All brand names and product names used in this book are trade names, service marks, trademarks or registered trademarks of their respective owners. The publisher is not associated with any product or vendor mentioned in this book.

Medical knowledge and practice change constantly. This book is designed to provide accurate, authoritative information about the subject matter in question. However, readers are advised to check the most current information available on procedures included and check information from the manufacturer of each product to be administered, to verify the recommended dose, formula, method and duration of administration, adverse effects and contraindications. It is the responsibility of the practitioner to take all appropriate safety precautions. Neither the publisher nor the author(s)/editor(s) assume any liability for any injury and/or damage to persons or property arising from or related to use of material in this book.

This book is sold on the understanding that the publisher is not engaged in providing professional medical services. If such advice or services are required, the services of a competent medical professional should be sought.

Every effort has been made where necessary to contact holders of copyright to obtain permission to reproduce copyright material. If any have been inadvertently overlooked, the publisher will be pleased to make the necessary arrangements at the first opportunity.

Inquiries for bulk sales may be solicited at: jaypee@jaypeebrothers.com

Ophthalmology Clinics-2 for Postgraduates: Basic Sciences, Instruments, Investigations, Imaging, Interpretation & Viva Voice

First Edition: 2020

Second Edition: **2025**

ISBN: 978-93-6616-127-3

Printed in India at Sterling Graphics Pvt. Ltd.

Dedicated to

*My parents, Mr Devendra Maharana and Mrs Binadini Maharana,
My wife Ritu Nagpal, My son Anay, and daughter Anayira*

—***Prafulla Kumar Maharana***

*My parents, Dr Ramesh C Sharma and Mrs Maitreyi Pushpa,
My husband Dr Subhash Chandra and daughter Vasavdatta*

—***Namrata Sharma***

*My late parents, Mr Sanat Kumar and Mrs Swarna Kumar,
My wife, Parul Kumar and children Aman and Arshi*

—***Atul Kumar***

Contributors

Aafreen Bari MD
Assistant Professor
Dr Rajendra Prasad Centre for Ophthalmic Sciences
All India Institute of Medical Sciences
New Delhi, India

Aayush Majumdar MBBS MD
Senior Resident
Dr Rajendra Prasad Centre for Ophthalmic Sciences
All India Institute of Medical Sciences
New Delhi, India

Abhipsa Sharma MD
Junior Ophthalmologist Consultant
LV Prasad Eye Institute
Visakhapatnam, Andhra Pradesh, India

Aditi Dubey MS
Associate Professor
Department of Ophthalmology
Gandhi Medical College
Bhopal, Madhya Pradesh, India

Alisha Kishore MD DNB
Assistant Professor
Government Medical College and Hospital
Chandigarh, India

Amber Bhayana MD
Assistant Professor
ESIC—Medical College and Postgraduate Institute of Medical Science and Research
New Delhi, India

Anin Sethi MD DNB FAICO
Consultant
Department of Glaucoma
Pediatric Ophthalmology and Strabismus
Dr Agarwals Eye Hospitals
Chandigarh, India

Ankit Singh Tomar MD
Consultant
Department of Ophthalmology
Tulane University School of Medicine
New Orleans Louisiana, USA

Anusha Sachan MD DNB FICO
Consultant
Department of Vitreoretina, Uvea, ROP and Cataract
EYE-Q Eye Hospitals
Hisar, Haryana, India

Arpit Sharma MD MRCS (Glasgow) FVRS FAICO
Assistant Professor
Geetanjali Medical College
Udaipur, Rajasthan, India

Asha Samdani MD (AIIMS, Delhi) DNB FICO
Consultant Ophthalmologist
Department of Squint, Oculoplasty and Cataract
Hyderabad, Telangana, India

Atul Kumar MD FAMS FRCS (Ed)
Medical Director
Department of Ophthalmology
AK Institute of Ophthalmology
New Delhi, India

Brijesh Takkar MD
Consultant
LV Prasad Eye Institute
Hyderabad, Telangana, India

Chandradevi Shanmugam MBBS MD
Clinical Ophthalmologist
Dr Rajendra Prasad Centre for Ophthalmic Sciences
All India Institute of Medical Sciences
New Delhi, India

Deepali Singhal
MD (AIIMS, Delhi) DNB FICO Fellowship
Refractive Surgery (Greece)
Director
Department of Cataract, Cornea, Refractive Surgery
AcktivVision EyeCare
Thane, Maharashtra, India

Contributors

Devesh Kumawat MD FRCOphth FRCS
Assistant Professor
Dr Rajendra Prasad Centre for Ophthalmic Sciences
All India Institute of Medical Sciences
New Delhi, India

Divya Agarwal MD DNB FICO
Medical Director
Vikalp Eye and Retina Centre
Bareilly, Uttar Pradesh, India

Gaurav Garg MD
Oculoplastic Fellow
Centre for Sight Superspecialty Eye Hospital
Hyderabad, Telangana, India
Former Professor
Department of Microbiology
Dr Rajendra Prasad Centre for Ophthalmic Sciences
All India Institute of Medical Sciences
New Delhi, India

Geeta Satpathy MD
Professor
Department of Microbiology
Dr Rajendra Prasad Centre for Ophthalmic Sciences
All India Institute of Medical Sciences
New Delhi, India

Gunjan Saluja MD DNB FRCS (Glasgow)
Director and Consultant
Bhatia Advanced Eye Care Centre
Bhilai, Chhattisgarh, India

Hannah Shiny R MD DNB FVRS
Assistant Professor
Sree Mookambika Institute of Medical Sciences
Kanyakumari, Tamil Nadu, India

Harika Regani MBBS MD
Director and Consultant
iFOCUS- The Eye and Esthetics, Superspeciality
Eye Hospital
Vijayawada, Andhra Pradesh, India

Jeewan Singh Titiyal MD
Professor
Dr Rajendra Prasad Centre for Ophthalmic Sciences
All India Institute of Medical Sciences
New Delhi, India

Jyoti Shakrawal MD
Assistant Professor
Department of Ophthalmology
All India Institute of Medical Sciences
Jodhpur, Rajasthan, India

Karthika Bhaskaran MD
Junior Resident, Ophthalmologist
Dr Rajendra Prasad Centre for Ophthalmic Sciences
All India Institute of Medical Sciences
New Delhi, India

Lohith Rambarki MD
Consultant
All India Institute of Medical Sciences
New Delhi
Visakha Eye Hospital
Visakhapatnam, Andhra Pradesh, India

Manasi Tripathi MD FRCS (Glasgow)
Senior Research Officer
Dr Rajendra Prasad Centre for Ophthalmic Sciences
All India Institute of Medical Sciences
New Delhi, India

Meenakshi Wadhwani MS PhD
Assistant Professor
Guru Nanak Eye Centre
Maulana Azad Medical College
New Delhi, India

Mohamed Ibrahime Asif
MD FRCOphth FRCS (Glasgow)
Consultant Ophthalmologist
Vasan Eye Care
Puducherry, India

Mohit Goyal MBBS MD
Senior Resident
Department of Ophthalmology
Government Medical College
Patiala, Punjab, India

Mousumi Bannerjee
MD FAICO (Retina and Vitreous)
Assistant Professor
Maharaja Agrasen Medical College
Agroha, Haryana, India

Namrata Sharma MD
Professor
Dr Rajendra Prasad Centre for Ophthalmic Sciences
All India Institute of Medical Sciences
New Delhi, India

Nasiq Hasan
MD (AIIMS) DNB FICO FICO (Vitreoretina)
FAICO (Vitreous & Retina)
Clinical Research Associate
University of Pittsburgh Medical Center
Pittsburgh, Pennsylvania, United States

Nawazish Shaikh MD
Research Officer
Dr Rajendra Prasad Centre for Ophthalmic Sciences
All India Institute of Medical Sciences
New Delhi, India

Nikita Gupta
MD MCh (Vitreoretinal Surgery) FICO FAICO
Consultant
Department of Retina and Uvea
Centre for Sight Hospital
New Delhi, India

Nishat Hussain Ahmed MD
Additional Professor
Department of Microbiology
Dr Rajendra Prasad Centre for Ophthalmic Sciences
All India Institute of Medical Sciences
New Delhi, India

Pallavi Shukla MD
Scientist B
Department of Community Ophthalmology
Dr Rajendra Prasad Centre for Ophthalmic Sciences
All India Institute of Medical Sciences
New Delhi, India

Pallavi Singh MD PhD (Community Ophthalmology)
Senior Resident
Dr Rajendra Prasad Centre for Ophthalmic Sciences
All India Institute of Medical Sciences
New Delhi, India

Prafulla Kumar Maharana MD DNB
Additional Professor
Dr Rajendra Prasad Centre for Ophthalmic Sciences
All India Institute of Medical Sciences
New Delhi, India

Pranita Sahay
MD (AIIMS Delhi) FRCOphth (London) FRCS (Glasgow)
FICO (Cornea) FAICO (Ref Sx) DNB
Assistant Professor
Guru Nanak Eye Centre
Maulana Azad Medical College
New Delhi, India

Praveen Vashist MD MSc (CEH)
Professor
Department of Community Ophthalmology
Dr Rajendra Prasad Centre for Ophthalmic Sciences
All India Institute of Medical Sciences
New Delhi, India

Priyanka MS
Senior Resident
Department of Ophthalmology
All India Institute of Medical Sciences
Bhopal, Madhya Pradesh, India

Priyanka Ramesh MD DNB FICO
Consultant Ophthalmologist
Ramesh Eye Clinic and Ophthalmic Microsurgical Center
Retina Institute of Karnataka
The Eye Foundation
Bengaluru, Karnataka, India

Rinky Agarwal MD DNB MNAMS
Consultant
The Sight Avenue
New Delhi, India

Ritu Nagpal MD
Senior Research Associate
Dr Rajendra Prasad Centre for Ophthalmic Sciences
All India Institute of Medical Sciences
New Delhi, India

Contributors

Rohan Chawla MD
Additional Professor
Dr Rajendra Prasad Centre for Ophthalmic Sciences
All India Institute of Medical Sciences
New Delhi, India

Sahil Agrawal MD FICO MRCSEd
Assistant Professor
Oculoplasty and Oncology Services
Dr Rajendra Prasad Centre for Ophthalmic Sciences
All India Institute of Medical Sciences
New Delhi, India

Saloni Gupta MS DNB MNAMS FICO
Consultant
Cornea and Cataract Services
Northern Railway Central Hospital
New Delhi, India

Sanjay Sharma MD
Professor
Department of Radiodiagnosis
Dr Rajendra Prasad Centre for Ophthalmic Sciences
All India Institute of Medical Sciences
New Delhi, India

Saurabh Verma MBBS
Senior Resident, Ophthalmologist
All India Institute of Medical Sciences
New Delhi, India

Savinay Kapur MD
Senior Resident
Department of Radiodiagnosis
Dr Rajendra Prasad Centre for Ophthalmic Sciences
All India Institute of Medical Sciences
New Delhi, India

Seema Kashyap MD
Professor
Department of Pathology
Dr Rajendra Prasad Centre for Ophthalmic Sciences
All India Institute of Medical Sciences
New Delhi, India

Shahnaz Anjum MD FRCS (Glasgow)
Consultant
Dr Rajendra Prasad Centre for Ophthalmic Sciences
All India Institute of Medical Sciences
New Delhi, India

Shipra Singhi MD
Consultant
Department of Ophthalmology
Medipulse Hospital
Jodhpur, Rajasthan, India

Shreya Nayak MD
Senior Resident
Dr Rajendra Prasad Centre for Ophthalmic Sciences
All India Institute of Medical Sciences
New Delhi, India

Siddhi Goel
MBBS MD (AIIMS – Gold Medalist) DNB FICO ICO (Cornea and External Disease)
Consultant and Head Unit-2 – Ophthalmology
Asian Institute of Medical Science
Faridabad, Haryana, India

Sitesh Kumar Bergaal MD
Consultant
Drishti Eye Hospital
Panchkula, Haryana, India

Sourabh Verma MD
Assistant Professor
Dr Rajendra Prasad Centre for Ophthalmic Sciences
All India Institute of Medical Sciences
New Delhi, India

Suman Lata MD DNB
Consultant
Department of Cornea, Cataract and Refractive
Grewal Eye Institute
Chandigarh, India

Suman Meena MD
Senior Resident
Dr Rajendra Prasad Centre for Ophthalmic Sciences
All India Institute of Medical Sciences
New Delhi, India

Suraj S Senjam MD
Additional Professor
Department of Community Ophthalmology
Dr Rajendra Prasad Centre for Ophthalmic Sciences
All India Institute of Medical Sciences
New Delhi, India

(Surg Capt) Srujana D MS
Professor and Senior Advisor
Department of Cornea, Lens and Refractive Surgery
Indian Naval Hospital Ship Asvini
Mumbai, Maharashtra, India

Talvir Sidhu MD DNB
Assistant Professor
Department of Ophthalmology
Government Medical College
Patiala, Punjab, India

Tanuj Dada MD
Professor
Dr Rajendra Prasad Centre for Ophthalmic Sciences
All India Institute of Medical Sciences
New Delhi, India

Vatika Jain MD FGS FAICO
Consultant Ophthalmologist
Tarabai Desai Charitable Eye Hospital
Jodhpur, Rajasthan, India

Vatsalya Venkatraman MD
Consultant Oculoplasty
ASG Eye Hospitals
Jodhpur, Rajasthan, India

Vivek Gupta MD
Assistant Professor
Department of Community Ophthalmology
Dr Rajendra Prasad Centre for Ophthalmic Sciences
All India Institute of Medical Sciences
New Delhi, India

Yogita Gupta MD
Assistant Professor
Lady Hardinge Medical College, Delhi
Senior Research Associate
All India Institute of Medical Sciences
New Delhi, India

Preface to the Second Edition

A Big Thank You to Everyone!

Dear readers, I am overwhelmed by the response our book has received from you all. A lot of hard work was involved while bringing out the first edition of this book. The best satisfaction is *"when hard work pays off"*.

The revised edition of the book has several additions. I have included new chapters on OCT Angiography, Wide-Field Imaging, Corneal Biomechanics and OCT in Glaucoma. In the instruments section, several new instruments including images have been included. I have included as many flowcharts and tables as possible to help the readers.

There were several errors in our earlier edition. I would like to thank the readers across India who communicated with me about these errors. I have tried our best to correct all the errors of the previous edition and to avoid any errors in the current edition.

The goal of this book is to help the Diploma/DNB/MS/MD (Ophthalmology) students appearing in various examinations across the world. I hope the revised edition will be helpful to the readers and it will receive the same appreciation as our previous edition.

Lastly, in spite of all the efforts, there may still be some errors, I request the readers to communicate with me so that I can make the necessary corrections.

All the Best

Prafulla Kumar Maharana
drpraful13@gmail.com

Preface to the First Edition

First of all, we thank the readers for the tremendous positive response to our earlier book *"Ophthalmology Clinics for Postgraduates"*. Just to reiterate "Postgraduate examination is one of the most difficult and stressful milestones in the medical profession. It entails a tremendous amount of stress on the candidates who appear for the examination." Our previous book was primarily targeted at the discussion on cases that are often given as long and short cases. However, any examination is not complete without going through the much difficult phase of viva based on the various investigations, their result and interpretation. Besides, investigations and their interpretation are an invaluable tool for diagnosis of common clinical problems seen in day-to-day practice.

Imaging in ophthalmology has dramatically advanced over the last decade. It is often difficult for a student to get information about all the investigation tools at one place. Similarly, a general practitioner often finds it difficult to interpret the outputs of so many investigating tools. This book attempts to present important investigative tools in a format that is exactly the same as required in the practical examinations and day-to-day practice for an ophthalmologist.

The primary focus is on principles of different investigative tools, and the clinical interpretation of their outputs. Special emphasis has been given to present the outputs in different clinical cases that are often encountered in day-to-day practice and postgraduate examinations. Every possible effort has been made to include photographs of all-important cases seen in the outpatient department (OPD), and given as cases in examinations.

A section on Basic Sciences such as Ocular Pathology, Ocular Microbiology, and Community Ophthalmology have been included. This will help the students to appear in viva examinations. A section on Orbital Imaging will help the students and practitioners to be able to diagnose the common clinical situations seen in day-to-day practice. In addition, a chapter on instruments has been included with every section, which is invariably a part of all postgraduate practical examinations. The editors and all the contributors have made sincere efforts to make things simple and concise to facilitate quick and thorough revision. Each chapter ends with a section on viva questions that will help the candidates to mentally prepare for the viva before the final examination.

Lastly, we remind the postgraduate students that the book is not a replacement for the standard textbooks, but it will make their understanding and application easier whenever there is some doubt or confusion.

The editors wish the best of luck to the students for their examinations!

Prafulla Kumar Maharana
Namrata Sharma
Atul Kumar

Contents

SECTION 1 — Appliances and Instruments

1. **Oculoplasty and Orbital Imaging** 3
   - 1.1 Exophthalmometry 3
     Pallavi Singh, Siddhi Goel
   - 1.2 Orbital Imaging Techniques 7
     Sanjay Sharma, Savinay Kapur
   - 1.3 A Pattern-based Approach to Radiologic Diagnosis in Ophthalmology: Part I 15
     Sanjay Sharma, Savinay Kapur
   - 1.4 A Pattern-based Approach to Radiologic Diagnosis in Ophthalmology: Part II 23
     Sanjay Sharma, Savinay Kapur
   - 1.5 Ultrasonography 31
     Asha Samdani, Aditi Dubey
   - 1.6 Appliances and Instruments in Oculoplasty 44
     Saloni Gupta, Sahil Agrawal, Pranita Sahay

2. **Cornea** 56
   - 2.1 Slit-lamp Biomicroscopy 56
     Rinky Agarwal, Sitesh Kumar Bergaal, Ritu Nagpal, Namrata Sharma
   - 2.2 Keratometer 68
     Ritu Nagpal, Siddhi Goel, Shipra Singhi, Prafulla Kumar Maharana
   - 2.3 Pentacam 72
     Prafulla Kumar Maharana, Siddhi Goel, Abhipsa Sharma, Pranita Sahay, Anin Sethi, Jeewan Singh Titiyal
   - 2.4 Aberrometers 88
     Prafulla Kumar Maharana, Deepali Singhal, Aafreen Bari, Siddhi Goel
   - 2.5 Anterior Segment Optical Coherence Tomography 99
     Sourabh Verma, Talvir Sidhu, Deepali Singhal, Manasi Tripathi, Namrata Sharma
   - 2.6 Specular Microscope 112
     Manasi Tripathi, Pranita Sahay, Mohamed Ibrahime Asif, Divya Agarwal, Prafulla Kumar Maharana
   - 2.7 Ultrasonic Pachymeter 122
     Pranita Sahay, Mohamed Ibrahime Asif, Manasi Tripathi, Namrata Sharma
   - 2.8 Orbscan 127
     Alisha Kishore, Pranita Sahay, Ritu Nagpal
   - 2.9 Corneal Biomechanics 135
     Ritu Nagpal, Chandradevi Shanmugam
   - 2.10 Appliances and Instruments in Cornea 142
     Pranita Sahay, Mohamed Ibrahime Asif, Devesh Kumawat, Namrata Sharma

3. Cataract 153

3.1 Intraocular Lens Master 153
Deepali Singhal, Alisha Kishore, Arpit Sharma, Prafulla Kumar Maharana

3.2 LenStar 159
Yogita Gupta, Deepali Singhal, Prafulla Kumar Maharana

3.3 A-Scan 162
(Surg Capt) Srujana D, Mohamed Ibrahime Asif, Pranita Sahay, Ritu Nagpal

3.4 Appliances and Instruments in Cataract Surgery 166
Pranita Sahay, Prafulla Kumar Maharana

4. Retina and Uvea 176

4.1 Ophthalmoscope 176
Alisha Kishore, Hannah Shiny R, Suman Meena, Pranita Sahay

4.2 Fundus Fluorescein Angiography 182
Nasiq Hasan, Priyanka, Brijesh Takkar, Rohan Chawla, Atul Kumar

4.3 Optical Coherence Tomography 192
Priyanka Ramesh, Nawazish Shaikh, Nasiq Hasan, Aayush Majumdar, Atul Kumar

4.4 Indocyanine Green Angiography 202
Anusha Sachan, Nasiq Hasan, Atul Kumar

4.5 Electroretinogram 204
Sourabh Verma, Lohith Rambarki, Divya Agarwal

4.6 Multispot Laser System 212
Anusha Sachan, Brijesh Takkar, Amber Bhayana

4.7 Adaptive Optics 215
Anusha Sachan, Divya Agarwal, Rohan Chawla

4.8 Amsler Grid 218
Ankit Singh Tomar, Saurabh Verma, Atul Kumar

4.9 Vitreoretinal Instruments 221
Devesh Kumawat, Pranita Sahay, Anusha Sachan, Atul Kumar

4.10 Optical Coherence Tomography Angiography 227
Aayush Majumdar, Nawazish Shaikh, Saurabh Verma

4.11 Ultra-widefield Imaging 237
Aayush Majumdar, Nawazish Shaikh, Saurabh Verma

5. Glaucoma 245

5.1 Gonioscopy 245
Talvir Sidhu, Tanuj Dada

5.2 Tonometry 256
Jyoti Shakrawal, Talvir Sidhu, Shahnaz Anjum

5.3 Optic Nerve Head Evaluation 264
Talvir Sidhu, Mohit Goyal, Tanuj Dada

5.4 Perimetry Part 1: Kinetic Perimetry—Goldmann Visual Field 274
Jyoti Shakrawal, Talvir Sidhu, Nikita Gupta

5.5 Perimetry Part 2: Static Perimetry—Humphrey Visual Field 280
Talvir Sidhu, Jyoti Shakrawal, Harika Regani, Tanuj Dada

5.6 Ultrasound Biomicroscopy and Anterior Segment
Optical Coherence Tomography in Glaucoma 296
Talvir Sidhu, Saurabh Verma, Tanuj Dada

5.7 Optical Coherence Tomography in Glaucoma—Interpretation 302
Talvir Sidhu, Jyoti Shakrawal, Ritu Nagpal, Tanuj Dada

5.8 Heidelberg Retina Tomograph 318
Gaurav Garg, Jyoti Shakrawal

5.9 Instruments Used in Glaucoma Surgeries...326
Vatsalya Venkatraman, Pranita Sahay, Jyoti Shakrawal

6. Squint and Neuro-Ophthalmology 330

6.1 Hess Chart/Lees Screen 330
Ritu Nagpal, Mousumi Bannerjee, Anin Sethi, Pallavi Singh

6.2 Synoptophore..337
Pallavi Singh, Vatika Jain, Pranita Sahay

6.3 Tests for Binocular Vision and Stereopsis...342
Pallavi Singh, Shreya Nayak, Pranita Sahay

6.4 Instruments for Squint Surgery 351
Pranita Sahay, Devesh Kumawat, Divya Agarwal, Karthika Bhaskaran

SECTION 2 — Basic Sciences

7. Pathology Basics 359
Seema Kashyap, Siddhi Goel, Suman Lata, Prafulla Kumar Maharana

8. Ocular Microbiology 375
Siddhi Goel, Nishat Hussain Ahmed, Geeta Satpathy

9. Community Ophthalmology 384

9.1 Blindness: Definition, Burden, Prevention, and Rehabilitation 384
Vivek Gupta, Pallavi Shukla, Suraj S Senjam, Meenakshi Wadhwani, Praveen Vashist

9.2 Survey Methods in Ophthalmology 395
Vivek Gupta, Meenakshi Wadhwani, Praveen Vashist, Suraj S Senjam

SECTION 3 — Interpretation of Images and Reports

10. Interpretation of Images 407
Pranita Sahay, Jyoti Shakrawal, Gunjan Saluja, Siddhi Goel

Index 429

SECTION 1: Appliances and Instruments

1. Oculoplasty and Orbital Imaging
2. Cornea
3. Cataract
4. Retina and Uvea
5. Glaucoma
6. Squint and Neuro-Ophthalmology

CHAPTER 1: Oculoplasty and Orbital Imaging

1.1 EXOPHTHALMOMETRY

Pallavi Singh, Siddhi Goel

INTRODUCTION

Disorders of the orbit are quite commonly seen in ophthalmic practice. These are often associated with displacement of the globe from its normal position in the orbit. Exophthalmometer is an instrument used for measuring the degree of displacement of the globe. It is used for measurement of both exophthalmos as well as enophthalmos.

PRINCIPLE

Exophthalmometry is the science of quantitatively assessing the position of the globe in the orbit, by measuring the distance of the anterior corneal apex from the lateral margins. There are three different types of clinical exophthalmometry:
1. *Absolute:* Comparison with the normal values seen in the general population
2. *Relative:* Comparison of one eye with the other
3. *Comparative:* Comparison of measurements of one eye over a period

TYPES OF EXOPHTHALMOMETER

Various types of exophthalmometers have been described over the years. The first such device, called ophthalmoprostatometer was developed by Cohn in 1865.[1] Perpendicular globe position was obtained by Zehender, by placing a mirror medial to the cornea and parallel to his ruler. A sighting device was placed lateral to the ruler and exactly opposite to the marked center of the mirror, to ensure perpendicular position of the globe. The Hertel exophthalmometer was introduced in 1905 and till date remains the most popular device used for clinical exophthalmometry. Luedde invented a pocket-sized device in 1938, which was an inexpensive and useful alternative to the previous devices. In 1970, Davanger sought to eliminate the error caused in measurement by parallax by introducing a prism, which moves forward and back. Naugle and Couvillion described their exophthalmometer in 1992, which uses superior and inferior orbital rims as reference points, thus enabling measurements in cases of lateral orbital wall fractures. Hertel's exophthalmometer has been variously modified to use the external auditory meatus as the point of reference (Yeatts) and with a fixation adapter to fixate on the forehead and nose (Kratky and Hurwitz). Computed tomography (CT) scans can be used to document the degree of proptosis accurately, however, they are expensive, time-consuming, and cause radiation exposure.[1]

TECHNIQUE

To use the Hertel's exophthalmometer, the examiner sits opposite the patient at eye level. The instrument is then placed at both the lateral orbital rims and the base distance between the two is noted. The examiner asks the patient to look straight ahead with eyelids wide open. Each eye is measured separately for proptosis by looking into the mirror (which has a millimeter scale marked on it) with one eye and moving the head side to side until the red fixation lines match up, thus eliminating any parallax. The examiner can now determine the position of the corneal apex of the patient from the millimeter reading.

NORMAL VALUES

The normal values in exophthalmometry are taken as 10–23 mm (average 16 mm) in whites, and 12–23 mm (average 18 mm) in blacks. On an average, in the Indian population, a value of greater than 21 mm or a difference of 2 mm or greater between two eyes is considered significant.[2,3]

VIVA QUESTIONS

1. What are the different types of exophthalmometry?

Ans. There are three different types of exophthalmometry:
1. *Absolute:* Comparison with the normal values seen in the general population
2. *Relative:*
   a. Comparison of one eye with the other
   b. Normal values are ≤2 mm
3. *Comparative:*
   a. Serial exophthalmometry readings of the same eye are compared over time.
   b. It is better to use the same instrument.
   c. Useful in Graves' disease
   d. Hertel preferred over Luedde

2. Name different types of exophthalmometers.

Ans. Hertel, Naugle, Luedde, Zehender, Davanger, and Gormaz are a few different types of exophthalmometers.

Hertel's (Figs. 1.1.1 and 1.1.2):
- It has a footplates (or yokes) "grooved arc" to fit over bony temporal margin of lateral orbital rim; a crossbar to establish baseline and to allow for binocular reading.
- It uses prisms (Marco's) or mirrors (B&L's or Lombart's) incline at 45° from sagittal plane.
- Overall dimensions are 25 × 7 × 2 cm. Weight is 117 g (4.1 oz)/light weight or 216 g (7.6 oz)/heavy duty.
- Scale for orbital wall goes from 75 to 121 mm.
- The scale to measure the proptosis ranges from 0 to 35 mm.

Luedde (Fig. 1.1.3):
- It is a transparent, plastic ruler that gives measurement in millimeters. It has a notch that conforms to angle of lateral orbital rim.

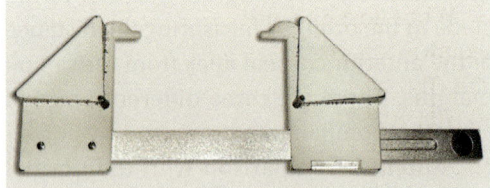

Fig. 1.1.1: Hertel's exophthalmometer.

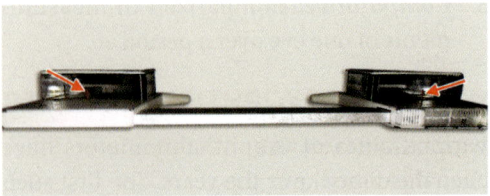

Fig. 1.1.2: Hertel's exophthalmometer with the red line used for parallax.

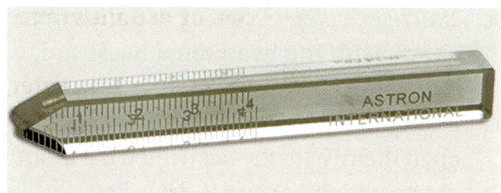

Fig. 1.1.3: Luedde exophthalmometer.

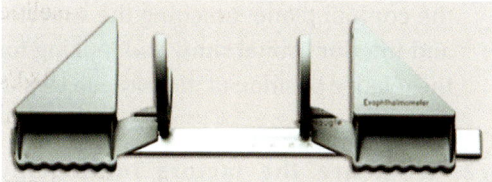

Fig. 1.1.4: Naugle's exophthalmometer.

- *Scale readings*: 0 mm (end of notch) to 40 mm
- Parallax is minimized by using scale on both sides of the rod (advantages of using Luedde over a standard ophthalmic millimeter ruler).

Naugle's exophthalmometer (Fig. 1.1.4): This is an inferior and superior rim-based instrument. It may be used when the lateral orbital rim is not intact.

3. What are the advantages of Hertel's exophthalmometer?

Ans. The advantages are:
- *Binocular reading:* It provides the ability to measure both eyes simultaneously and the measurement of the distance between lateral orbital rims.
- *Baseline for sequential readings:* It is also useful for serial follow-ups of the same patient.
- Best for comparative exophthalmometry

4. What are the disadvantages of Hertel's exophthalmometer?

Ans. The disadvantages are:
- Parallax error while performing measurements—tilting of instrument leading to minor deviations in position result in gross variations in reading.
- Difficulty of visualizing the scale under conditions of low illumination, which may result in inaccurate readings.
- Variations in the distance between the two halves of the instruments lead to displacement of the footplate, which considerably affects the measurement.
- It is also a relatively expensive instrument.
- Induced error may occur when measuring globes that are not horizontally at the same level.
- Narrow base on Hertel—difficult setting up
- Facial bone deformity—may cause unreliable measurements due to unparallel placement of device while measuring globes that are not horizontally at the same level.
- Poor fixation or convergence can lead to unreliable measurement.

5. What are the advantages of Luedde's exophthalmometer over Hertel's?

Ans. The advantages are:
- Luedde's exophthalmometer measures degree of proptosis of each eye separately, thus is useful in cases of *facial asymmetry*.
- It is pocket-sized, portable, and easily stored.
- It is easier to clean and sterilize.
- It is cheaper as compared to the Hertel's exophthalmometer.
- It can be used in presence of *strabismus*.

6. What are the advantages of Naugle's exophthalmometer over Hertel's?

Ans. Advantages are:
- Naugle's exophthalmometer uses a prism that can move backward and forward, which *eliminates parallax*.
- It utilizes superior and inferior orbital rims for measurement, thus can be used in cases of *lateral orbital rim fractures*.

- It also has the advantage of measuring hyperophthalmos and hypo-ophthalmos with a vertical gradient scale.

7. What is the definition of exophthalmos/enophthalmos?

Ans. Exophthalmos is a protrusion of the eyeball due to an increase in orbital contents in a normal bony orbit. Protrusion of the eyeball >21 mm or a difference of 2 mm between both the eyes is defined as proptosis/exophthalmos. Enophthalmos is abnormal posterior displacement of globe (sinking of eyeball into orbit).

8. What are the causes of pseudoproptosis?

Ans. Causes are:
- Facial asymmetry
- Unilateral high myopia
- Buphthalmic eye
- Lid retraction
- Enophthalmos of the other eye

9. What is exorbitism?

Ans. Exorbitism is a protrusion of the eyeball due to a decrease in capacity of the orbital container, with a normal orbital content volume, as seen in Crouzon's syndrome.

10. How is proptosis measured on CT scan?

Ans. The method described by Hilal and Trokel is most commonly used.[4] In a midaxial CT scan, a line is drawn connecting the tips of the orbital rims. The perpendicular distance from this line to each corneal apex is measured. Proptosis is present if either line measures greater than 21 mm or the difference between the two eyes is >2 mm.

11. What are clinical ways to assess exophthalmos?

Ans. The various examination techniques are:
- *Worm's eye view:* Looking at the patient from down below, when the head is tilted backward to look for protrusion of the eyeball
- *Naffziger's view:* Looking at patient from above, with the head tilted backward, to look for eyeball protrusion; alternatively, asking the patient to close eyes and then open them, with the head tilted backward, to see which cornea is seen first on eye opening
- *Ruler method:* Placing a ruler parallel to the coronal plane, touching the superior and inferior orbital rims, and looking for the relative position of the corneal apex to the ruler.

12. What are the factors influencing exophthalmometry reading?

Ans. Several factors can influence exophthalmometry reading such as:[3]
- *Age:* Lower readings are recorded for children (average 14 mm). In children and teenagers mean exophthalmometric measurements increase with age.[5]
  - <4 years old (13.2 mm)
  - 5-8 years old (14.4 mm)
  - 9-12 years old (15.2 mm)
  - 13-17 years old (16.2 mm)
- *Sex:* Males have higher readings (~1 mm)
- *Posture:* In supine position, normal eyes sink back 1-3 mm in Graves' disease, eyes are not affected by this phenomena.
- *Ethnicity:* Blacks have higher reading. Asians have smaller ranges.
- *Spherical equivalent:* Negatively correlated.[3]
- *Axial length (AL):* Positively correlated.[3]

REFERENCES

1. Genders SW, Mourits DL, Jasem M, Kloos RJ, Saeed P, Mourits MP. Parallax-free Exophthalmometry: a comprehensive review of the literature on clinical exophthalmometry and the introduction of the first parallax-free exophthalmometer. Orbit. 2015;34(1):23-9.
2. Karti O, Selver OB, Karahan E, Zengin MO, Uyar M. The Effect of Age, Gender,

Refractive Status and Axial Length on the Measurements of Hertel Exophthalmometry. Open Ophthalmol J. 2015;9:113-5.
3. Ramli N, Kala S, Samsudin A, Rahmat K, Abidin ZZ. Proptosis: Correlation and Agreement between Hertel Exophthalmometry and Computed Tomography. Orbit. 2015;34(5):257-62.
4. Hilal SK, Trokel SL. Computerized tomography of the orbit using thin sections. Semin Roentgenol. 1977;12(2):137-47.
5. Dijkstal JM, Bothun ED, Harrison AR, Lee MS. Normal exophthalmometry measurements in a United States pediatric population. Ophthalmic Plast Reconstr Surg. 2012;28(1):54-6.

1.2 ORBITAL IMAGING TECHNIQUES

Sanjay Sharma, Savinay Kapur

ORBITAL RADIOGRAPHS

Standard projections for the bony orbit include posteroanterior (PA) **(Fig. 1.2.1A)**, lateral **(Fig. 1.2.1B)**, and optic foramen view **(Fig. 1.2.1C)**. The patient can either be seated, standing or semiprone. The PA projection also called the occipitofrontal view is done with a 20° caudal tilt, with the central beam exiting at the nasion. On the radiographs, the innominate line **(Fig. 1.2.1A**, black arrows) should cross the greater wing of sphenoid on the temporal side of the orbit. For the lateral view, the patient is positioned with the mid sagittal plane of the skull placed parallel to

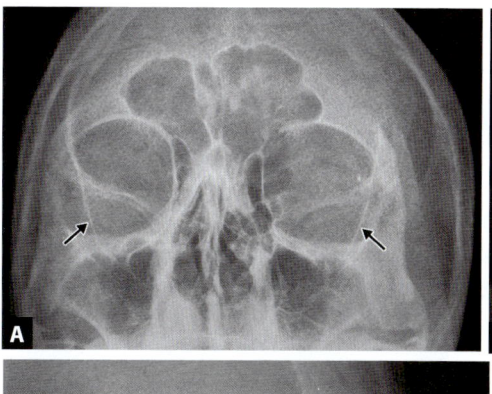

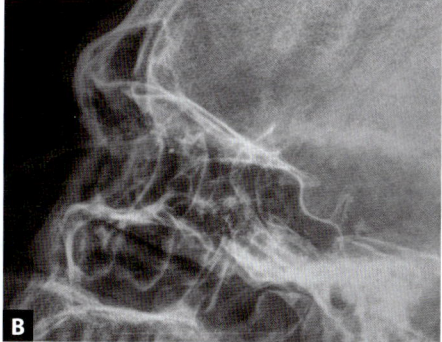

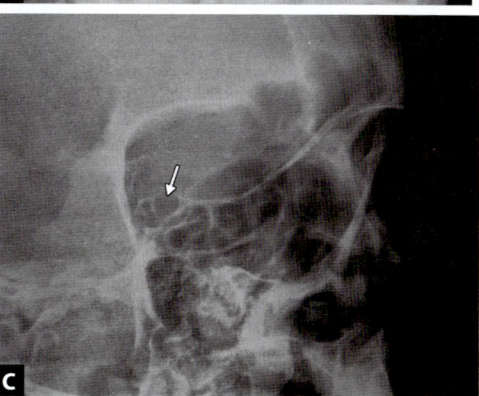

Figs. 1.2.1A to C: Different commonly done normal orbital radiographs views. (A) Anteroposterior (AP) view; (B) lateral view; and (C) optic foramen view (marked by a white arrow). Black arrows mark the innominate line.

the image receptor. The beam is centered at a point 2.5 cm posterior to the outer canthus. To evaluate whether a radiograph is true lateral or not, look at the superimposition of the floor of the anterior cranial fossa on both sides. For visualizing the optic foramen, Rhese projection is used. Here the head is placed on the detector face first such that cheek, nose, and chin touch the detector, with orbit in center. The head is tilted in a manner that the orbitomeatal line is perpendicular to the detector, keeping the midsagittal plane at an angle of 53° to the image receptor. Beam is centered 2.5 cm superior and 2.5 cm posterior to the upper external auditory meatus. The superior orbital fissure and optic foramen are well seen on this view as are the margins of the orbit. With the increasing use of modern cross-sectional imaging this view is not commonly requested. The current use of orbital radiographs are limited to patients with trauma or suspected intraorbital foreign body. In many centers, it is now restricted only to exclude foreign body prior to a magnetic resonance imaging (MRI) examination.

ULTRASOUND

Nowadays, ultrasound is considered as an extension of physical examination due to its easy availability and noninvasive nature. It is the first line of investigation for evaluation of ocular and orbital pathology. Its main utility lies in evaluation of intraocular lesions, especially when the media is opaque. It also acts as a problem-solving tool after CT/MRI as it allows for differentiation of cystic from solid lesions. Also, being a dynamic modality, it can be used to assess intraorbital pathologies and extraocular muscles (EOMs) in various stages of contraction. However, an inherent limitation of ultrasound is the trade-off between image resolution and depth of evaluation. High-frequency probes permit high-resolution imaging, but allow only limited depth of evaluation. Hence, its utility for evaluation of deep-seated orbital pathologies is limited. Both A (amplitude) and B (brightness) **(Fig. 1.2.2A)** mode scans are used. The A-mode scan is mainly used by ophthalmologists where spikes are produced by the returning echoes from different interfaces within the eye. B-mode scan of the eyeball is done with a linear high-resolution array transducer with frequency between 7.5 and 10 MHz. For evaluation of the orbit, a lower frequency probe with 5–7.5 MHz bandwidth is used. To maintain an air-free interface, coupling gel is applied over closed eyelids. In a normal individual, the anterior and posterior chambers are cystic (no echoes seen within anechoic) with an echogenic lens present between the two. Posterior to the globe, echogenic fat **(Fig. 1.2.2A)** is seen with a central hypoechoic linear structure representing the optic nerve sheath complex (ONSC) **(Fig. 1.2.2A)**. A color Doppler evaluation may be done to evaluate the blood flow in suspected persistent hyperplastic primary vitreous (PHPV) **(Fig. 1.2.2B**, shown

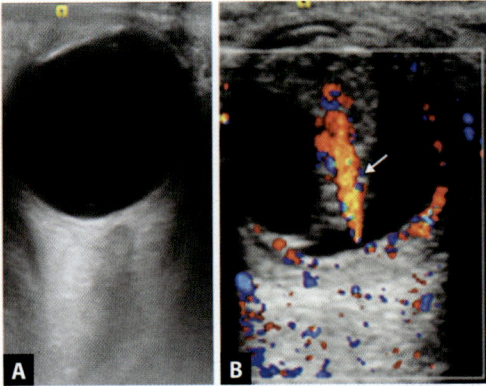

Figs. 1.2.2A and B: (A) Normal orbital ultrasound; (B) Doppler in a child with persistent hyperplastic primary vitreous (PHPV) showing embryonic vascular channel marked by a white arrow.

by a white arrow) tumors and vascular malformations. In vascular lesions such as arteriovenous malformation (AVM) and caroticocavernous fistula, spectral trace can be obtained to confirm the arterial or venous nature of flow. This information has an important therapeutic implication. Another new tool, which can add to the evaluation of intraocular masses is contrast-enhanced ultrasound. Microbubble-based ultrasound contrast agents stay within the intravascular compartment and hence differentiate masses from pseudomasses [like retinal detachment (RD)/hemorrhage] as well as can potentially help to characterize masses as these tend to have different contrast kinetics. Ultrasound elastography is a yet another tool that evaluates the elasticity of a tissue that may find applications in times to come. Ultrasound biomicroscopy (UBM) is another exciting application for the evaluation of anterior chamber. It uses a high >30 MHz transducer to produce high-resolution two-dimensional grayscale images of the anterior chamber.

■ COMPUTED TOMOGRAPHY

Computed tomography is a main orbital imaging modality which utilizes X-rays to generate cross-sectional images (slices). This volumetric cross-sectional information is used by software techniques to provide multiplanar images [along axial **(Fig. 1.2.3A)**/coronal **(Fig. 1.2.3B)**/sagittal/curved planes] as well as volume-rendered imaging (3D dataset, **Fig. 1.2.3C**).

Computed tomography scanning is based on the following principles:
- The images are acquired by a 360° rapid rotation of the X-ray tube around the patient. In modern CT scanners, the table moves horizontally through the gantry,

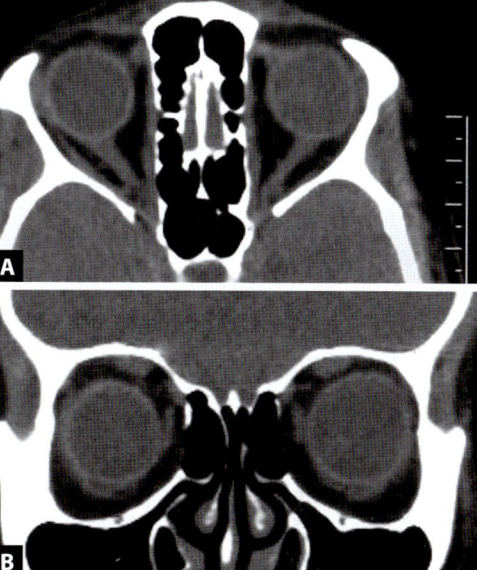

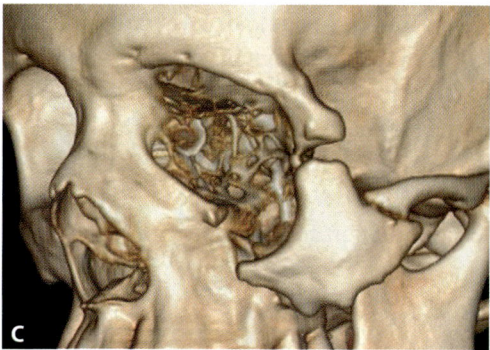

Figs. 1.2.3A to C: Normal orbital computed tomography (CT) sections; (A) axial; and (B) coronal; (C) A 3D volume-rendered view in an adult with left tripod fracture.

which houses the X-ray source and the detectors to generate helical (spiral) dataset.
- As the X-rays pass through the patient, they are attenuated depending on the radiographic density (attenuation coefficient) of tissues through which they pass. The scattered and transmitted radiation is then measured by a ring of sensitive detectors located in the gantry around the patient.

- Hence, each point in the body is imaged by a number of X-ray beams at different angles which allows for depth assessment (third dimension). The final image is reconstructed from multiple X-ray projections depending on the attenuation coefficients of the tissues through which beam passes.
- Filtered back projection is the most commonly used method by which attenuation data is converted to an image.
- The attenuation value of tissues is expressed on a scale named *Hounsfield units (HU)* with a range of 3,000 HU. Cortex of bones generally has an attenuation value of around +800 to +1,000 HU (white on the CT image), air has an attenuation value in the range of –800 to –1,000 HU (black on the CT image), muscles and soft tissues have an attenuation value of +40 to +80 HU while fat has an attenuation of –40 to –80 HU. Water is defined by having zero attenuation as a standard reference.

CONTRAST-ENHANCED COMPUTED TOMOGRAPHY IMAGING

Contrast-enhanced CT (CECT) imaging of the orbit and brain is obtained following intravenous injection of an iodinated contrast medium. Enhancement of various tissues following contrast administration depends on their blood flow and vascular permeability. Iso-osmolar-iodinated contrast media like iohexol (Omnipaque) and iodixanol (Visipaque) are used routinely with iodine concentration between 300 and 350 mg I/mL. Orbital fat provides an intrinsic background contrast against which some orbital pathologies can be visualized without requiring a contrast medium.

ACQUISITION AND INTERPRETATION OF COMPUTED TOMOGRAPHY

The first step in acquisition of CT scans is obtaining a scout image/scannogram/localizer. For orbital CT, a lateral scout view is obtained, which is a low-dose X-ray projection where there is no gantry rotation around the patient but taken with a fixed position of the X-ray source and detectors. The use of a scannogram is to plan the acquisition and specify the craniocaudal extent of the scan. Volumetric data is now obtained with overlap between slices of the helix so that 3D reconstruction can be obtained.

Contrast can be given hand-injected or by a pressure injector. For routine CECT, a hand injection is a safer, cheaper, and acceptable technique. Generally 50 mL of contrast in adults (2 mL/kg for children) would suffice for most indications. However, in cases where CT angiogram is required a pressure injector must be used. Angiograms are arterial phase images to evaluate arterial anatomy/supply (like in suspected AVMs and sometimes caroticocavernous fistula).

On hard copy CT films, the scannogram is usually displayed as the first image on the CT film, preceding the series of axial images. The scout view not only gives an overview, but also allows confirmation of the fact that the entire region of interest has been included in the scanned area.

MAGNETIC RESONANCE IMAGING

Principle

Hydrogen is the most abundant element in human body. It has unpaired protons in their nuclei and therefore behaves as tiny magnet. These protons precess about their axis and as a result have a very small associated magnetic field. However, as they precess in different directions and are randomly oriented inside the body, the net magnetization vector is nullified. However, it changes when the human body is placed in a strong external magnetic field. The protons inside the hydrogen atoms act like tiny dipoles and get aligned along the direction of magnetic field, being either parallel or antiparallel to the field (longitudinal magnetization). They also rotate around their axes following the strength of the magnetic field. When a radiofrequency pulse is applied, these tiny dipoles are tilted off the equilibrium and start to precess in phase with one another in a direction perpendicular to the axis of the main magnetic field (transverse magnetization). When external pulse is switched off, the longitudinal magnetization is regained with time (T1 relaxation). There is also a loss of the transverse magnetization (T2 relaxation). T1 and T2 relaxation times (time needed to regain 66% of longitudinal magnetization and lose 66% of transverse magnetization, respectively) depend upon the composition of the tissue and also the environment in which the tissue is situated. Hence, different magnetic resonance (MR) sequences can be designed to make use of this difference in T1 and T2 relaxation times to display difference in composition of different tissues. These sequences can have different T1 and T2 weighting to display contrast between tissues, which have different T1 and T2 relaxation times.

Magnetic Resonance Imaging Contrast Media

Most commonly used compounds for contrast enhancement are gadolinium-based. These are also extracellular agents like CT contrast media and are distributed in the intravascular and interstitial tissues depending on the blood flow and permeability. They shorten the T1 relaxation times and hence are bright on T1-weighted (T1W) images. Because fat is also bright on T1W images it needs to be suppressed so that enhancement is not masked due to bright signal of fat. Hence, postcontrast images are generally fat suppressed.

When to Choose MRI Over CT?

- Higher contrast resolution needed—characterization of masses and soft-tissue lesions
- To assess intracranial pathologies including cranial nerves and cavernous sinus pathologies
- To see intracranial extent/spread of extra-cranial pathologies like fungal sinusitis
- Children.

Basic Image Sequences in MRI

T1-Weighted Images
(Figs. 1.2.4A and 1.2.5A)

Tissues with shorter T1 relaxation times such as fat appear brighter than those with longer T1 relaxation times such as water, vitreous, and cerebrospinal fluid (CSF).

It is the best sequence for studying anatomy.

Substances bright on T1 images:
- Fat
- Melanin
- Gadolinium
- Soft calcium
- Methemoglobin (subacute hemorrhage)
- High protein/exudative fluid like in craniopharyngiomas/posterior pituitary

T2-Weighted Images
(Figs. 1.2.4B and 1.2.5B)

Tissues with longer T2-relaxation like water, vitreous, and CSF appear brighter than tissues with shorter T2-relaxation such as blood products.

Fluid Attenuation Inversion Recovery (Fig. 1.2.5C)

Signals from free fluid can be suppressed using the fluid attenuation inversion recovery (FLAIR) sequence. FLAIR is especially useful in demyelinating conditions where white matter hyperintensities on T2W images are better appreciated when the bright signal from the adjacent CSF in the ventricles is nulled.

It is the best sequence for studying in brain pathology.

Fat-Suppressed Images (Figs. 1.2.4B and C)

Bright signals from intraorbital fat can mask the signal and enhancing pathologies. This problem can be overcome by suppressing the signal of fat by unique fat suppression sequences. It is an ideal sequence for identifying intraorbital pathology along with postcontrast T1W images.

Postcontrast Images (Figs. 1.2.4C and 1.2.5D)

Gadolinium does not cross the blood–brain barrier (BBB) and hence does not cause enhancement in the brain when BBB is intact. When the BBB is disrupted, gadolinium diffuses into the interstitial spaces resulting in their enhancement.

> *Normally enhancing structures in orbit*:
> - Lacrimal glands, EOMs, and uveal tract:
>   - Structure which never enhances normally:
>   - Optic nerve

Diffusion-Weighted Images

Primary application of diffusion-weighted images (DWI) in the brain is to look for acute infarcts. When there is cytotoxic edema, the cells swell and there is a restriction of diffusion in the extracellular space. This is reflected as a bright signal on DWI and low signal on apparent diffusion coefficient (ADC) maps. Always look at ADC maps to differentiate true diffusion restriction from "T2 shine through" (T2 bright areas may appear bright on DWI

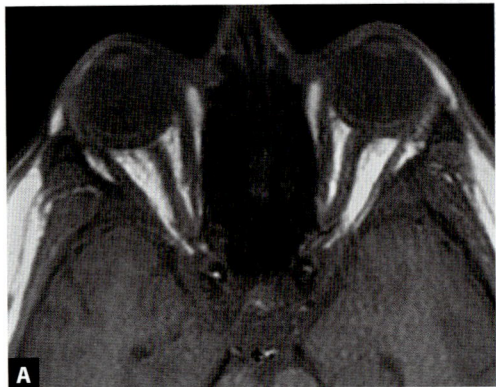
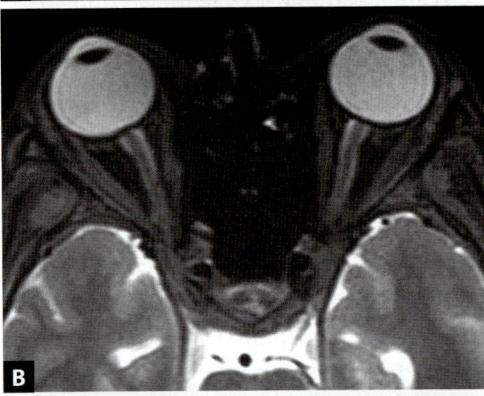
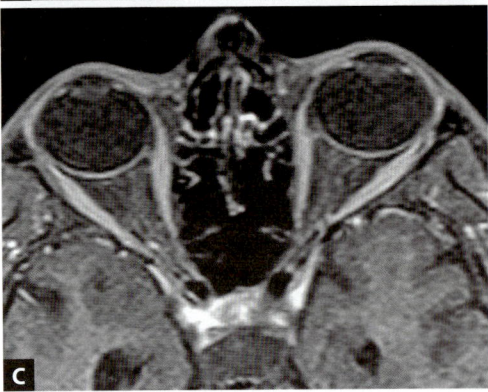

Figs. 1.2.4A to C: Routine normal magnetic resonance imaging (MRI) sequences of orbit in axial plane. (A) T1-weighted; (B) T2-weighted fat suppressed; (C) T1-weighted postcontrast images.

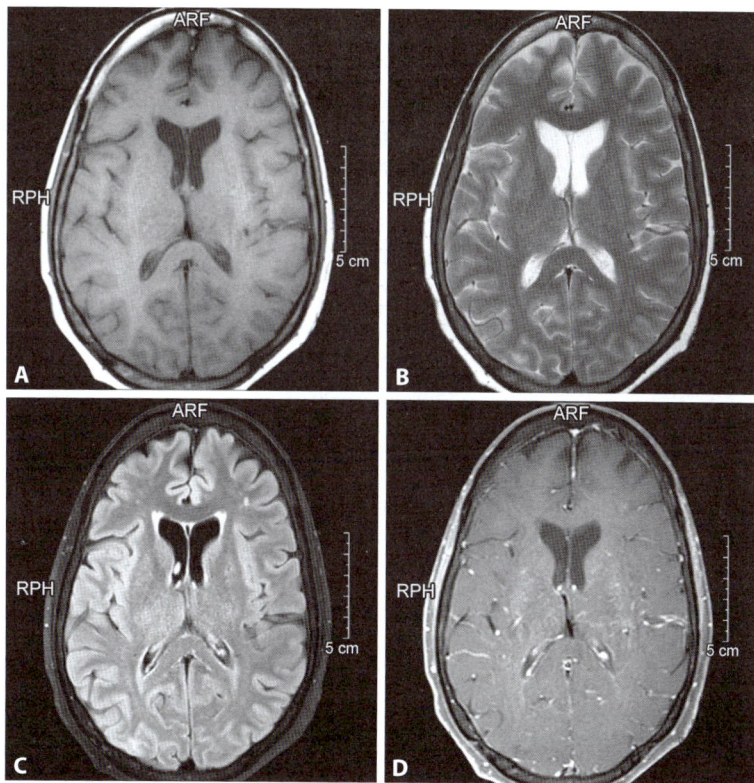

Figs. 1.2.5A to D: Routine normal magnetic resonance imaging (MRI) sequences of brain in axial plane. (A) T1-weighted; (B) T2-weighted; (C) Fluid attenuation inversion recovery (FLAIR); (D) T1-weighted postcontrast images. (ARF: acoustic radiation force; RPH: relative peak height)

images without having diffusion restriction, however these are bright on ADC images as well).

Susceptibility-Weighted Images

Magnetic resonance imaging sequences can either be spin echo or gradient echo sequences. The technique of gradient echo images is beyond the scope of this book. However, it is important to know the utility of these images **(Table 1.2.1)**. Susceptibility-weighted images (SWIs) are very sensitive to local field inhomogeneities and hence are therefore best to look for calcification and deoxyhemoglobin (hemorrhage).

Standard brain protocol—routine sections are taken at 5 mm.

Basic protocol:
- Axial T2
- Sagittal T2
- Axial T1
- Axial FLAIR

Extended protocol:
- SWI
- DWI
- Post-gadolinium—axial/sagittal/coronal images

Orbit protocol:
- Thin (3 mm sections) T2 axial
- Thin T1 axial
- Thin T2 fat saturation axial, coronal (oblique sagittal on the side of pathology)
- Thin T1 fat saturation postcontrast images in all three planes

TABLE 1.2.1: Appearances (signal) of various tissues on standard MRI sequence.

Tissues	T1WI	T2WI	FLAIR/fat saturation
Free water (like in cysts/CSF)	Dark	Bright	Suppressed (dark)
Fat	Bright	Bright	Suppressed (dark)
Interstitial fluid secondary to increased vascular permeability in inflammatory/neoplastic pathology	Dark	Bright	Bright

Note: The terminology used to describe images is as follows:
Dark = Hypointense
Bright = Hyperintense
(On CT, dark = hypodense, bright = hyperdense)
(CSF: cerebrospinal fluid; CT: computed tomography; FLAIR: fluid attenuation inversion recovery; MRI: magnetic resonance imaging; T1WI: T1-weighted image; T2WI: T2-weighted image)

For brain lesions, intensity is defined with respect to gray matter. Any lesion with signal intensity higher than the cortex (brighter) is said to be hyperintense and lesions darker than gray matter are hypointense by definition.

EMISSION COMPUTED TOMOGRAPHY

Emission CT is a form of scintigraphy wherein a radioactive tracer substance is injected intravenously. The tracer substance acts as a source of radiation for imaging. However, the spatial resolution is lower compared to CT as well as MRI. With single-photon emission computed tomography (SPECT), the radionuclides emit gamma and X-rays, and the images are obtained using a rotating gamma camera. This technique allows detection of disturbances of BBB as well as abnormalities of cerebral blood flow. *Positron emission tomography (PET)* on the other hand utilizes a β+ emitting nuclide (^{11}carbon and ^{18}fluorine) and is based on the concept of positron annihilation. It is frequently employed when there is suspicion of a systemic disease coexisting with orbital disease.

VIVA QUESTIONS

1. When to order a CECT scan?
Ans. The following clinical situations require an additional injection of a contrast medium:

- *Mass lesions*: Benign/malignant tumors
- *Vascular lesions*: Caroticocavernous fistula (CT angiogram)/cavernous sinus pathology
- *Inflammatory conditions*: Optic neuritis, cysticercosis, panophthalmitis/orbital cellulitis, especially if suspecting an abscess

2. (More importantly) when to order a noncontrast-enhanced CT scan?
Ans.
- Where the clinical indication is for detection and localization of foreign bodies or trauma where assessment of bony fractures/EOM entrapment is of primary concern.
- To differentiate between acute hemorrhage and mass lesions as both would be bright on contrast-enhanced images (blood is hyperdense on NCCT scan, most mass lesions are not).
- As a complimentary tool for detection of calcification/bony destruction in masses already being evaluated by MRI.
- When there is a contraindication to iodinated contrast media—renal function derangement/known contrast allergy.
- Thyroid ophthalmopathy to evaluate anatomy of EOMs and crowding at orbital apex.

1.3 A PATTERN-BASED APPROACH TO RADIOLOGIC DIAGNOSIS IN OPHTHALMOLOGY: PART I

Sanjay Sharma, Savinay Kapur

▪ INTRODUCTION

Most orbital pathologies can be divided into six basic imaging patterns:
1. *Intraocular:* Retinoblastoma (RB), melanoma, metastasis, and endophthalmitis
2. *Intraconal:* Cavernous malformation, venous varix, lymphoproliferative disease and metastasis, and venolymphatic malformation
3. *Extraconal:* Dermoid, lacrimal gland masses, bone lesions, venolymphatic malformation, schwannoma, hemangiopericytoma, capillary hemangioma, sinonasal masses with orbital extension, postseptal infection, and lymphoproliferative lesions *(subperiosteal space is separate from extraconal compartment)*
4. *ONSC lesions:* Meningioma, glioma, sarcoidosis, optic neuritis, idiopathic orbital inflammation (IOI), and lymphoproliferative disease *(these are intraconal lesions)*
5. *Conal (EOM enlargement of various etiologies):* Thyroid-associated orbitopathy, IOI, carotid-cavernous fistula (CCF), sarcoidosis, lymphoproliferative disease and metastasis, myocysticercus, and traumatic contusion
6. *Infiltrative diseases:* Metastasis, IOI, lymphoproliferative disease, cellulitis, sarcoidosis, plexiform neurofibroma (PNF), and rhabdomyosarcoma (RMS)

Pearl:
- Three most common intraorbital pathologies—thyroid orbitopathy, lymphoproliferative disorders, and IOI
- Three most common transcompartmental orbital lesions—IOI, capillary hemangioma, and venolymphatic malformation

▪ INTRACONAL LESIONS

Cavernous Hemangioma (A Slow-Flow Venous Malformation)

Typical presentation: Painless, progressive proptosis in a middle-aged woman.

Imaging findings: They appear as well-defined (pathologically encapsulated), oval to round, and homogeneous masses with a density somewhat greater than that of the muscle. They are typically located within the intraconal space (especially laterally), but larger lesions may extend outside the muscle cone. Bone remodeling is seen with large and longstanding lesions. Small foci of calcification are sometimes present which represent phleboliths. Enhancement is generally moderate owing to the low vascular flow. The lesion enhances progressively with homogeneous enhancement on delayed images **(Fig. 1.3.1)**. On MRI, the lesion is

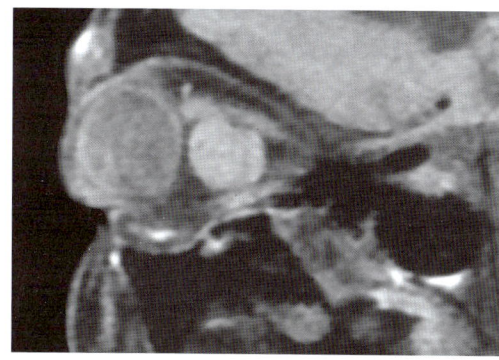

Fig. 1.3.1: Oblique parasagittal T1-weighted (T1W) fat suppressed postcontrast magnetic resonance imaging (MRI), with *cavernous hemangioma,* showing an ovoid enhancing soft-tissue intraconal mass separate from the optic nerve.

hypointense on T1, hyperintense on T2WIs. Intralesional hemorrhage is uncommon (cf. cerebral cavernous malformation and lymphatic malformation).

Lymphangioma (Venolymphatic Malformation)

Typical presentation: Gradual, painless progressive proptosis in a child, often painful when sudden in onset.

Imaging findings: They appear as irregular heterogeneous masses, which are poorly defined (pathologically unencapsulated) and insinuate along normal orbital structures. They are known to cross anatomic boundaries such as the orbital septum and fascial layers. They can be macrocystic or microcystic. The macrocystic variant has multiple low-density cystic areas while in the microcystic variants the cysts are too small (to be seen on imaging) and hence look like a soft-tissue mass. There is mild or no contrast enhancement. The wall and septae may show patchy enhancement, typically less than capillary hemangioma. Larger lesions may cause bone remodeling with extension into preseptal or infratemporal fossa through the inferior orbital fissure. MR is the investigation of choice for evaluating the extent of lesion. Signal characteristics depend on the presence or absence of proteinaceous contents/blood products within the lesion. In the absence of these, the cystic areas are hypointense on T1 and hyperintense on T2. Blood–fluid levels are characteristically seen in the setting of recent intralesional hemorrhage **(Fig. 1.3.2)**.

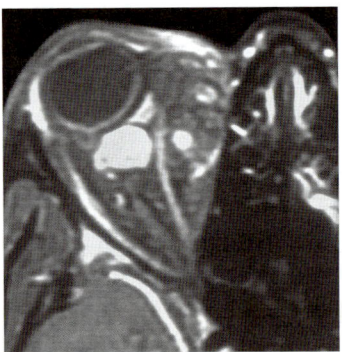

Fig. 1.3.2: Axial T1-weighted (T1W) fat suppressed postcontrast magnetic resonance imaging (MRI), with *lymphangioma (synonym: venolymphatic malformation)* showing a transcompartmental ill-circumscribed mass lesion with foci of hemorrhage and fluid–fluid levels.

Venous Varix

Typical presentation: Painless, progressive proptosis that increases on stooping forward/Valsalva.

Imaging findings: Orbital varix represents a form of hamartoma, with thin-walled distensible venous channels that communicate with the normal orbital venous vasculature. Ultrasound is a highly useful modality for their diagnosis as it allows for dynamic assessment. The dilated venous channels collapse in the upright posture or at rest, but on straining, the increased blood flow with dilation of channels becomes obvious. On CT, the varices appear as an irregular or smooth variably enhancing lesion located at the orbital apex, which significantly increases in size with straining. However, as the study requires dynamicity and straining CT and MRI are seldom used for diagnosis. Once it is thrombosed, patients may present with acute-onset retro-orbital pain and proptosis. CT at this time shows no change on straining and absence of enhancement. The lesion may appear hyperdense on NCCT due to hemorrhagic contents. MRI done at this time will show a well-defined T1/T2 heterogeneously hyperintense lesion due to hemorrhagic contents.

Pearl: Orbital varices can be a difficult radiologic diagnosis (on CT/MRI), as the discrete venous channels are seldom visualized.

Lymphoproliferative Disease and Intraconal Metastasis

These are difficult to differentiate from other intraconal masses and need evidence of a primary elsewhere to make this diagnosis. Rapid increase in size may be a pointer. Systemic work is warranted.

■ EXTRACONAL LESIONS

Dermoid Cyst

Typical presentation: Child or young adult with a mass near the frontozygomatic/frontoethmoid suture often with globe dystopia.

Imaging findings: It typically appears as a round to oval, well-defined lesion, located in the anterior superotemporal orbit. It is almost always extraconal and has a cystic center with areas of fat within **(Fig. 1.3.3)**. A fat–fluid level may be present. Denser foci within the lesion represent flecks of keratin and sebum. The cyst is surrounded by a thin rim of tissue that may be partially calcified. Adjacent bone commonly shows remodeling/sutural widening. Occasionally, the cystic cavity extends into the temporal fossa or the intracranial space. Contrast administration may produce mild enhancement of cyst rim, but not its center. On MRI, the lesion tends to be heterogeneously hyperintense on T2WI and hypointense on T1WI, however, areas of T1 hyperintensity are seen within the mass, which show signal dropout on fat-suppressed images.

Orbital Schwannoma

Typical presentation: Painless, progressive proptosis along with symptoms due to mass effect on surrounding structures. This may be present acutely with painful proptosis in cases of hemorrhage into the lesion.

Imaging findings: They are typically extraconal though they can be intraconal or extraconal or both. They commonly involve the frontal branches of the ophthalmic division of the trigeminal nerve. Schwannomas have a heterogeneous T2 signal **(Fig. 1.3.4)** and variable patterns of enhancement with homogeneous or ring enhancement being most common.

> Orbital schwannomas can show delayed homogeneous enhancement like cavernous malformations, but do not follow the centripetal enhancement pattern of the latter.

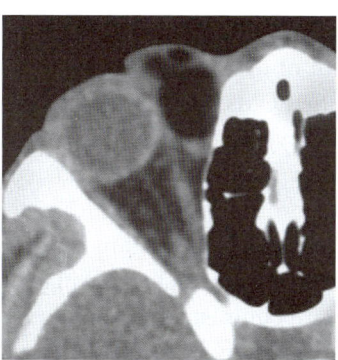

Fig. 1.3.3: Axial noncontrast computed tomography (CT), with right medial angular *dermoid*, showing a well-defined mass of fat attenuation.

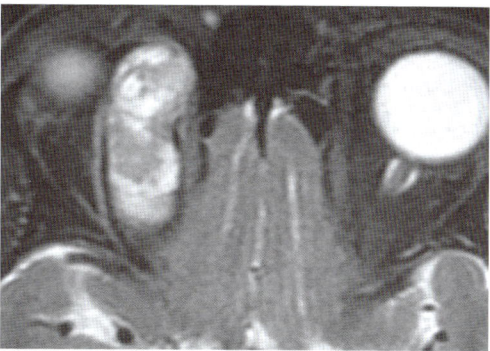

Fig. 1.3.4: Axial T2-weighted (T2W) fat-suppressed magnetic resonance imaging (MRI), with right *intraorbital schwannoma* showing an elongated extraconal heterogeneous well-defined mass lesion with foci of necrosis and hemorrhage.

Hemangiopericytoma (Solitary Fibrous Tumor of Orbit)

Hemangiopericytoma appears as homogeneous to heterogeneous, rounded or elongated masses of moderate density in an extraconal location most commonly along the paranasal sinuses. The borders are smooth and well-circumscribed, similar to cavernous hemangioma. Calcification may be seen in up to one-fourth of cases. Bone erosion is unusual, but some degree of cortical disruption is sometimes seen along with rare periosteal reaction. Following contrast administration, enhancement is moderate to mark. Dynamic CT may show prominent early enhancement with rapid washout. The MRI image shows a round-to-oval tumor with well-defined borders. On the T1WI, the signal is isointense to cortical gray matter and muscle, and hypointense to fat. On the T2WI, the lesion is hyperintense to fat. Low-intensity signal voids represent large vessels with rapid blood flow. Moderate, diffuse, and homogeneous enhancement is seen with gadolinium.

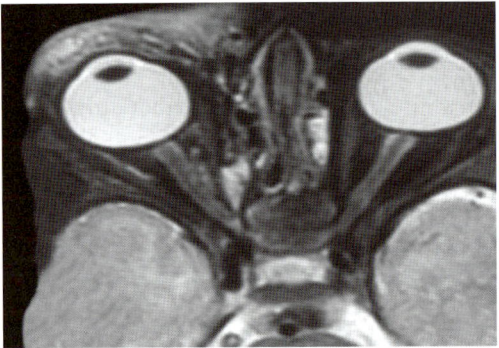

Fig. 1.3.5: Axial T2-weighted (T2W) fat suppressed magnetic resonance imaging (MRI), with right *orbital capillary hemangioma*, showing an ill-defined transcompartmental mass with areas of flow void. It showed marked contrast enhancement (in another section not shown).

Capillary Hemangioma

Typical history: Cutaneous discoloration or leash of vessels on the lids, periocular soft tissues; present at birth during infancy, grows with the child say up to 5–7 years age, and disappear by 10 years.

Imaging findings: They appear as ill-defined to irregularly marginated, lobulated, infiltrating masses most commonly located anterior to the globe in the eyelid. They show moderate to marked contrast enhancement.

Longstanding lesions in young children may cause expansion of bony orbital volume. Rarely occur as intraosseous lesions forming expansile masses with intact tables. In its proliferative phase, the mass shows intense and early enhancement (in arterial phase) with multiple flow voids on T1W/T2W images. However, in its involuting phase or if it does not involute completely, they tend to have heterogeneous high-signal intensity on T1W and T2W **(Fig. 1.3.5)** with heterogeneous enhancement on contrast images.

Rhabdomyosarcoma

These lesions appear as irregular, moderate to well-defined soft-tissue masses, mostly occupying the extraconal space, with about half extending into the intraconal space. Two-thirds of tumors arise in the superonasal quadrant of orbit. The density is similar to that of the EOMs, but may be heterogeneous due to intervening focal areas of hemorrhage. The tumor may conform to adjacent bony walls and orbital structures such as the globe. Bony erosion or destruction is unusual, but with larger lesions can be seen in up to 40% of cases. With contrast administration, mild-to-moderate uniform enhancement is observed.

Pearl: Most common malignancy of the orbit (head and neck region) in a child.

Lacrimal Gland Lesions

Benign neoplasms like pleomorphic adenoma present as indolent painless enlargement of the gland. Malignant and inflammatory lesions present with a shorter history and pain. They are broadly divided into epithelial and nonepithelial lesions. Epithelial lesions arise from the acini and tend to be neoplastic while nonepithelial lesions are predominantly inflammatory or infiltrative in nature. Adenoid cystic carcinoma is the most common malignancy of the lacrimal gland with propensity for perineural spread. CT scan of these lesions shows a heterogeneous mass in the lacrimal gland fossa area **(Fig. 1.3.6)**. They can be irregular in shape with poorly demarcated margins or be round to oval in shape with well-defined borders. Larger tumors may extend along the lateral orbital wall to reach up to the orbital apex.

Foci of calcification are frequently present within the lesion. Destruction or sclerosis of adjacent bone is a common phenomenon, especially with large tumors. Contrast administration shows areas of marked and focal enhancement.

On MR, pleomorphic adenoma is typically isointense to muscle with bright enhancement. Lymphomas on the other hand have a homogeneous T2 hypointense signal higher than muscle. Lacrimal glands are the second most common location for IOI.

Pearl: Idiopathic inflammatory inflammation and lymphomas are the two most common masses of lacrimal gland.

Bony Orbital Lesions

Orbital bone lesions are malignant or benign. Metastatic lesions are more common than primary malignancy. In children, the common causes are Ewing's and neuroblastoma **(Fig. 1.3.7)** while in adults metastases are common from lung, breast, and prostate. Meningiomas of the greater wing of sphenoid cause intraosseous growth, which may cause narrowing of intraorbital foramina. This sclerosis can be more easily seen on the CT images while on MR, there is increase in the dark signal of the bone. Non-neoplastic benign fibro-osseous lesions include fibrous dysplasia (FD) and ossifying fibroma. FD is seen in patients <30 years of age.

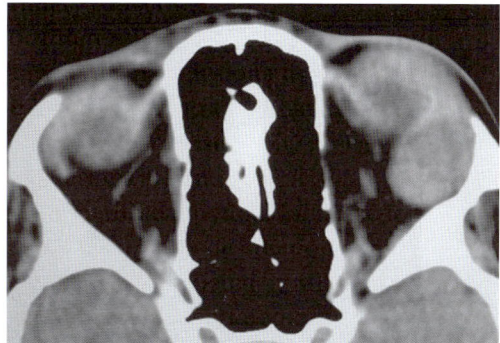

Fig. 1.3.6: Axial contrast computed tomography (CT), with a left *lacrimal gland mass* (pleomorphic adenoma), showing heterogeneous enhancement, remodeling of the adjacent bone, and abaxial proptosis.

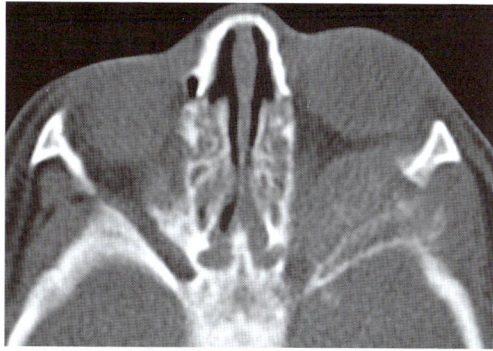

Fig. 1.3.7: Axial computed tomography (CT) (bone window), in a 2-year-old child with *metastatic neuroblastoma*, showing a destructive left sphenoid bone lesion with spiculated periosteal reaction and abaxial proptosis.

On CT, characteristic ground-glass density is seen, with T1/T2 hypointensity on MR. Sagittal and oblique planes are helpful for evaluating the orbital apex and optic canal.

> Ossifying fibromas may have internal mineralization, which can mimic that of FD on CT. However, ossifying fibroma usually has borders that are better defined than those of FD, which tends to have a poorly defined transition zone.

Mucocele

Long-standing lesions appear as masses opacifying one or more paranasal sinuses, extending into the orbit. The most common sinuses to get involved are frontal and ethmoid. The intervening bone may be expanded or remodeled or dehiscent around the cyst. This is best evaluated in bone window settings. Orbital structures are displaced, usually laterally or inferiorly. The cystic cavity is usually filled with a homogeneous, low-density mucoid material. The lesion lacks contrast enhancement unless contains pus. Long-standing inspissated secretions and proteinaceous contents appear T1 hyperintense and hyperdense on NCCT **(Fig. 1.3.8)** despite their cystic character.

INTRAOCULAR MASS

Metastases

In half of these cases, the intraocular metastases are asymptomatic, but in the other, they may present with vision loss or scotoma.

Uvea is the most common site for intraocular metastasis, mostly localized to the choroid. These tend to occur as flatter/broad-based lesions (posterior to the equator) **(Fig. 1.3.9)**, compared to melanoma, which tend to be mushroom-shaped. The most common primary tumors responsible for intraocular metastases are lung for men and breast for women. The prevalence of orbital metastases ranges from 2 to 5%. Few tumors have a propensity to metastasize to particular tissues (prostate to bone, melanoma to EOMs, breast to fatty tissue, and EOMs). The overall distribution of orbital metastases is in a ratio of 2:2:1, bone:fat:muscle.

Retinal Detachment

Retinal detachment typically begins with posterior vitreous detachment (PVD) and is typically a clinical diagnosis based on

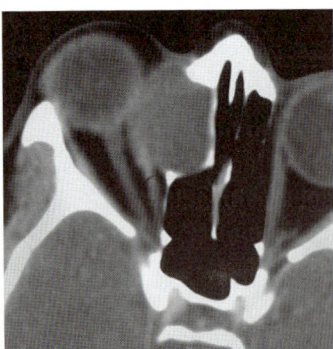

Fig. 1.3.8: Axial contrast computed tomography (CT), with right *ethmoid mucocele*, showing an expansile hyperattenuating lesion centered in the right anterior ethmoid sinus seen breaking into the orbit through the dehiscent lamina papyracea and causing abaxial proptosis.

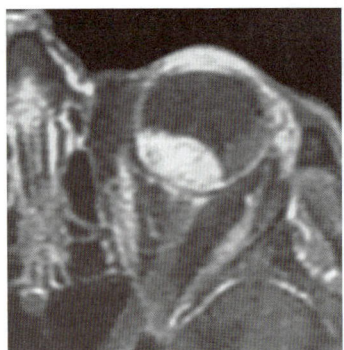

Fig. 1.3.9: Axial T1-weighted (T1W) fat suppressed magnetic resonance imaging (MRI), with left intraocular *metastatic lung cancer* showing bright homogeneous enhancement and retinal detachment.

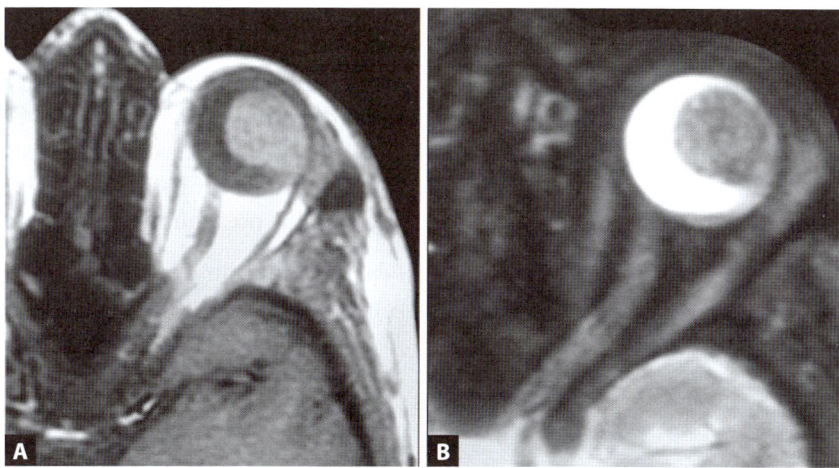

Figs. 1.3.10A and B: Axial T1-weighted (T1W) (A) and T2-weighted (T2W) (B) fat-suppressed magnetic resonance imaging (MRI), in an elderly man, with a polypoidal left intraocular mass, a *uveal melanoma*, which is bright on T1W and dark on T2W images.

history and examination. On imaging, there is a characteristic V-shaped area of abnormal density in the posterior globe, which is limited by the anterior attachment of the retina, in contradistinction to suprachoroidal collections, which extend anteriorly to the level of the ciliary body.

Pearl: Ultrasound is the best radiologic modality for its detection. A CT may completely miss the RD.

Uveal Melanoma

Uveal melanoma is the most common primary intraocular malignancy in adults, constituting 5–6% of melanoma diagnoses with up to 50% of patients developing distant metastases. It may arise in any part of the uvea, including the ciliary body, iris, or choroid (most common). Cross-sectional imaging is of use when ocular opacities limit assessment. MRI is the investigation of choice with characteristic findings of melanoma being marked hyperintensity on T1WIs and hypointensity on T2WIs **(Figs. 1.3.10A and B)**, which makes this a unique tumor. It enhances brightly on contrast-enhanced CT and MR, however subtraction MR imaging may be needed to demonstrate enhancement as the tumor is bright on T1 images as well. MR is also useful for distinguishing the tumor from associated hemorrhage.

Pearl: Ultrasound should be the first-line radiologic modality for the evaluation of suspected intraocular masses, and MRI later, if required. Systemic workup is necessary for staging.

Retinoblastoma

Child typically presents with white reflex or strabismus. It is the most common intraocular malignancy in childhood. It is considered a clinical diagnosis supported by ultrasound. MRI is required for the larger tumors for local staging. Ultrasonography (USG) and MRI can both be useful to distinguish RB from other differential diagnoses, viz., Coats' disease, PHPV, retinopathy of prematurity (ROP)

(Fig. 1.3.11) or toxocariasis. CT is only considered a problem-solving tool due to the radiation risk, CT is an excellent modality to detect small calcifications, which may be diagnostic in doubtful cases **(Fig. 1.3.12A)**.

However, an A-mode ultrasound is a popular modality to evaluate calcification in the tumors. MRI is the preferred imaging modality for delineating the morphology and extent of the tumor, especially extraocular spread and optic nerve involvement **(Fig. 1.3.12B)**. RB has characteristic low T2 signal, because of its high cellular density and variable postcontrast MR enhancement.

Pearl: Evaluation of white reflex in a child is a common and difficult clinical problem. The diagnosis is often not apparent even after thorough clinically evaluation and radiology.

Endophthalmitis

Endophthalmitis occurs either following surgery or trauma due to local inoculation or even secondary to hematogenous spread of infection from a distant anatomic site. Although usually a clinical diagnosis, the role of imaging remains detection of complications like formation of intraorbital abscess, RD, cavernous sinus involvement, and development of phthisis bulbi.

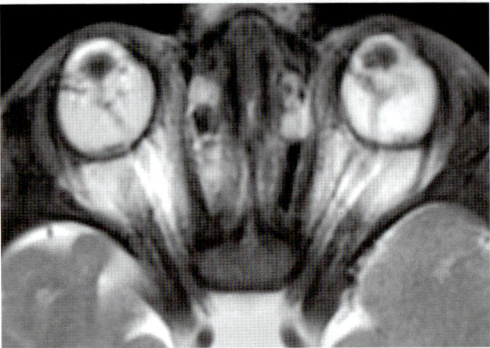

Fig. 1.3.11: Axial T2-weighted (T2W) magnetic resonance imaging (MRI), in a premature child who received oxygen in neonatal care for 2 weeks, having *retinopathy of prematurity*, showing bilateral microphthalmia, retinal detachment, and bilateral intraocular hemorrhage but no mass.

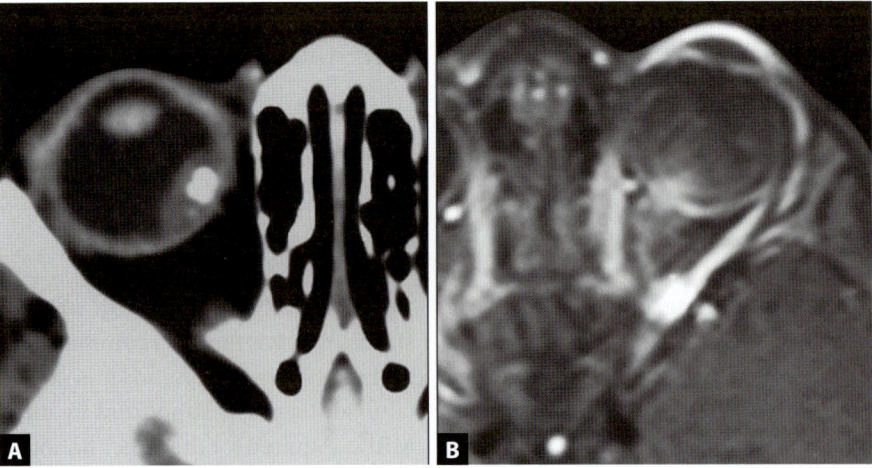

Figs. 1.3.12A and B: Axial noncontrast computed tomography (CT) (A) and T1-weighted (T1W) fat-suppressed contrast-enhanced (CE) magnetic resonance imaging (MRI) (B) in another child with *retinoblastoma* showing calcified right intraocular mass (A) and enhancing left intraocular mass with optic nerve involvement up to the apex.

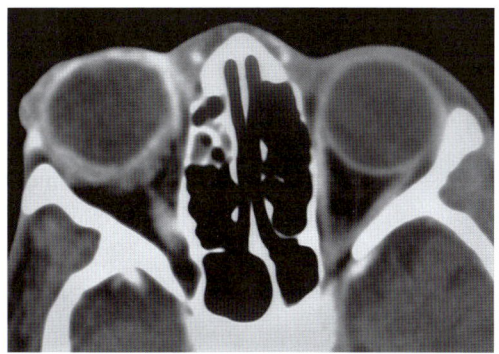

Fig. 1.3.13: Axial contrast computed tomography (CT), with right metastatic *endophthalmitis*, showing diffuse thickening of right ocular coats but no fluid collection or abscess. An active abdominal sepsis was presumed to be the cause of his disease.

The ocular coats are seen to be diffusely thickened **(Fig. 1.3.13)**. Abscesses can also occur in both the suprachoroidal space and the subretinal space. On CT and MR, abscesses are peripherally enhancing layers of predominantly fluid attenuation. On T2WI, the high signal of vitreous may obscure pathology; however, the inflamed uveal tract can be clearly seen separately from the vitreous on FLAIR imaging. Contrast MRI may be useful in demonstrating abscesses.

1.4 A PATTERN-BASED APPROACH TO RADIOLOGIC DIAGNOSIS IN OPHTHALMOLOGY: PART II

Sanjay Sharma, Savinay Kapur

OPTIC NERVE SHEATH COMPLEX LESIONS

Optic Glioma

Typical presentation: Decreased visual activity, visual field defect, proptosis, and relative afferent pupillary defect (RAPD).

Imaging findings: These are glial tumors, which in the brain arise from the parenchyma of white matter, but often also involve the adjacent gray matter. The Dodge classification divides these tumors into just three groups based on anatomical localization:
1. *Stage 1:* Optic nerves only
2. *Stage 2:* Chiasm involved (with or without optic nerve involvement)
3. *Stage 3:* Hypothalamic involvement and/or other adjacent structures

> Neurofibromatosis type 1 (NF1) associated—more likely to involve the optic nerve. Sporadic—more likely to involve the chiasm.

In patients of neurofibromatosis (NF), these lesions appear on CT as hypodense and poorly defined masses. The optic nerve cannot be seen separate from the mass; hence, the nerve appears tubular, tortuous, and kinked. Minimal or no enhancement is seen in the lesion. Sporadic gliomas tend to have solid cystic appearance similar to pilocytic astrocytomas. The solid areas are generally T2 hyperintense and show contrast enhancement **(Fig. 1.4.1)**.

Pearls: If unilateral, NF1 in 20% patients; if bilateral—pathognomonic of NF1.

Optic Nerve Sheath Meningioma

Typical presentation: Insidious vision loss over months to years.

Imaging findings: The typically appear as smooth tubular enlargement of the optic nerve. Less commonly, they may be fusiform

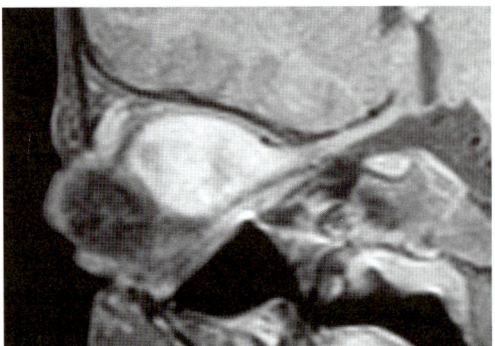

Fig. 1.4.1: Oblique sagittal T1-weight (T1W) post-contrast magnetic resonance imaging (MRI) of *optic nerve glioma* showing a fusiform-enhancing tumor not separate from the optic nerve.

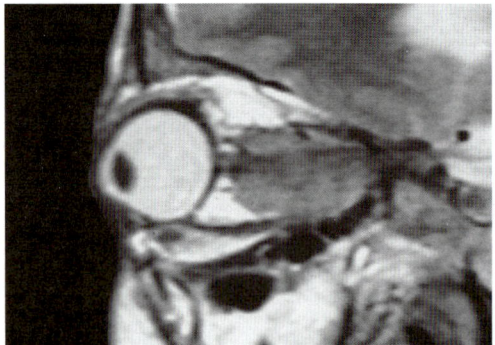

Fig. 1.4.2: Oblique sagittal T2-weight (T2W) magnetic resonance imaging (MRI) with *optic sheath meningioma* showing a fusiform intermediate signal intensity neoplasm encasing the optic nerve. Note that the neoplasm is seen distinct from the optic nerve.

or globular in appearance in case the dura is breached. The lesion appears iso to hyperdense on CT and may show foci of calcification in 20–50% of cases. There is marked and homogeneous contrast enhancement of the mass, often with a linear central zone of reduced density representing the normal optic nerve (tram-tracking sign). Expansion of bony orbital walls is seen in case the tumor is longstanding. Meningiomas generally produce isointense signals on T1W images with respect to normal optic nerve and cortical gray matter. The T2W image is heterogeneous and varies from being slightly hypointense to slightly hyperintense **(Fig. 1.4.2)** with respect to the gray matter. The fibroblastic stromal elements give meningiomas their characteristic hypointense signal. The post-gadolinium T1W image shows marked enhancement of the tumor surrounding an optic nerve of lower signal intensity with a dural tail. This is best distinguished on fat suppression sequences. A subtle intracranial extension may only be visible on the contrast image.

Pearl: Think of NF2, if multiple or associated with other neoplasms like schwannomas or ependymomas.

Optic Neuritis

Typical presentation: Unilateral rapid onset of vision loss; eye pain worsened with eye movements.

Imaging findings: Optic neuritis is a MRI diagnosis; CT has no role. Key imaging sequences—axial, coronal T2 FS, and T1 FS postcontrast are required. Optic nerve involvement may be segmental or diffuse. Optic neuritis manifests as increased T2 signal and bulk of the nerve, which may be associated with abnormal enhancement.

Pearls

First pearl: Always image the brain if optic neuritis presents as there is 25% risk of multiple sclerosis. Can also be seen with neuromyelitis optica (NMO).

Second pearl: Hence screening of cervical spine with short inversion time inversion recovery (STIR) sequence may be done.

Third pearl: If bilateral **(Fig. 1.4.3)**, then think of infectious causes, such as viral prodrome in children.

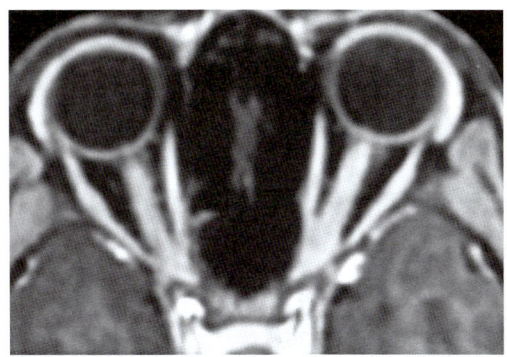

Fig. 1.4.3: Axial postcontrast fat-suppressed T1-weight (T1W) magnetic resonance imaging (MRI) with *bilateral optic neuritis* showing a marked enhancement of both optic nerves. Note that the normal optic nerves never enhance as brightly as the extraocular muscles (EOMs), as in this case.

Idiopathic Orbital Inflammation

Typical presentation: Unilateral more common than bilateral, rapid onset pain ± diplopia ± vision loss and redness.

Imaging findings: Orbital inflammation may be seen in a variety of orbital conditions, however, about 5–15% have no discernible cause and hence classified as idiopathic. Also called orbital pseudotumor, idiopathic orbital pseudotumor, or nonspecific orbital inflammation. Many patients would have underlying systemic vasculitis as a cause. It may be related to immunoglobulin G4 (IgG4) disease. Here the optic nerve sheath is involved instead of the optic nerve itself. There is frequent involvement of retrobulbar fat, EOMs, lacrimal glands, and optic nerve. The masses are ill-defined on CT. On MRI, they are T1 intermediate, T2 dark, and show variable enhancement.

Radiological differential diagnosis—lymphoproliferative disease/sarcoidosis (neither has a similar clinical presentation), systemic vasculitis, and IgG4-related orbital disease.

Lymphoproliferative Disease

Lymphoproliferative disease includes lymphoma (most common), lymphoid hyperplasia and atypical lymphoid hyperplasia, and ocular adnexal lymphoma.

Around a quarter of all masses in patients older than 60 years are lymphomas. Non-Hodgkin's lymphoma, specifically the mucosa-associated lymphoid tissue (MALT) form, is the most common primary orbital lymphoma.

Sarcoidosis

Presentation is similar to inflammatory pseudotumor. Most common site of involvement is the uvea or lacrimal gland. On MRI, involvement of the optic nerve sheath may show linear tram-track enhancement. On imaging, if there is isolated optic nerve involvement, it may be indistinguishable from the above two conditions. Laboratory investigations [serum calcium and angiotensin-converting enzyme (ACE) levels] are supportive, besides the systemic workup for the evidence of the disease elsewhere in the body to help make the diagnosis.

CONAL (EXTRAOCULAR MUSCLE ENLARGEMENT)

Thyroid-associated Orbitopathy

Typical presentation: Bilateral painless axial proptosis.

Imaging findings: This is the most common extrathyroidal manifestation of Graves', disease (25–50% patients). This is caused by accumulation of glycosaminoglycans in the orbital soft tissues and increased fat volume. On CT, enlargement of EOMs is the imaging hallmark of the disease and is best appreciated on axial and coronal scans **(Figs. 1.4.4A and B)**. The enlarged muscles are sharply

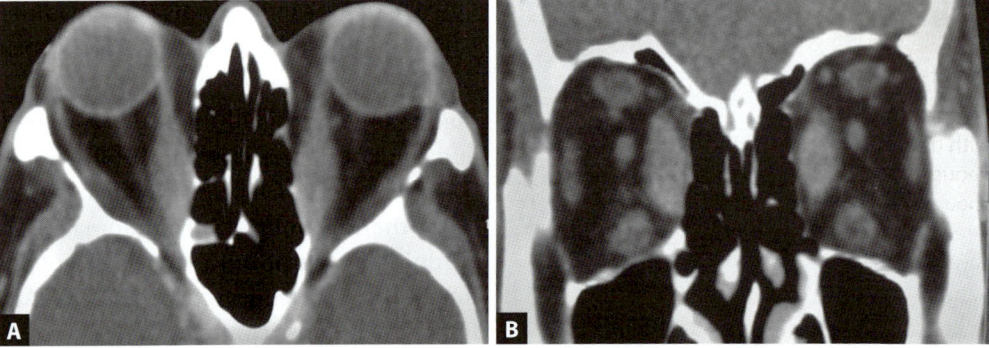

Figs. 1.4.4A and B: Axial (A) and coronal (B) contrast-enhanced computed tomography (CECT) scan in *thyroid-associated orbitopathy* shows bulky bellies of bilateral extraocular muscles (EOMs) especially inferior and medial recti. Note the typical tendinous sparing.

defined, sometimes demonstrating increased density. There may be focal areas of low density, reflecting fatty infiltration. Typically, only the muscle bellies are involved, with relatively normal tendinous insertion referred to as the "coca-cola" sign seen on axial images (cf. pseudotumor). The inferior and the medial rectus muscles are the most frequently involved ones. The superior ophthalmic vein may be enlarged as a result of apical compression. The bulky EOMs are isointense on T1 and slightly hyperintense on T2W images. The thickened tensor intermuscularis appears as a prominent curved band between the superior and lateral rectus muscles. Contrast administration is not necessary for imaging to make a diagnosis. Up to 8% of patients with thromboangiitis obliterans (TAO) develop dystrophic optic neuropathy (DON) likely secondary to optic nerve compression by the enlarged EOMs. The presentation may sometimes be asymmetric (unilateral) or even antedate the clinical disease.

Idiopathic Orbital Inflammation

Typical presentation: Pain, ocular dysmotility, and redness.

Imaging findings: Myositis is one of the most common orbital manifestations of IOI. In contradistinction to TAO, IOI of the EOMs is typically unilateral, painful, and rapid in onset (hours to days). However, some patients may have an atypical presentation, with a relatively painless manifestation, or bilateral disease (25% of patients, common in children). On imaging, the differentiation is based on involvement of tendinous insertion with inflammation in the adjacent fat.

Carotid-Cavernous Fistula

Carotid-cavernous fistulas have been variously classified by their hemodynamics (high or low flow), cause (spontaneous or posttraumatic), or vascular anatomy (direct or indirect; **Table 1.4.1**).

Computed tomography scan in these cases demonstrates proptosis with the prominence of the orbital vasculature. The superior ophthalmic vein is dilated in most cases. Low density, nonenhancing areas within the vessel or the cavernous sinus represent thrombosis. Symmetrical enlargement of EOMs from vascular engorgement is commonly seen.

TABLE 1.4.1: Direct and indirect carotid-cavernous fistula (CCF).	
Direct CCF	**Indirect CCF**
Frequently associated with trauma (spontaneous may be to aneurysm rupture) and direct flow from CCA to cavernous sinus	Dural shunting of arterial flow from branches of ICA/ECA/both into the cavernous sinus
Progresses rapidly	Insidious onset
High flow	Low flow

(CCA: cavernous carotid artery; ECA: external carotid artery; ICA: internal carotid artery)

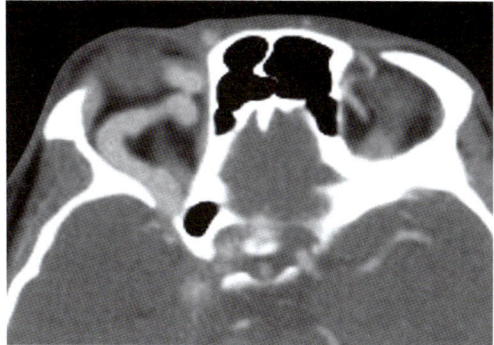

Fig. 1.4.5: Axial contrast-enhanced computed tomography (CECT) in a young male with *caroticocavernous fistula* showing engorged right superior ophthalmic vein. The swelling of left extraocular muscles is not seen in this section.

Enlargement of cavernous sinus may be appreciated, and in long-standing cases, the superior orbital fissure can be widened. Contrast CT is generally diagnostic in most cases **(Fig. 1.4.5)**. However, invasive digital subtraction angiography (DSA) may be necessary occasionally, especially to demonstrate an indirect fistula or for interventional radiological treatment of CCF. On MR, vessels with fast-flowing blood show a signal void on both T1W and T2W images and these can be demonstrated on gadolinium-enhanced magnetic resonance angiography (MRA) images.

Sarcoidosis

Involvement of the EOMs by sarcoidosis is unusual and can have a variety of presentations. There may be involvement of multiple muscles on one side or bilateral, painful or indolent, with or without involvement of other orbital soft tissues such as the lacrimal gland. It may spare or involve the tendinous insertions, and hence is difficult to differentiate from TAO or IOI by physical examination and imaging, especially if there is no evidence of systemic sarcoidosis.

Lymphoproliferative Disease and Metastases

Intramuscular metastases and lymphoma are rare. Metastases and lymphoma or other lymphoproliferative diseases occurring in the EOMs have been reported only sporadically in the literature. Carcinoma (predominantly breast), melanoma, non-Hodgkin lymphoma, and neuroendocrine tumors such as carcinoid are better known primaries. Breast carcinoma may sometimes involve the EOMs in a bilateral symmetric pattern with sparing of the tendons, which may be difficult to distinguish from TAO on imaging.

INFILTRATIVE DISEASES

Metastasis

Most common primary malignancy to metastasize to the orbits is breast carcinoma. Diffuse intraconal disease is one of many imaging patterns that may be seen in breast cancer, in addition to intramuscular or osseous masses. Infiltrative scirrhous breast carcinoma may cause enophthalmos, because fibrous tissue replaces the normal orbital fat.

Idiopathic Orbital Inflammation

Diffuse involvement of the orbital fat is less common than involvement of other orbital structures such as the lacrimal gland or EOMs **(Fig. 1.4.6)**. The eponym "Tolosa–Hunt syndrome" applies when there is predominantly involvement of the orbital apex or cavernous sinus.

Lymphoproliferative Disease

Similar to IOI, lymphoproliferative disease such as lymphoma may present with an infiltrative pattern, involving any orbital structure. However, in contrast to IOI, lymphoproliferative disease presents with minimal or no pain and with gradual progression. In some series, diffuse ill-defined orbital disease was found to be more common than a well-circumscribed round or oblong mass. On MRI, T2W signal isointense or hypointense to muscle is typical of lymphoproliferative disease and restricted diffusion may also be seen.

Orbital Cellulitis

Involvement of the soft tissues posterior to the orbital septum is the imaging hallmark of orbital cellulitis (cf. preseptal cellulitis). It is important to make this distinction as orbital cellulitis has a higher complication rate and may be associated with optic neuropathy, encephalomeningitis, cavernous sinus thrombosis, sepsis, and intracranial abscess. Orbital cellulitis in early stages is characterized by eyelid edema and sinusitis on CT images. Postcontrast scans show marked increased in enhancement. More typically inflammation is seen in the medial or superomedial orbit adjacent to the opacified sinus, associated with fat stranding, i.e., heterogeneity in the retrobulbar fat **(Fig. 1.4.7)**. An orbital abscess appears as a well-defined mass with a low-density necrotic center, and an enhancing rim. On MRI, orbital inflammation and edema produce a diffuse signal that is isointense to muscle. On the T2W image, a fluid level may be visible as a layered hyperintense signal in an abscess or sinus. The inflammatory exudate remains hypointense. The necrotic abscess center remains dark, but there is an enhancement of the peripheral rim.

Plexiform Neurofibroma

Plexiform neurofibroma (PNF) occurs in about one-third of patients with NF1

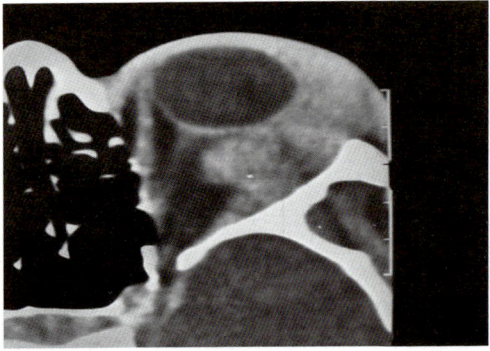

Fig. 1.4.6: Axial contrast-enhanced computed tomography (CECT) in a middle-aged woman with *idiopathic orbital inflammation* showing the infiltrating multicompartmental soft-tissue mass involving left lateral rectus, lacrimal gland, retrobulbar fat, and preseptal soft tissues.

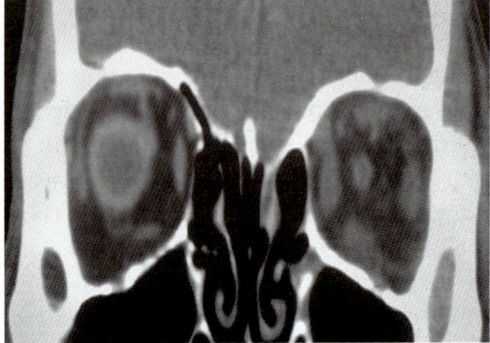

Fig. 1.4.7: Coronal contrast-enhanced computed tomography (CECT) in left *orbital cellulitis* showing swollen left extraocular muscles and fat stranding.

(**Fig. 1.4.8**). It commonly affects the trigeminal nerve, especially the ophthalmic and maxillary divisions. PNF has a multispatial growth pattern, similar to venous and lymphatic malformations that follow vessels. The patient's age and relevant history are the key to the correct diagnosis. On imaging, PNF follows the distribution of the involved nerves through fascial boundaries with a characteristic targetoid appearance on T2W images.

Rhabdomyosarcoma

Rhabdomyosarcoma is the most common soft-tissue sarcoma of the head and neck in childhood (mean age is 8 years), with 10% of all cases involving in the orbit. Proptosis and blepharoptosis are common presenting symptoms of orbital RMS. Pain is uncommon and may indicate an advanced tumor. Typically, it presents as an extraconal well-defined mass without osseous destruction, however more advanced cases can be both extra- and intraconal and infiltrative with bone destruction. It can involve any part of the orbit, including the EOMs. On NCCT, the mass is isodense to muscle. On MRI, RMS is typically T2 hyperintense with areas of high T1 signal secondary to hemorrhage, with some contrast enhancement.

■ MISCELLANEOUS PATHOLOGIES

Intraocular/Intraorbital Foreign Body

Noncontrast CT scan is the imaging modality of choice for evaluation of suspected intraorbital foreign bodies. It has an advantage over the plain radiographs owing to its superior spatial resolution; it can often identify nonmetallic foreign bodies like wood also. Helical CT scans allow precise localization of the foreign body and delineation of its relationship with the surrounding structures (**Fig. 1.4.9**). MRI is contraindicated for evaluating metallic intraorbital foreign bodies.

Cysticercosis

Ultrasound is often the first-line imaging modality for evaluating suspected cysticercus (**Figs. 1.4.10A and B**), especially if intraocular. MRI is preferred over CT for identification of myocysticercosis. Orbital cysticercosis on

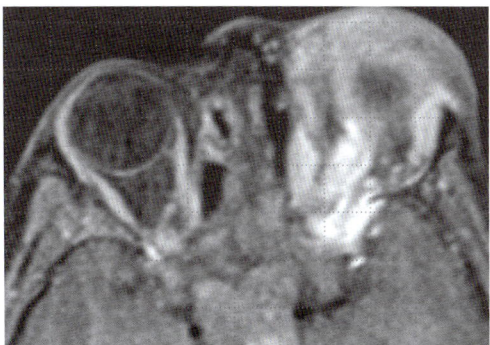

Fig. 1.4.8: Axial postcontrast fat suppressed T1-weighted (T1W) magnetic resonance imaging (MRI) with left orbital *plexiform neurofibroma* showing an infiltrating enhancing soft-tissue mass in a patient with neurofibromatosis type 1 (NF1).

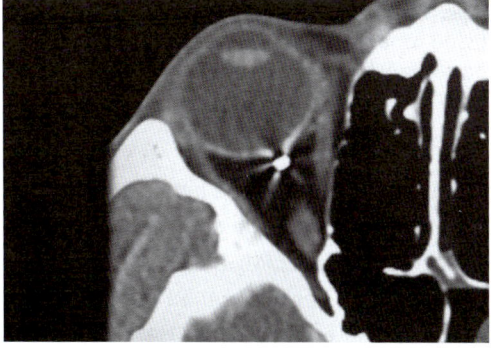

Fig. 1.4.9: Axial noncontrast computed tomography (NCCT) shows a tiny *metallic foreign body* just behind the right globe, adjacent to the optic disc. It clearly shows that it is lying in extraocular location.

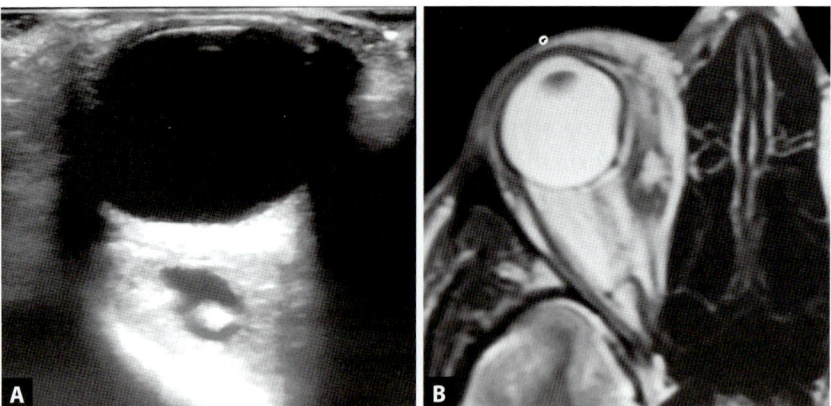

Figs. 1.4.10A and B: Ultrasound (A) and axial T2-weighted (T2W) magnetic resonance imaging (MRI) (B) in *myocysticercus* showing a cystic intraorbital lesion in the lateral rectus with a hyperechoic center suggesting a scolex (A); another patient showing a swollen medial rectus with a cyst and nodule.

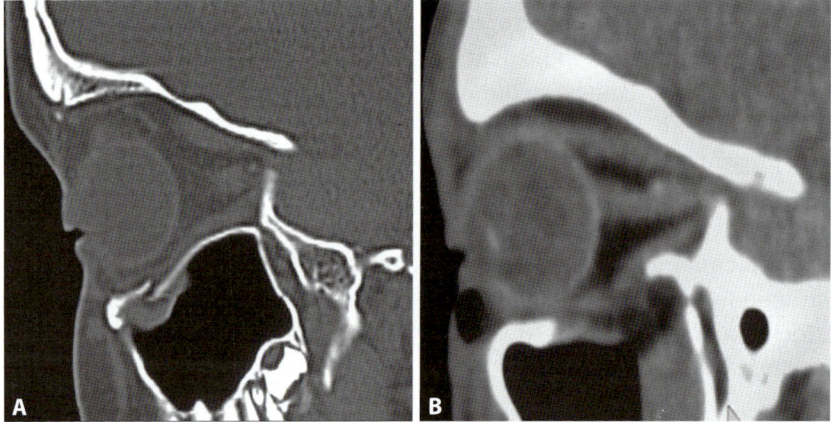

Figs. 1.4.11A and B: Oblique sagittal computed tomography (CT) reconstruction, bone window (A) soft-tissue window (B), in two different patients of *blowout fracture* of the orbit. Note clearly the orbital floor fractures with normal inferior rectus (IR) and teardrop-shaped hemorrhage pouting in the maxillary sinus in (A) and entrapped swollen IR in (B).

MRI scans appears as a T2 hyperintense cystic lesion often with an eccentric hypointense scolex within the EOM. The muscle itself may be bulky with perilesional T2 hyperintensity suggestive of edema **(Figs. 1.4.10A and B)**. CECT may show a ring-enhancing lesion in one of the EOMs with an eccentric focus of enhancement or calcification representing the scolex.

Orbital Trauma

Computed tomography is the preferred imaging modality for evaluation of orbital and cranial fractures because of its ability to provide detailed bony images in high spatial resolution. An NCCT with bone and soft-tissue windows with multiplanar reconstruction is employed **(Figs. 1.4.11A and B)**. Diffuse hyperdense areas suggest acute intraorbital bleed while air pockets represent orbital emphysema. A "blowout" orbital fracture involving the medial wall and floor is a frequent injury. In a pure blowout fracture of the orbital floor, it is displaced downward into the maxillary sinus **(Figs. 1.4.11A and B)**. In children, due to resilient bones, there is often a minimal bony displacement and herniation of orbital contents but inferior rectus may still get entrapped, referred to as "trapdoor fracture". The muscle may be bulky, heterogeneous with a rounded contour suggesting hematoma or contusion. Medial wall fractures show displacement of the lamina papyracea into the ethmoid air cells often with opacification of the sinus. The medial rectus muscle with intraorbital fat may also be displaced into the fracture site.

Axial images are best for the evaluation of the maxillary antrum, pterygoid plates, zygomatic arches, and the medial and lateral orbital walls. Coronal images are more useful for evaluation of orbital rims, the orbital floor and roof, the cribriform plate, and the skull base. Reformatted images in the orthogonal sagittal and oblique planes are helpful for evaluating subtle orbital apex and optic canal fractures.

Pearl: MRI may miss fractures as the bony structures are not quite conspicuous.

1.5 ULTRASONOGRAPHY

Asha Samdani, Aditi Dubey

■ INTRODUCTION

Ultrasonography has broad application in ophthalmology. In 1793, Lazzaro Spallanzani (Italy) discovered that bats orient themselves with the help of sound whistles while flying in darkness. This was the basis of modern ultrasound application. Two types of devices, are used diagnostically, i.e., A-scan and B-scan. *A-scan* is a one-dimensional amplitude modulation scan commonly used for measurement of AL and pachymetry.

Along with B-scan, it is used to determine the ultrasonic properties such as internal reflectivity, and dimensions of posterior segment masses. *B-scan* is a two-dimensional, cross-section brightness scan. Its use is primarily to evaluate posterior segment and orbital pathology when the ocular media are cloudy, and a direct view is not possible. High-resolution B-scan or *UBM* uses higher frequency probes (20–50 MHz vs. the standard 10 MHz) to provide detailed images of anterior segment structures such as the angle, iris, and ciliary body. This chapter deals with B-scan USG primarily.[1-3]

For sound to be considered ultrasound, it must have a frequency of greater than 20,000 oscillations per second, or 20 KHz, rendering it inaudible to human ears. USG of the eye is an indispensable noninvasive tool in the diagnosis and management of various ocular orbital diseases. It was first used in ophthalmology in 1956 by Mundt and Hughes as A-scan. Baum and Greenwood introduced the first B-scan in 1958. Coleman in the 70s developed the first commercially available B-scan.

■ PRINCIPLE

Ophthalmic ultrasound **(Figs. 1.5.1 and 1.5.2)** uses high-frequency ultrasound waves,

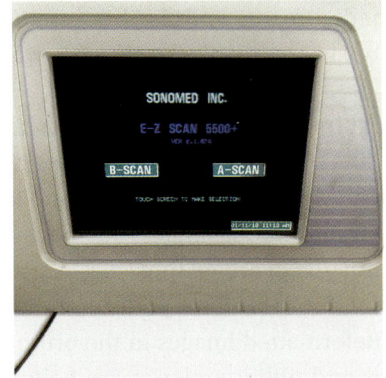

Fig. 1.5.1: Ultrasonography display.

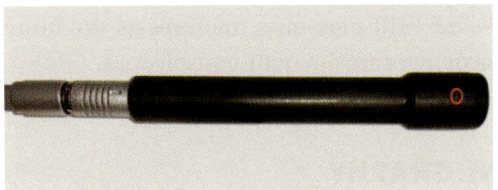

Fig. 1.5.2: Ultrasonography probe.

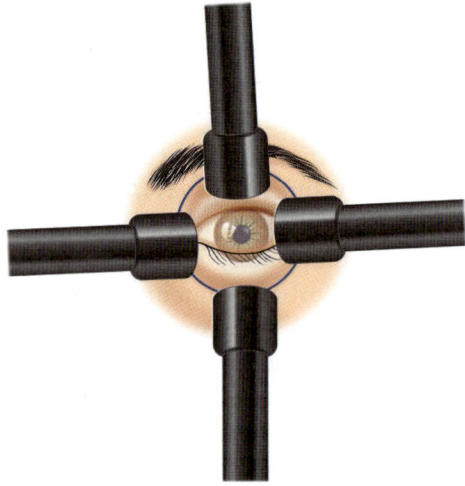

Fig. 1.5.3: Orientation of ultrasonography (USG) probe while performing scanning.

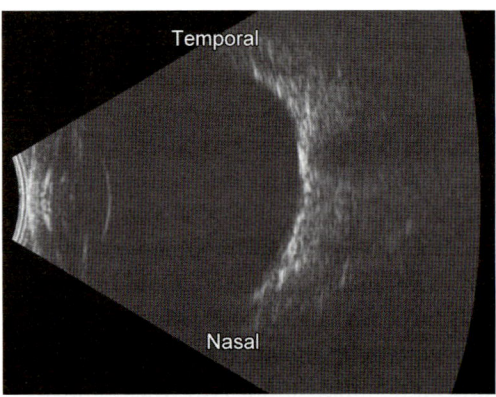

Fig. 1.5.4: Orientation.

which are transmitted from probe to eye. Tissue penetration is directly proportional to resolution and inversely to frequency. That is why USG probes used for ocular USG are of higher frequency (10 MHz) as it needs much less tissue penetration. As the sound waves strike intraocular structures, they are reflected back to the probe and converted into an electric signal. These signals are subsequently reconstructed as an image on a monitor.

The ophthalmic B-scan probe has high frequencies of 10 MHz and contains piezoelectric crystal. Marker on probe helps in the understanding orientation of the image on the screen **(Fig. 1.5.2)**. The orientation of the marker **(Fig. 1.5.3)** is directly correlated to the sound beam orientation. Wherever the marker is directed on the eye *represents the upper portion* of the echogram **(Fig. 1.5.4)** and, in most instances, the probe is placed opposite the area of the eye to be examined.

Velocity depends on the density of the medium. Sound travels faster through solids than liquids in aqueous and vitreous = 1,532 m/s, and in cornea and lens = 1,641 m/s **(Table 1.5.1)**.

Reflectivity is higher when the echoes are stronger and thus producing brighter dots.

The angle of incidence of the probe is critical. When the probe is held perpendicular

TABLE 1.5.1: Velocity of sound in various media.	
980	Silicone intraocular lens (IOL)
986	Silicone oil
1480	Fresh water
1532	Aqueous, vitreous
1550	*Solid tissue:* Intraocular and orbital soft-tissue blood
1640	Clear crystalline lens

to the area of interest, more of the echo is reflected directly back into the probe tip and sent to the display screen. When held oblique to the area imaged, part of the echo is reflected away from the probe tip, and less is sent to the display screen the higher the perpendicularity.

Absorption: The density of the solid lid structure results in absorption of part of the sound wave when B-scan is performed through the closed eye, thereby compromising the image of the posterior segment.

Shadowing reduction in echo amplitude posterior to a strongly reflecting or attenuating surface can also lead to poor quality of the image.

Gain: The amplification of the display can be altered by adjusting the gain, which is measured in decibels (dB). When the gain is high, weaker signals are displayed, such as vitreous opacities and PVDs. When the gain is low, the weaker signals disappear, and only the stronger echoes, such as the retina, remain on the screen.

BASIC SCREENING TECHNIQUE

Probe positions: The probe can be used in the following positions:

- *Transverse position:* Most commonly used; the probe is positioned parallel to limbus (on opposite scleral surface). It demonstrates the lateral extent of pathology (approximately 6 o'clock hours) **(Fig. 1.5.4)**.
- *Longitudinal position:* The probe is perpendicular to the limbus. It represents the radial extent of pathology and proximity to the optic nerve and demonstrates only 1 o'clock hour that represents optic nerve to the periphery.
- *Axial position:* Patient is fixating in primary gaze, probe face centered on the cornea. Displays the lens and the optic nerve. Horizontal axial scan-marker is toward the patient's nose. Vertical axial scan-marker is toward the 12 o'clock position.
- *Oblique position:* The patient is asked to look at various gazes and probe is placed at the oblique axis.

An examination performed when there is no view into the eye because of opaque media, and the determination of the status of the posterior segment is required. The highest gain setting must be used to visualize any weak signals, such as vitreous opacities and PVDs, or to gauge the extent of vitreous hemorrhages. If any pathology such as retinal or choroidal detachments (CDs) is found, then the gain may be reduced for better resolution of the stronger signals from these structures. The entire globe must be examined, from the posterior pole out to the far periphery.

Using a limbus-to-fornix approach, the four major quadrants include the 12 o'clock, 3 o'clock, 6 o'clock, and 9 o'clock positions, and each centered on the right side of the echogram in transverse approaches are evaluated. The posterior pole with a horizontal axial scan is evaluated, which incorporates both the optic nerve and the macula in one echogram. If no additional pathology is detected, these five echograms complete the examination.

In case of any posterior pathology is detected during basic screening, it should be centered on the right side of the echogram to achieve the highest resolution. This is accomplished by determining the clock hour represented in the transverse scan where it was discovered. Once determined, the patient should be instructed to redirect his or her gaze to that meridian, with the probe then placed on the opposite scleral surface. The gain is now reduced until the highest resolution is achieved, and photographic documentation is produced.

Macular localizing: The four methods of localizing and centering of the macula are horizontal, vertical, transverse, and longitudinal. In the horizontal and vertical method, the probe is on the corneal vertex and should be aimed straight ahead to center the macula with marker directed nasally in horizontal method while the marker is in the 12 o'clock position in the vertical method. In the transverse and longitudinal method, patient fixating slightly temporally and the probe is placed onto the nasal sclera with the marker at the 12 o'clock position in transverse method while toward the limbus or temporally toward the macula in the longitudinal method. These scans bypasses the lens, thereby preventing absorption or reverberation artifacts from an intraocular lens.

Indications for B-scan

- *Opaque ocular media:*
  - Anterior segment: For example, corneal opacification, hyphema or hypopyon, miosis, cataract, pupillary or retrolenticular membrane
  - Posterior segment: For example, vitreous hemorrhage or inflammation
- *Clear ocular media:*
  - Anterior segment: For example, iris lesions, ciliary body lesions
  - Posterior segment: Tumors, CD, RD, optic disc abnormalities
- *Intraocular foreign bodies:* For detection and localization

■ VIVA QUESTIONS

1. What are the different examination modes of USG?

Ans. Various examination modes in ophthalmic USG are:
- *A-scan:* Amplitude modulation scan
- *B-scan:* Brightness modulation scan
- Vector A-scan
- Doppler USG
- UBM (high-frequency ultrasound)

A-scan: Amplitude modulation scan—salient features are:
- AL
- Time-amplitude scan
- Pressure, falsely low AL
- It can also be used for pachymetry.
- The frequency of the probe is around 8 MHz.
- *Quantitative USG:*
  - Helps to determine the texture of lesion
  - Based on reflectivity
- It is semiquantitative **(Table 1.5.2)**.

B-scan (brightness modulation scan):
- Multiple A-scans
- As internal emitter is rapidly swept back and forth
- Two-dimensional

TABLE 1.5.2: A-scan amplitude.

Category	Spike height (%)
Extremely low	0–5
Low	5–40
Medium	40–60
Medium to high	60–80
High	80–100

- Topographic examination for shape, border, location, and extent
- *Kinetic USG:* Mobility, after movements, vascularity (Valsalva)
- It can assess:
  - Vitreoretinal status
  - Macula
  - Optic nerve head (ONH)
  - Anterior two-thirds of orbit
  - EOM

Doppler ultrasound:
- Using frequency shifts from acoustic reflections to measure movements, flow conditions within vessels is detected.
- Presentation as false color based on the frequency
- Three-dimensional reconstructions.

2. **Give differences between RD, CD, and PVD.**

Ans. Refer to **Table 1.5.3**. Other important points include:
- *Retinal detachment:* It appears as a highly reflective, attached to the ora serrata anteriorly and the optic nerve (**Fig. 1.5.5**). It has moderate mobility and translucent subretinal space. It maintains 100% reflectivity even on low gain.
- There is a gradual separation of the membrane from the ocular wall unlike in CD.
- Attachment at disc is broad and at the periphery of the disc.
- Persists at low gain
- Thickness corresponds to proliferative vitreoretinopathy (PVR).
- Configuration—convex rhegmatogenous retinal detachment (RRD), concave tractional RD (TRD), double-layer sign in giant retinal tear (GRT)
- The configuration of funnel (**Figs. 1.5.6 and 1.5.7**), retinoschisis

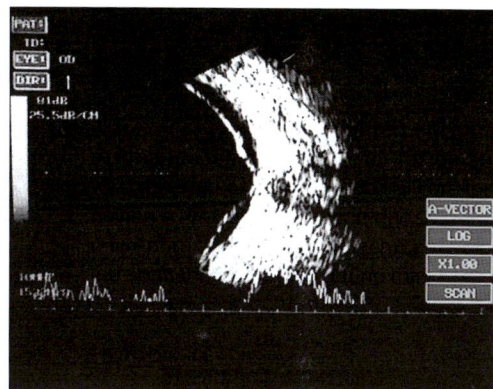

Fig. 1.5.5: Retinal detachment.

TABLE 1.5.3: Differences between RD, CD, and PVD.

	CD	RD	PVD
Topography	Dome-shaped	Linear, V	V, U
Location	Periphery (pre-equator)	Variable	Variable
Attachment to optic disc	No	Yes	Variable
Others	Kissing choroids, vortex vein	Folds, breaks	Inferior, thicker
Quantitative (A)			
Spike height	90–100%	80–100%	40–90%
Spike peak	Double	Single	Single
Kinetic (A and B)			
Mobility	Minimal	Moderate	Marked
After movement	Absent	Minimal to moderate	Marked

(CD: choroidal detachment; PVD: posterior vitreous detachment; RD: retinal detachment)

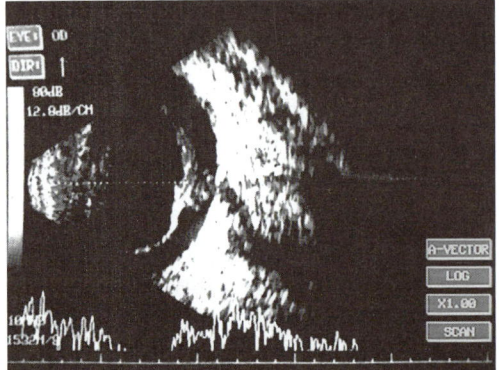

Fig. 1.5.6: Open funnel retinal detachment (RD).

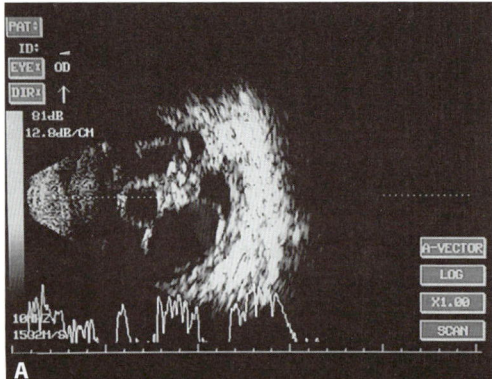

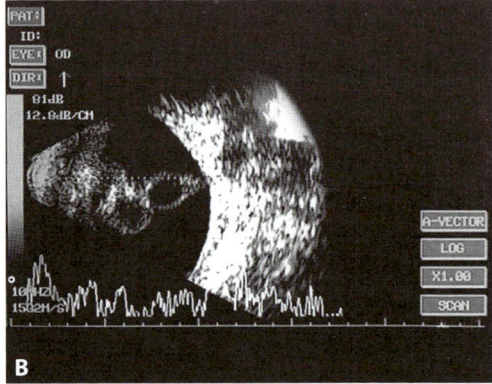

Figs. 1.5.8A and B: Retinal cyst in old retinal detachment (RD).

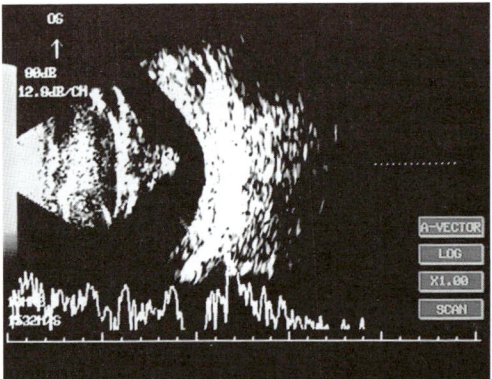

Fig. 1.5.7: Closed funnel retinal detachment (RD).

- Coexisting findings can be peripheral retinal looping, cyst formation in long-standing RD **(Figs. 1.5.8A and B)**.
- Tractional retinal detachment (TRD), common finding in vascular retinopathies caused by strong adhesion **(Fig. 1.5.9)** and subsequent traction leading to detached retina with concave appearance.
- GRTs appear as large tears with rolled out tissue and clear breach.
- *Posterior vitreous detachment*: In PVD with the normal eye, the reflectivity is very low, high gain (90 dB) setting is

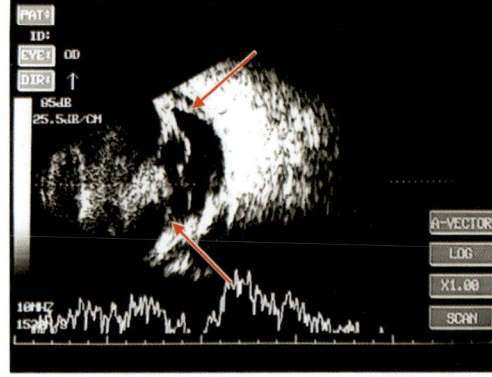

Fig. 1.5.9: Tractional retinal detachment (TRD).

required **(Fig. 1.5.10)**. The reflectivity disappears on lowering the gain under 70 dB. Kinetic echography typically

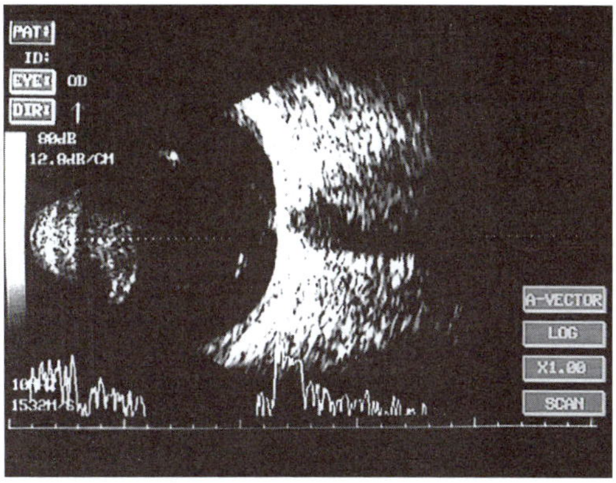

Fig. 1.5.10: Posterior vitreous detachment.

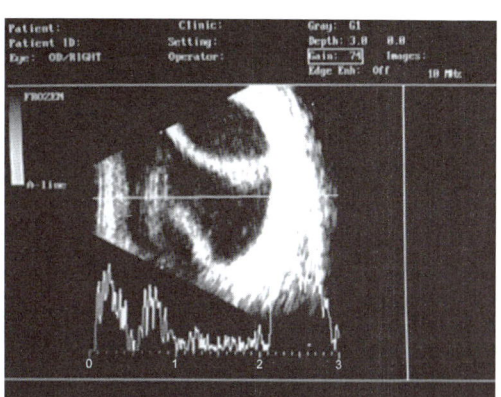

Fig. 1.5.11: Choroidal detachment.

shows a very undulating movement that continues after the eye movements stop:
- Attachment at disc narrow or none
- About 40–90% spike height decreasing anteriorly
- The height of PVD generally more superiorly
- Thick PVD spike may persist at low gain.
- How to differentiate from RD? Measure the difference in decibels between the 50% spike height of membrane and sclera

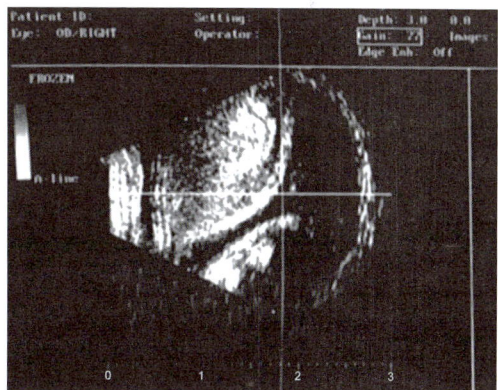

Fig. 1.5.12: Hemorrhagic choroidal detachment (CD) with kissing choroids.

- *Choroidal detachment:* CD is smooth, dome-shaped and thick, no movement seen with eye movement **(Fig. 1.5.11)**. When extensive, one can see multiple dome-shaped detachments, which may "kiss" in the central vitreous cavity.
    - *Serous* CD has anechoic suprachoroidal space.
    - *Hemorrhagic* CD has dispersed opacities **(Fig. 1.5.12)**.
- Seen as thick bright opacity even at low gain
- Sometimes thin stretched cord-like opacity extending between the wall and detached choroidal layer presumed to be vortex vein.

3. Describe vitreous hemorrhage.

Ans. Vitreous hemorrhage is a fresh mild hemorrhage that appears as small dots or linear areas of low reflective mobile vitreous opacities **(Fig. 1.5.13)**. Old vitreous hemorrhage appears vitreous filled with multiple large opacities that are higher in their reflectively and membranes as the blood organizes.

Differentiation between vitreous hemorrhage and asteroid hyalosis: Asteroid hyalosis is calcium deposits in vitreous cavity and appears as bright round signals on B scan with echo-free space in front of the retina.

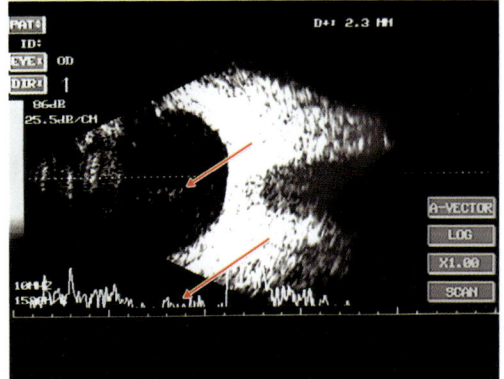

Fig. 1.5.13: Vitreous hemorrhage.

Asteroid hyalosis is highly echogenic, and they are still visible when the gain setting is reduced up to 60 dB whereas vitreous hemorrhage which usually disappears by 60 dB.

4. **Describe USG appearance of endophthalmitis.**

Ans. It depends on the degree and severity of infection and extent of vitreous involvement.
- Low-to-moderate cases—hyper-reflective opacities noted
- Severe cases—moderate or coarse opacities with membrane formation **(Figs. 1.5.14A and B)**

5. **Describe USG appearance of persistent fetal vasculature.**

Ans. It is a congenital abnormality when the fetal hyaloid artery does not resorb. Very thin persistent hyaloidal vessel coursing from the disc to the lens can be seen. Globe size is usually small **(Fig. 1.5.15)**.

6. **Describe USG appearance of intraocular foreign body.**

Ans:
- A-scan:
  • Steeply rising wide echo spike along the baseline between the initial spike and ocular wall spike

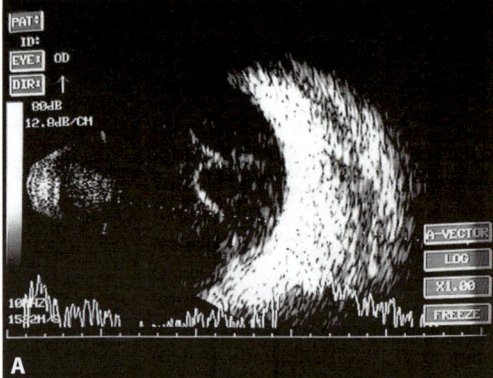

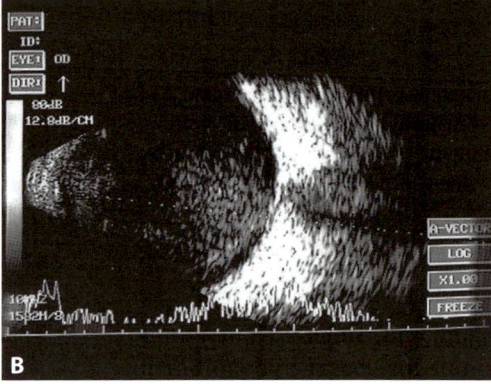

Figs. 1.5.14A and B: Endophthalmitis.

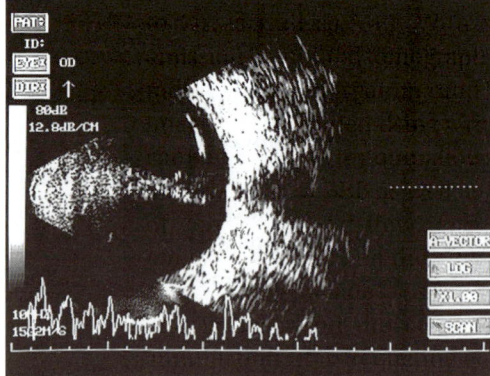

Fig. 1.5.15: Persistent fetal vasculature.

- Extremely high reflectivity (100% spike), which persists on low gain **(Figs. 1.5.16A and B)**.
- The distance between the intraocular foreign body and the adjacent sclera is

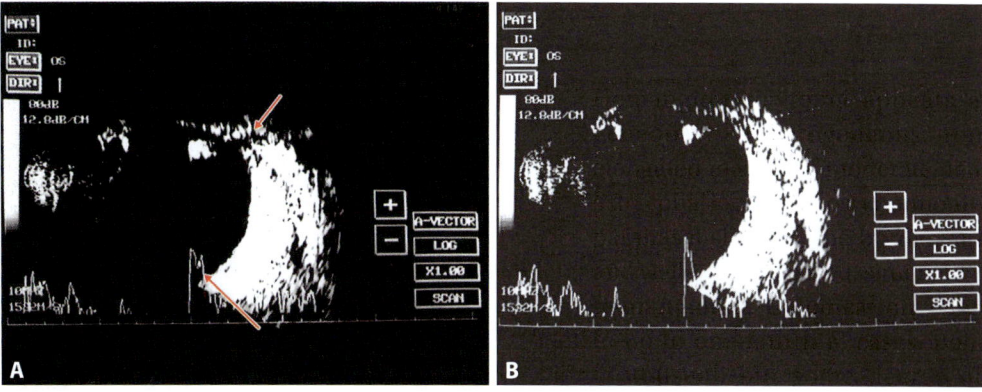

Figs. 1.5.16A and B: Intraocular foreign body.

accurately measured at lower system sensitivity.
- Sound attenuation is very strong.
- B-scan:
  - Acoustically opaque contrasting with the acoustically clear vitreous
  - Persists even when the system sensitivity is decreased by 20–30 dB.
  - Topographic and kinetic echography will show if the foreign body is adherent to the retina or if it is floating in the vitreous.
  - Sound attenuation is very strong.
  - Shadowing of the ocular and orbital tissues behind it as it totally reflects the sound beams preventing its propagation within tissues behind it **(Figs. 1.5.16A and B)**.
  - Associated findings like vitreous hemorrhage, vitreous bands, fibrosis, RD, CD, and even scleral entry wounds can be assessed.

7. Describe USG appearance of posterior staphyloma.
Ans. This appears as a shallow excavation of posterior pole with smooth edges in highly myopic eyes (focal area of thinned sclera) **(Fig. 1.5.17)**.

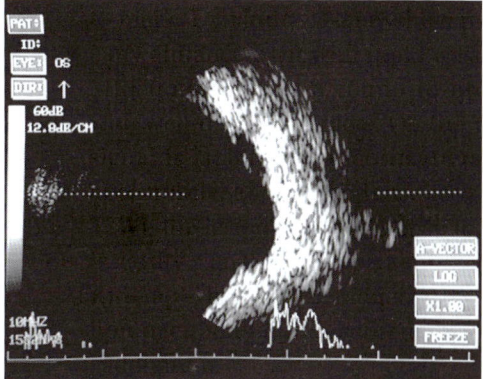

Fig. 1.5.17: Posterior staphyloma.

8. Describe USG appearance of posterior scleritis.
Ans. The degree of scleral thickening can vary from mild to severe. It is commonly, associated edema adjacent to the sclera. This manifests itself as an echolucent area in the tenon space, it forms a "T-sign" USG is the best modality for diagnosis **(Figs. 1.5.18A and B)**.

9. Describe USG appearance of optic nerve pathologies.
Ans.
- Optic disc drusen—appears as an echogenic focus within or on the surface

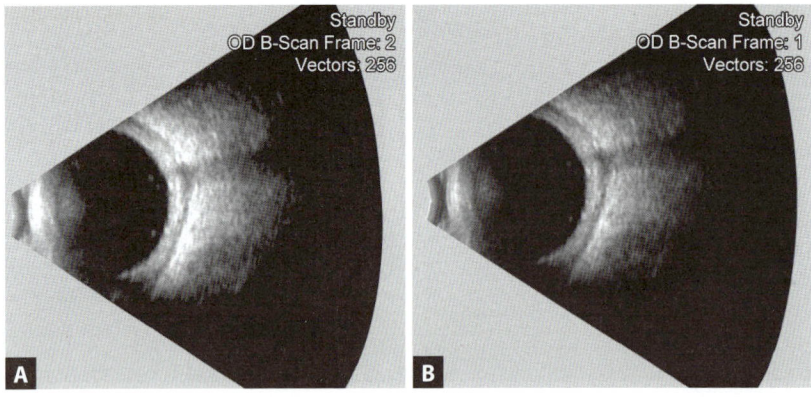

Figs. 1.5.18A and B: Posterior scleritis. (A) "T" sign in the right eye; (B) left eye.

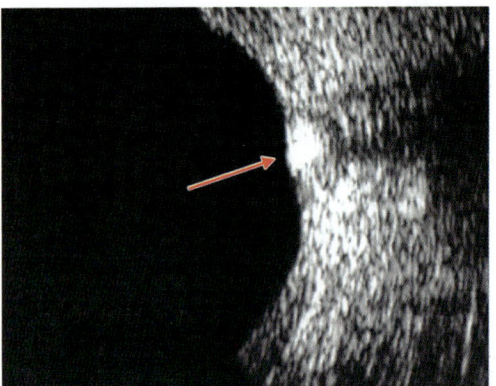

Fig. 1.5.19: Optic disc drusen.

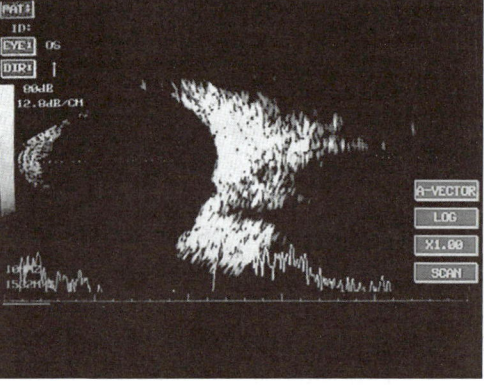

Fig. 1.5.20: Early optic nerve head cupping.

of the ONH **(Fig. 1.5.19)**. Posterior acoustic shadowing may be present with larger lesions. Astrocytic hamartomas may confuse with drusen and can be differentiated by following points:
- Seen in patients with tuberous sclerosis or NF
- Usually unilateral
- Usually larger
- Associated with RD

- ONH cupping—appears as an excavation of the disc **(Figs. 1.5.20 and 1.5.21)**. It is important to note that USG can detect cupping reliably only in advanced cases.

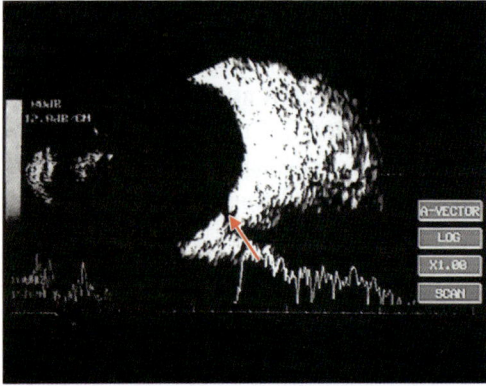

Fig. 1.5.21: Advanced optic nerve head cupping.

CHAPTER 1: Oculoplasty and Orbital Imaging 41

TABLE 1.5.4: Common intraocular tumors in ultrasonography (USG).			
	Melanoma	*Metastasis*	*Hemangioma*
Shape	Domed, mushroom	Domed/bi-domed, irregular	Domed
Location	Variable	Near macula	Near disc
Associated RD	Variable	Common	Rare
Growth	Variable	Rapid	Slow
Quantitative (A)			
Reflectivity	Low/medium	Variable	High
Internal structure	Regular	Irregular	Regular
Sound attenuation	Strong	Variable	Weak
Kinetic (A)			
Vascularity	Present	Absent	Absent
(RD: retinal detachment)			

10. Describe USG appearance of intraocular tumors.

Ans. Ultrasonographic appearance of intraocular tumors has been summarized in **Table 1.5.4**.

- *Choroidal melanoma:*
  - Mushroom shape is caused by tumor growth through a break in Bruch's membrane.
  - Choroidal excavation (produced by dome-shaped fundus lesions in ultrasound beam path)
  - Solid mass with shadowing (**Figs. 1.5.22A and B**)
  - The scleral extension should be watched for.
- *Choroidal metastasis:* The tumor has an irregular outline and heterogeneous internal structure.
- *Hemangioma:* A scan honeycomb spikes, spikes do not touch baseline.

11. Describe USG appearance of cysticercosis extraocular muscle.

Ans. Extraocular muscle cysticercosis manifests as a well-demarcated cyst in relation to the right recti muscle with a central echodense, highly reflective structure within the sonolucent cyst, corresponding to

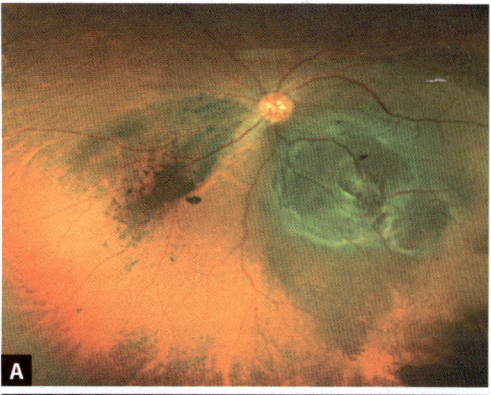
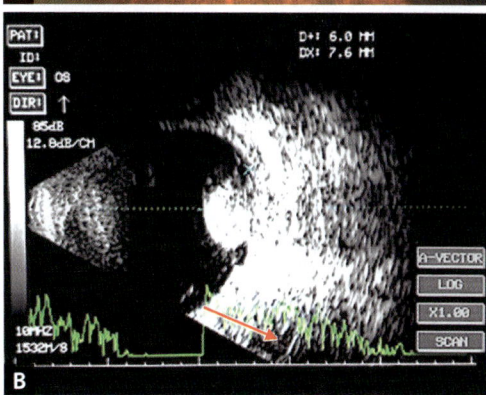

Figs. 1.5.22A and B: Choroidal melanoma.

the scolex (**Fig. 1.5.23**). EOM involvement is the most common variety of orbital cysticercosis. The subconjunctival space is the next common site, followed by the eyelid, optic nerve, retro-orbital space, and lacrimal gland. All the EOMs are involved in myocysticercosis. However, the lateral rectus, medial rectus, and the superior oblique muscles have been found to be affected to a greater extent.

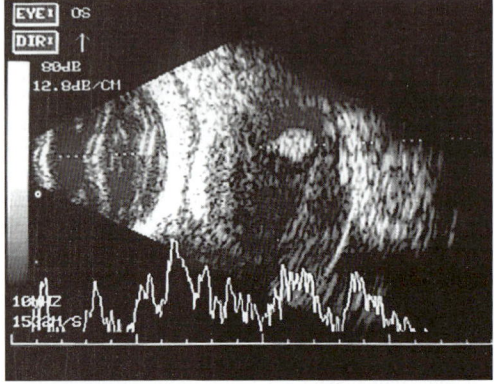

Fig. 1.5.23: Cysticercosis extraocular muscle.

12. **Describe USG appearance ROP.**
Ans.
- Multiple membranes in the periphery
- RD
- Focal fibrovascular fonds
- Open funnel RD
- Closed funnel RD

13. **Describe Coats' disease.**
Ans.
- Unilateral
- RD, turbid SRF

14. **Give features of retinoblastoma.**
Ans.
- Solid tumor
- Calcification
- Moderate internal reflectivity
- *If necrosis, calcification:* High reflectivity

(**Figs. 1.5.24A to C**).

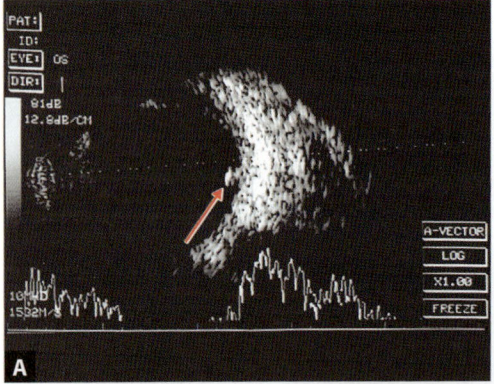

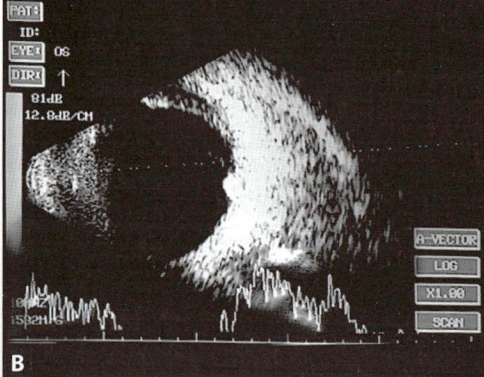

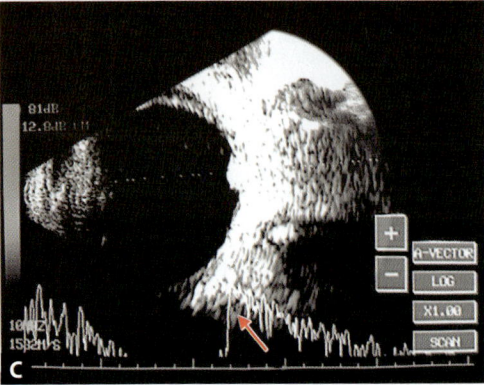

Figs. 1.5.24A to C: Retinoblastoma.

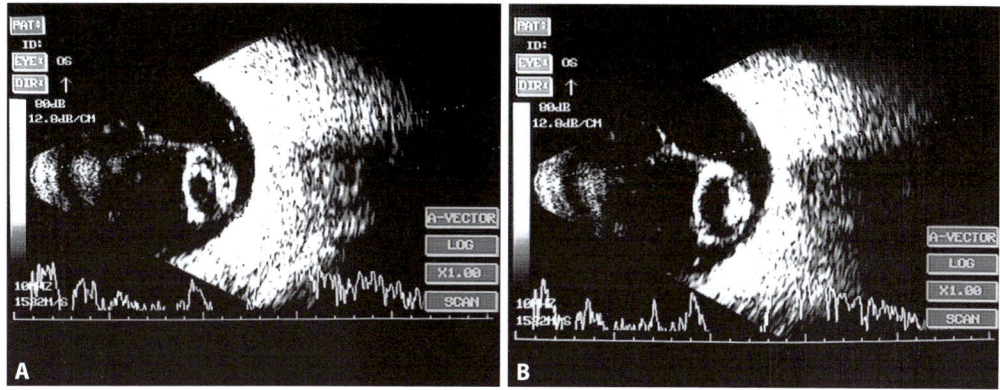

Figs. 1.5.25A and B: Nucleus drop.

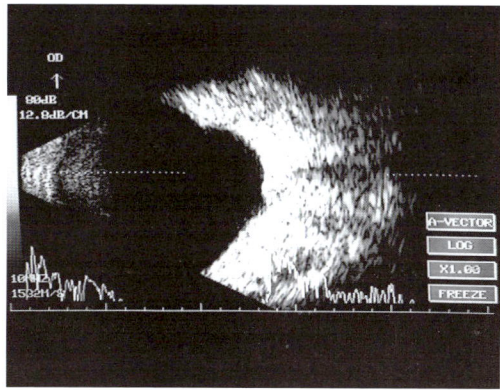

Fig. 1.5.26: Choroidal coloboma.

- Sound attenuation moderate to high
- *If glaucoma:* Globe enlarged

15. Describe nucleus drop.
Ans.
- Biconvex-shaped structure **(Figs. 1.5.25A and B)**
- Surrounding mild-to-moderate spikes suggesting vitritis

16. What are the findings in choroidal coloboma?
Ans.
Following findings can be there:
- Excavation of posterior layer **(Fig. 1.5.26)**
- Cyst
- RD **(Figs. 1.5.27A to C)**
- Small eyeball

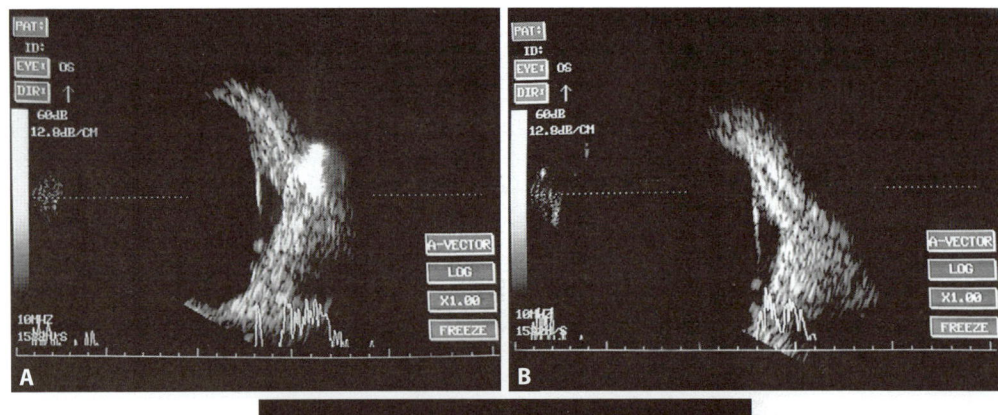

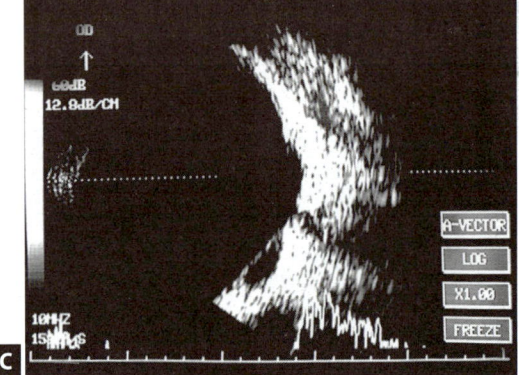

Figs. 1.5.27A to C: Choroidal coloboma with retinal detachment (RD).

REFERENCES

1. Aironi VD, Gandage SG. Pictorial essay: B-scan ultrasonography in ocular abnormalities. Indian J Radiol Imaging. 2009; 19(2):109-15.
2. Coleman JD, Silverman RH, Lizzi FL, Rondeau MJ. Ultrasonography of eye and orbit, 2nd edition. Philadelphia: Lippincott Williams and Wilkins; 2005. pp. 47-122.
3. Pushker N, Bajaj MS, Chandra M, Neena. Ocular and orbital cysticercosis. Acta Ophthalmol Scand. 2001;79(4):408-13.

1.6 APPLIANCES AND INSTRUMENTS IN OCULOPLASTY

Saloni Gupta, Sahil Agrawal, Pranita Sahay

INTRODUCTION

The commonly used instruments in oculoplasty surgery include the following:

- Lid clamp or Snellen's entropion clamp **(Fig. 1.6.1)**
- Jaeger's lid spatula **(Fig. 1.6.2)**
- Epilation forceps **(Fig. 1.6.3)**

CHAPTER 1: Oculoplasty and Orbital Imaging

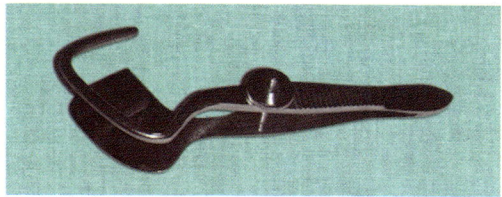

Fig. 1.6.1: Lid clamp or Snellen's entropion clamp.

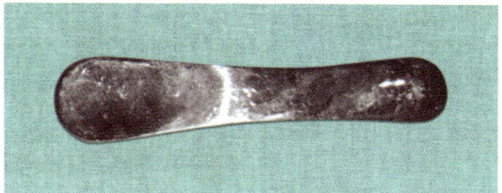

Fig. 1.6.2: Jaeger's lid spatula.

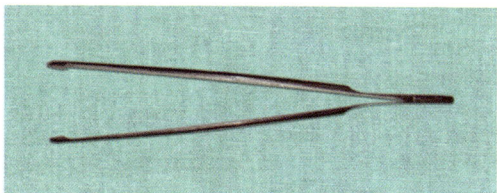

Fig. 1.6.3: Epilation forceps.

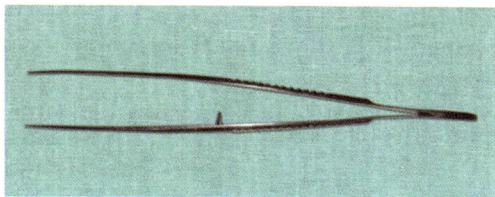

Fig. 1.6.4: Plain forceps.

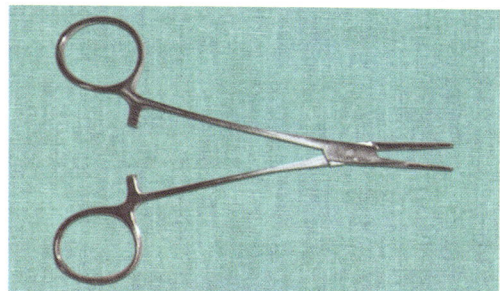

Fig. 1.6.5: Artery (hemostatic) forceps.

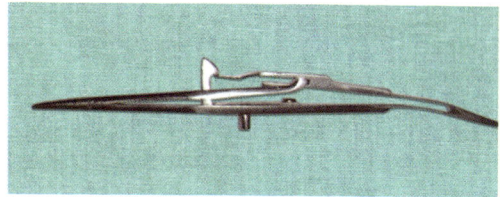

Fig. 1.6.6: Arruga's needle holder.

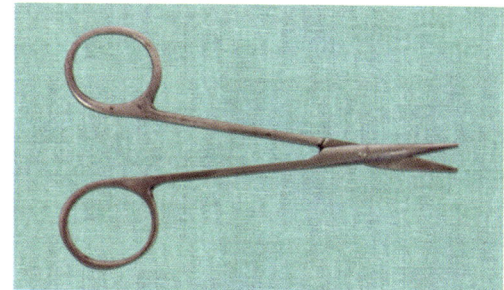

Fig. 1.6.7: Stevens tenotomy scissors.

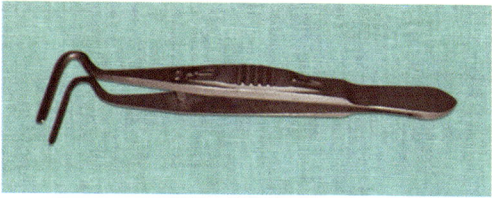

Fig. 1.6.8: Berke's ptosis clamp.

- Plain forceps **(Fig. 1.6.4)**
- Artery (hemostatic) forceps **(Fig. 1.6.5)**
- Arruga's needle holder **(Fig. 1.6.6)**
- Stevens tenotomy scissors **(Fig. 1.6.7)**
- Berke's ptosis clamp **(Fig. 1.6.8)**
- Wells enucleation spoon **(Fig. 1.6.9)**
- Enucleation scissors **(Fig. 1.6.10)**
- Mules evisceration spatula **(Fig. 1.6.11)**
- Evisceration curette **(Fig. 1.6.12)**
- Chalazion clamp **(Fig. 1.6.13)**
- Chalazion scoop **(Fig. 1.6.14)**
- Nettleship punctum dilator **(Fig. 1.6.15)**
- Bowman lacrimal probe **(Fig. 1.6.16)**
- Freer periosteal elevator **(Fig. 1.6.17)**

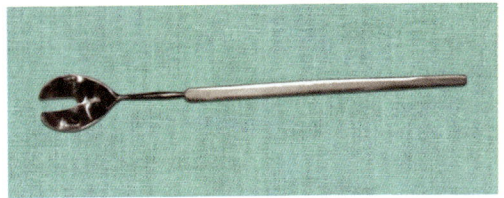

Fig. 1.6.9: Well's enucleation spoon.

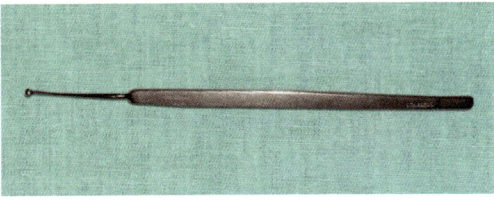

Fig. 1.6.14: Chalazion scoop.

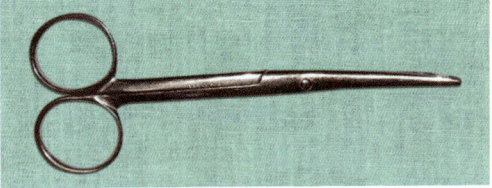

Fig. 1.6.10: Enucleation scissors.

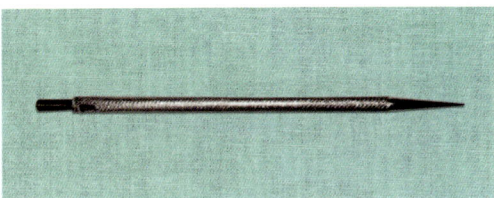

Fig. 1.6.15: Nettleship's punctum dilator.

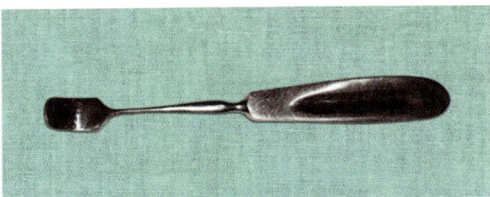

Fig. 1.6.11: Mule's evisceration spatula.

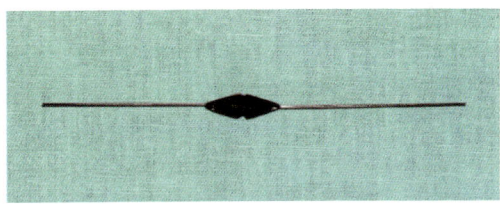

Fig. 1.6.16: Bowman lacrimal probe.

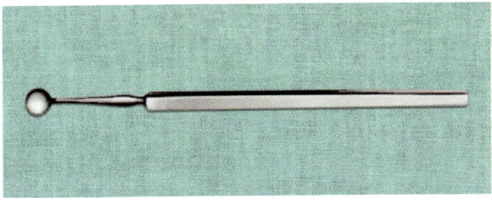

Fig. 1.6.12: Evisceration curette.

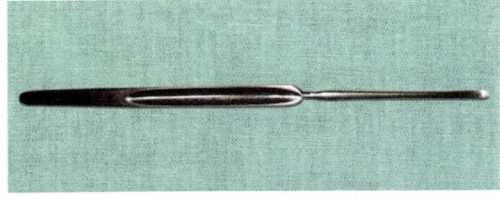

Fig. 1.6.17: Freer periosteal elevator.

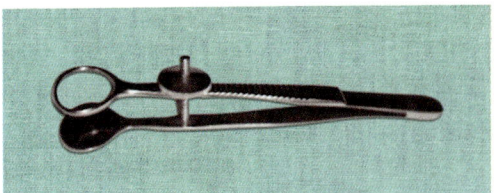

Fig. 1.6.13: Chalazion clamp.

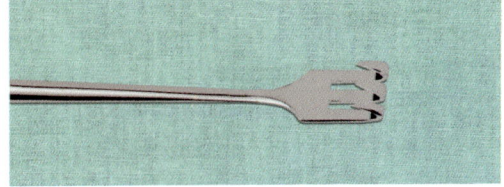

Fig. 1.6.18: Cat's paw lacrimal wound retractor.

- Cat's paw lacrimal wound retractor (**Fig. 1.6.18**)
- Lacrimal sac dissector and curette (**Fig. 1.6.19**)
- Kerrison bone punch (**Fig. 1.6.20**)
- The details of the abovementioned instruments have discussed in Ophthalmology Clinics for Postgraduates.

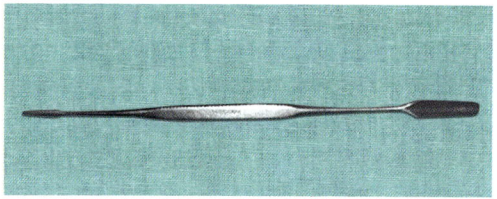

Fig. 1.6.19: Lacrimal sac dissector and curette.

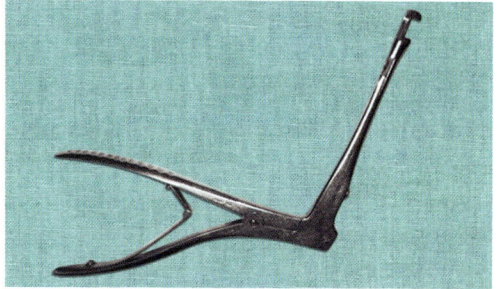

Fig. 1.6.20: Kerrison bone punch.

PTOSIS

The three categories of surgical procedures most commonly used in ptosis are:
1. *External approach*: Transcutaneous levator advancement
2. *Internal approach*: Levator/tarsus/Müller muscle resection (*Putterman Müllerectomy, Fasanella-Servat procedure*)
3. Frontalis muscle suspension using sling

The most common determining factors in the choice of the surgical procedure for ptosis repair are:
- The amount and type of ptosis
- Levator function
- Surgeon's comfort level and experience with various procedures

Surgical correction of the levator aponeurosis is preferred in cases with good levator function.
- *External (transcutaneous)* levator advancement surgery is most commonly used when levator function is normal and the upper eyelid crease is high. In this setting, the levator muscle itself is normal, but the levator aponeurosis (its tendinous attachment to the tarsal plate) is stretched or disinserted, thus requiring advancement. It also allows the surgeon to simultaneously remove excess eyelid skin.
- For repair of minimal ptosis (2 mm)— Putterman Müllerectomy if 2.5% phenylephrine test is positive or *Fasanella-Servat procedure* (requires removal of the superior tarsus).
- Frontalis muscle suspension techniques done in cases where levator function is poor or absent.

Amount of Resection

- Berke's rule:

Levator function	Intraoperative lid height
2–3 mm	At upper limbus
4–5 mm	1–2 mm overlap
6–7 mm	2 mm overlap
8–9 mm	3–4 mm
10–11 mm	5 mm overlap

- Beard's rule:

Preoperative margin to reflex distance	Amount of resection
10–13 mm	3–4 mm
14–17 mm	2–3 mm
18–22 mm	1–2 mm
>23 mm	0–1 mm

Complications of Ptosis Surgery

- Overcorrection
- Undercorrection
- Lid contour abnormalities
- Lid lag and lagophthalmos
- Lid crease and fold asymmetry
- Keratopathy

- Infection and/or inflammation
- Hemorrhage

Complications of Ptosis Clamp

- Oculocardiac reflex (Aschner phenomenon or Aschner–Dagnini reflex) is a known complication. Compression, traction, or any manipulation of the EOMs can lead to a sudden decrease in pulse rate/bradycardia.
- Afferent pathway is ophthalmic branch of the Vth cranial nerve via the ciliary ganglion.
- Efferent pathway is the vagus nerve.
- The reflex is mediated by visceral motor nucleus of the vagus nerve in the brain stem, stimulation of which leads to decreased output of the sinoatrial (SA) node of heart causing bradycardia, junctional rhythm, and asystole. Most commonly seen in neonates and children during strabismus correction surgery. However, it can occur with other ocular surgeries and adults.

Management

- Immediate removal of the stimulus can result in the restoration of normal sinus rhythm.
- If not, the use of atropine or glycopyrrolate can revert the attack.
- In severe cases, such as asystole, cardiopulmonary resuscitation (CPR) is required.
- Surgery can be continued if the attack can be reversed successfully.

Materials for Sling Surgery

- *Autologous tissue:*
  - Fascia lata (both autologous and preserved)
  - Palmaris longus tendon
  - Temporalis fascia
- *Synthetic material*: Silicone nonabsorbable sutures, Gore-Tex strips (polytetrafluoroethylene), polypropylene (Prolene), polyester mesh, monofilament nylon, and Supramid Extra (polyfilament and nylon).

Management of Residual Ptosis

- The moderate-to-severe cases of residual ptosis were tackled by levator resection by skin approach, which has all the advantages like ease of the proper exposure of levator and its dissection, availability of adequate amount of levator muscle for resection after cutting the horns, and proper lid fold formation is possible.
- The cases of mild ptosis with faint lid folds were managed by proper lid fold formation.

Nonsurgical Management of Ptosis

A dropped eyelid can be managed nonsurgically by:
- External mechanical devices (skin-taping, adhesives, or spectacle-based lid crutches) to retract the upper lid
- Stimulating Müller's muscle (topical eye drops)
- Weakening orbicularis muscle tone (injectable botulinum toxin)

ENUCLEATION

- *Current indications of enucleation:*
  - Intraocular malignancy (uveal melanoma and RB)
  - Trauma
  - Painful blind eye
  - Sympathetic ophthalmitis
  - Microphthalmos.
- *Evisceration versus enucleation:* **Table 1.6.1** shows difference between evisceration and enucleation.

CHAPTER 1: Oculoplasty and Orbital Imaging

TABLE 1.6.1: Differences between evisceration and enucleation.

	Evisceration	Enucleation
Definition	Surgical technique of removing the intraocular contents, at the same time preserving the remaining scleral shell, extraocular muscle attachments, and surrounding orbital adnexa	Surgical procedure of removal of the entire globe and its intraocular contents, while preserving all other periorbital and orbital structures
Indications	• Endophthalmitis • Penetrating ocular trauma • Painful blind eye	• Intraocular malignancy (uveal melanoma and retinoblastoma) • Trauma • Painful blind eye • Sympathetic ophthalmitis • Microphthalmos
Advantages	• Shorter duration of surgery • Less complex procedure • Less disruption of orbital tissues • Improved postoperative prosthesis motility and better orbital volume • In cases of infection, less chance of spread to central nervous system (CNS) • Less painful more cost-efficient	• Lesser risk of sympathetic ophthalmitis • Lesser risk of intraocular tumor dissemination

- *Causes of bleeding during enucleation:*
  - Bleeding from central retinal vessels following optic nerve transection
  - Bleeding from anterior ciliary arteries during muscle transection
- *Hemostasis during enucleation:*
  - Retrobulbar injection of lignocaine and adrenaline preoperatively can help in intraoperative hemostasis.
  - Small amount of bleeding can be controlled by firm digital pressure.
  - Use of cautery is rarely required and should be used with caution near the orbital apex to prevent damage to EOMs and oculomotor nerves.
  - Postoperatively a pressure patch for the first 48 hours helps in maintain hemostasis.
- *Types of enucleation:*
  - *Based on technique:*
    - Conventional (imbrication) technique of enucleation
    - Myoconjunctival technique of enucleation—where EOMs are attached to the respective fornices instead of imbricating over the implant.
  - *Modifications of conventional:*
    - 4-petal technique
    - Double-petal technique
    - Scleral patch/orbital fat over porous implants
  - Based on primary or secondary implant.
- *Best approach to achieve optimal optic nerve length in RB:*
  - Gentle traction is applied to cause subluxation of globe out of rim.
  - Use of blunt 15° curved tenotomy scissors from the *lateral* aspect to transect the nerve
- *Complications of enucleation:*
  - *Intraoperative:*
    - Damage to or loss of EOMs
    - Hemorrhage

- Extensive dissection and mishandling of conjunctiva and tenons, leading to poor closure
- Improper implant sizing
- *Postoperative:*
  - Infection
  - Hemorrhage
  - Wound dehiscence
  - Extrusion of the conformer
  - Contraction of the fornices
  - Exposure, extrusion or migration of the implant
  - Ptosis
  - Hollow or deep superior sulcus
  - Poorly fitting prosthesis
  - Enophthalmos
  - Socket contracture
  - Postenucleation socket syndrome
  - Orbital cellulitis.
- *Calculate the size of implant:*
  - Formula for enucleation implant size: Implant diameter = AL – 2 mm
  - Subtract 1 mm from the above implant diameter for evisceration or hyperopia.
  - With a proper-sized implant, almost no chances of superior sulcus deformity or enophthalmos
  - The implant replaces the volume, leaving space for prosthesis 1.5–2.5 mL.
- *Types of implant:*
  - Nonintegrated [silicone, acrylic, and semi-integrated implants (Universal and Iowa) polymethyl methacrylate (PMMA)] and integrated (hydroxyapatite, porous polyethylene, and bioceramic)
  - Buried and exposed implants
- *Exenteration:* Exenteration is a surgical procedure involving removal of the entire globe and its adnexa (including muscles, fat, nerves, and eyelids). Types of exenteration are shown in **Table 1.6.2**.

TABLE 1.6.2: Types of exenteration.

Types	Contents removed
Anterior exenteration/extended enucleation	Globe, posterior lamella of eyelid, and conjunctival sac
Lid-sparing exenteration/subtotal exenteration	Orbital contents including periosteum of orbital walls
Total exenteration/eyelid sacrificing	Orbital contents, periorbita and lids
Radical/extended exenteration	Dissection involves paranasal sinuses, face, jaw, palate, and skull base

EVISCERATION

- *Current indications of evisceration:*
  - Blind painful eye
  - Endophthalmitis
  - Phthisis bulbi
  - Staphylomatous globe
  - Severe traumatic injury
  - End-stage glaucoma
- *Difference between enucleation and evisceration:* This is shown in **Table 1.6.1**.
- *Causes of bleeding during evisceration:* From retained uveal tissue
- *Hemostasis during evisceration:*
  - Subconjunctival injection of lignocaine and adrenaline preoperatively can help in intraoperative hemostasis.
  - Complete removal of uveal tissue adherent to scleral shell.
  - Inner side of empty scleral cup should be cleaned with sponge soaked in absolute alcohol aids in removing residual uveal tissue.
  - Small amount of bleeding can be controlled by firm digital pressure.
  - In case of excessive bleeding, cautery can be used.
- *Types of evisceration:* Two-flap technique and four-flap technique

- What is anophthalmic socket?
  - Anophthalmic socket is defined as the absence of the globe and ocular tissue from the orbit.
  - The majority of cases of anophthalmos are seen following evisceration or enucleation. Congenital anophthalmos, although seen rarely, happens due to the arrest of embryogenesis during formation of the optic vesicle.
- *Types of implant:* Refer to topic enucleation.

CHALAZION

- *Nonsurgical management of chalazion (Fig. 1.6.21):*
  - Warm compresses and lid hygiene
  - Tetracycline class of antibiotics [non-antimicrobial effects—inhibiting polymorph degranulation, reducing meibomian secretion viscosity, decreasing collagenase production, and inhibiting matrix metalloproteinase-9 (MMP-9) activity]
  - Topical steroids—to prevent the chronic inflammatory response
  - Local intralesional injection of a steroid (triamcinolone or methylprednisolone)—reduces inflammation and cause regression of the chalazion
- *Intralesional steroid:* Agents, dose, technique, indication, and complication:
  - Local intralesional injection of a steroid (triamcinolone or methylprednisolone) 0.2 mL of 40 mg/mL into the chalazion's center
  - *Indications:*
    - As an alternative first-line treatment when biopsy is not required
    - When the lesion is located near the lacrimal drainage system
    - Where an incision could cause complications involving tear flow

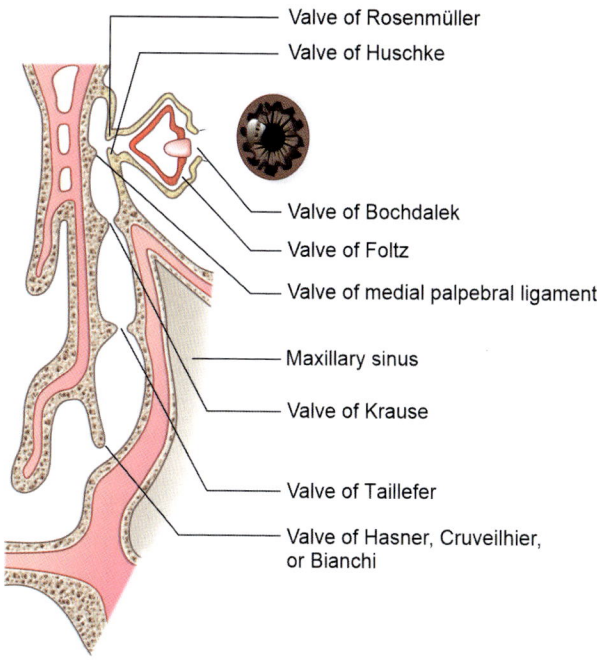

Fig. 1.6.21: Chalazion.

- Complications: Hypopigmentation and atrophy of the area, a visible depot of medication, corneal perforation, traumatic cataract, elevated intraocular pressure, and bacterial or viral infections
- How to prevent recurrence following chalazion excision?
    - Adequate curettage and drainage may prevent recurrences
    - Cauterization of the meibomian gland with a hyfrecator, phenol or trichloroacetic acid, and helps in preventing recurrences
    - Long-term low-dose tetracycline class therapy frequently has also been shown to prevent recurrence.
- *Approaches for excision:*
    - Transconjunctival vertical incision—to avoid damage to nearby glands
    - External (skin) horizontal incision—if a chalazion threatens to break through the skin or has drained through.

DACRYOCYSTORHINOSTOMY

- *Valves in nasolacrimal duct (NLD) system and their clinical importance:*
    - *Valves in NLD system*: The mucous membrane folds in the lacrimal pathways form a type of valve and serve to block the backward tear outflow.
    - *Valve of Rosenmüller*: It is a fold of mucosa at the junction between common canaliculi and lacrimal sac. It prevents reflux of tear from sac back into canaliculi.
    - *Valve of Hasner*: It is located at the junction of the opening of duct into inferior meatus of nose. It prevents sudden blast of air entering the lacrimal sac while blowing the nose.
    - *Other valves*: Valve of Huschke, Bochdalek, Folta, Krause, Hyrtl, Taillefer
- Lengths/distance of surgically important landmarks in NLD system:
    - The NLD is located, on average, 24.6 ± 3.56 mm posterior to the anterior nasal spine.
    - The marginal vessels lie medial to medial canthus while angular vein lies 8 mm medial to medial canthus. Thus, it is important to plan the skin incision and dissect tissues carefully.
    - The uncinate process is attached just posterior to the NLD, which is only 4 mm anterior to the maxillary sinus ostium.
    - Maxillary sinus ostium is also an important landmark to determine the location of the NLD.
- What is false passage in probing?
  At the time of probing, lacrimal probe may pierce through and go into a different track instead of NLD system creating a false passage.
- What is the size of probes preferred in congenital nasolacrimal duct obstruction (NLDO)?
  Size: 0–00
- *Lacrimal sac dimensions and parts:*
    - *Lacrimal sac:*
        - Length 15 mm
        - Breadth 5–6 mm
        - Volume 20 mm^3
    - Parts:
        - Fundus (3–5 mm)—portion above the opening of canaliculi
        - Body (10–12 mm)—middle part
        - Neck—lower small part
- What is lacrimal pump **(Fig. 1.6.22)**?
    - Lacrimal pump is a system helping in tear drainage.
    - In the relaxed state, the puncta lie in the tear lake.

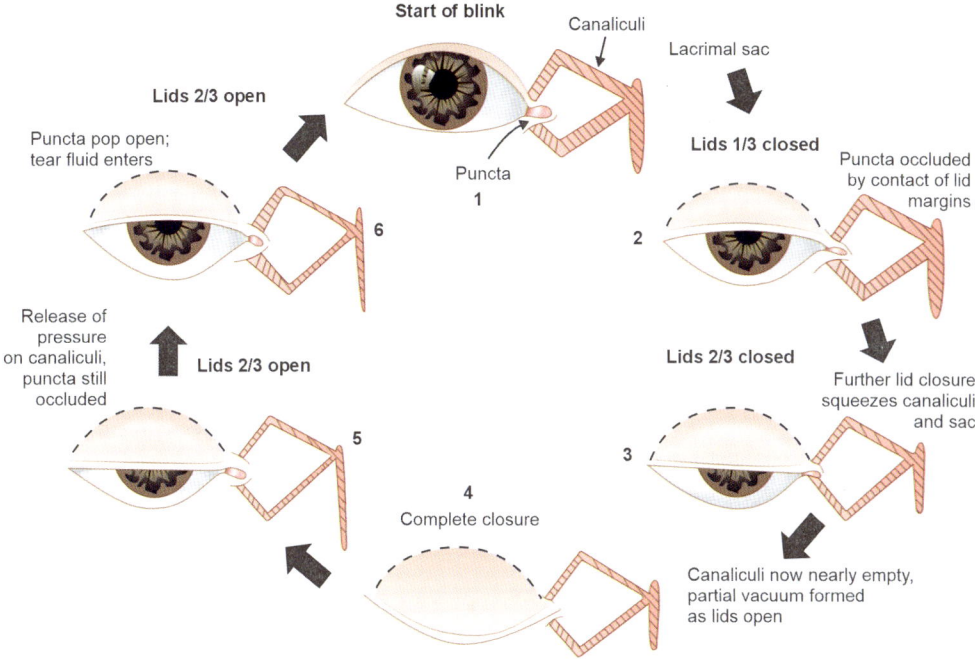

Fig. 1.6.22: Lacrimal pump.

- With eyelid closure, the orbicularis oculi muscle contracts. The pretarsal orbicularis squeezes and closes the puncta and canaliculi. The preseptal orbicularis, which inserts into the lacrimal sac, pulls the lacrimal sac open and draws the tears into the sac by creating a negative pressure within sac.
- With eyelid opening, the orbicularis relaxes, the puncta open, and the lacrimal sac collapses, propelling tears down the duct. Simultaneously, with the puncta opened, the canaliculi refill, completing the cycle.
  - *Muscles of lacrimal pump mechanism:*
    - *Horner's muscle (pars lacrimalis):* Fibers of pretarsal portion arising from lacrimal fascia and upper part of posterior lacrimal crest. They help in draining tears by lacrimal sac.
    - *Muscle of Riolan (pars ciliaris):* Fibers of pretarsal portion, which run along lid margins behind ciliary follicles; they keep lid in close opposition to globe.
  - What is percentage of tear drainage through upper and lower puncta?
    70% tear enter the lower canaliculus while 30% enter the upper.
  - *Types of dacryocystorhinostomy (DCR):*
    - External DCR
    - Endonasal DCR
    - Transcanalicular endoscopic DCR
    - Conjunctival DCR
    - Canalicular DCR
  - *Advantage and disadvantage of endoscopic DCR:* The advantage and disadvantage of endoscopic DCR are shown in **Table 1.6.3**.
  - *Site of ostium in DCR:*
    - The bony ostium is initiated at the junction of lacrimal bone and lamina papyracea.
    - *Extension:*

TABLE 1.6.3: Advantages and disadvantages of endoscopic dacryocystorhinostomy (DCR).

Advantages	Disadvantages
No external scar	Requires extensive knowledge of endonasal anatomy
Endonasal anatomy is directly visualized	Requires skills
In cases of primary failure, scar tissue under direct visualization can be easily mended	Increased operative time
If indicated concomitant sinus surgery performed	Expensive equipment

- *Superiorly:* About 2 mm above the medial canthal tendon (MCT)
- *Inferiorly:* Till the upper edge of NLD
- *Posteriorly:* Including the lamina papyracea
- *Anteriorly:* Till 3–4 mm above the level of anterior crest

- What is sump syndrome?
  - Lacrimal sump syndrome occurs as result of incomplete opening of inferior portion of the lacrimal sac, or the bone adjacent to the inferior sac, such that dependent fluid continues to collect in the sac. It can also result when mucosal healing leads to reapproximation of cut surfaces.
  - It is an uncommon cause of failed DCR.
- *Indications of intubation DCR:* Not indicated in uncomplicated DCR as tube-induced granulation tissue formation can itself cause closure of anastomosis. Indications of intubation DCR are as follows:
  - Canalicular stenosis
  - Fibrosed sac with inadequate mucosal flaps
  - Repeat DCR
  - Loss of mucosal flaps during surgery
- *Different types of intubation tubes (stents):* Two main types of stents are bicanalicular and monocanalicular.
  1. *Bicanalicular stent:* Pass through both the upper and lower canaliculus; e.g., Crawford stent, Ritleng stent, Pigtail/Donut stent, and Kaneka LacriFlow stent
  2. *Monocanalicular stents:* Do not provide a closed loop system, only intubating either the upper or lower canaliculus. Types include Mini-Monoka stent and Jones tube.
- *CSF rhinorrhea in DCR:*
  - CSF leakage or rhinorrhea is a very rare complication of DCR.
  - The cause of CSF leak after external DCR can either be the direct or indirect mode of bone injury. Inadvertent extension of the osteotomy to the anterior part of the base of the skull can produce direct injury.
  - With the development of new surgical procedures such as endoscopic DCR, the incidence of iatrogenic CSF rhinorrhea has increased.
  - It is more likely to occur during a pediatric DCR as children have low-lying cribriform plate as compared to adults.
  - Most of the iatrogenic CSF leaks resolve within 7–10 days with conservative management. The main goal of management of CSF rhinorrhea is to prevent ascending meningitis.
- *Rate of failed DCR:* The failure of DCR in most series is <10% of cases.
- *Difference between DCR and dacryocystectomy (DCT):*

- DCT is a surgical procedure of complete extirpation of the lacrimal sac.
- It was the standard of care for management of dacryocystitis and lacrimal fistulas before the advent of DCR.
- Indications for DCT include fibrotic sac, lacrimal sac tumor, tuberculosis (TB) of lacrimal sac, and NLDO associated with atrophic rhinitis.

- *Appropriate age for massage, probing, and DCR in congenital NLDO*:
  - Conservative management (Crigler's sac massage) of congenital NLDO up to 6–12 months of age
  - *NLD probing (therapeutic)*:
    - 12–18 months if conservative treatment fails.
    - Before 1 year in special cases (mucocele, prior to intraocular surgery, and repeated episodes of dacryocystitis)
  - DCR—after at least three trial of failed probing

- How to confirm that regurgitated fluid is from sac not canaliculus?
  - Regurgitated fluid from canaliculus is clear fluid whereas from sac is mucoid/pus.
  - It can be confirmed by dacryocystography.

CHAPTER 2

Cornea

2.1 SLIT-LAMP BIOMICROSCOPY

Rinky Agarwal, Sitesh Kumar Bergaal, Ritu Nagpal, Namrata Sharma

■ INTRODUCTION

Ocular diseases can involve any part of the eye starting from adnexa to optic nerve and numerous instruments can aid in their diagnosis. Naked eye examination with a bright light projected from a torch forms the most basic part of ocular examination. However, this being limited by lack of magnification leads to overlooking of minute, but extremely important details required for diagnosis of several ocular pathologies. Gullstrand combined principles of microscope and illumination in a single instrument and introduced slit lamp in early 20th century to aid enthusiastic ophthalmologists obtain a magnified as well as detailed view of various ocular parts.[1] Mawas later on introduced the word *biomecroscopy* and defined it as examination of living eye by means of corneal microscope and a slit lamp.

Modern-day slit-lamp biomicroscopy (SLB) with its auxiliary devices forms an indispensable tool for complete examination of the eye. It not only provides a magnified view of every part of the eye from adnexa to cornea to retina, but also allows clinical photography for documentation. In addition to qualitative assessment, quantitative measurement of intraocular pressure (IOP), pupil size, corneal thickness, endothelial cell morphology, and anterior chamber (AC) depth can also be obtained with modern-day SLB.

■ PARTS OF SLIT LAMP

Slit lamp, in a simplified language is a horizontally mounted microscope with provision for bright light, especially designed for ophthalmic use **(Fig. 2.1.1)**.

Observation System (Microscope)

The observation system, essentially composed of two optical elements, an objective lens

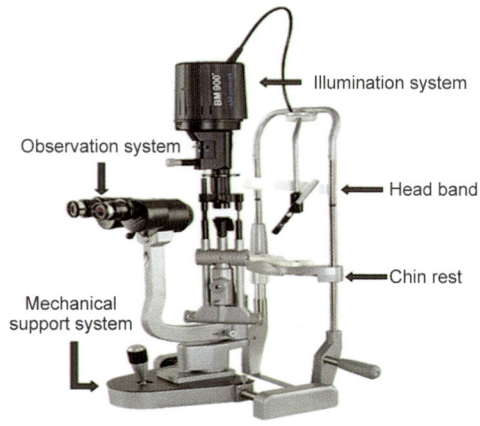

Fig. 2.1.1: Parts of a slit lamp (Haag Streit).

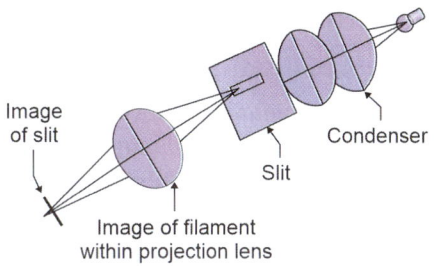

Fig. 2.1.2: Optical principle of slit lamp.

(providing a power of +22 D by two plano-convex lenses) and an eyepiece (power of +10 D), presents an enlarged but inverted image of near object to the observer, a problem overcome by use of prisms between objective and eyepiece. Two eyepieces are independently adjustable to match observer's interpupillary distance and refractive error **(Fig. 2.1.2)**.

Modern-day slit lamps provide a range of magnifications from 6× to 40×. Three types of magnification systems used in different models of slit lamps comprise:
1. Czapskiscope with rotating objectives (different objectives placed in a turret type of arrangement)
2. Littmann Galilean telescope principle of magnification
3. Zoom system

Nowadays, observation arm has a high-quality digital camera, connected to a computer, incorporated for real-time photographic and videographic documentation of ocular details permitting future references and teaching.[2]

Illumination System

The Gullstrand's illumination system is designed to provide a bright, evenly illuminated, finely focused, and highly malleable slit of light. It is composed of a light source, which provides an illumination of 2×10^5 to 4×10^5 lux and a condenser lens system with a couple of plano-convex lenses with their convex lenses in apposition to focus light on the desired object. A projection lens provided in the system ensures a high-quality image of slit at the eye by decreasing aberrations and increasing its depth of focus. A mirror or prism placed perpendicular to the projection system allows latter to pass easily from one side of the microscope to the other. Whenever required for examination of fundus, illumination system can be made to coincide with the viewing axis without obstructing the field of view by use of a narrow prism or mirror.

Adjustment of height and width of the slit and its rotation in both vertical and horizontal meridian is facilitated by use of different knobs specifically provided for this purpose. Various filters like cobalt blue filter and red-free filter attached to the illumination system provide enhanced view of iron lines and corneal epithelial defects and blood vessels, respectively.

Mechanical Support System

Thorough ocular examination requires a confident clinician, a comfortable patient, and a long working distance between observer and patient's eye. The former is an art learnt with time, patience, and perseverance while the latter two are supplemented by an ergonomically supportive mechanical system, which has changed little over the years.

Mechanical coupling of microscope and illumination system allows them to rotate along a common axis that coincides with their focal planes. This safeguards parfocality between slit beam and microscope for adequate illumination of patient's eye while examination. Slight decentration may, however, be required while performing added procedures like gonioscopy and fundoscopy with accessory lenses.

Back and forth, side-by-side, and up-down movement of microscope and illumination system is facilitated by joystick provided in the slit lamp. Movement of the instrument relative to chinrest (to accommodate individuals of all sizes and age) and movement of chinrest relative to patient's face are aided by a screw device fitted in the mechanical system. A movable fixation target in accordance with clinician's requirement and a black mark on the chinrest coinciding with the eyebrow of the patient allows an unimpeded ocular examination.

BASIC PRINCIPLES OF SLIT-LAMP ILLUMINATION

Three specific types of illumination provided by slit lamp enhance examiner's ability to see details of ocular structure examined.
1. *Focal illumination*, achieved by narrowing the slit beam horizontally or vertically permits examination of specific areas without any extraneous light outside area of examination.
2. *Oblique illumination*, obtained by projecting light oblique to the tissue examined, is essential for examining different layers of ocular structures.
3. *Optical slit section*, which makes the instrument unique, is used to examine internal details of all layers of ocular structure examined. Importance of slit beam of light cannot be overemphasized in revolutionizing ophthalmologic expansions. Incorporation of this simple idea in intraoperative microscope has reformed clinician's ability to objectively judge intraoperative depth of a lesion tremendously.[3] Newer devices like Orbscan also utilize slit scanning technology for assessment of corneal topography.

TECHNIQUE OF BIOMICROSCOPY

Methods of Illumination

- *Diffuse illumination:* Diffuse illumination is facilitated by use of widest slit beam (medium-to-high illumination and medium-to-high magnification), the intensity of which can made more endurable to the patient with the aid of a neutral density diffuse filter and shortest examination time possible to avoid phototoxicity of retina. The maximum beam height ranges from 8 to 14 mm depending on the model of slit lamp. This height is still less for examination of adnexa in entirety; therefore beam has to be moved up and down and side to side to overcome omission of any additional details **(Figs. 2.1.3 and 2.1.4)**.
- *Direct focal slit illumination:* Direct focal examination of ocular structure is enabled by projecting a narrow-slit beam at an angle to coincide with exact focus of the microscope **(Figs. 2.1.5 and 2.1.6)**. This can be done as an optical section, as parallelepiped beam or conical beam. Narrowing the slit beam, although it reduces the amount of illumination available for examination, helps clinician

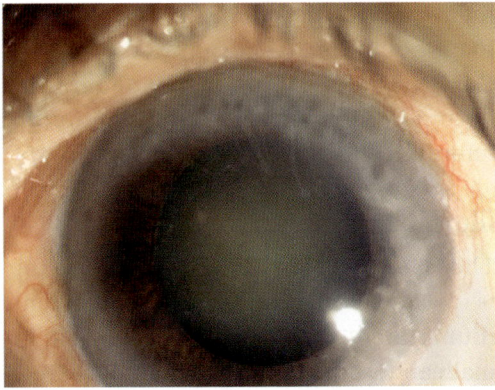

Fig. 2.1.3: Target sign seen on diffuse illumination in pseudoexfoliation syndrome.

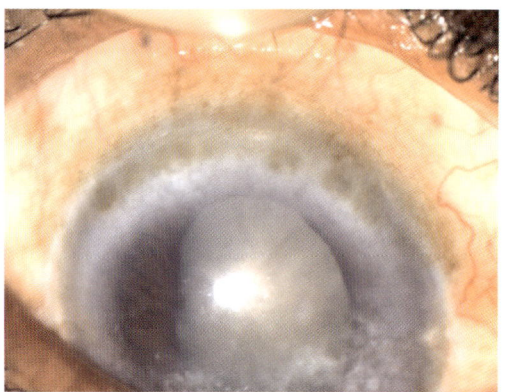

Fig. 2.1.4: Herbert's pits seen superiorly diffuse illumination in healed trachoma.

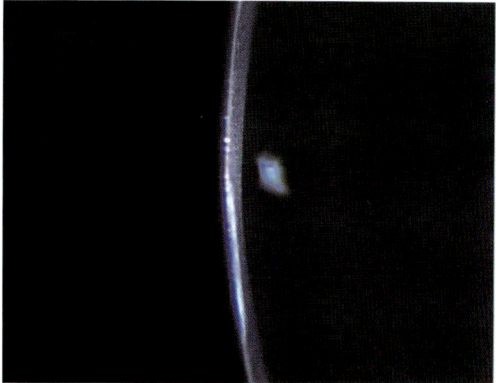

Fig. 2.1.6: Magnified slit view of **Figure 2.1.5** also showing anterior stromal scarring.

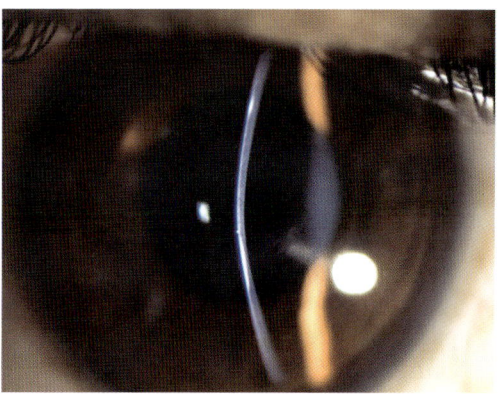

Fig. 2.1.5: Central steepening and thinning of cornea in keratoconus as seen on direct slit illumination.

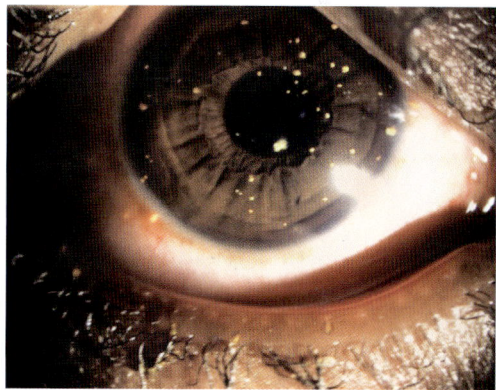

Fig. 2.1.7: Multiple corneal foreign bodies seen on scleral scatter.

acquire comprehensive information about various layers of cornea. The problem of low illumination can be overcome by maintaining dim background lights. This makes examiner's eyes more sensitive to low illumination of light.

A special form of direct focal illumination called *broad tangential illumination*, attained by reflecting light at an extremely oblique illumination angle, helps in diagnosing surface abnormalities of cornea and in corneal photography.

- *Sclerotic scatter:* Examination of faintest corneal opacities can be heightened by technique of scleral scatter, where light beam focused at one side of scleral limbus emerges from entire circumference of limbus by utilizing principle of *total internal reflection* (provided cornea is transparent) **(Fig. 2.1.7)**. Complete loss of parfocality between illumination and microscope for this technique is ensured by focusing broad beam of light at 3 or 9 o'clock scleral limbus (till halo of light appears around entire limbus) and examining cornea independently by microscope.

- *Retroillumination:* Retroillumination, as the name implies, means inspection of

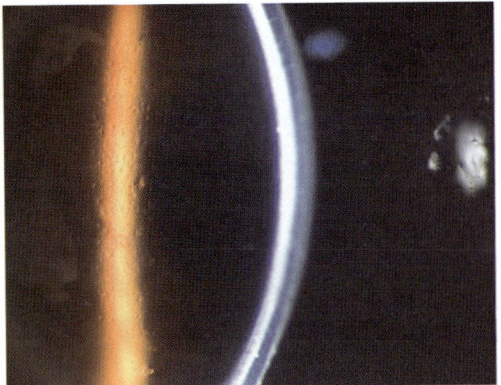

Fig. 2.1.8: Recurrence of spheroidal degeneration at interface postlamellar keratoplasty appreciated on retroillumination from iris.

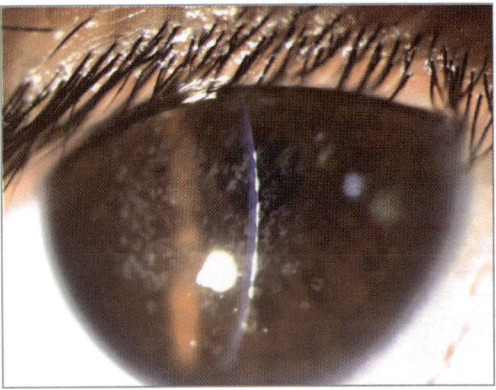

Fig. 2.1.10: Hyaline deposits of granular dystrophy seen on proximal illumination.

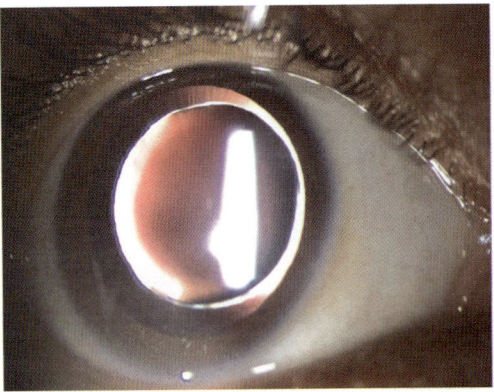

Fig. 2.1.9: Crystalline lens in microspherophakia best appreciated on retroillumination from fundus.

any pathological area with the aid of light reflected from structure posterior to it. A corneal or lenticular abnormality can be assessed by broad illuminating light reflected by iris **(Fig. 2.1.8)** or fundus [red reflex emerging from retinal pigmented epithelium (RPE) and choroid] **(Fig. 2.1.9)** under either direct illumination (pathology is seen against illuminated background) or indirect illumination (as light is at right angle to observed pathology, it is seen against dark background).

- *Proximal (indirect) illumination:* Proximal illumination, a technique that syndicates sclerotic scatter and retroillumination, can be employed to assess any pathological area by directing light adjacent to the area under examination. Indirect illumination permits visualization of additional details of any abnormality by preventing dazzling light from masking underlying structures **(Fig. 2.1.10)**. When a moderately wide beam of light is directed adjacent to a particular area, transparency of that area causes light to travel effortlessly within it whereas any opacity reflects it back to the observer, permitting its enhanced identification.

- *Specular reflection:* Specular reflection, based on principle of *Snell's law*, is a method used to examine planar surfaces by means of total internal reflection. Clinically, this principle is largely used to scrutinize corneal endothelial cells **(Fig. 2.1.11)**. When light is incident on endothelial layer, dazzling reflex of light reflected from zone of discontinuity leads to specular reflection. For this patient is instructed to look 30° temporally and light is incident from opposite side such that angle between microscope and light is 60°. A parallelepiped beam under high

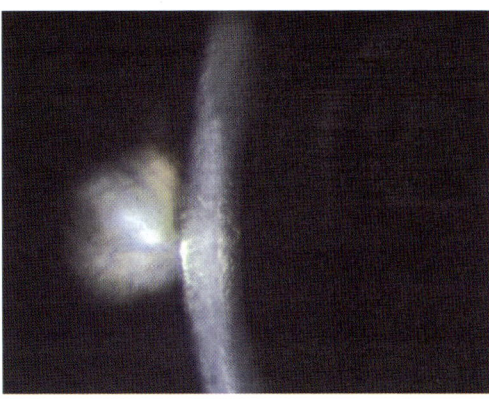

Fig. 2.1.11: Specular endothelium at endothelium shows presence of guttae.

illumination and high magnification is required for this purpose.[4]

All these techniques are mentioned comprehensively in **Table 2.1.1**.[5]

DYNAMIC SLIT-LAMP BIOMICROSCOPY

Slit-lamp biomicroscopy is a dynamic process in which examiner constantly integrates various types of illumination techniques to obtain an accurate, three-dimensional, fully detailed, and complete mental image of ocular structures examined. Every clinician

TABLE 2.1.1: Different techniques of slit-lamp examination.[5]

Method of slit-lamp examination		Angle between microscope and illumination	Slit beam	Structures/lesions seen
Diffuse illumination		30°–45°	Diffuse	Generalized view of adnexa, lids, ocular surface, and anterior segment
Direct focal illumination	Optical section	30°–45°	Narrow slit beam	• Cornea • Epithelial layer (dark), Bowman's membrane (bright), stroma (gray), Descemet's membrane (brightest) • Crystalline lens • Anterior capsule, anterior cortical layer, nucleus, cortical layer, posterior capsule • Anterior one-third of vitreous
	Parallelopiped section	30°–45°	2–3 mm wide slit beam	Corneal scars and infiltrates (appear brighter than surroundings because of more density)
	Conical beam	45°–60°	Semi-circular pattern	• Flare—gray or milky haze in anterior chamber • Cells—white dots
	Broad tangential illumination	70°–80°	Wide beam	• Anterior surface irregularities of cornea like band-shaped keratopathy (BSK), punctate keratopathy • Posterior corneal surface irregularities like Descemet's folds

Contd...

Contd...

Method of slit-lamp examination		Angle between microscope and illumination	Slit beam	Structures/lesions seen
Retro-illumination	Iris (undilated pupil)	60° slightly rotated off-axis	Moderately broad beam	Epithelial microcysts, refractile materials like Salzmann's nodules and amyloid deposits, stromal infiltrates, blood vessels, pigmented deposits and Descemet's excrescences
	Fundus (dilated pupil)	Slit beam is coaxial to microscope and centered in the pupil	Moderately broad beam	• Corneal scars, epithelial basement membrane and lattice corneal dystrophy, guttae, ridges in Descemet's membrane, oil droplet reflex in keratoconus • Lenticular opacities like blue dot cataract, posterior subcapsular cataract
Sclerotic scatter		15° slightly decentered	Maximum slit height, moderate width	Faintest of corneal opacities like subepithelial infiltrates, epithelial edema, stromal edema
Indirect illumination		>45°	2–3 mm height, 0.2 mm broad, decentered beam	Corneal infiltrates, microcysts and vacuoles
Specular reflection		60°	40× magnification, 3–4 mm height, 0.5 mm wide beam	Tear film abnormalities, corneal endothelial cells

must establish an individualized protocol for a systematic, multidirectional, and unbiased examination to gather every possible data within a single, if required repeated, examination **(Fig. 2.1.12)**.

- A semi-dark room ensures adaptation of examiner to low sensitivities of light for a comprehensive examination of fine details.
- Key step for an unhindered examination is adjustment of instrument according to comfort of both patient and the clinician. Clinicians should adapt to an

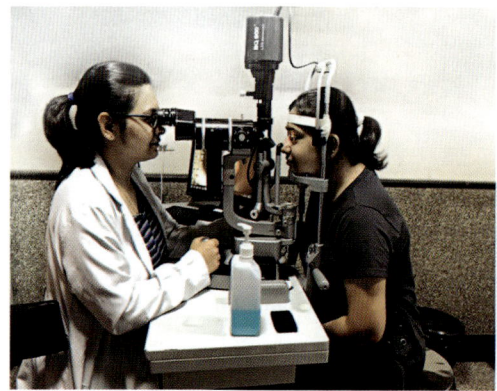

Fig. 2.1.12: Dynamic slit-lamp biomicroscopy.

erect posture owing to ill-effects of bad ergonomics on clinician's spine and muscles in the long run.
- Slit-lamp examination begins with diffuse examination of both eyes at lowest magnification with filtered slit beam to locate any gross abnormalities. This is followed by detailed examination of each eye under high magnification.
- Sclerotic scatter from temporal limbus is used to identify faintest of corneal opacities. Direct focal and indirect illumination of affected area is followed by visualization of internal details of abnormality against retroillumination of iris and fundus. Two or three scans across cornea with light beam projected from nasal, temporal, superior, and inferior directions guarantee complete impression of extent and severity of any abnormality if present.
- Examination of lens and anterior vitreous against red reflex of fundus, direct and indirect illumination methods follow evaluation of cornea.
- Clinicians should make it a habit to constantly move the instrument from anterior to posterior part of eye to encompass every single detail piecemeal and later on reconstruct the mental image in toto on a drawing using color coding for repeated interpretation of details **(Table 2.1.2)**.[6]
- Application of any vital dyes, medications, or accessory procedures are performed after an unhindered primary examination described above.

ACCESSORY DEVICES

The addition of accessory devices to slit lamp allows performance of various specialized

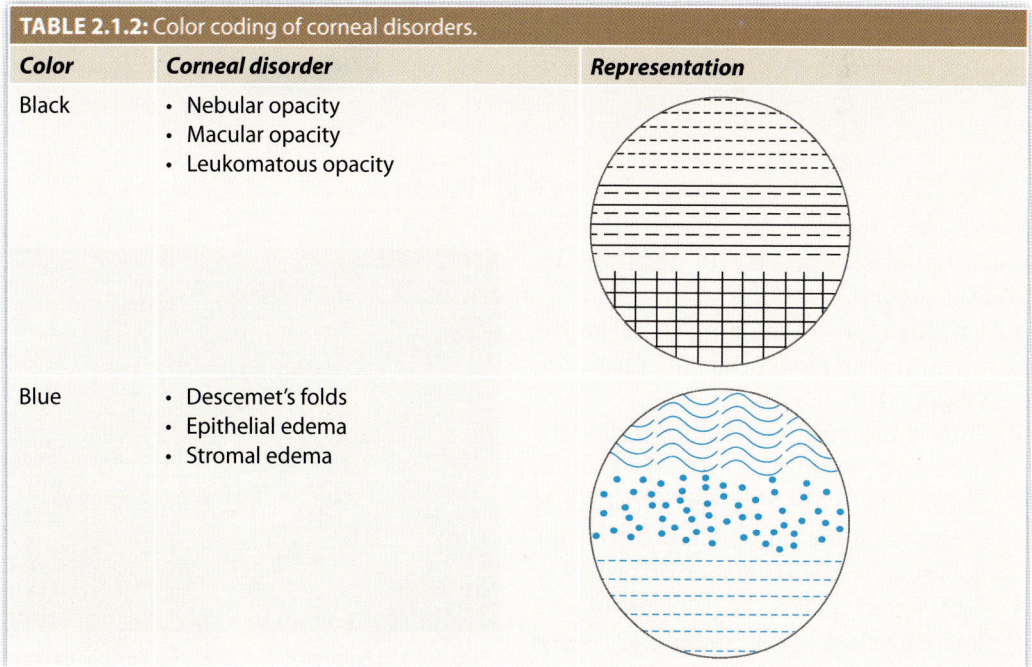

TABLE 2.1.2: Color coding of corneal disorders.

Color	Corneal disorder	Representation
Black	• Nebular opacity • Macular opacity • Leukomatous opacity	
Blue	• Descemet's folds • Epithelial edema • Stromal edema	

Contd...

Contd...

Color	Corneal disorder	Representation
Red brown	• Iron pigmentation • Deep intrastromal blood vessel—straight lines extending till limbus • Superficial conjunctival blood vessels—dotted lines extending beyond limbus • Intracorneal blood	
Yellow	• Keratic precipitates • Hypopyon • Infiltrate	
Green	• Filaments • Punctate staining • Epithelial defect	

examinations necessary to substantiate clinical findings.

- Various types of staining to diagnose, measure, and monitor treatment success **(Fig. 2.1.13)**
- One of the most commonly performed accessory examinations; applanation tonometry with a prism particularly designed for this purpose is presently the gold standard for estimation of the IOP.
- Gonioscopy utilizes the principle of total internal reflection to examine angle recess by means of an accessory convex lens **(Figs. 2.1.14A and B)**. Fundoscopy with

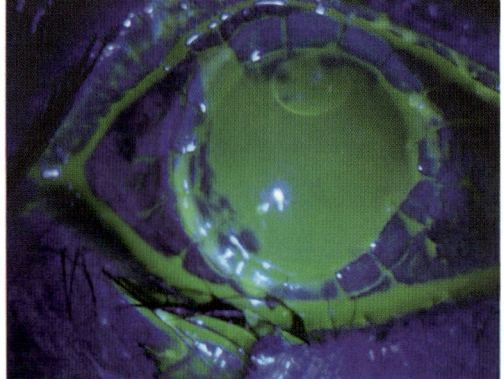

Fig. 2.1.13: Epithelial defect as seen under cobalt blue light after fluorescein staining.

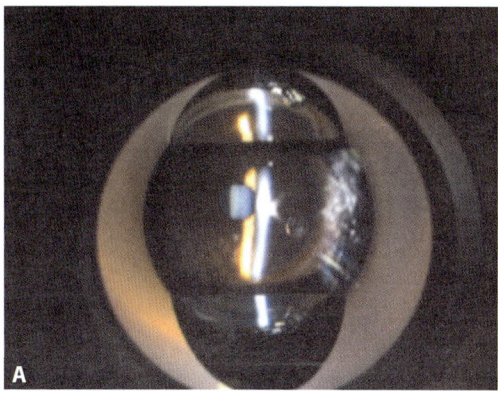
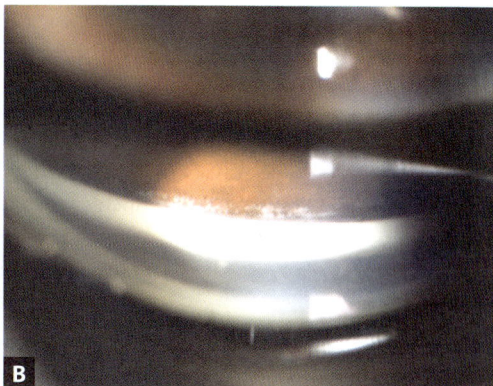

Figs. 2.1.14A and B: (A) Gonioscopy procedure being performed with Goldmann two mirror lens; (B) Widened ciliary body band seen on gonioscopy in angle recession.

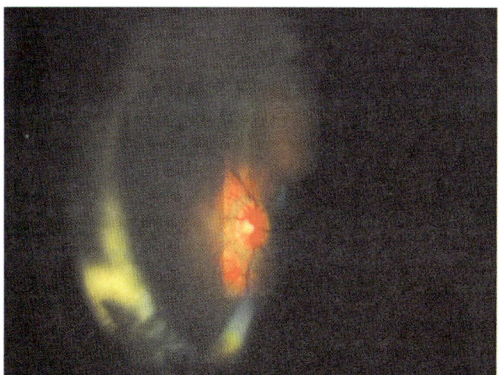

Fig. 2.1.15: Magnified disc details appreciated on slit-lamp biomicroscopy examination with 90D.

highly convex (90 D) or concave (Hruby lens) lens provides magnified slit view of macula and disc **(Fig. 2.1.15)**.
- In contact lens (CL) users, SLB plays a paramount role in assessment of CL fitting, centration, and movement (by means of tear film formation between CL and cornea after fluorescein staining) along with inspection of any secondary effects and aftercare at every follow-up.
- Accessory laser delivery devices attached to slit lamp can be used to perform laser capsulotomy, iridotomy, trabeculoplasty, and retinal photocoagulation as out-patient procedures.
- Laser interferometry and potential acuity meter also exploit slit lamp for gauging visual potential of a patient.

■ VIVA QUESTIONS

1. What are the different filters in a slit lamp? Enumerate their clinical uses.
Ans. Refer to **Table 2.1.3**.

2. Describe dyes used for corneal staining along with their specific uses, staining property, advantages, and disadvantages.
Ans. Refer to **Table 2.1.4**.

3. How to mark the axis, preoperatively for toric intraocular lens (IOL) on slit lamp?
Ans.
- There are various markers available for preoperative toric axis marking such as Gimble marker (ASICO) and the Nuits/Lane Pre-op Toric Reference Marker (bubble), Neuhann-Nuijts One-Step Toric Marker, AXsys™ One Step Electronic Toric Marking Device, and pendulum-attached marker.
- Manual marking can also be done accurately. The eye should be marked while the patient is sitting upright and fixing with the other eye at a distant target

TABLE 2.1.3: Different filters in a slit lamp.

Filter	Use
Cobalt blue filter	• Fluorescein staining • Goldmann applanation tonometry • Fleischer ring
Yellow filter	Increases contrast enhancement when using cobalt blue filter
Red-free/green filter	• Rose Bengal staining • Blood vessels • Hemorrhages
Diffuser and white filter	Generalized examination of eye and adnexa
Neutral density filter and gray filter	Decrease brightness for photophobic patients
Heat absorbing	Decreases patient discomfort

TABLE 2.1.4: Dyes used for corneal staining.

Dye	Staining property	Advantages	Disadvantages
Sodium fluorescein	• Yellow color water-soluble dye • Stains epithelium bright green as seen under cobalt blue filter, diffuses into intercellular spaces, does not stain devitalized tissue	Can be used for assessment of ocular surface integrity and function, tear film breakup time (TBUT), corneal epithelial defects, rigid contact lens fitting, applanation tonometry, Seidel's test, Jones dye test, fluorescein dye disappearance test (FDDT)	Can exhibit pseudoflare, stain soft contact lens and promote growth of *Pseudomonas aeruginosa* in solution
Rose Bengal	Red color under red-free/green filter, stains dead or degenerated cells and mucus strands	For staining of conjunctiva and evaluation of herpetic keratouveitis, true dendrites, superficial punctate keratitis	Intrinsic cellular toxicity to corneal epithelial cells, patient discomfort, particularly stinging upon instillation
Lissamine green	• Green color under white light • Preferentially stains dead and devitalized cells, does not stain normal ocular surface	• Detects dead or degenerate conjunctival cells • Minimal effect on corneal epithelial cells and minimal stinging on application	

to avoid cyclotorsion. Make slit lamp's illuminating column coaxial with viewing column. For 0°–180° reference marking, a narrow-slit beam can be focused on the cornea and the axis can be marked. Maintain steady fixation of the patient by closing contralateral eye and asking patient to look straight ahead into the slit lamp. Mark axis on peripheral cornea using gentian violet marker pen or a 26G sterile needle on a 2-mL syringe at the point where slit beam cuts limbus.

TABLE 2.1.5: Clinical grading on aqueous cells on slit lamp.

Standardization of Uveitis Nomenclature (SUN) classification of cells grading

Grade	Cells*	Flare
0	<1	None
0.5+	1–5	
1+	6–15	Faint (barely detectable)
2+	16–25	Moderate (iris/lens details clear)
3+	26–50	Marked (iris/lens details hazy)
4+	>50	Intense (fibrin/plastic aqueous)

*Slit-lamp beam field size is 1 × 1 mm^2, preferably 16× magnification.

TABLE 2.1.6: Grading of flare on slit lamp.

Grade	Description	Findings
0	None	
1+	Faint	Mild anterior chamber turbidity
2+	Moderate	Iris and lens details clear
3+	Marked	Iris and lens details hazy
4+	Intense	Fibrin or plastic aqueous

This type of marking uses the first Purkinje image principle.

4. How to calculate magnification in SLB with 90 D?

Ans. Image magnification factor for emmetropic eye = 60/90 D × magnification of slit lamp.

5. Describe color coding in corneal ulcer.

Ans. Refer to **Table 2.1.2**.

6. How to perform specular microscopy?

Ans.
- Instruct the patient to look straight ahead.
- Project slit beam from onto the central cornea from temporal side.
- Shorten the size of the beam (3–4 mm height and 0.5 mm width) and increase magnification (25× or 40×).
- Coincide slit beam with light reflected from nasal iris and first catoptric/Purkinje image (it has rectangular shape of the slit-lamp mirror).
- Paving stone pattern consisting of hexagonal endothelial cells with dark center and bright borders can be appreciated.

7. Describe the method for grading cells and flare.

Ans. Refer to **Tables 2.1.5 and 2.1.6**. Laser flare/cell photometry is based on measurement of light [incoming laser (helium–neon/diode) beam] scattered in AC. ASOCT-based measurements like aqueous-to-air relative intensity (ARI) index method to examine retrolental cells have also been described.

REFERENCES

1. Timoney PJ, Breathnach CS. Allvar Gullstrand and the slit lamp 1911. Ir J Med Sci. 2013;182(2):301-5.

2. Martin R. Cornea and anterior eye assessment with slit lamp biomicroscopy, specular microscopy, confocal microscopy, and ultrasound biomicroscopy. Indian J Ophthalmol. 2018;66(2):195-201.
3. KA. Biomicroscopie du Cristallin. Arch Ophthalmol. 1931;5(1):154.
4. Bourne WM, Kaufman HE. Specular microscopy of human corneal endothelium in vivo. Am J Ophthalmol. 1976;81(3): 319-23.
5. Krachmer JH, Mannis MJ, Holland EJ. Cornea. St Louis Missouri: Mosby/Elsevier; 2011. p. 1967.
6. Waring GO, Laibson PR. A systematic method of drawing corneal pathologic conditions. Arch Ophthalmol. 1977;95(9): 1540-2.

2.2 KERATOMETER

Ritu Nagpal, Siddhi Goel, Shipra Singhi, Prafulla Kumar Maharana

INTRODUCTION

Keratometer **(Fig. 2.2.1)** is a device used to measure the anterior curvature of the central 3 mm of cornea. It is an essential tool for biometry of cases undergoing cataract surgery. Besides, it is useful for CL trial and diagnosis of irregular astigmatism. Although new-generation videokeratography devices have superseded its role, it is still considered as the gold standard for calculation of keratometry before cataract surgery.

PRINCIPLES

The keratometer assumes that the cornea is a perfect, thin, dry, and inelastic sphere and calculates the corneal power using the following principles:[1-3]

- The cornea is a convex refracting surface.
- In order to find the refracting power of the cornea, we need to reflect an object of a known size at a known distance to the corneal surface.
- Keeping the distance between the eye and keratometer fixed, the corneal radius is directly proportional to the size of the reflected image, which is nothing but the first Purkinje image and indirectly proportional to the size of the object.
- The anterior corneal curvature is then calculated using the convex mirror formula. The size of the reflecting image is determined with a measuring telescope, and the refractive power of the cornea is calculated based on the refractive index of $n = 1.3375$ (this may vary depending upon the type of instrument).
- The corneal power is calculated based on Snell's law of refraction:

$$\text{Surface power formula: } D = n_2 - n_1/R$$

D = The dioptric power of the cornea
n_1 = Refractive index of the first medium (air–cornea)

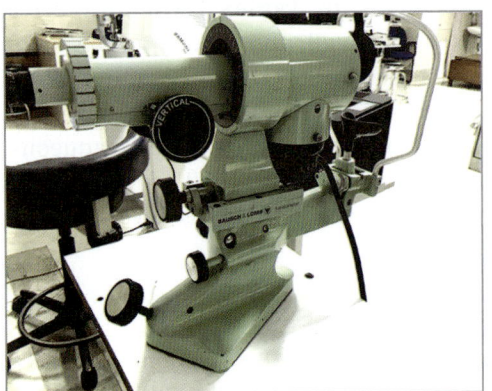

Fig. 2.2.1: Bausch and Lomb keratometer.

n_2 = Refractive index of the second medium (cornea–aqueous)
R = The radius of curvature of the cornea in meters
- The keratometer does not take into account the power of posterior corneal curvature, instead adjusts the index of refraction (1.3375 vs. 1.376) to account for the posterior corneal power.
- *Doubling principle:* Due to involuntary eye movements, the image formed on cornea will not be stable. To overcome this Ramsden developed the doubling technique where a prism is introduced into the optical system so that two images are formed, and the prism is moved until the images touch each other.

TYPES OF KERATOMETER

Keratometer can be classified based on:
- *Principles of keratometer:*[4]
  - *Javal–Schiotz keratometer:* Fixed image size with variable object size (fixed doubling); here, Wollaston prisms are used.
  - *Bausch and Lomb keratometer:* Fixed object size with variable image size (variable doubling); there are two prisms, one prism in the horizontal direction and the other in the vertical direction. There are two apertures through which whatever the rays are passing; they are undeviated.

  Other keratometers described includes:
  - *Helmholtz doubling principle keratometer:* It consists of two rotating prisms that create an angle with each other.
  - *Original American optical keratometer:* Here, biprisms are used.
- *Depending upon the need to rotate the prism:*
  - *One-position keratometer:* Horizontal and vertical meridian can be assessed without rotation because it consists of horizontal and vertical direction prism. Examples include Bausch and Lomb keratometer and Appa Swamy keratometer.[4]
  - *Two-position keratometer:* In this type, horizontal meridian is assessed first following which the keratometer is rotated 90° apart to assess another meridian. Here, Wollaston prism is used, e.g., Javal–Schiotz keratometer.[4]
- *Depending upon working:*
  - Automated
  - Manual

PARTS OF KERATOMETER

- Telescope
- Eyepiece at one end (near to examiner)
- Objective (near to the patient)
- Knobs for adjustment of vertical and horizontal curvature on the telescope
- Knobs adjusting the height of telescope
- Chinrest-adjusting knobs
- Bulb for illumination
- Knob for focusing of mires
- Model cornea with the occluder

Performing Keratometry

- Looking through the eyepiece of the keratometer, use the eyepiece to focus the crosshair.
- The patient can comfortably put the chin and forehead on the appropriate rests.
- Use the occluder attached to the keratometer to cover the eye not being measured.
- Then use the height adjustment knob of the keratometer to position the light reflections at the level of the cornea **(Figs. 2.2.2 and 2.2.3)**.

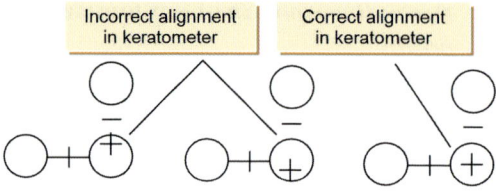

Fig. 2.2.2: Correct and incorrect alignment in keratometer.

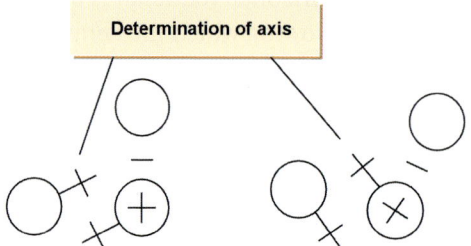

Fig. 2.2.3: Determination of steep and flat axis.

INTERPRETATION

Measurement Range

- The measurement range is 36–52 D
- Its lower limit can be extended up to 30 D by interposing –1.0 D in front of the objective of the telescope.
- Its upper limit can be extended up to 61 D by interposing a lens of +1.25 D in front of the objective of the telescope.
- *Normal keratometry*:
  - The cornea contributes for two-thirds of the refractive power of the eye.
  - Around 98% of the population has a corneal power between 40 and 48 D.[2]
  - Around 68% have a cornea power between 42 and 45 D.[2]

Limitations

- Keratometer measures only two points at the 3–4 mm zone, and does not provide information about the cornea central or peripheral to these points.
- It assumes that the cornea is sphero-cylindrical and symmetric with a major and minor axis separated by 90°, which is not always true thus it ignores spherical aberration (SA).
- Focusing and misalignment errors
- Cannot accurately measure irregular corneas
- It does not measure the posterior corneal surface that contributes approximately 0.4 D of against-the-rule astigmatism to the total corneal power. This is important when calculating the amount of total corneal astigmatism for toric IOL implantation and refractive lens exchange with multifocal IOL implantation.

SOURCES OF ERRORS IN KERATOMETRY

There are many factors that can lead to inaccuracies in measurement, as follows:[2,3]

- *Diurnal variations in corneal physiology*: The refractive index of the cornea shows diurnal fluctuations due to variations in corneal hydration. Although not that significant, repeated measurements should be done at the same time of the day when some research is planned.
- *CL wearers*: CL can cause temporary alterations in the curvature of the cornea. Patients must discontinue CL wear for 2 weeks for soft CLs and 4 weeks for rigid CLs before measurement of keratometry.
- *Nonsphericity of the cornea*: A keratometer assumes that the cornea is thin, inelastic, and a perfect sphere. On the contrary, the normal cornea has some thickness, is spherocylindrical, and elastic.
- *Improper calibration*: Steel balls are used to calibrate manual keratometers. Routine calibration is a must to avoid any error.
- *Failure to focus eyepieces*: To achieve focus, first, the eyepieces are turned

anticlockwise and then slowly turned clockwise until the mires are in sharp focus. The observer's refractive error must be neutralized to avoid any erroneous measurements.
- *Tear film breakup:* Disruptions of the corneal surface, either due to dry eye, corneal scarring or due to insufficiencies in the tear film can lead to errors. One drop of artificial tear drop before the examination can abolish this error.
- *Previous refractive surgery:* Keratometers assume that the Gullstrand ratio, i.e., relation between the front and back surface of the cornea is similar in corneas of different patients. However, corneal laser surgery results in changes in the relationship between the curvature of the anterior and posterior surfaces of the cornea and thus the posterior corneal power cannot be ignored in such cases.
- Drooping eyelids
- *Irregular cornea:* Inaccuracies can be avoided by repeat keratometry, if:
  - Corneal curvature >47 D or <40 D
  - The difference in the corneal cylinder is >1 D between eyes.

■ VIVA QUESTIONS

1. What are the types of keratometry?
Ans. Refer to text.

2. How to calibrate keratometer?
Ans. The keratometer is calibrated using steel balls. A steel ball of known radius of curvature is placed before the keratometer and its value is set on the dial. The mires are focused by rotating the eyepiece by trial-and-error method. When the mires are focused, calibration is said to be complete.

3. What is the principle of keratometer?
Ans. Refer to text.

4. Give disadvantages of keratometer.
Ans. Refer to text, limitations of keratometer.

5. Can you measure the central K in keratometer?
Ans. No.

6. What is the normal range of keratometer?
Ans. The normal range is 36–52 D.

7. How can the range of measurements be increased?
Ans. Refer to text.

8. Which equipment can give you an accurate estimation of posterior corneal surface power?
Ans. Pentacam.

9. Which equipment can give you total astigmatism?
Ans. Cassini (based on ray tracing principle) and Pentacam (total power map).

10. State the conditions where posterior corneal power cannot be ignored.
Ans. Postrefractive surgery and postradial keratotomy.

■ REFERENCES

1. Friedman NJ, Kaiser PK. Optics/Refraction. Case Reviews in Ophthalmology, 2nd edition. New York: Elsevier; 2017. pp. 1-46.
2. Elliott DB. Determination of the refractive correction. Clinical Procedures in Primary Eye Care, 3rd edition. Edinburgh: Butterworth–Heinemann; 2007. pp. 83-150.
3. Embleton SJ. Pre-operative biometry and intraocular lens calculation. Cataract. Edinburgh: Butterworth–Heinemann; 2008. pp. 33-72.
4. Chowdhury PH, Shah BH, Tiwari N. Keratometer: Easy to Understand. J Ophthalmol. 2018;3(S1):000S1-016.

2.3 PENTACAM

Prafulla Kumar Maharana, Siddhi Goel, Abhipsa Sharma, Pranita Sahay, Anin Sethi, Jeewan Singh Titiyal

■ INTRODUCTION

Cornea is the principal refractive element of the human eye. Out of around 58–60 D, cornea contributes around 42–45 D or almost two-thirds of the total power of the eye. The anterior surface of the cornea accounts for the maximum refraction that occurs in the eye. The considerable difference in the refractive index of air and cornea accounts for this (air $\mu = 1$; corneal $\mu = 1.37$). Thus, evaluation and characterization of the corneal surface is an essential component for the diagnosis, planning, treatment, and postoperative follow-up of many corneal disorders such as keratoconus (KC) and other ectatic disorders, refractive surgery, and CL fitting.

Corneal topography refers to the graphic representation of the geometrical properties of the cornea whereas corneal tomography includes three-dimensional (3D) characterization of the cornea. Nowadays, various corneal topographic and tomographic systems are available which are noninvasive and easy to operate and interpret **(Table 2.3.1)**. Further discussion in this chapter would be on the Pentacam system **(Fig. 2.3.1)**.

■ PRINCIPLE

The Pentacam is based on the Scheimpflug principle, introduced by Theodore Scheimpflug,[1] a cartographer of the Austrian naval forces. This was initially used for topographic imaging for military purposes with cameras attached to the gliders or hot air balloons with the prototype devices. The Scheimpflug law states that "In order to get a higher depth of focus, the picture plane, the objective plane, and the film plane should be moved in such a way that they cut each other in one line or one point of intersection, known as the Scheimpflug intersection" **(Fig. 2.3.2)**. Typically, in a camera, the lens plane, the image plane, and the plane of focus are parallel to each other, resulting in a decreased depth of focus. Scheimpflug-based imaging system provides a high depth-of-focus, sharp images of the anterior as well as posterior corneal surface, iris, and lens.

TABLE 2.3.1: Various corneal topographers/tomographers.

Principle	Device
Placido-based	• Placido disc • Videokeratoscope
Slit scanning system	Orbscan
Slit scanning system + Placido	Orbscan II
Scheimpflug	• Pentacam • Sirius • Galilei
Ray tracing	Cassini

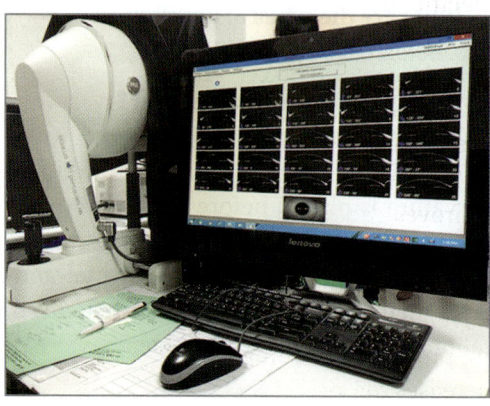

Fig. 2.3.1: Pentacam.

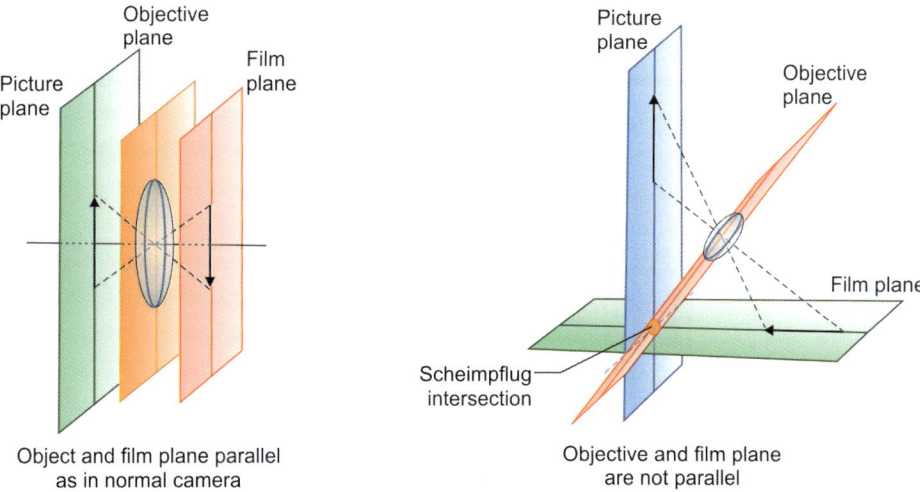

Fig. 2.3.2: Image formation in a normal camera versus Scheimpflug principle.

The depth of penetration though depends upon the media transparency and pupillary diameter.[2]

EXAMINATION METHODS

The Pentacam uses a combination of a rotating Scheimpflug camera and a static camera. It uses a monochromatic slit-light, ultraviolet (UV) free blue light-emitting diode (LED), of wavelength 475 nm. The camera takes a total of 50 images in maximum 2 seconds, from 0° to 180°, with each of the photographs is an image of the cornea at a specific angle. The software combines all these images and provides a 360° image of the anterior segment consisting of as many as 25,000 (in case of Pentacam HR it is 138,000) true elevation points.

The addition of the second camera improves the reproducibility of Pentacam significantly when compared to other corneal topography systems. It detects any eye movement of the fixating eye and corrects the position accordingly. This significantly increases the reliability and repeatability of Pentacam.

INTERPRETATION

As shown in **Figure 2.3.3**, the Pentacam output consists of corneal, AC parameters on the left side, and the "quad map" on the right side. The quad map consists of the anterior curvature sagittal map, the anterior and posterior elevation maps, and the pachymetry map. However, the display can be modified as per the need of the investigator.

CURVATURE MAPS

Curvature maps give information about pattern, symmetry, and skewing of the axis of the anterior surface of the cornea. The usual pattern is the symmetric bowtie (SB), where the two segments are equal in size and their axes are aligned **(Fig. 2.3.3)**. The SB represents regular astigmatism. This can be with-the-rule, against-the-rule (ATR) or oblique depending upon the orientation of the bowties. Various other patterns include **(Figs. 2.3.4 and 2.3.5)**:
- Round—steepest part of the cornea is round but decentered.
- Oval—steepest part is oval and it can be centered or decentered.

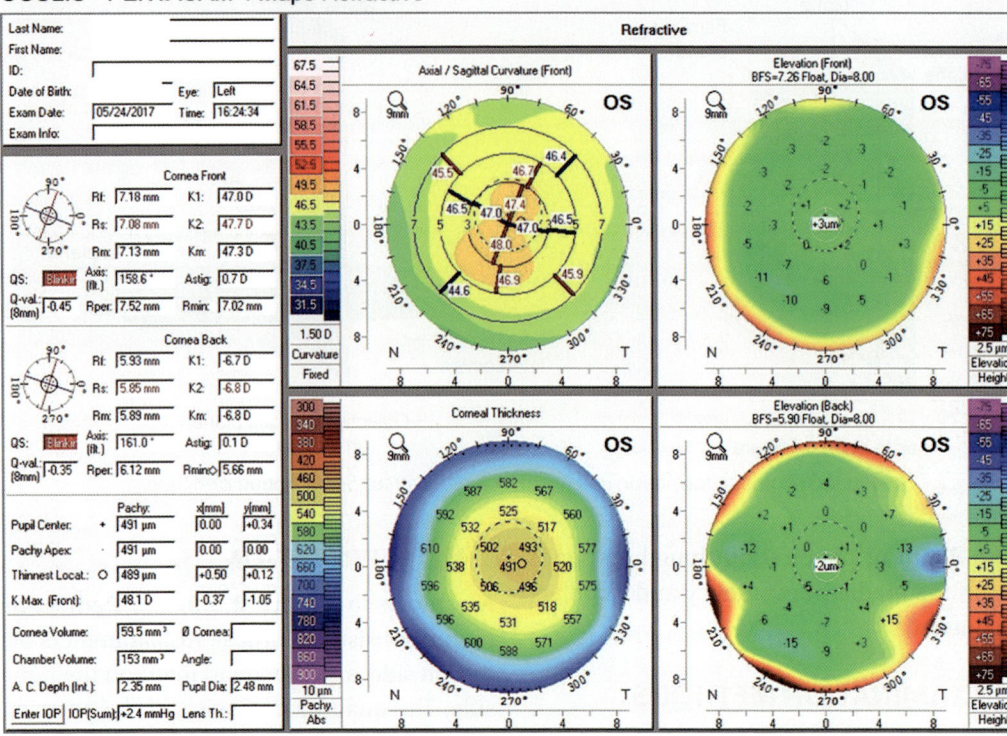

Fig. 2.3.3: Corneal tomography. On the left is the table of corneal parameters and on the right is the four-view refractive composite map.

- Superior steep—steepest part is located in the superior quadrant
- Inferior steep—steepest part is located in the inferior quadrant
- Irregular—no particular shape
- Abnormal SB:
  - *SB with skewed radial axis (SB/SRAX):* The angle between the axes of the two lobes is >22°.
  - *Asymmetric bowtie with inferior steepening (AB/IS):* The IS difference is >1.5 D.
  - *Asymmetric bowtie with superior steepening (AB/SS):* The SI difference is >2.5 D.
  - *Asymmetric bowtie with skewed radial axis (AB/SRAX):* The angle between the axes of the two lobes is >22°.
- Butterfly
- Claw pattern or "kissing birds"—seen in pellucid marginal degeneration (PMD)
- Junctional (vertical D)—circular shape, where two segments are connected laterally
- Smiling face—may be an indicator of KC and postoperative ectasia.
- Vortex—the steep and flat segments are distributed in a vortex pattern. It is an indicator of corneal instability.

A phenomenon occasionally exists in some individuals; the sagittal map in one eye appears as a mirror shape of that in the other eye, this is known as "enantiomorphism". When this phenomenon is seen, borderline irregularities can be considered normal.

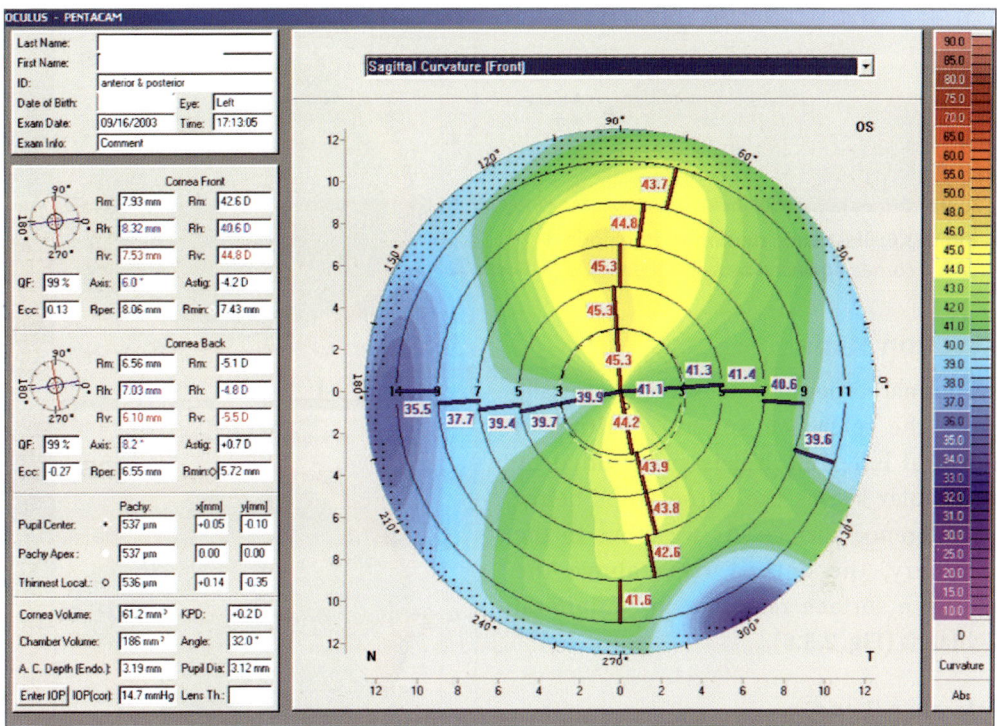

Fig. 2.3.4: Anterior sagittal map showing symmetric bowtie pattern.

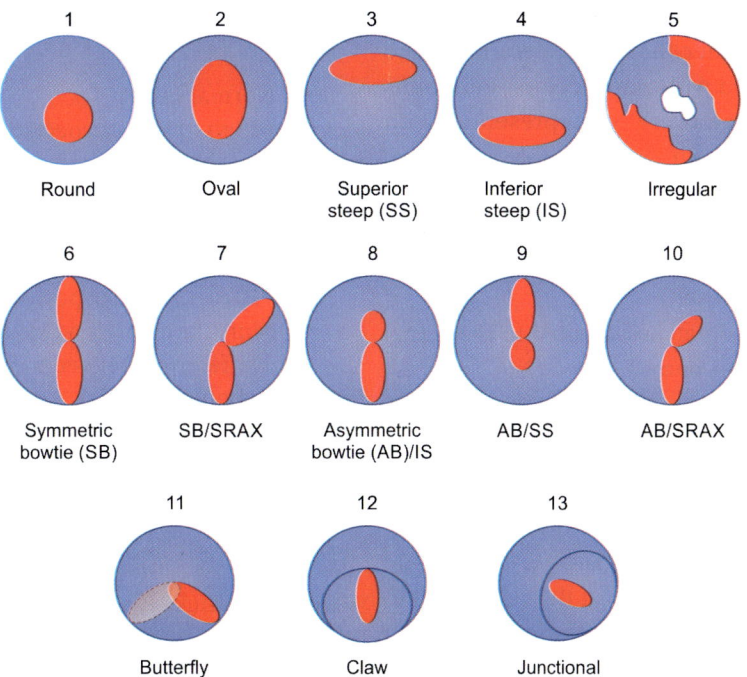

Fig. 2.3.5: Various patterns of the anterior sagittal map. (SRAX: skewed radial axis)

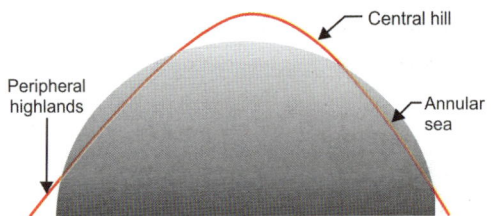

Fig. 2.3.6: Illustration demonstrating normal cornea against a best-fit sphere.

Elevation Maps

The normal cornea is prolate; it rises centrally above the reference sphere resulting in a central hill. This hill is surrounded by an annular sea as the cornea dips below the reference surface. As we move to the periphery, the cornea rises above the reference surface resulting in peripheral highlands **(Fig. 2.3.6)**.

Reference Plane

Various points on the corneal surface are compared against a reference plane and any point higher than the reference plane is represented with warm colors and points lower than reference are represented with cooler colors. Three selectable reference bodies are available:
1. *Best-fit toric ellipsoid (BFTE)*—matches perfectly to astigmatic corneas (most frequently used)
2. *Ellipsoid*—matches optimal to the actual shape of the cornea
3. *Best-fit sphere (BFS)*—comparable to Orbscan

The Pentacam displays both the front and back elevation maps **(Fig. 2.3.7)**.
- *Elevation on the front surface:* While interpreting, we look at the values within the central 5 mm circle on the map in BFTE mode. Clinical interpretation is as follows:

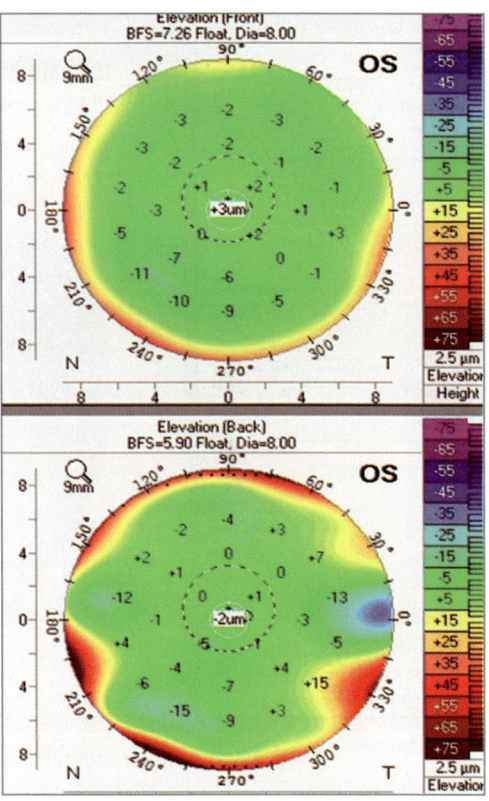

Fig. 2.3.7: Front and back elevation maps.

- Normal <+12 μ
- +13 to +15 μ—suspected
- More than +15 μ is a risk factor
- *Elevation at the back surface:* Clinical interpretation is as follows:
  - Normal—<+17 μ
  - +18 to +20 μ—suspected
  - More than 20 μ is a risk factor

The difference between front and back surfaces should be <+5 μ. Any isolated island on either the anterior or posterior surface is suspicious even in the presence of normal values.

Thickness/Pachymetry Maps

The true thickness of the cornea is the difference between the anterior and posterior elevations **(Fig. 2.3.8)**. The Pentacam generates 25,000 data points to describe the

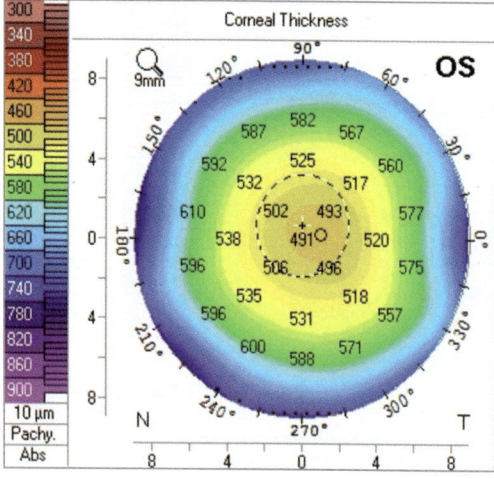

Fig. 2.3.8: Corneal pachymetry map.

true thickness whereas a standard ultrasound pachymetry can only image one single data point. Pachymetry is important for the diagnosis of ectatic disorders and preoperative planning of various corneal procedures like laser-assisted in situ keratomileusis (LASIK), small-incision lenticule extraction (SMILE), Intacs, and corneal crosslinking. Clinical interpretation is as follows:

- Inferior steepening ratio compares the superior and inferior values at 5 mm circle. A difference of >30 µ is suspicious.
- Difference between thinnest pachy and pachy at apex should be <10 µ.
- The difference of thinnest pachy between the two eyes should be <30 µ.
- If the thinnest point is decentered from apex by >500 µ, suspect KC.

Asphericity of Cornea

If the rays passing through the corneal periphery are refracted more than the rays passing through the central part, then it will give rise to SA. Therefore, in the case of an oblate cornea where the radius of curvature becomes smaller toward the periphery, stronger SAs are encountered.

On the contrary, in case of a prolate cornea, the radius of curvature increases toward the periphery and thus SA decreases.

The corneal asphericity is described in terms of Q value. Q value of normal cornea is −0.26 to 0.35. Q value is negative when the cornea is prolate as the rays from corneal periphery would fall behind the central rays. On the contrary, Q value is positive in the oblate cornea as the peripheral rays would fall ahead of the central rays.

Belin/Ambrósio Enhanced Ectasia Display

Belin/Ambrósio enhanced ectasia display (BAD) is a screening tool that combines elevation-based mapping and progression analysis of corneal pachymetry **(Fig. 2.3.9)**. This is an extremely important tool for early diagnosis of corneal ectasia and hence frequently used for screening of cases for KC before any refractive surgery.

Corneal Thickness Progression Analysis

The corneal thickness progression analysis (CTPA) is measured by taking the thickness of cornea at multiple concentric rings, starting from the thinnest point and 2, 4, 6, 8, and 10 mm. Corneal thickness spatial profile (CTSP) is calculated by measuring the corneal thickness at the thinnest location and the averages of the points on 22 imaginary circles centered on the thinnest point with increased diameters at 0.4 mm steps. Corneal-volume distribution is calculated by measuring the corneal volume is within diameters from 1.0 to 7.0 mm with 0.5 mm steps centered on the thinnest point.[3] In the CTSP graph the following things can be seen:

- *Vertical axis:* It represents the percentage of thickness increment.

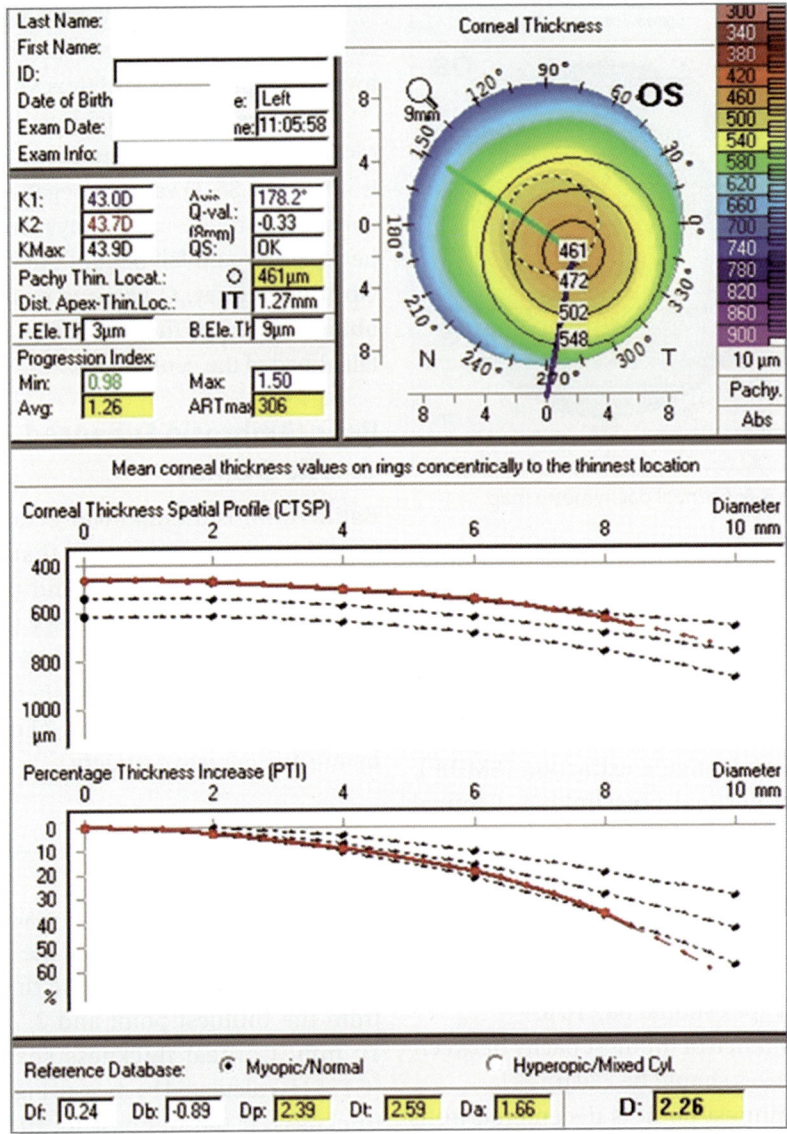

Fig. 2.3.9: Pentacam map with Belin/Ambrósio enhanced ectasia display (BAD).

- *Horizontal axis:* It represents the location as circles centered on the thinnest location.
- *Red color line:* It represents the curve of the examined cornea.
- *Black dashed line:* It represents the result of the standard value study.
- *The upper and lower line:* Both these lines represent the double standard deviation (SD) (95%) of the corneal thickness.

Interpretation

The red curve must fall within the normal range, and its course should be parallel to

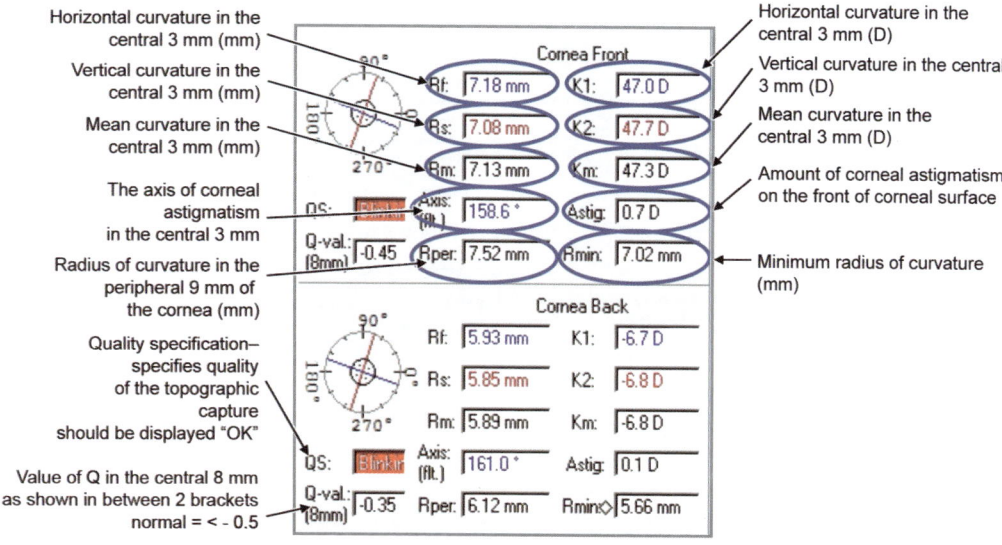

Fig. 2.3.10: Corneal parameters.

the normal range. If the red curve deviates as or after the 6 mm circle, it is normal. A quick downward deviation is a risk factor as it means that the corneal center is relatively thin in relation to the periphery.

Advantages

As the measurements are centered on the thinnest point rather than the anatomical corneal center, the thickness profile change is abrupt from center to the periphery. This is especially important for early detection of corneal ectasia.

D Value

Five new terms (Df, Db, Dp, Dt, Dy) have been added.
1. *Df* for the front surface
2. *Db* for the back surface
3. *Dp* for pachymetric progression
4. *Dt* for the thinnest point
5. *Dy* for thinnest point displacement.

Each of these and their final D number are depicted as the SD from the mean with the help of colors in the interpretation map.

The parameter is indicated in the following colors:

- *White color:* D <1.6 SD, suggests normal
- *Yellow color:* D >1.6 SD, suggests suspicious
- *Red color:* D >2.6 SD, suggests abnormal

Figures 2.3.10 and 2.3.11 display various other parameters studied on the Pentacam.

CLINICAL APPLICATIONS AND EXAMPLES

Indications of Pentacam

When to get it done:
- Complain of frequent change of glasses
- Defective vision even with refraction
- Patients with a history of long-standing vernal keratoconjunctivitis (VKC) or allergic conjunctivitis
- Basic refractive surgery workup
- Abnormal keratometry
- Slit-lamp examination suggestive of thinning.

Why to get it done:
- Diagnosis and baseline topography

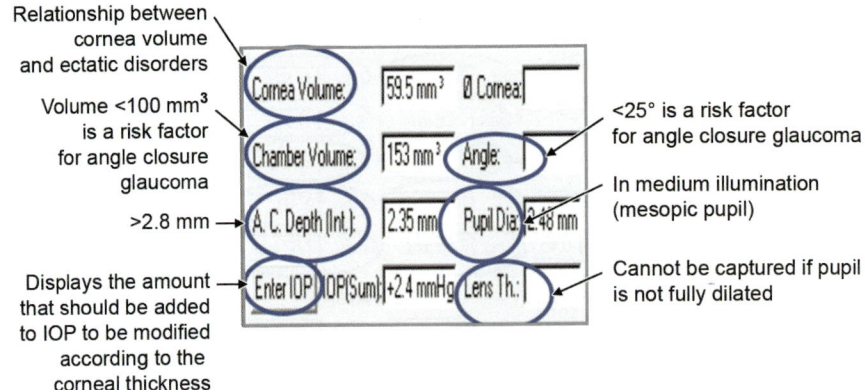

Fig. 2.3.11: Anterior chamber parameters. (IOP: intraocular pressure)

- Progression of the ectasia
- Classification of the disease

Applications

Screening and Diagnosis of Ectatic Disorders

The Pentacam system helps in identifying forme fruste keratoconus (FFKC) and aids in diagnosis and grading progression of KC and other ectatic disorders like PMD and Terrien marginal degeneration (TMD). The global consensus on KC and ectatic diseases[4] identified the following findings as mandatory to diagnose KC:

- Abnormal posterior elevation
- Abnormal corneal thickness distribution
- Clinical noninflammatory corneal thinning

Other findings suggestive of KC are increased area of corneal power surrounded by concentric areas of decreasing power, inferior–superior power asymmetry and skewing of the steepest radial axes (AB/SRAX). The AB/SRAX pattern only occurs in 0.05%[5] of the healthy patient population, but it is almost universal in patients with KC. **Figures 2.3.12** and **2.3.13** show the Pentacam quad map and BAD display of a patient with KC.

Box 2.3.1 summarizes the points that point toward a diagnosis of early KC.[6]

In cases of PMD, the classic topographic pattern is of IS, which is most dramatic between the 4 and 8 o'clock positions, with superior flattening; described as a "crab-claw" or "lobster-claw" pattern. The thinnest point does not coincide with the point of maximal steepening **(Fig. 2.3.14)**. However, the claw-shaped topography is not diagnostic of PMD; it can also be seen in cases of KC.

Refractive Surgery

Corneal topography has become an indispensable tool for pre- and postrefractive surgery corneal evaluation. They help in identifying individuals with high risk of developing post-LASIK ectasia, thus helping us to counsel them and provide other alternatives like phakic IOLs. Important risk factors include:[7]

- Abnormal topography
- *Abnormal pachymetry:* Residual corneal bed thickness
- Percentage tissue altered (PTA) >40% [PTA = (FT + AD)/CCT], where FT is flap thickness; AD is ablation depth; and CCT is preoperative central corneal thickness.
- Young age

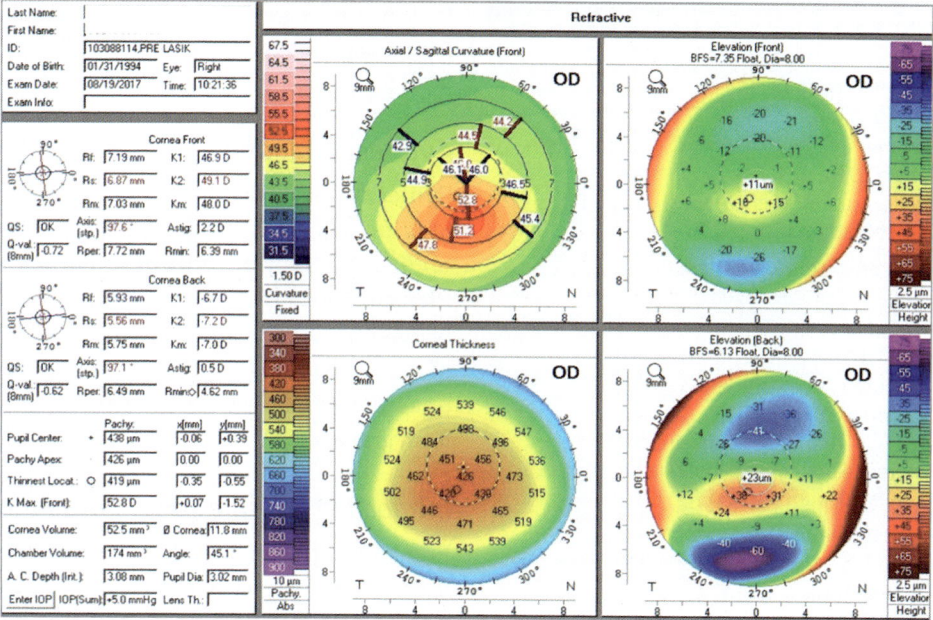

Fig. 2.3.12: The curvature map demonstrating corneal astigmatism with inferior steepening, elevation maps with abnormal anterior and posterior elevation and pachymetry map showing corneal thinning.

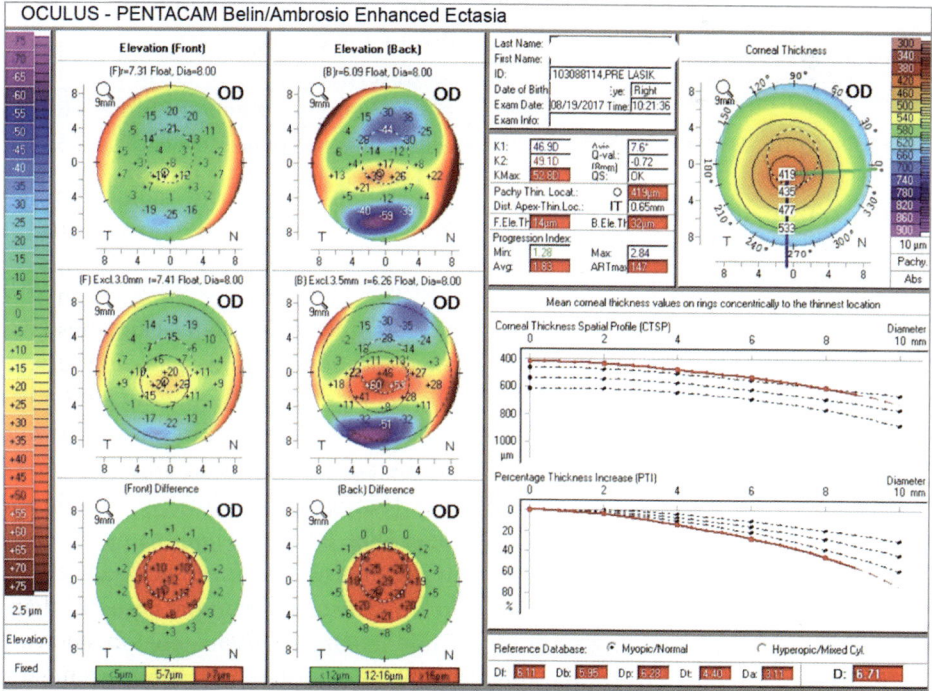

Fig. 2.3.13: The Pentacam Belin/Ambrósio enhanced ectasia display (BAD) showing corneal graph lying outside 2 standard deviation (SD) with abnormal D value.

> **BOX 2.3.1:** Pentacam parameters for diagnosis of early keratoconus (KC)/forme fruste KC (FFKC).
>
> *Findings on the sagittal map:*
> - Central K-readings ≥48 D
> - SRAX ≥22°
> - Superior–inferior difference (S-I) on the 5 mm circle ≥2.5 D
> - Inferior–superior difference (I-S) ≥1.5 D
> - Corneal astigmatism ≥6 D
>
> *Findings on the thickness map:*
> - Thinnest location <470 μ
> - Y-coordinate value of the thinnest location ≥−500 μ
> - Pachymetry apex-thickness at thinnest location ≥10 μ
> - Superior–inferior at 5 mm circle ≥30 μ
> - Difference in thickness between both eyes at thinnest locations ≥30 μ
>
> *Findings on the elevation maps:*
> - Isolated focal island of ectasia (BFS mode) on either surface
> - Values ≥12 μ within the central 5 mm on the anterior elevation map (BFTE mode)
> - Values ≥15 μ within the central 5 mm on the posterior elevation map (BFTE mode)

(BFS: best-fit sphere; BFTE: best-fit toric ellipsoid; FFKC: forme fruste keratoconus; SRAX: skewed radial axis)

- The topographic asymmetry between two eyes

Figure 2.3.15: Illustrates a case of a myopic patient who developed ectasia after undergoing LASIK.

Glaucoma Evaluation

Various parameters like anterior chamber depth (ACD) (both central and peripheral), AC volume, CCT, and inbuilt IOP correction formulae can be used for glaucoma screening **(Fig. 2.3.11)**.

Contact Lens Fitting

The Pentacam helps in the improved fitting of CL is irregular corneas. Topography helps to identify the corneal apex, cone diameter, corneal astigmatism, thereby helping the diagnostic lens selection. Various preprogrammed CL fitting software is available.

Cataract Evaluation

Pentacam also has the Pentacam Nucleus Staging (PNS) Module, which helps in objective quantification of lens opacities (densitometry) in 2D and 3D and graduation of lens opacities.[8] It also helps in visualization of lens opacities and posterior capsular opacities (PCOs). Cataract can be graded from grade 0 to 5.

Intraocular Pressure Power Calculation

Previously, postmyopic LASIK, overestimation of keratometry led to an underestimation of IOL power resulting in hyperopic outcomes and vice versa. The Holladay report[9] incorporated in the Pentacam software helps in calculating optimal IOL refractive power for postrefractive surgery patients. It determines total corneal power, as equivalent keratometry readings (EKRs) for different zones of the cornea. These EKRs can be entered in the IOL calculation formulae to get a correct IOL power.

Corneal Optical Densitometry Display

Scheimpflug images alone can never give the exact location of corneal pathologies because the ocular structures often do not lie within a flat plane and structures at similar depths in the cornea appear at different depths in the tomography.[2] Corneal densitometry map **(Fig. 2.3.16)** is handy in such cases as it presents all structures located at the same relative distance from the corneal surfaces.[2] Thus, making it a useful tool for assessing the depth and position of scattering phenomena occurring within the cornea.[2]

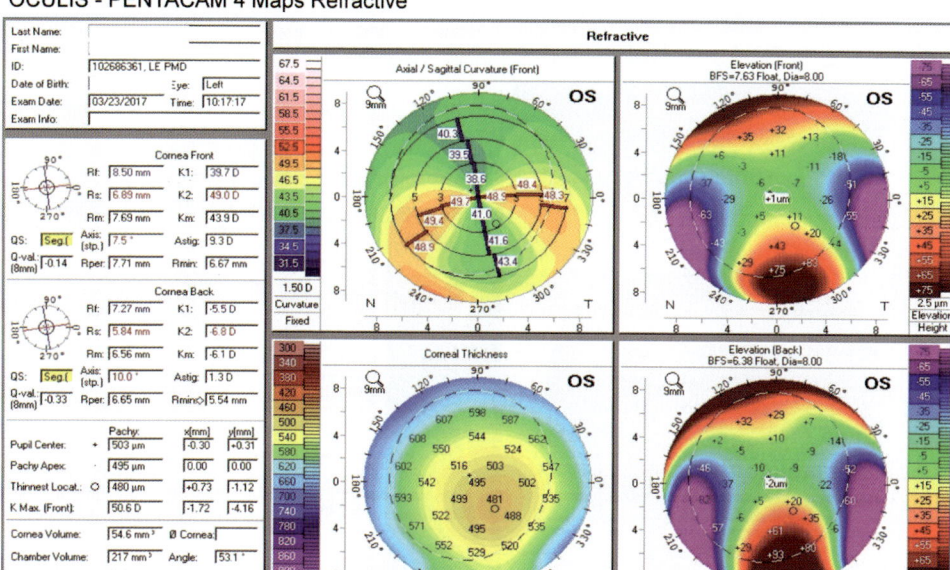

Fig. 2.3.14: Pentacam quad map of a patient of pellucid marginal degeneration (PMD) with crab-claw appearance. Note that the thinnest point does not coincide with the point of maximal steepening.

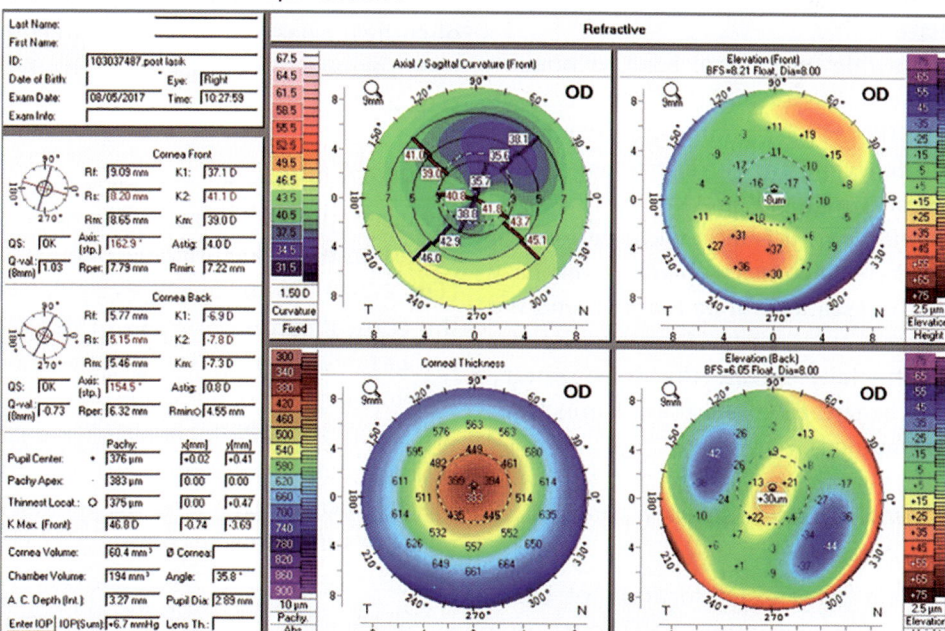

Fig. 2.3.15: Post-LASIK ectasia. Note the abnormal posterior elevation.

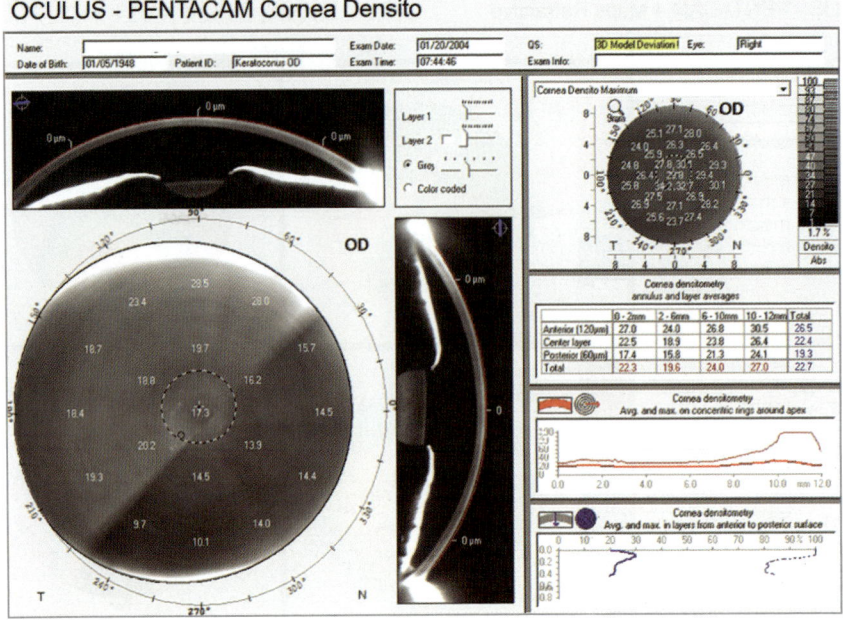

Fig. 2.3.16: Corneal optical densitometry display.

Clinical utility of corneal densitometry includes:
- Reproducible measurements of corneal haze
- Following up corneal haze or opacity (objective assessment) in patients post-LASIK or post-photorefractive keratectomy (PRK), or with infectious keratitis, corneal dystrophy, and KC.

Limitations: It is difficult to perform in cases where the cornea is opaque or very hazy as the backscatter will be too high and the measurements unreliable. Scleral backscatter can artificially elevate the densitometry values near the limbus (10–12 mm from central fixation).

Intracorneal Ring Segments Implantation

Pentacam gives exact location of cone, higher-order aberrations (HOAs) (fitting of corneal rings in reference to the axis of the coma) as well as corneal thickness at 5–7 mm zone, hence useful for preoperative as well as postoperative follow-up of cases of corneal ectasia undergoing intracorneal ring segments (ICRS) (Intacs or Kerra) **(Fig. 2.3.17)**.

Corneal Aberration

Pentacam provides Zernike analysis of the cornea based on the principle of ray tracing **(Fig. 2.3.18)**. It provides the calculation of the corneal wavefront (WF) of the entire cornea (anterior and posterior surface) and is thus independent of the shape of the cornea [e.g., post-LASIK, PRK, lamellar keratoplasty (LKP), penetrating keratoplasty (PKP), etc.].[2] Besides, it can be shown for the anterior and posterior surfaces of the cornea.

Uses:
- Selection of aspheric IOLs for correction of corneal SAs (Z4.0)

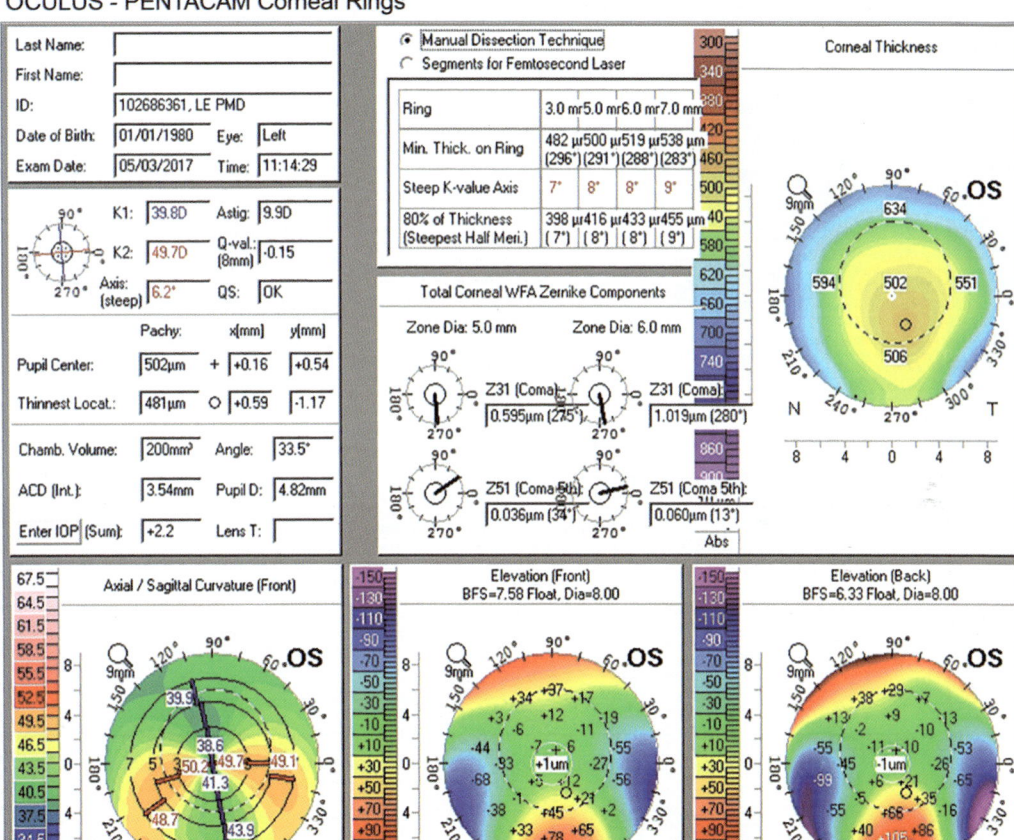

Fig. 2.3.17: Corneal rings in Pentacam.

- Fitting of corneal rings in reference to the axis of the coma
- Determination of low- and high-order aberrations[2]

CONCLUSION

The Pentacam topography system is a rapid-scanning, reproducible, and easy-to-use imaging system. It helps in a comprehensive evaluation of the anterior segment of the eye making it a useful tool for both diagnosis and surgical planning.

VIVA QUESTIONS

1. What are the Pentacam parameters for diagnosis of early KC/FFKC?
Ans. Refer to **Box 2.3.1**.

2. What is the difference between Pentacam and Orbscan?
Ans. Refer to **Table 2.3.2**.

3. What is the clinical utility of corneal densitometry?
Ans. Refer to text.

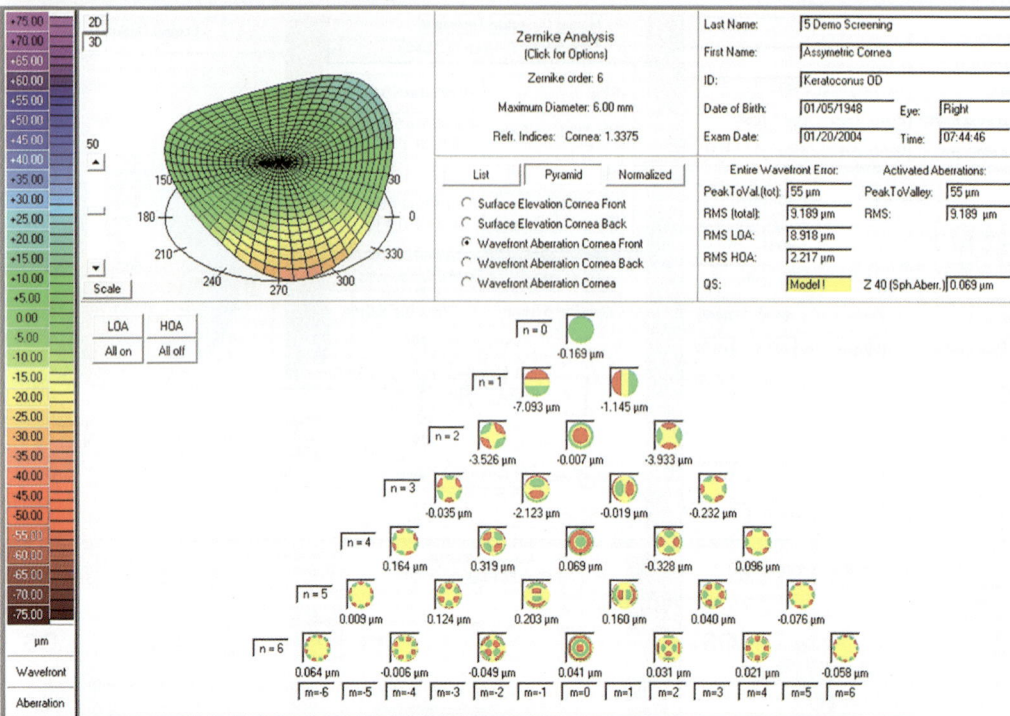

Fig. 2.3.18: Zernike analysis of the cornea in Pentacam.

TABLE 2.3.2: Pentacam versus Orbscan.

Pentacam	Orbscan
Based on Scheimpflug principle	Based on scanning slit and Placido disc system
Maintains the central point (the thinnest point) of each meridian; thus, can reregister these central points and eliminate the effect of eye movements; thus, it is 10 times more accurate than Orbscan	Takes multiple vertical images, which have no common point; thus, it cannot reregister for any eye movement
Posterior elevation data are more accurate	Less accurate

4. State the difference between Pentacam and Galilei.

Ans. The Pentacam Scheimpflug analyzer (Oculus Optikgeräte GmbH, Wetzlar, Germany) uses a single Scheimpflug camera to acquire multiple photographs of the anterior segment of the eye. The Galilei dual-Scheimpflug analyzer (V4.01 Ziemer, Port, Switzerland) uses dual Scheimpflug cameras and a Placido disc to improve the accuracy of corneal power and pachymetric measurements. Both the instruments show good correlation in all measured parameters except AC angle, AC volume, and average pupil diameter.[10] It is important to remember that these devices cannot be used interchangeably.

5. What is Pentacam AXL?

Ans. The Pentacam AXL determines the axial length of the eye as well as the data of the anterior eye segment, from the anterior corneal surface to the posterior surface of the crystalline lens, all in a single measurement. In doing so it makes combined use of the Pentacam technology and an equally proven interferometry-based biometry technique. Various functions of Pentacam AXL are:

- IOLs calculator for:
    - Both treated and untreated eyes
    - Spherical, aspherical multifocal, and toric IOL calculation
    - Toric IOL calculation based on the total corneal refractive power
- Fast screening report
- Belin/Ambrósio enhanced ectasia display (BAD)
- Topographical keratoconus classification (TKC)
- *Qualitative assessment of the cornea:*
    - Topography and elevation maps of the anterior and posterior corneal surface
    - Overall pachymetry
    - Corneal optical densitometry
- *Glaucoma screening:*
    - Pachymetry-based IOP correction
    - Chamber angle and chamber volume
- Elevation data
- PNS and 3D cataract analysis
- Premium IOL selection in four steps
- Comparative displays for follow-up
- Comparison and superimposition of Scheimpflug images
- CL fitting

REFERENCES

1. Scheimpflug T. Der photoperspektrograph und seine anwendung. Photogr Korr. 1906;43: 516-31.
2. Pentacam. Interpretation guideline: 3rd edition. [online] Available from https://www.pentacam.com/fileadmin/user_upload/pentacam.de/downloads/interpretations-leitfaden/interpretation_guideline_3rd_edition_0915.pdf [Last accessed October, 2024].
3. Ambrósio R, Alonso RS, Luz A, Coca Velarde LG. Corneal-thickness spatial profile and corneal-volume distribution: tomographic indices to detect keratoconus. J Cataract Refract Surg. 2006;32(11):1851-9.
4. Gomes JA, Tan D, Rapuano CJ, Belin MW, Ambrósio R Jr, Guell JL, et al.; Group of Panelists for the Global Delphi Panel of Keratoconus and Ectatic Diseases. Global Consensus on Keratoconus and Ectatic Diseases. Cornea. 2015;34(4):359-69.
5. Matalia H, Swarup R. Imaging modalities in keratoconus. Indian J Ophthalmol. 2013; 61(8):394-400.
6. Sinjab MM. Classifications and Patterns of Keratoconus and Keratectasia. Berlin, Heidelberg: Springer; 2012. pp. 13-58.
7. Randleman JB, Woodward M, Lynn MJ, Stulting RD. Risk assessment for ectasia after corneal refractive surgery. Ophthalmology. 2008;115(1):37-50.
8. Nixon DR. Preoperative cataract grading by Scheimpflug imaging and effect on operative fluidics and phacoemulsification energy. J Cataract Refract Surg. 2010;36(2): 242-6.
9. Holladay JT, Hill WE, Steinmueller A. Corneal power measurements using scheimpflug imaging in eyes with prior corneal refractive surgery. J Refract Surg. 2009;25(10): 862-8.
10. Baradaran-Rafii A, Motevasseli T, Yazdizadeh F, Karimian F, Fekri S, Baradaran-Rafii A. Comparison between two Scheimpflug anterior segment analyzers. J Ophthalmic Vis Res. 2017;12(1):23-9.

2.4 ABERROMETERS

Prafulla Kumar Maharana, Deepali Singhal, Aafreen Bari, Siddhi Goel

■ INTRODUCTION

An aberrometer is a device that measures the ocular aberrations. Based on the principle used, they can be categorized into the following types:[1]
- Hartmann–Shack aberrometry
- Tscherning's aberrometry
- Ray tracing aberrometry
- Automated retinoscope

Based on the ray projection type aberrometers can be classified into:[2]
- *Backward or outgoing projection type:* Hartmann–Shack aberrometer
- *Forward or ingoing projection type:* Ray tracing aberrometer, Tscherning's aberrometer, and automated retinoscope

■ iTRACE SYSTEM

The iTrace aberrometer (Tracey Technologies, Houston, Tx) is a combination of Placido disc corneal topography and ray tracing aberrometry **(Fig. 2.4.1)**. It measures the total aberrations of the eye. It is a serial, double pass, and forward projection type retinal image aberrometer. A topographer is added in the same unit as the aberrometer to measure the corneal aberrations.

Principle of iTrace[3]

Ray-tracing aberrometry is a more physiological method of measuring the aberrations since it measures the forward aberrations of the light going through the eye that is analyzing along the natural trajectory of the light. **Figure 2.4.2** shows a diagram of the ray-tracing technique.

This method uses a laser beam parallel to the line of sight through the pupil. It measures the exact site where the laser beam reaches the retina utilizing the retroreflected light captured by reference lineal sensors. An unexpanded laser beam is scanned so that it enters the eye sequentially through different pupil locations. One marginal (dotted line) and the principal ray (solid line) are shown. Each retinal image (A, O) is projected onto a charge-coupled device (CCD) camera (A,' O'). The displacement of the image with respect to a reference (A,' O'), is proportional to the local derivative of the wave aberration. Local aberrations in the path of the laser beam through the cornea and the internal structures cause a shift in the location on the retina. Once the first position has been determined the laser beam is shifted to another position, which is then located in the retina. This process continues until several distinct points are projected into the entrance pupil and reconstruction of the real WF error is done.

The iTrace uses this principle of ray tracing where a series of infrared rays (on the order of 100 microns and a 785 nm

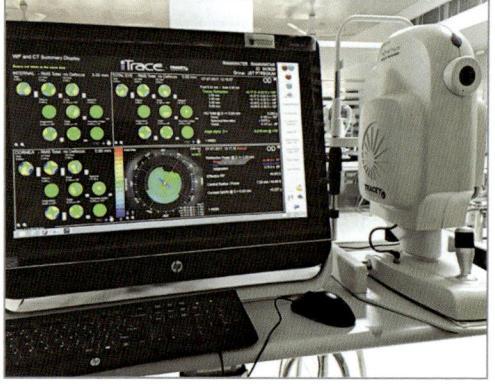

Fig. 2.4.1: The iTrace aberrometer.

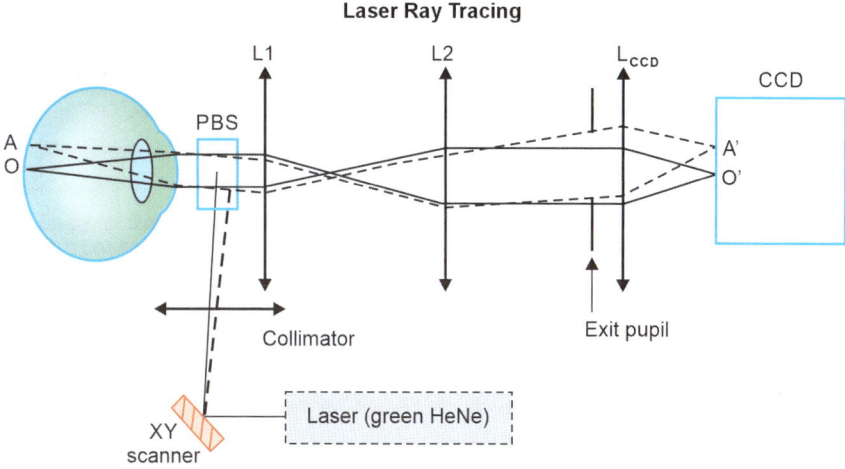

Fig. 2.4.2: Wavefront verification display showing the retinal spot diagram (RSD) (bottom left) with the horizontal point profile and the vertical point profile in the center. (CCD: charge-coupled device; PBS: pellicle beamsplitter)

wavelength each) are projected sequentially through pupil parallel to the eye's line of sight. 64 laser beams are projected through the pupil four times each (256 points) at a high speed (approximately 250 ms). All 256 points would be concentrated at a single point in the fovea in an emmetropic eye.

INTERPRETATION/DATA ANALYSIS[4]

- Wavefront analysis
- Topographic analysis

Wavefront analysis: WF analysis is based on the concept of retinal spot diagram (RSD), which consists of a set of points projected through the pupil onto the retina. RSD provides all relevant information related to refraction, aberrations, and point spread function (PSF) of the patient. RSD is used to find the modulation transfer function (MTF) and PSF. The size of the RSD is inversely proportional to the concentration of photons that reaches the retina.

Point spread function shows the image of a point source of light formed in the retina. A sharper and smaller PSF is considered to be better. The MTF measures the transfer of contrast from the subject to the image by an optical system at different spatial frequencies. It measures how accurately the details from the object are transferred to the image produced by the lens. Thus, RSD simulates the vision of the patient.[5]

Interpretation/Basic Data Graphs

Reading an iTrace map should be done in the following manner:[5]

- *Wavefront verification display:* This display shows the data on limbus-to-limbus diameter, pupil size, and scan diameter. The pupil diameter can be selected manually to determine the aberrations. The left side of this display shows the RSD, which shows the retinal image of all the points projected. In an emmetropic eye, all 256 points should be concentrated on the fovea, which will be seen as a single-point RSD. In the center of this display, the horizontal and the vertical point profile are seen.

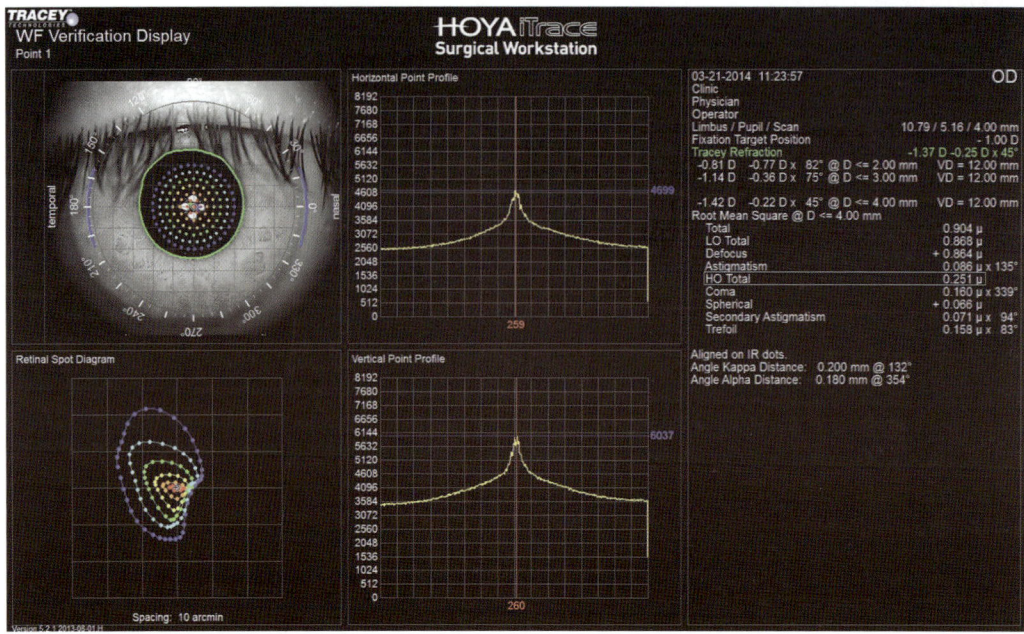

Fig. 2.4.3: Wavefront verification display showing the retinal spot diagram (RSD) (bottom left) with the horizontal point profile and the vertical point profile in the center.

They show the position of each point reflected on the retina, taking the center of each profile in the X- and Y-axis. It represents the quality of the signal captured, and the measurement is not accurate if it is irregular **(Fig. 2.4.3)**. The top right of this display shows the multizone refraction analysis depending on the size of the pupil. This iTrace refraction has been reported to be highly correlated with the manifest refraction.[6]

- *Wavefront map total and HOAs:* This is a color-coded map that shows the WF aberrations of the eye in microns. Warm colors on this map show that the WF is in front of the reference plane and cool colors show the retardation. This indicates what kind of aberrations are the main causes of low vision.
- *The root mean square (RMS):* This map gives the magnitude of aberrations. Total aberrations of the eye are measured as the RMS value. It also displays the total lower and HOAs separately along with a specific value for each Zernike term or component of the eye aberrations **(Fig. 2.4.4)**.
- *Total refractive and HOA refractive maps:* This map displays the refractive power of the eye in diopters referring to the whole eye and not just the corneal power. Emmetropia is represented in green, while myopia in red and hypermetropia in blue.
- *PSF total and HOA-PSF:* This represents the quality of an image of a point source of light at the retina. Greater aberrations show a higher defocus effect on the image **(Fig. 2.4.5)**.
- *Snellen letters total and HOA:* This represents the actual simulation of the patient's vision in the form of Snellen's E letter **(Fig. 2.4.6)**.

CHAPTER 2: Cornea

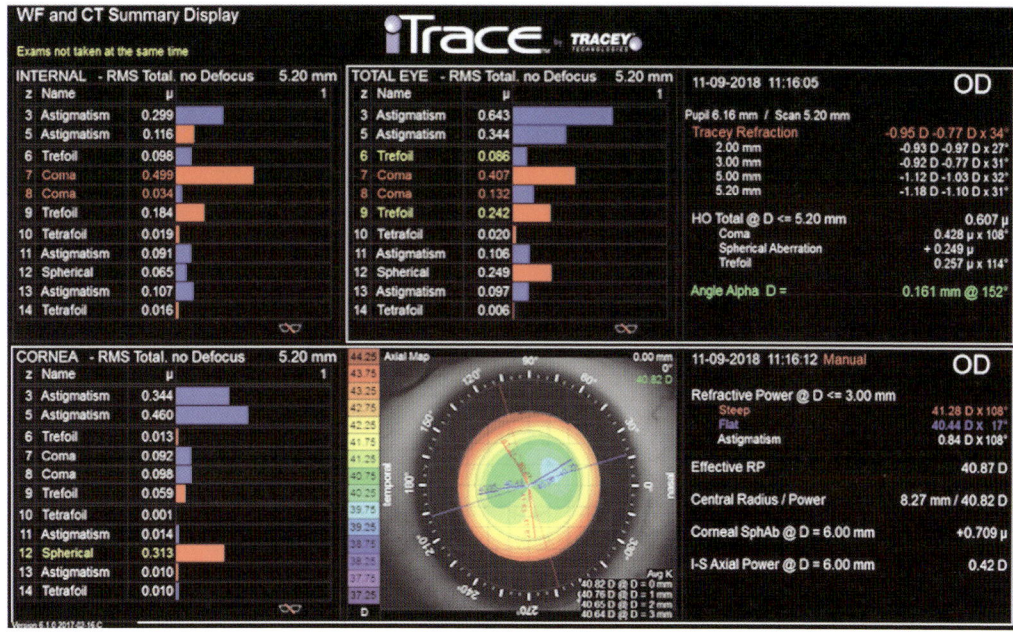

Fig. 2.4.4: Total root mean square (RMS) values, total lower-order aberration (LOA) and total higher-order aberration (HOA) (bottom right), and decomposition in each of the Zernike polynomials represented in red and blue bars depending on the value of the sign.

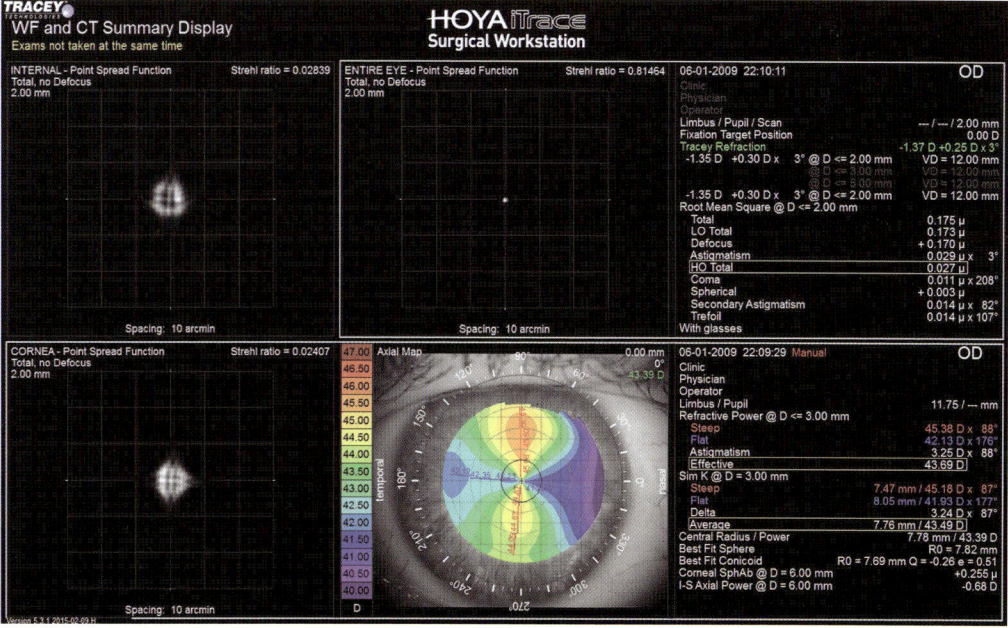

Fig. 2.4.5: Point spread function of a patient showing the compensation of corneal aberrations with internal optics.

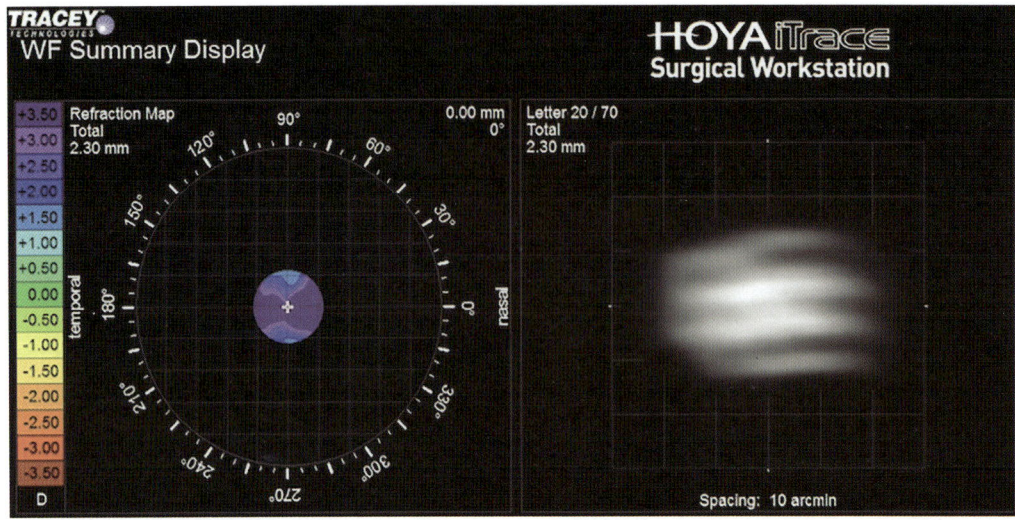

Fig. 2.4.6: Snellen letter equivalent of a patient with cataract reporting blurring of vision with glare.

- *Zernike polynomials bar graph:* This bar graph gives a detailed analysis of all total, corneal, and internal aberrations. iTrace shows the Zernike polynomials up to the 6th order (27 items).

Optical Alignment for Premium Intraocular Lenses

Angle alpha is the angle between the center of the limbus and the visual axis, whereas angle kappa is the angle between the center of the pupil and the visual axis **(Fig. 2.4.7)**. Angle alpha is less commonly used since it is more difficult to measure. Premium IOLs are being used increasingly to achieve an excellent refractive outcome after cataract surgery, which requires good centration relative to the visual axis.[7] Thus, angle alpha is an important determinant to decide whether these IOLs can be used or not. iTrace can be used to measure angle alpha and kappa with color coding. An angle ≤0.3 mm is green, 0.3–0.5 mm is yellow, and >0.5 mm is red. A green angle alpha has the maximum chances that the patient will be looking through the center of the central optic zone, as intended. It is not preferable to use these IOLs in cases with red angle alpha.

Cornea or Lens?

iTrace can separate the total aberrations between corneal and internal aberrations. Any significant internal aberrations indicate dysfunction of the lens. Thus, it helps to identify dysfunctional lens syndrome that is characterized by difficulty in seeing at a distance or at near due to congenital ametropia or due to aging and progressive presbyopia, respectively. It also provides the dysfunctional lens index (DLI) that is calculated based on a number of factors like internal HOAs, pupil size, and contrast sensitivity. In patients with this syndrome and without any significant corneal aberrations, it would be advisable to perform a refractive lens exchange for a better outcome.

Wavefront Analysis Screens

- *Visual function analysis (VFA) summary display:* This includes the WF higher-order

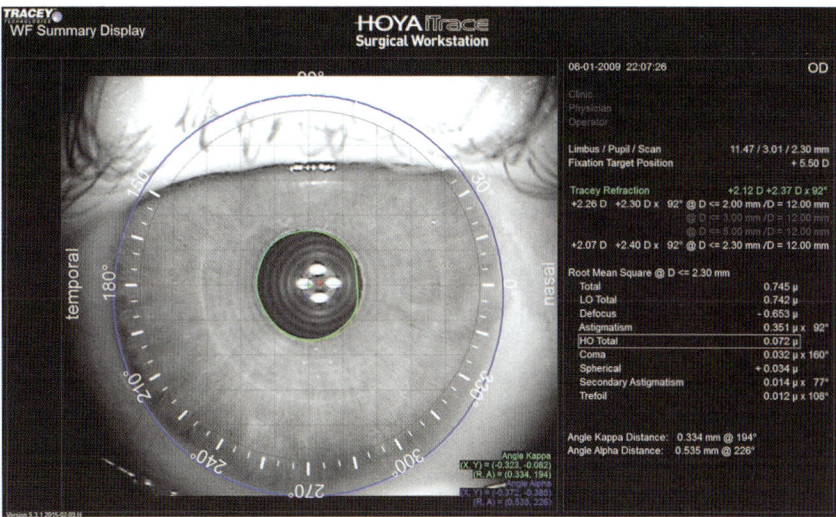

Fig. 2.4.7: Optical alignment using iTrace. The iTrace measures the distance between the visual axis, as estimated by the center of the first Purkinje reflex (red crosshair), and the center of the pupil (green crosshair), which is useful for laser-assisted in situ keratomileusis (LASIK). The angle alpha is the distance from the visual axis to the center of the limbus (blue crosshair), which is useful for intraocular lens (IOL) implantation.

(HO) total or the refraction map HO total along with refraction in diopters, the RMS, Snellen letter, PSF, and potential visual complaints (nocturnal myopia, glare, halos, defocus, and double vision).
- *Wavefront comparison map:* This display is used to compare the two WF maps in a patient. It can be used to compare the status of the aberrations before and after refractive surgery and also to measure accommodation.

Uses of Aberration Analysis

- In case of high total aberrations, it helps to decide that refractive procedure would be better in cornea or lens.
- Pre- and post-cataract surgery analysis help to study the effect on the aberrations induced or compensated by the IOL.
- It also helps to identify which type of IOL will be suitable and to analyze different types of IOL.
- The contribution of an opacified lens in total ocular aberrations can be measured.
- Measurement of angle alpha and angle kappa to plan for premium IOLs
- To evaluate the corneal and total astigmatism
- Planning of toric IOL **(Fig. 2.4.8)**

CORNEAL TOPOGRAPHIC ANALYSIS (COMPUTED TOMOGRAPHY)

Corneal topographic analysis is based on a Placido disc format named as Vista, which covers up to 10 mm of peripheral cornea.[5] This provides:
- Standard keratometric readings at 3 mm zone
- Refractive power of cornea in central 3 mm zone
- Inferior–superior asymmetry corneal index (I-S)
- *Topographic maps*:
  - Standard axial map
  - Tangential curvature map
  - Refractive map

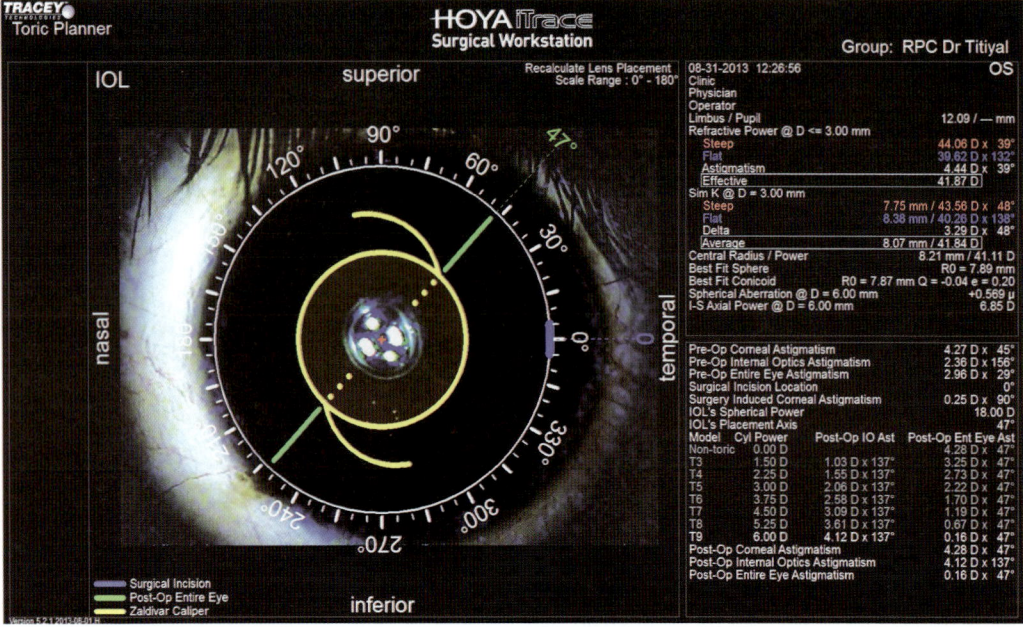

Fig. 2.4.8: Toric intraocular lens (IOL) planning with iTrace.

- Elevation map
- Corneal WF map

ADVANTAGES OF RAY-TRACING ABERROMETRY

- Ray-tracing aberrometry allows sequential capture of data with each point being processed separately and sequentially to avoid any confusion.
- The pattern of laser beams projected adjusts to the pupil size.
- Highly accurate and has a high resolution since each point is measured separately using linear detectors.
- iTrace is less susceptible to eye motion and tear film artifacts.

CLINICAL EXAMPLES

Case 1: Lenticonus

Here we analyze a case of Alport syndrome with anterior lenticonus showing a distorted RSD with the refraction of –4.37 D sphere with astigmatism of +2 D, and RMS HOA total of 1.5 microns **(Fig. 2.4.9)**. On analyzing further to know from where the astigmatism is coming from the WF, and computed tomography (CT) summary display shows that the significant contribution of all lower-order aberration (LOA) and HOA is from the internal optics or the lens **(Fig. 2.4.10)**. Similar results are seen with total Snellen eye **(Fig. 2.4.11)**, thus this patient would benefit from a lens-based procedure.

Case 2: Corneal Astigmatism

Hereby we analyze a WF and CT summary display of a case with against the rule astigmatism. On separating the aberrations of cornea and lens, it is seen that the main contribution of astigmatism is from the cornea **(Fig. 2.4.12)**.

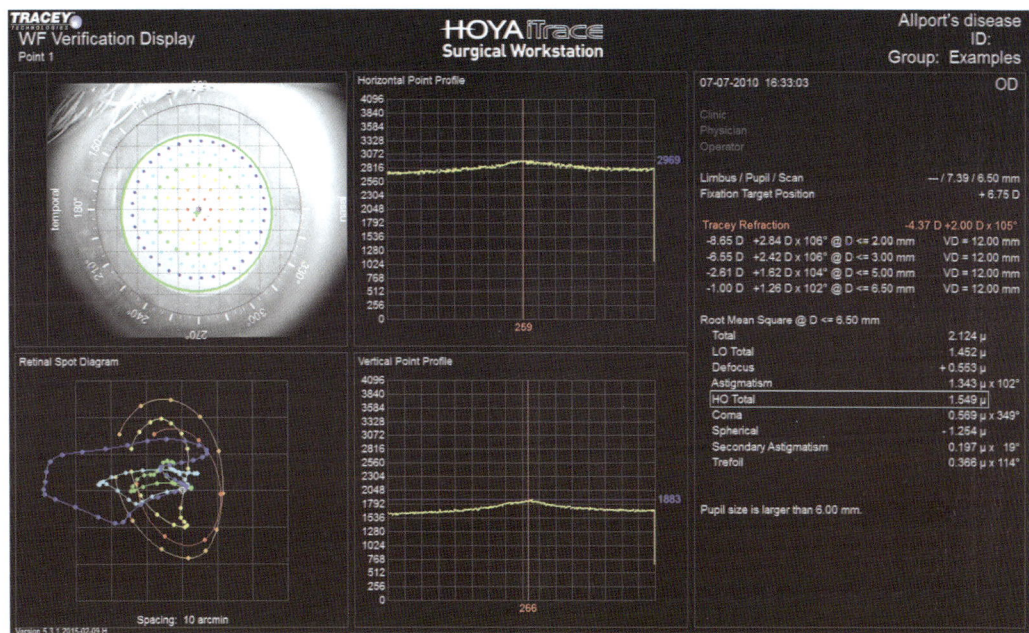

Fig. 2.4.9: Wavefront verification display of a case of Alport syndrome with anterior lenticonus showing the distorted RSD (bottom left) with the refraction of −4.37 D sphere and +2 D cyl, and RMS HOA total of 1.5 microns.

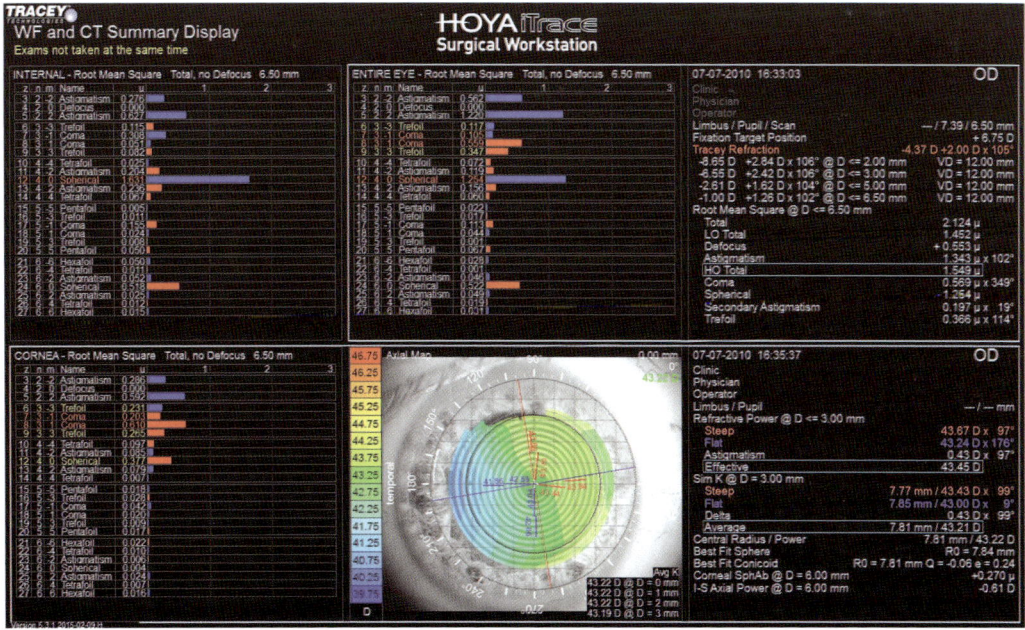

Fig. 2.4.10: Computed tomography display of a case of Alport syndrome with anterior lenticonus showing that there is a significant contribution of internal (lenticular) HOA to the total eye HOA mainly spherical aberration.

SECTION 1: Appliances and Instruments

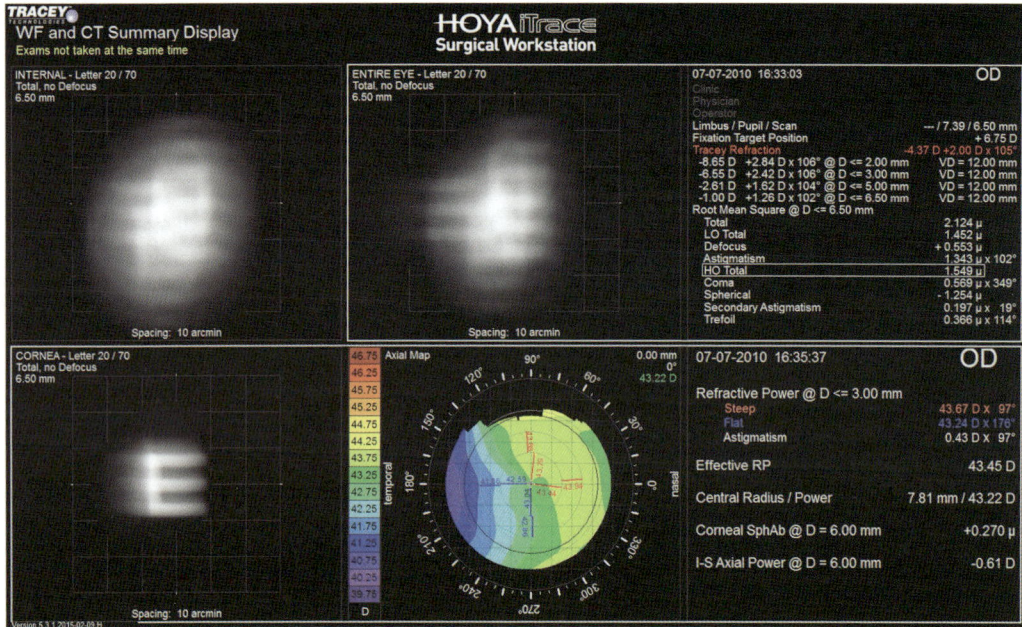

Fig. 2.4.11: Computed tomography display of a case of Alport syndrome with anterior lenticonus showing that major contribution of the distortion in Snellen E letter is due to internal aberrations and not due to corneal.

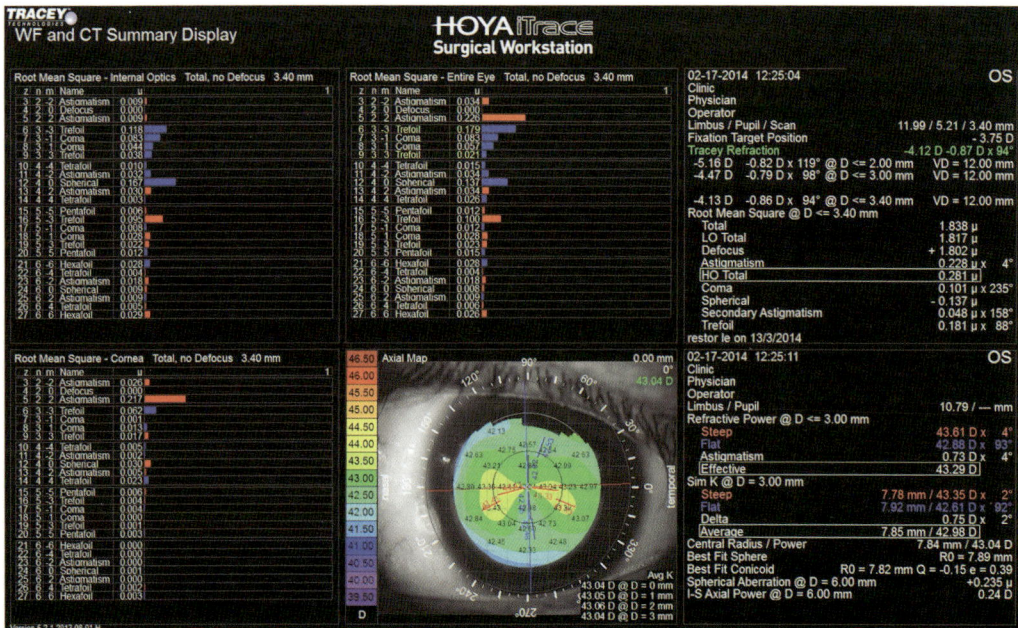

Fig. 2.4.12: A wavefront (WF) and computed tomography (CT) display of a case of corneal astigmatism showing that the main contribution of total eye aberrations is from corneal aberrations, especially astigmatism.

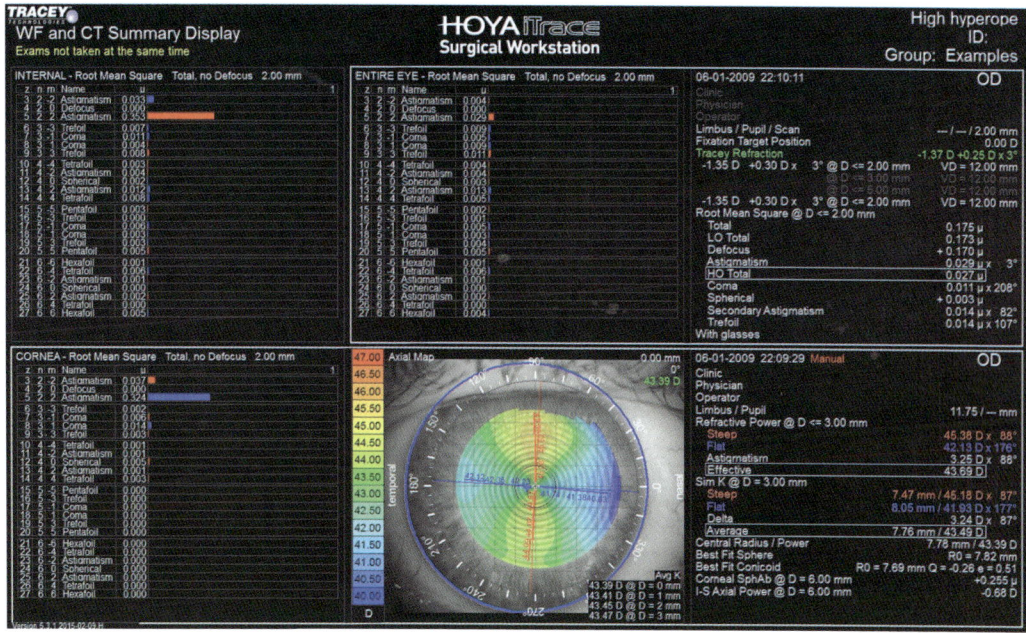

Fig. 2.4.13: A wavefront (WF) and computed tomography (CT) summary display of a case showing that the internal eye aberrations are compensated with the corneal aberrations.

Case 3: Balancing of Corneal and Internal Optics

This WF and CT summary display show that the internal aberrations compensate the corneal aberrations. Thus, the visual quality may get worsened if any procedure is done **(Fig. 2.4.13)**.

Case 4: Astigmatism

This case has an against the rule astigmatism of −1.5 D, which is the leading cause of blurring of vision. On analyzing the WF summary map, we can see that the axial map of corneal topography (bottom right) does not correspond to the map of the entire eye. However, the internal optics maps correspond to that of the entire eye suggesting that the main contribution of astigmatism and HOAs is from the lens **(Fig. 2.4.14)**. Thus, this patient would benefit from a lens-based procedure.

■ CONCLUSION

Thus, ray-tracing aberrometry is an important tool that helps the surgeon at all stages of patient management. This includes preoperative planning and evaluation to achieve the best possible outcome along with evaluating the postoperative performance. At the same time, it can also help to find out the cause of low vision in a dissatisfied patient. Moreover, this technology being user-friendly has made the understanding of a complex science easy and widely applicable.

■ VIVA QUESTIONS

1. What is aberration?
Ans. Aberration originates from the Latin "aberrātiō", which means going offtrack or deviating. Aberration is the difference between an ideal image and that achieved with the actual optical system. WF aberrations are most commonly specified by Zernike

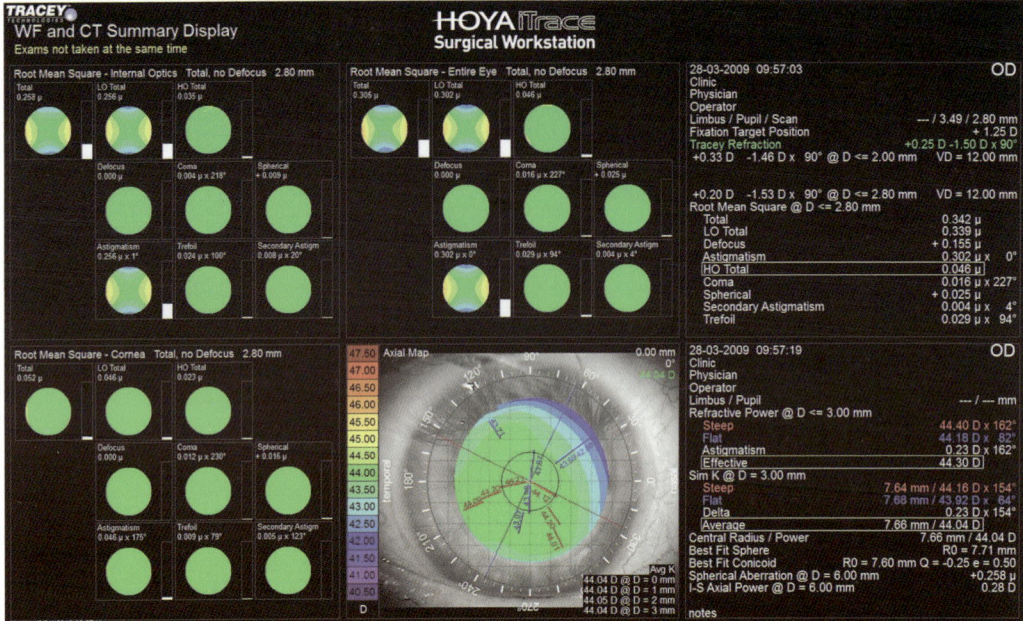

Fig. 2.4.14: The wavefront summary map of a case with astigmatism of 1.5 D on manifest refraction showing that the axial map of corneal topography (bottom right) does not correspond to the map of the entire eye and the main contribution of astigmatism is from internal eye or the lens.

polynomials, and these may be positive or negative in value leading to predictable alterations in the image quality. The magnitude of these aberrations is expressed as an RMS error that is the deviation of the WF averaged over the entire WF. The higher the RMS value, the greater the overall aberration for a given eye. Majority of the population has a total RMS value of <0.3 µm.

2. Till what grade aberration can be corrected?

Ans. Aberrations can be corrected surgically till 4th order that is SAs.

3. What type of aberration is seen most commonly in KC?

Ans. The most common aberration seen in KC is vertical coma.

4. Mention the type of aberration in following: Cataract, aging, and myopia.

Ans.
- *Cataract:* In the case of cortical cataract, the most common type of aberration reported is SA while in nuclear cataract it is coma.[8]
- *Aging:* With aging, the major changes occur in HO and SAs only. This is mainly contributed by the changes in the lens with age, while there is a minimal contribution by the cornea. So, cornea does not affect significantly the changes in ocular aberrations seen with aging. In a young patient, the corneal aberrations are compensated by internal optics. Since the cornea has a positive SA, it is partially compensated by the negative SA of the clear lens. As age increases, the SA of the lens becomes less negative leading to a net increase in the total ocular SA. Also, there is an increase in the horizontal coma and other third-order aberrations

as well. Thus, HOAs increase with age due in part to a decoupling of cornea and lens. In particular, lateral coma remains compensated in most of the older eyes due to angle kappa remaining stable with age and the lens shape factor only experiencing small changes.[9,10]

- *Myopia:* In eyes with myopic astigmatism, primary horizontal trefoil, SA, and primary vertical coma are the predominant HOAs in descending order of frequency. A significant correlation has been seen between spherical equivalent refractive error and primary horizontal coma and the RMS of SA.[11]

REFERENCES

1. Maeda N. Clinical applications of wavefront aberrometry: a review. Clin Exp Ophthalmol. 2009;37:118-29.
2. Thibos LN. Principles of Hartmann-Shack aberrometry. J Refract Surg. 2000;16:S563-5.
3. Molebny VV, Panagopoulou SI, Molebny SV, Wakil YS, Pallikaris IG. Principles of ray tracing aberrometry. J Refract Surg. 2000;16:S572-5.
4. Wakil JS, Padrick TD, Molebny S. The iTrace combination corneal topography and wavefront system by Tracey technologies. In: Wang M (Ed). Corneal Topography in the Wavefront Era. Thorofare, NJ: SLACK Inc.; 2006. pp. 177-88.
5. Gomez AC, Rey AVD, Bautista CP, Ferrándiz AE, MD4; González DC, OD5; Burgos SC. Principles and clinical applications of ray-tracing aberrometry (part I). J Emmetropia. 2012;3:96-110.
6. Wang Li, Wang Nan, Koch DD. Evaluation of refractive error measurements of the WaveScan Wavefront system and the Tracey wavefront aberrometer. J Cataract Refract Surg. 2003;29:970-9.
7. Park CY, Oh SY, Chuck RS. Measurement of angle kappa and centration in refractive surgery. Curr Opin Ophthalmol. 2012;23(4):269-75.
8. Rocha KM, Nosé W, Bottós K, Bottós J, Morimoto L, Soriano E. Higher-order aberrations of age-related cataract. J Cataract Refract Surg. 2007;33(8):1442-6.
9. Athaide HV, Campos M, Costa C. Study of ocular aberrations with age. Arq Bras Oftalmol. 2009;72(5):617-21.
10. Berrio E, Tabernero J, Artal P. Optical aberrations and alignment of the eye with age. J Vis. 2010;10(14):34.
11. Karimian F, Feizi S, Doozande A. Higher-order aberrations in myopic eyes. J Ophthalmic Vis Res. 2010;5(1):3-9.

2.5 ANTERIOR SEGMENT OPTICAL COHERENCE TOMOGRAPHY

Sourabh Verma, Talvir Sidhu, Deepali Singhal, Manasi Tripathi, Namrata Sharma

INTRODUCTION

Huang et al. first described optical coherence tomography (OCT) as high-resolution imaging modality for cross-sectional analysis of retina.[1] Since its conception, OCT technology has dramatically improved resulting in more accurate and detailed reconstruction of images, which has revolutionized our understanding of retinal pathologies. More recently, a modification of OCT technology known as anterior segment optical coherence tomography (ASOCT) was described by Izzat et al. as a useful diagnostic tool for analyzing more anterior structures such as cornea, angle anatomy, association between iris and lens, intraocular masses and tumors, abnormalities of lens, etc.[2]

Anterior segment OCT is a noncontact and noninvasive optical imaging modality with a resolution much higher than ultrasound or ultrasound biomicroscopy (UBM). It is done in sitting position and requires no anesthesia. Currently, most commonly available commercial models include Visante (by Carl Zeiss Meditec) and slit-lamp OCT, which are time domain (TD) OCT and CIRRUS HD-OCT 5000/500 (Carl Zeiss Meditec, Inc. Dublin, USA), CASIA SS-1000 OCT (by Tomey, Japan), which is a SS-OCT.

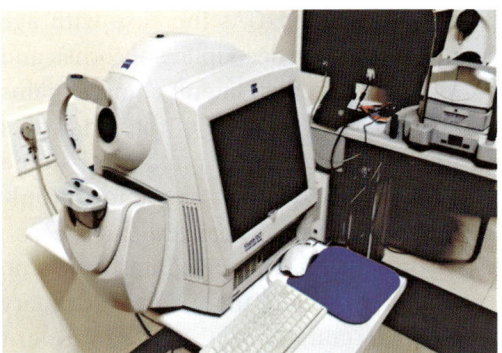

Fig. 2.5.1: Visante anterior segment optical coherence tomography (time domain).

PRINCIPLES AND SPECIFICATIONS

Anterior segment OCT is based on principle of low coherence interferometry. A two-dimensional image of anterior structures of eye is produced by scattering of light by internal tissue microstructures. It makes use of longer wavelength (1,310 nm; Visante) or shorter wavelength (810 or 840 nm; Optovue). This results in less scattering through opaque media and deeper penetration through limbus and sclera.

Visante **(Fig. 2.5.1)** has a 16 mm scan width and 6 mm scan depth, which is more than spectral domain-OCT (SD-OCT) systems in which only a small component of anterior segment is captured. It has an axial resolution of 15–20 microns.

CASIA ASOCT **(Fig. 2.5.2)** uses a single detector and a rapidly tunable laser, taking about 30,000 A-scans per second. It can achieve an axial and transverse resolution of 10 and 30 microns, respectively. CASSIA is also capable of producing a 360° image of angle in 128 cross-sections in about 2.4 seconds. SD-OCT devices have a horizontal scan width of 3–6 microns and lesser scan depth than TD-OCT devices.

Ultrahigh-resolution OCT **(Fig. 2.5.3)** has been recently introduced with axial resolution up to 1–3 microns, but they are

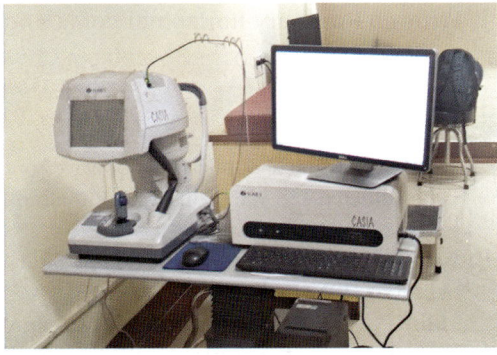

Fig. 2.5.2: CASIA anterior segment optical coherence tomography (ASOCT) (Fourier domain).

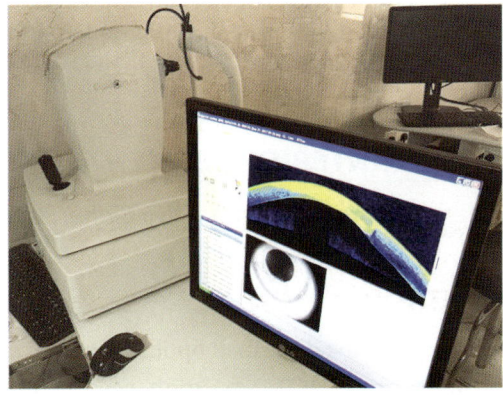

Fig. 2.5.3: Ultrahigh-resolution anterior segment optical coherence tomography.

used mostly for research purposes and are yet to find widespread clinical use. These devices have a scan depth of 5–12 microns.

INDICATIONS OF ANTERIOR SEGMENT OPTICAL COHERENCE TOMOGRAPHY

Anterior segment OCT is most useful for glaucoma and cornea specialists to diagnose, treat, and follow patients.

Applications in Corneal Conditions

Corneal Opacity

Corneal opacity can be used for determining depth and extent of corneal opacities. Such information is of great help when deciding for the level of LKP procedure **(Figs. 2.5.4 and 2.5.5)**. In addition, residual cornea opacities can be evaluated in postoperative period **(Fig. 2.5.6)**.

Penetrating Keratoplasty

It has been used to study wound apposition and healing postpenetrating keratoplasty (PK). Any graft host junction malposition can be picked up. Studies have shown that such malposition can result in postoperative astigmatism, myopia, and faulty IOP measurements. ASOCT has been used for studying wound healing patterns in various configurations of femto-assisted PKs and zigzag configuration has been found to be most stable with minimum astigmatism. It has also been used for evaluating postoperative complications. ASOCT-based studies have proved that incomplete excision of Descemet's membrane can result in postoperative glaucoma.

Anterior Lamellar Keratoplasty

Anterior LKP offers several advantages over PK such as lesser chances of graft rejection and a closed globe procedure. Based on level of abnormality, different types of anterior lamellar procedures such as superficial anterior lamellar keratoplasty (SALK) and automated lamellar therapeutic keratoplasty (ALTK) can be done **(Fig. 2.5.6)**. In deeper

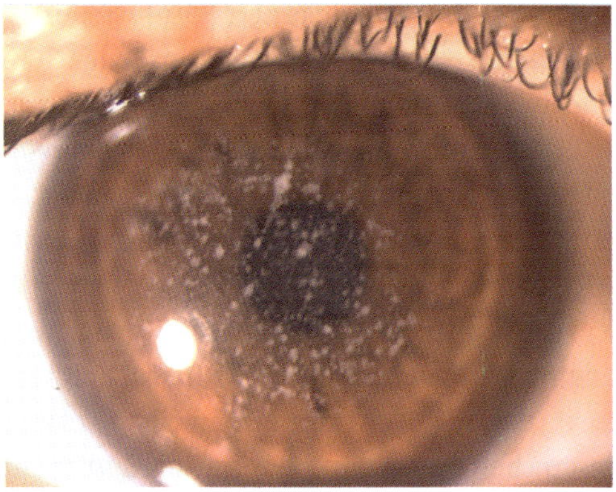

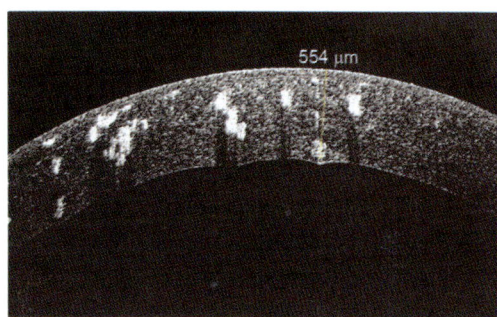

Fig. 2.5.5: Anterior segment optical coherence tomography showing multiple stromal cornea opacities in granular corneal dystrophy.

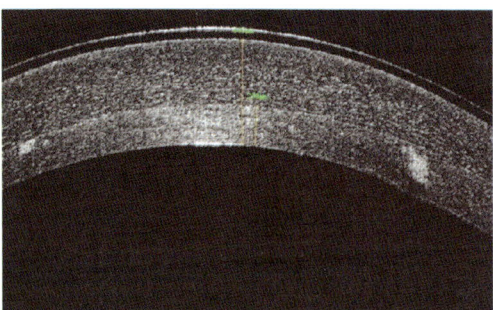

Fig. 2.5.6: Anterior segment optical coherence tomography (ASOCT) image posterior-anterior lamellar therapeutic keratoplasty clearly showing graft host junction and residual opacity in host cornea outside the visual axis.

Fig. 2.5.4: Diffuse slit-lamp corneal image of granular corneal dystrophy.

opacities and ectatic conditions, procedure such as deep anterior lamellar keratoplasty (DALK) can produce similar outcome as PK with minimal complications. Not only ASOCT helps in decision-making, but it also helps in diagnosing possible complications like Descemet's membrane detachment, double or triple AC, and interface keratitis.[3]

Endothelial Keratoplasty

The corneal stroma must be free from opacity, scarring, or haze to achieve optimal postoperative outcomes after endothelial keratoplasty (EK) for corneal decompensation. Preoperative assessment using ASOCT can effectively evaluate stromal clarity, thereby aiding in the appropriate selection of cases for EK. In postoperative period, ASOCT helps identify adequate apposition between donor and host corneal components, presence of any fluid pockets or debris in the graft–host interphase and retained Descemet's membrane and monitors resolution of corneal edema. Complications such as donor graft dislocation, epithelial ingrowth, interface opacities, and persistent interphase fluid can also be diagnosed.[3]

Eye Bank

Eye bank can also be used for screening eyes for evidence of any previous refractive procedure, which is a contraindication for being used as donor tissue.

Infective keratitis: ASOCT proves to be of great utility in cases with infective keratitis. With the application of this modality, clinicians can objectively assess the depth and extent of infiltrates. Stromal infiltrates appear as hyperreflective areas with ill-defined margins on ASOCT scans, which may or may not be associated with posterior shadowing **(Fig. 2.5.7)**. Endothelial plagues can also be identified and characterized on ASOCT. Additionally, response to treatment can be monitored by sequentially assessing the above parameters.

Intraoperative Optical Coherence Tomography

Intraoperative OCT (iOCT) can be used to confirm apposition between lamellae in lamellar procedures and analyze the interface. Intraoperative Descemet's membrane detachment can be visualized and effectively managed with intracameral air or gas injections. The iOCT-based studies have shown that an optimal donor–host apposition reached within minutes after Descemet stripping automated endothelial keratoplasty (DSAEK) thus reducing time for positioning in operation theater (OT).

Others

Keratoconus eyes have demonstrated donut-shaped configuration of epithelial thickness profile when examined through ultrahigh-resolution OCT. Epithelium over cornea is thinned, but epithelium in surrounding 3-4 mm zone is thickened. Other features, which are seen, include hyper-reflectivity and interruptions in Bowman's membrane, stromal thinning, and scarring in advanced cases. Descemet's membrane tear and corneal hydration can be visualized in cases with corneal hydrops **(Fig. 2.5.8)**.

Vanathi et al. used ASOCT to monitor acute hydrops in a patient with PMD.[4] Igbree et al. used it to measure AC cells.[5] Corneal re-epithelization can be monitored with the help of ASOCT with epithelium being hyper-reflective **(Fig. 2.5.9)**.

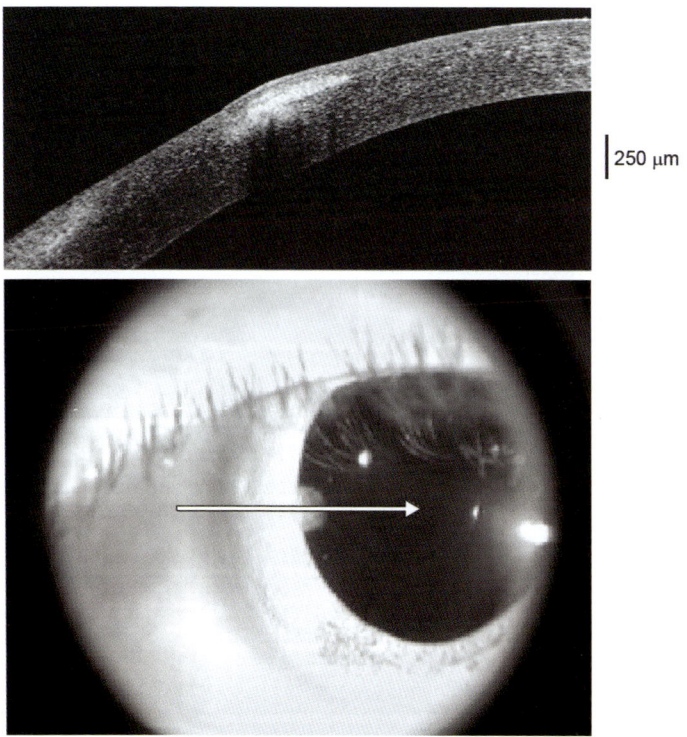

Fig. 2.5.7: Subepithelial corneal infiltrate as seen on anterior segment optical coherence tomography.

Applications in Ocular Surface Diseases

Conjunctival Diseases

In conjunctivochalasis, it can be used to measure cross-sectional area of prolapsed tissue in tear meniscus. Pterygium and pinguecula appear as hyper-reflective wedge-shaped masses with thinned out epithelium. In lymphoma, hyper-reflective uninvolved epithelium and hyporeflective subepithelial lesion is seen. In conjunctival melanoma and nevi, hyper-reflectivity at basal epithelial layer and cysts can be seen.

Anterior Segment Tumors

Anterior segment OCT has been extensively used to evaluate ocular surface squamous neoplasia (OSSN). The extent of OSSN can be determined by hyper-reflective thickened epithelium of lesion and its abrupt transition to normal epithelium in uninvolved area. Depth of lesion can also be determined; however, UBM has proved to be superior in this regard. Deep intraocular penetration can warrant enucleation in place of medical management. Normalization of epithelial appearance has been seen with resolution of OSSN with medical management. Tumors of iris, angle, and ciliary body can be visualized but UBM has proved to be superior and a more reproducible modality to image and follow-up response to treatment.

Dry Eye

Studies using ASOCT have shown that it is a useful tool for evaluation of tear film thickness, tear meniscus height, and can be

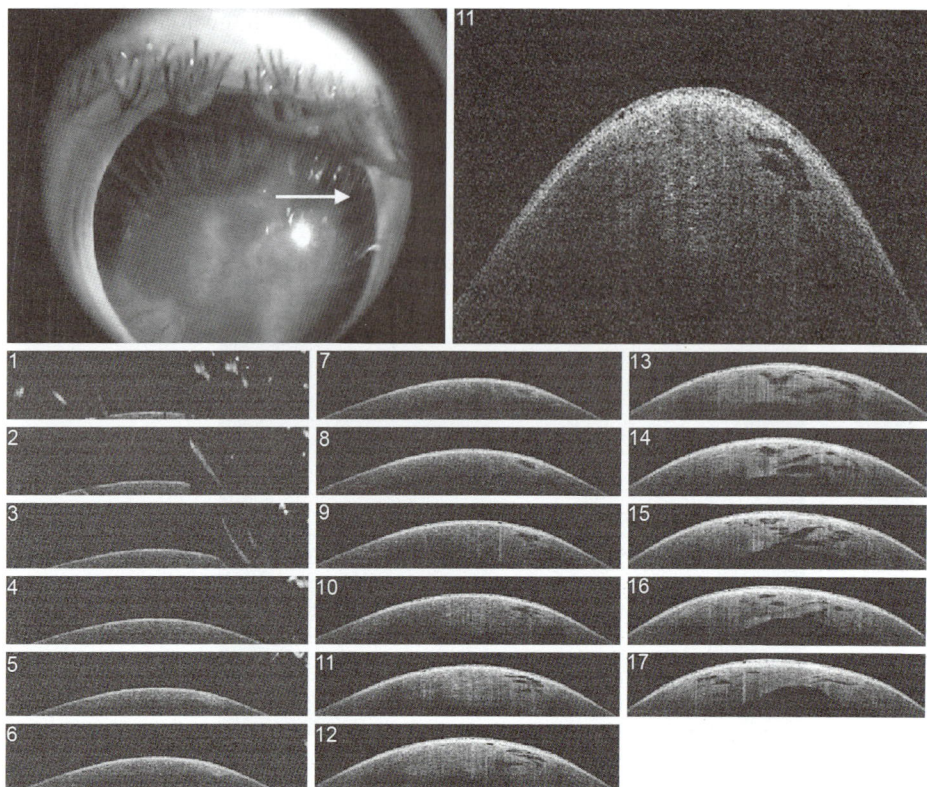

Fig. 2.5.8: Anterior segment optical coherence tomography image of corneal hydrops showing multiple stromal fluid clefts and markedly increased corneal thickness.

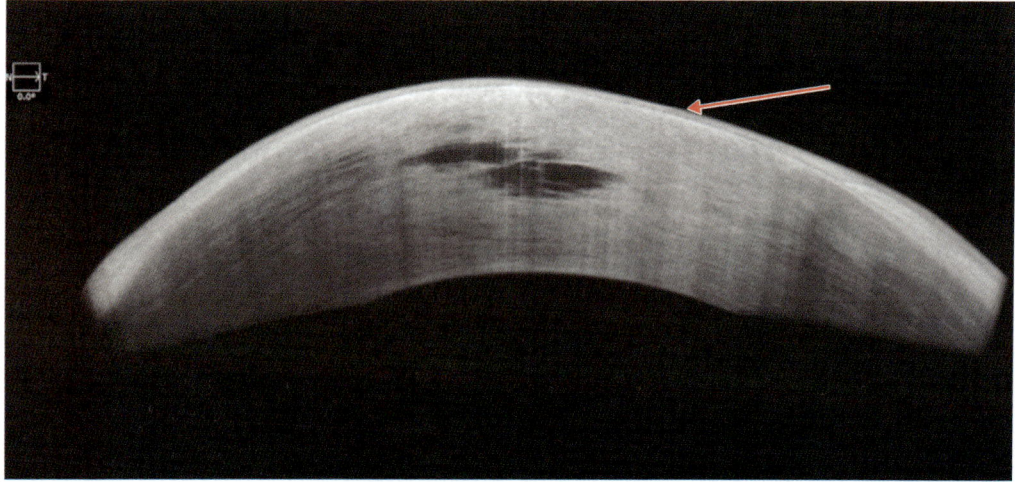

Fig. 2.5.9: Anterior segment optical coherence tomography (ASOCT) showing completely epithelialized surface as shown by red arrow.

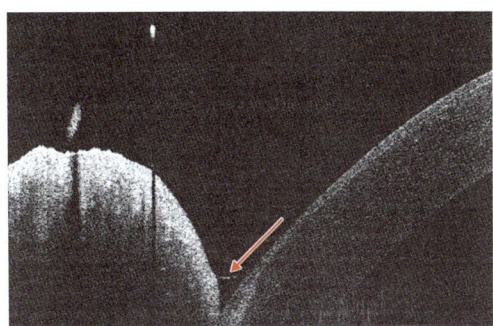

Fig. 2.5.10: Tear meniscus as visualized on anterior segment optical coherence tomography (red arrow).

used to follow-up response of management of dry eye **(Fig. 2.5.10)**. Recently, it has been used to reconstruct three-dimensional images of meibomian glands, thus proving its potential worth in managing meibomian gland disorders.

Anterior Segment Trauma

History of any ocular trauma or a suspected open globe injury is a contraindication for any contact procedure. ASOCT can be used to examine any corneal or scleral perforations and determining size, shape, and position of any intraocular foreign body in anterior segment of eye. It is useful for determining the extent of injury in case of media opacity and monitoring response to medical management or amniotic membrane graft (AMG) in cases with thermal or chemical injuries.

Applications in Refractive Surgeries

Anterior segment OCT enables precise measurement of corneal thickness, flap thickness, and residual stromal bed thickness. This is especially useful in cases where a LASIK enhancement is planned and can avoid any postoperative ectasia.

It has been used to evaluate corneal wound healing responses, interface smoothness, and apposition after manual and laser-assisted LASIK. It can be used in diagnosis and management of postrefractive surgery complications. Interface fluid syndrome is a flap-related complication of LASIK, which is characterized by fluid collection in interface, flap edema, and haze.[6]

Anterior segment OCT is also used for preoperative assessment of ACD prior to planning for phakic IOL. ACD ≥2.8 mm is recommended for myopic phakic IOLs, while ACD ≥3 mm is recommended for hyperopic phakic IOLs. In postoperative period, ASOCT can objectively measure phakic IOL vault. Ideal lens vault varies between 250 microns and 750 microns; anything beyond this range may warrant a replacement procedure **(Fig. 2.5.11)**.

The ASOCT can also be utilized in the preoperative planning and postoperative assessment of patients undergoing intracorneal ring segments.

Applications in Cataract Surgeries

It can be used for evaluation of corneal biometry, lens, AC, and angle structures. Corneal power as measured with ASOCT can be used for calculating IOL power. Tang et al. showed that in patients with previous myopic laser correction, IOL power calculation with ASOCT-based biometry is equally or more accurate than current standard.[7]

Lens density measurement with ASOCT is highly reproducible and correlates well with lens opacity classification system III (LOCS III). It has been used to study corneal incisions and epithelial remodeling after cataract surgeries. Localized Descemet's membrane detachments can be visualized at incision sites, which are otherwise very difficult to observe clinically.[6]

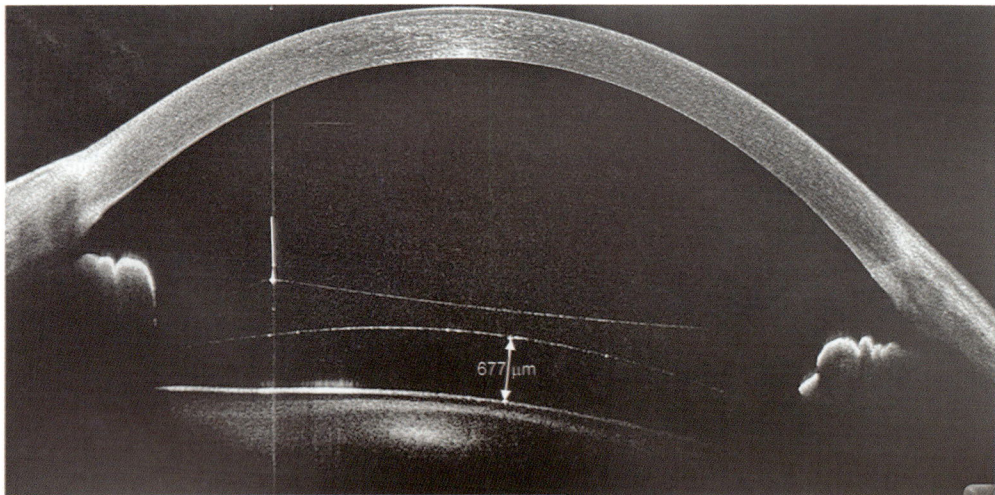

Fig. 2.5.11: Anterior segment optical coherence tomography (ASOCT) showing high vault in a patient who underwent ICL implantation. (ICL: implantable collamer lens)

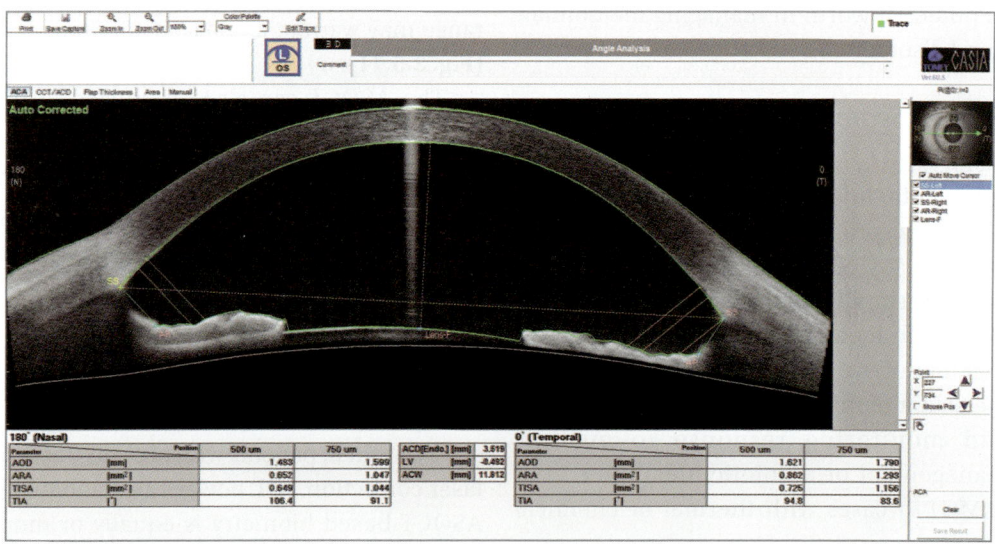

Fig. 2.5.12: Angle details on anterior segment optical coherence tomography.

Applications in Glaucoma

Anterior segment OCT is useful in quantifying angle closure glaucoma and important landmarks include scleral spur, Schlemm's canal, Schwalbe's line, and trabecular meshwork **(Fig. 2.5.12)**. ASOCT can help in identifying occludable angles and quantifying extent of peripheral anterior synechiae. Pre- and post-laser peripheral iridotomy (LPI) ASOCT shows opening up of angles due to posterior falling of iris. It can also be used to confirm patency of peripheral iridotomies and study its healing response.

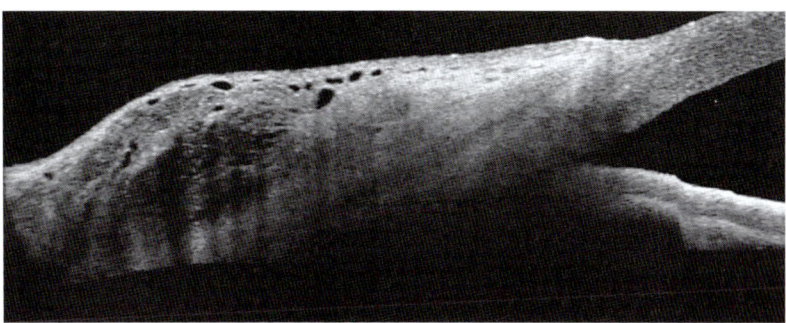

Fig. 2.5.13: Elevated bleb with microcysts.

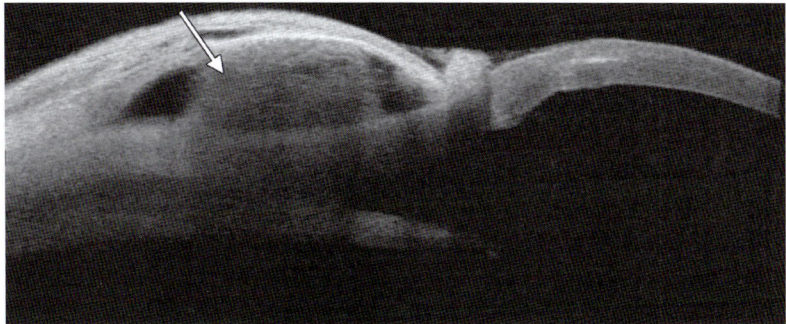

Fig. 2.5.14: Bleb with subconjunctival ologen (arrow).

Pigment dispersion syndrome is characterized by open angle and posterior bowing of peripheral iris giving a typical "S-shaped configuration". "Sinusoidal configuration" of iris in plateau iris syndrome can be picked up. Opening up of AC angle after cataract surgery and IOL implantation can be seen on ASOCT.

It can also be used to study bleb morphology. It can visualize bleb dimensions, bleb wall thickness, flap, bleb cavity, patency of ostium, cysts within the bleb **(Fig. 2.5.13)**, and Ologen implant **(Fig. 2.5.14)**. It can help in identification of failing bleb and its cause so that timely management is possible.

Failing bleb can show occlusion of ostium, apposition of conjunctiva and episclera to sclera, and absence of bleb wall thickening (bleb wall thickening is a sign of successful bleb). In cases where glaucoma drainage devices (GDDs) have been used, it can be used to know the position, patency, and state of drainage of GDD tube. Any excessive contact with iris or cornea can be picked up and appropriate management can be done.[8] Biodegradable collagen implants **(Fig. 2.5.13)** can be visualized in situ with ASOCT and has been used to study implant–tissue interaction.

Use in Squint Surgery

Ocular muscle insertions cannot be evaluated by ocular sonography or by computed tomography. ASOCT can be used to look at the anterior part of the ocular muscles and muscle insertion. The distance of muscle insertion or absence may be accurately determined using ASOCT.[9-11]

LIMITATIONS

- Inability to visualize beyond iris; it is of no use in conditions where ciliary body imaging is required for diagnosis such as ciliary body tumors, misdirected ciliary processes, etc.
- It is unable to visualize beyond densely opaque media.
- Upper and lower eyelid interferes in imaging of superior and inferior angles thus reducing the amount of data obtained
- Limited cost-effectiveness

VIVA QUESTIONS

1. Describe role of ASOCT in early detection of KC.

Ans. Refer to text.

2. Describe ASOCT classification of KC.

Ans. Keratoconus can be classified into five distinct stages based on Fourier-domain OCT findings as proposed by Sandali et al.[12]

1. *Stage 1:* Thinning of apparently normal epithelial and stromal layers at the conus
2. *Stage 2:* Hyper-reflective anomalies occurring at the Bowman's layer level with epithelial thickening at the conus
3. *Stage 3:* Posterior displacement of the hyper-reflective structures occurring at the Bowman's layer level with increased epithelial thickening and stromal thinning.
4. *Stage 4:* Panstromal scar
5. *Stage 5:* Corneal hydrops:
   a. *Stage 5a, acute onset:* Descemet's membrane rupture with separation of collagen lamellae with large fluid-filled intrastromal and fluid-filled cysts
   b. *Stage 5b, healing stage:* Panstromal scarring with a remaining aspect of Descemet's membrane rupture

3. State the difference between TD and SD.

Ans. Refer to **Table 2.5.1**.

4. What is swept source OCT and its role in anterior segment imaging?

Ans. Refer to text.

TABLE 2.5.1: Difference between time domain and spectral domain ASOCT.

Characteristics	Visante anterior segment OCT	Cirrus HD-OCT [RTVue-OCT (Optovue)]
Wavelength	1,310 nm	840 nm
Scanning	• 6 mm depth by 16 mm width • 256 A-scan per B-scan • 3 mm depth by 10 mm width 512 A-scan per B-scan • 2,048 A-scans per second	• *Cube:* 4 × 4 mm, 512 A-scan • *5-line raster:* 3 mm, 4,096 A-scans • 26,000 A-scans per second
Resolution	Transverse—60 µm; vertical—18 µm	Transverse—5 µm; vertical—8 µm
Advantage	Can penetrate deeper into the sclera, iris, and cornea than FD-OCT, owing to longer wavelength of its detector	High scan speed, improved resolution, significantly reduces motion artifacts, and increases signal-to-noise ratio
Principle	Time-domain OCT	Fourier-domain OCT

(ASOCT: anterior segment optical coherence tomography; FD-OCT: frequency domain optical coherence tomography; OCT: optical coherence tomography)

5. Describe the role of ASOCT in corneal dystrophy classification.

Ans. ASOCT imaging has been included in 2015 update of International Committee for Classification of Corneal Dystrophies (IC3D) classification of corneal dystrophies. It is useful in determining depth and extent of corneal opacities and depositions.

6. Describe the role of ASOCT in tear film assessment.

Ans. Refer to text.

7. What are DISCOVER and PIONEER studies and their impact in anterior segment surgeries?

Ans. Determination of feasibility of Intraoperative Spectral domain microscope combined/integrated OCT Visualization during En face Retinal and ophthalmic surgery (DISCOVER) study examined microscope-integrated OCT systems in ophthalmic surgery.[13] It concluded that real-time iOCT can influence decision-making during Descemet's membrane endothelial keratoplasty (DMEK) and is especially useful for novice surgeons. iOCT findings resulted in additional surgical maneuvers in 41% of patients and around 50% of cases, the iOCT provided information that was discordant to surgeon impression.

Prospective Intraoperative and Perioperative Ophthalmic ImagiNg with Optical CoherEncE TomogRaphy (PIONEER) established the feasibility of microscope-mounted portable OCT system.[14] PIONEER study evaluated use of iOCT in both anterior and posterior segment surgeries like lamellar corneal procedures and membrane peeling and concluded that it can influence decision-making in both types of surgeries. This technology helps in confirming correct graft orientation, ruling out any interface separation and reduces need of resurgeries.

iOCT identified residual persistent fluid in 48% of eyes that resulted in additional surgical maneuvers. In 18% of cases, the surgeon believed there were residual fluids but iOCT confirmed complete apposition, mitigating the need for additional maneuvers.

8. Describe the role of ASOCT postcorneal crosslinking (CXL) of cornea.

Ans. ASOCT has been used to evaluate depth of demarcation line (DL) created after corneal corneal crosslinking procedures. Depth of DL does not depend upon osmolarity of riboflavin. Average depth of DL after epithelium off CXL using Dresden protocol or accelerated protocol is around 300 microns. In transepithelial procedures, it is much shallower and lies at around 100 microns' depth.

9. Describe the role of ASOCT in corneal hydrops.

Ans. In corneal hydrops, ASOCT can be used to assess corneal edema, rolled edges, and extent of Descemet detachment. It can be used to monitor resolution of corneal edema and attachment of Descemet's membrane after intracameral gas or air injection.

10. Describe ASOCT finding in pigment dispersion syndrome.

Ans. Wide open angle with posterior bowing of iris can be seen on ASOCT (**Fig. 2.5.15**).

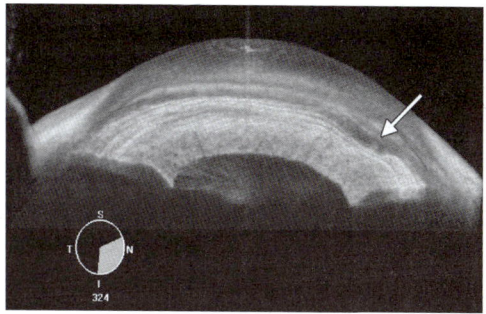

Fig. 2.5.15: Pigment dispersion syndrome showing wide-open angle with posterior bowing of iris.

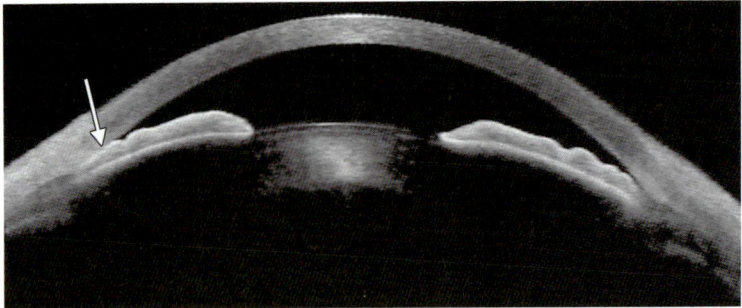

Fig. 2.5.16: Appositional angle closure in primary angle-closure glaucoma (PACG) (arrow).

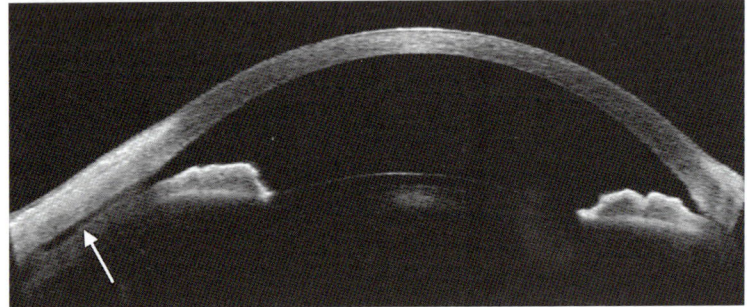

Fig. 2.5.17: Shallow choroidal detachment after trauma (arrow).

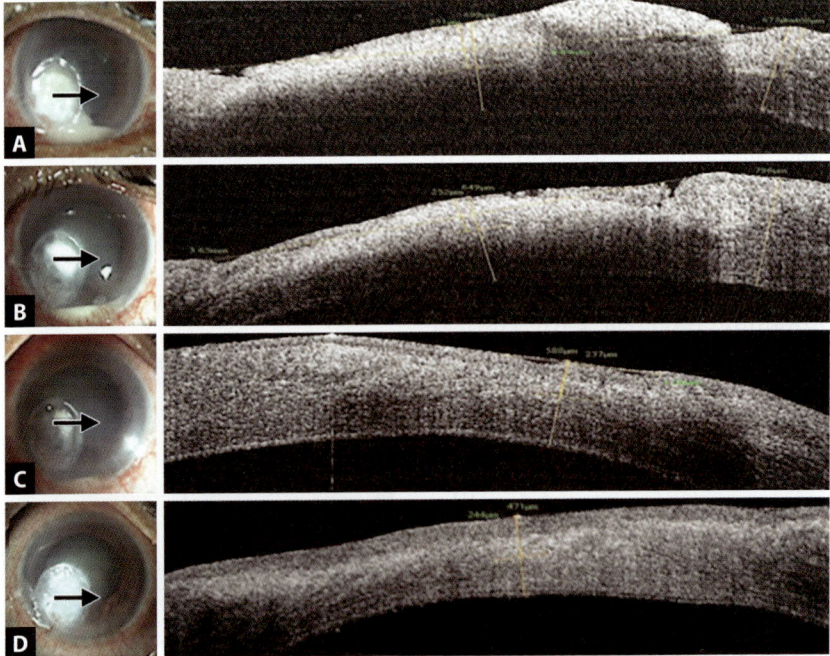

Figs. 2.5.18A to D: Location and extent of corneal infiltrate, thinning, and monitor of healing on anterior segment optical coherence tomography.

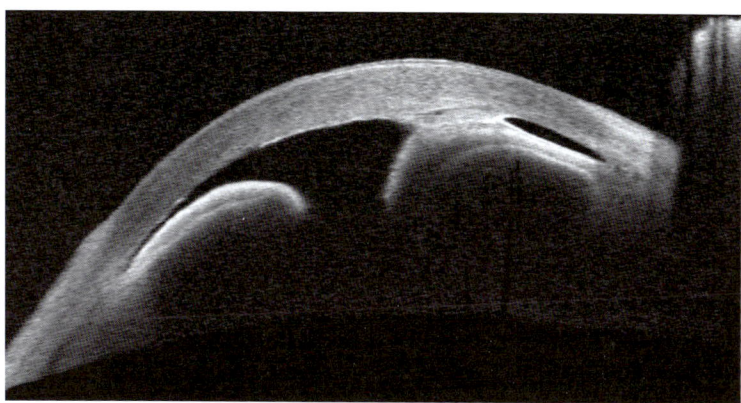

Fig. 2.5.19: Sequel of corneal ulcer such as adherent leukoma visualized on anterior segment optical coherence tomography.

11. Describe the role of ASOCT in detecting lens-induced secondary angle closure glaucoma.

Ans. Thick lens can push iris anteriorly causing narrowing of angle predisposing to angle closure that can be visualized by ASOCT **(Fig. 2.5.16)**.

12. Describe the role of ASOCT in supraciliary effusion.

Ans. ASOCT can be used to detect supraciliary effusion as shown in **Figure 2.5.17**.

13. Describe the role of ASOCT in keratitis.

Ans. ASOCT can be used to assess the depth and extent of corneal infiltrates in keratitis. It can be used to determine location and extent of corneal thinning and monitor healing **(Figs. 2.5.18A to D)**. Sequelae of corneal ulcer such as adherent leukoma can be visualized on ASOCT **(Fig. 2.5.19)**.

REFERENCES

1. Huang D, Swanson EA, Lin CP, Schuman JS, Stinson WG, Chang W, et al. Optical coherence tomography. Science. 1991; 254(5035):1178-81.
2. Izatt JA, Hee MR, Swanson EA, Lin CP, Huang D, Schuman JS, et al. Micrometer-scale resolution imaging of the anterior eye in vivo with optical coherence tomography. Arch Ophthalmol. 1994;112(12):1584-9.
3. Nesi TT, Leite DA, Rocha FM, Tanure MA, Reis PP, Rodrigues EB, et al. Indications of Optical Coherence Tomography in Keratoplasties: Literature Review. J Ophthalmol. 2012;2012: 1-6.
4. Vanathi M, Behera G, Vengayil S, Panda A, Khokhar S. Intracameral SF6 injection and anterior segment OCT-based documentation for acute hydrops management in pellucid marginal corneal degeneration. Cont Lens Anterior Eye. 2008;31(3):164-6.
5. Igbre AO, Rico MC, Garg SJ. High-speed optical coherence tomography as a reliable adjuvant tool to grade ocular anterior chamber inflammation. Retina. 2014;34(3):504-8.
6. Han SB, Liu YC, Noriega KM, Mehta JS. Applications of anterior segment optical coherence tomography in cornea and ocular surface diseases. J Ophthalmol. 2016; 2016:4971572.
7. Tang M, Wang L, Koch DD, Li Y, Huang D. Intraocular lens power calculation after previous myopic laser vision correction based on corneal power measured by Fourier-domain optical coherence tomography. J Cataract Refract Surg. 2012;38(4):589-94.
8. Maslin J, Barkana Y, Dorairaj SK. Anterior segment imaging in glaucoma: an updated review. Indian J Ophthalmol. 2015;63(8): 630-40.

9. Paciuc-Beja M, Salcedo-Villanueva G, Quiroz-Mercado H. The accuracy of anterior segment optical coherence tomography (AS-OCT) in localizing extraocular rectus muscles insertions. J AAPOS. 2015;19(5): 489-90.
10. Park KA, Lee JY, Oh SY. Reproducibility of horizontal extraocular muscle insertion distance in anterior segment optical coherence tomography and the effect of head position. J AAPOS. 2014;18(1):15-20.
11. Pihlblad MS, Erenler F, Sharma A, Manchandia A, Reynolds JD. Anterior segment optical coherence tomography of the horizontal and vertical extraocular muscles with measurement of the insertion to limbus distance. J Pediatr Ophthalmol Strabismus. 2016;53(3):141-5.
12. Sandali O, El Sanharawi M, Temstet C, Hamiche T, Galan A, Ghouali W, et al. Fourier-domain optical coherence tomography imaging in keratoconus: a corneal structural classification. Ophthalmology. 2013;120(12):2403-12.
13. Ehlers JP, Goshe J, Dupps WJ, Kaiser PK, Singh RP, Gans R, et al. Determination of feasibility and utility of microscope-integrated optical coherence tomography during ophthalmic surgery: The DISCOVER Study RESCAN Results. JAMA Ophthalmol. 2015;133(10):1124-32.
14. Ehlers JP, Dupps WJ, Kaiser PK, Goshe J, Singh RP, Petkovsek D, et al. The Prospective Intraoperative and Perioperative Ophthalmic ImagiNg with Optical CoherEncE TomogRaphy (PIONEER) study: 2-year results. Am J Ophthalmol. 2014;158(5): 999-1007.

2.6 SPECULAR MICROSCOPE

Manasi Tripathi, Pranita Sahay, Mohamed Ibrahime Asif, Divya Agarwal, Prafulla Kumar Maharana

■ INTRODUCTION

Specular microscope **(Fig. 2.6.1)** images light that is reflected in a mirror-like fashion off the tissue interface from the incident light.[1] When light strikes a surface it can undergo three types of changes namely reflection, transmission, or absorption. In general, it undergoes a combination of all the three effects. Specular reflection occurs when the angle of reflection is equal to the angle of incidence. This reflected light is captured by the microscope. As the reflection can occur from any surface, there are multiple interfaces such as corneal epithelium, stroma, endothelium, and lens. The most important surface for evaluation is between endothelium and aqueous.

David Maurice in 1968[2] described the first specular microscope, which was later modified by Laing et al.[3] Subsequently various designs have been introduced that varies in the light projected (stationary slit, moving slit,

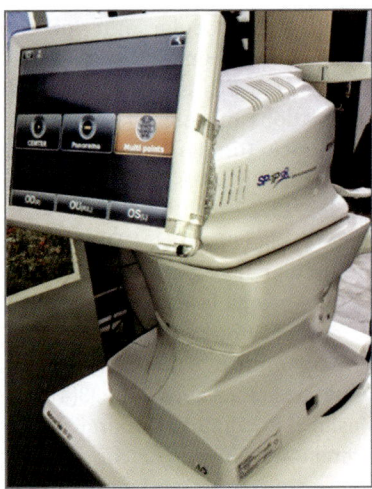

Fig. 2.6.1: Specular microscope.

and moving spot) or optical design (confocal or non-confocal) or the interface (contact or noncontact).

OPTICAL PRINCIPLE

As discussed specular reflection occurs when the angle of the incident light is equal to the angle of the reflected light at the interface (**Fig. 2.6.2**).[4] The reflected light is estimated to be about 0.02% of the incident light at the endothelium and aqueous interface. Reflected light from epithelium and stroma can obscure the reflected light from endothelial surface; hence, a narrow slit-beam of light is used for illumination. Laing described that specular microscopy yields image with three or four distinct zones depending on the width of the illuminating slit such as:[3,4]

- *Zone 1:* Epithelium/lens-coupling fluid
- *Zone 2:* Corneal stroma
- *Zone 3:* Corneal endothelium
- *Zone 4:* Aqueous humor

The boundary between zones 2 and 3 is usually bright called "bright boundary", and the boundary between zones 3 and 4 is almost dark and is termed as "dark boundary".

TYPES OF SPECULAR MICROSCOPES

- *Contact specular microscope:* A CL with coupling fluid of refractive index similar to the cornea is needed to eliminate the corneal surface reflection. In such arrangements, corneal thickness also includes CL thickness.
  Advantage: It provides good resolution and magnification.
  Disadvantages: These include patient discomfort, the risk of spread of infection, and artifacts are produced during manipulation.
  Example: HAI Labs, Inc. Lexington (CL-1000xyz), Heidelberg Engineering Vista-confocal contact immersion (corneal module HRT), Nidek Fremont-confocal contact immersion (Confoscan 4).
- *Noncontact specular microscope:* In this, the reflection from the anterior corneal surface is eliminated by increasing the angle of incidence, so the reflection is moved to the side covering less of specular reflection from endothelium.
  Advantages: These include greater patient comfort, no risk of corneal trauma/infections, and a broader field of view.
  Disadvantages: These include decreased resolution and magnification due to uncontrolled eye movements.
  Example: CEM-530, confoscan 4.
- *Wide-field specular microscope:* Standard specular microscope is modified using a scanning mirror, which increases the field to 800 microns diameter with no loss in contrast.
  Advantages: The advantages are 10–15 times increased field of view, improved resolution of endothelium, endothelial

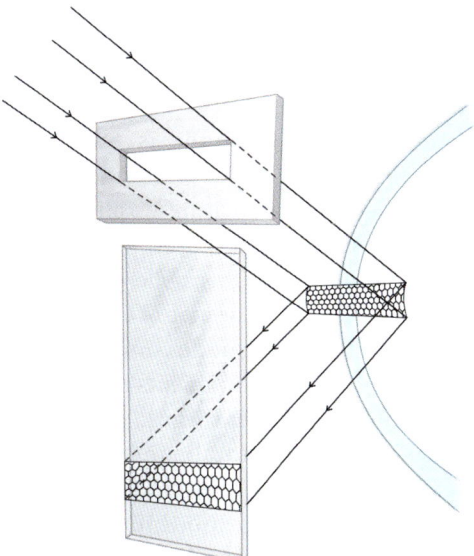

Fig. 2.6.2: Specular reflection.

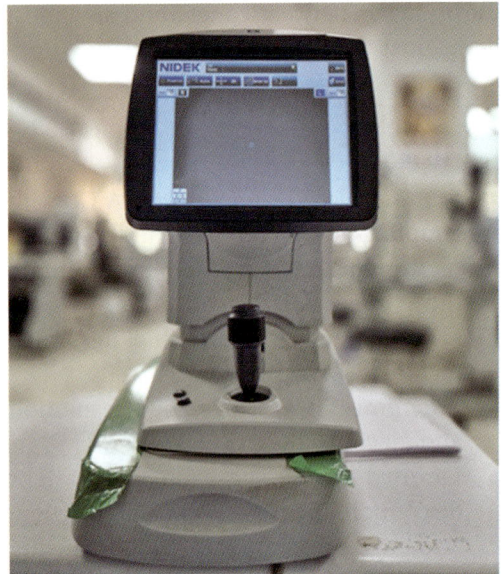

Fig. 2.6.3: Example of a horizontal specular microscope.

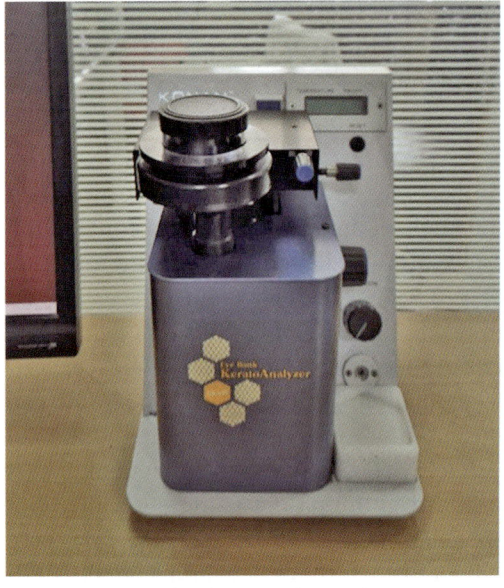

Fig. 2.6.4: Example of a vertical specular microscope used in eyes banks for evaluation of donor corneal tissues.

topography is more easily evaluated with easier visualization of a specific region, and improved optics so decreased annoying reflections.

Apart from this classification, specular microscopes can also be categorized as horizontal or vertical specular microscopes. Horizontal specular microscopes are utilized in clinical settings for the diagnosis and monitoring of corneal disorders **(Figs. 2.6.1 and 2.6.3)**. In contrast, vertical specular microscopes are used in eyebanks to assess the health of donor corneal tissues **(Fig. 2.6.4)**.

■ PROCEDURE

The patient is explained about the procedure. Then, the patient is seated comfortably, which is very important to obtain a good scan. In noncontact, the patient is asked to blink so that the corneal surface remains wet and smooth before capturing image. If using contact microscope, topical anesthesia is employed. Once contacted, punctate epithelial erosions can be seen; however, they disappear within a few hours. An internal fixation target is used to keep the patient's eye straight.

The image can be captured in three ways, such as:

1. *Automated*: This mode is quick and requires virtually no training as both alignment, and auto firing are automated. It is convenient for any user.
2. *Semi-automated*: In this mode, the user has better control over the area of examination while automatic mode simplifies the capture. It is useful in patients with fixation difficulty or irregular cornea.
3. *Manual*: Offers total control to the examiner as both alignment and firing are manual. This mode is useful in corneas with weak reflection or other anomalies.

Analytic Measurements

The qualitative examination involves analysis of the cell borders, configuration, cell intersections, guttae, intracellular bodies, vacuoles or bleb.[3,4]

Quantitative analysis includes calculation of cell area, density, polymegathism, and pleomorphism.[3,4]

Qualitative Analysis

Cell conformation: Normal endothelium is quasi-hexagonal/quasi-regular with side lengths equal and angle of intersection approximately 120°.

Cell boundaries: Often boundaries appear as dark, narrow lines.

Quantitative Analysis

- *Endothelial cell density (ECD):* ECD is calculated as cells/mm². This can be determined by various methods like:
  - *Comparison method:* By comparing cells imaged with a standard set of hexagonal cell size design.
  - *Frame method:* All cells within a frame are counted and are expressed as cells/mm². The problem is the need for adjustment of cells overlying the border by counting partial cells as full cells on two adjacent frames. It can be a fixed-frame or a variable-frame method **(Figs. 2.6.5A and B)**.
  - *Corner method:* Cell border corners are taken into account to determine cell area from a polygon digitization.
  - *Center method:* The center of contiguous cells is marked to facilitate counting.

Endothelial cell density does not reflect the status of endothelial function accurately. This is evidenced by a clear cornea, even with ECD as low as 500 cells/mm². Theoretically, coefficient of variation (CV) and percentage of hexagonal cells are a better indicator for corneal endothelium dysfunction.

The CV: Mean cell area is measured as μm²/cell. The CV is determined by measuring the areas of a population of cells and calculating the coefficient of variance, which is the SD of mean cell area divided by mean cell area. Normal CV is 0.40. Anything above 0.4 is considered abnormal.

Pleomorphism: It is usually measured as a percentage of six, less than six or more than six-sided cells. Percentage of hexagonal cells endothelial mosaic in a healthy cornea is around 70–80% **(Fig. 2.6.6)**.

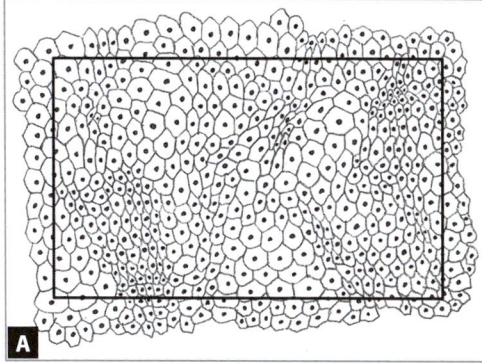 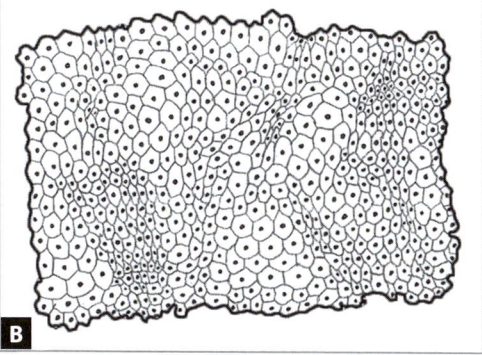

Figs. 2.6.5A and B: (A) Fixed frame analysis; (B) Variable frame analysis.

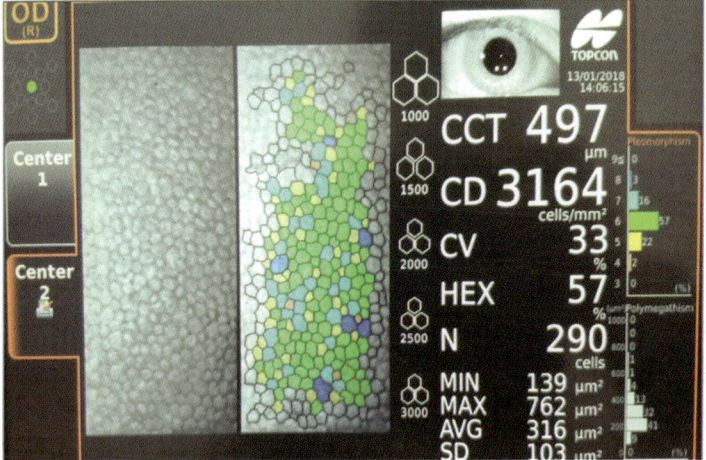

Fig. 2.6.6: Specular microscopy of a normal corneal endothelium.

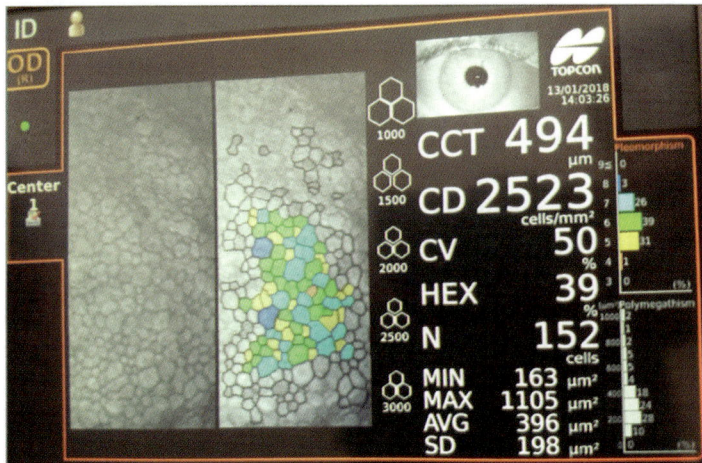

Fig. 2.6.7: Specular microscopy of a case with abnormal findings.

SOURCES OF ERRORS IN MEASUREMENT

- Missed cell(s)
- Counting a cell twice
- Including unanalyzable area in frame
- Failure to trace cells borders automatically
- In vertical microscopes, large corneoscleral rims of certain donor tissues may hamper optimal visualization of endothelial cells.

CLINICAL APPLICATIONS

- Specular microscopy is useful in the following:
  - *Diagnosis of diseases*: For example, Fuchs endothelial dystrophy, posterior polymorphous dystrophy (PPMD) **(Fig. 2.6.7)**, and bullous keratopathy
- *Research and monitoring of endothelium:* For assessment of changes in the endothelium associated with:
  - Aging

- Surgical procedures like keratoplasty, cataract surgery, and LASIK
- Pathological conditions like glaucoma, uveitis, and trauma
- CL use
- Endothelial cell culture
- Comparison of different surgical procedures.

■ *Eye banking:* For assessment of endothelium in donor corneas and the effect of preservation—Grading of donor cornea in eye bank is done based on ECD of the donor cornea. Prior to assessment, the donor tissue should be brought to room temperature/25°C for optimum visualization of endothelial cells **(Fig. 2.6.8)**. A minimum of 2,000 cells/mm² is required to grade a donor cornea as an optical grade. A higher ECD is required for EK (2,300–2,500 cells/mm²) **(Fig. 2.6.9)**.

■ *Surgery: Decision-making*—for example:
  - ECD <1,000 may be a relative contraindication for cataract surgery.
  - Less than 1,500 is a contraindication for putting an anterior chamber intraocular lens (ACIOL).
  - Less than 2,500 is a contraindication for phakic IOL (ICL)

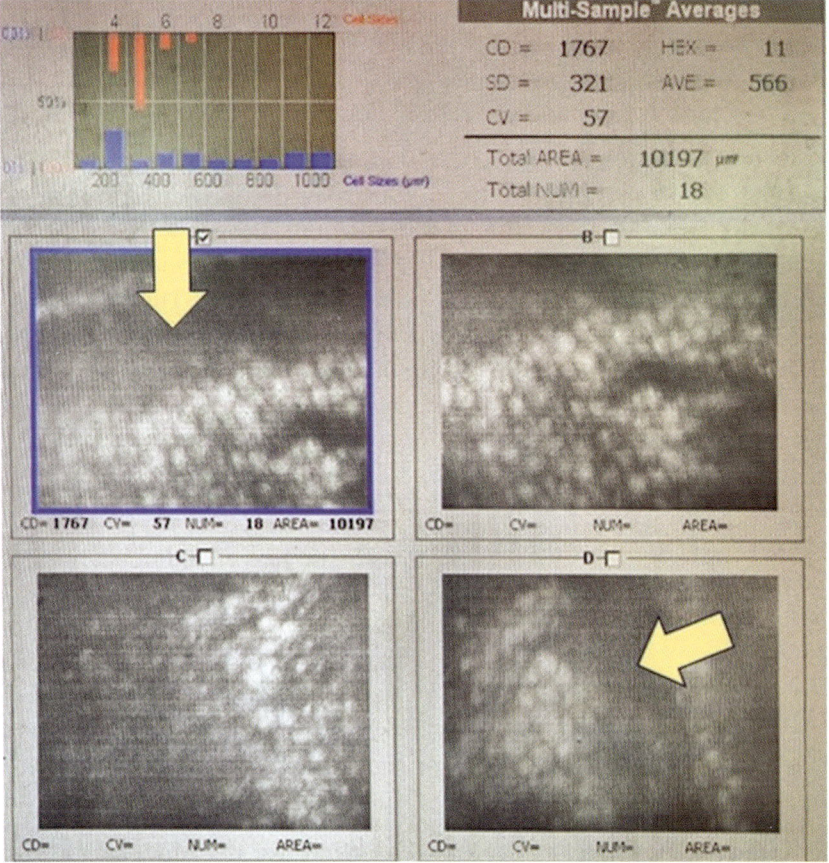

Fig. 2.6.8: Specular microscopy of a therapeutic-grade corneal donor tissue; note the low cell count, cell dropouts, and Descemet's membrane (DM) folds (yellow arrow).

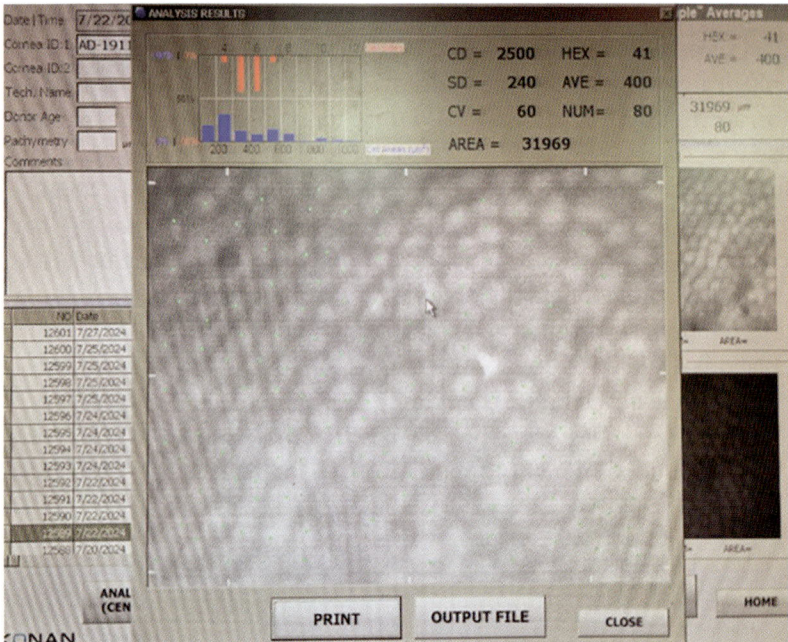

Fig. 2.6.9: Specular microscopy of a healthy corneal donor tissue.

- Less than 800 is an indication to go for DSAEK triple in cases of Fuchs endothelial corneal dystrophy (FECD) with cataract.
- *For assessment of the long-term effect of surgeries:* Efficacy of cataract surgery; comparison of different forms of EK (DSAEK versus DMEK, PKP versus DALK)
- *For measuring the corneal thickness (with contact type)*
- *For assessment of epithelium and lens; common conditions and their specular findings:* This has been summarized in **Table 2.6.1**.

VIVA QUESTIONS

1. What is the principle of a specular microscope?

Ans. Refer to text.

2. What is the normal endothelial cell count at birth and amount of loss with aging?

Ans. Normal ECD at birth is around 6,000 cells/mm^2. The count falls by 26% in the first year of life and a further decrease of 26% over the next 11 years. This rapid loss is partly due to the enlarging globe. It stabilizes from the age of 20 years through 50 years. After 60 years, on an average endothelial loss is approximately 0.5% per year.

3. What is bi-exponential decay model for endothelial cell loss?

Ans. The loss of endothelial cells follows a bi-exponential decay, i.e., a phase of rapid loss followed by a phase of the slow rate of endothelial loss.[5] Although this theory is not well established, it is supported by the results of most of the studies exploring endothelial cell loss. The proposed rates have been described in **Table 2.6.2**.

4. What are the different rates of endothelial loss following ocular surgeries?

Ans. Refer to **Table 2.6.3**.[6-13]

TABLE 2.6.1: Common conditions and their specular findings.

Conditions	Specular findings
Keratoconus	Stretched cells with long axis in the direction of the apex of the cone; dark bodies inside normal appearing cell can also be seen
Lattice corneal dystrophy	Branching criss-cross lines in the stroma, which are believed to be amyloid deposits; a crater form appearance has also been described
Posterior polymorphous corneal dystrophy	Vesicles with dark, thick border yielding doughnut appearance, appears to lie anterior to undistorted endothelial cells
Fuchs endothelial corneal dystrophy	Guttae (excrescences) with adjacent distorted endothelial cells; they appear as dark spots sometimes with central bright corneal reflections
Iridocorneal endothelial syndrome	ICE/ICE-berg cells look like PPMD vesicles within endothelium. There is loss of cellular definition and increased granularity and can eventually become completely blacked out areas. A reversal pattern may develop with black central and white borders
Glaucoma	Decreased endothelial count
Intraocular inflammation	Mononuclear inflammatory cells are seen between endothelial cells. Endothelial cells are generally unharmed
Contact lens wear	• Within minutes—small dark endothelial blebs occur but disappear quickly if lens is removed • Long-term-increased polymegathism that does not reverse, depends on duration and type of contact lens use
Diabetes	• Decreased cell density with age, increased polymegathism and pleomorphism and decreased hexagonality • Topical aldose reductase inhibitor reverses this morphologic changes

(ICE: iridocorneal endothelial syndrome; PPMD: posterior polymorphous corneal dystrophy)

TABLE 2.6.2: Phases of endothelial loss.

Condition	Rapid	Slow
Age	14–15 years	Rest of the life
Cataract	6 months	21 years
Penetrating keratoplasty	4 years	26 years

5. What are the parameters measured using a specular microscope and its significance?

Ans. Refer to text.

6. What are different methods of estimating endothelial cell count?

Ans. Refer to text.

7. What are the changes seen in specular microscopy in Fuchs corneal dystrophy?

Ans. Specular microscopy of FECD demonstrates the following changes.[14]

- *Stage 1*: Characterized by the presence of guttae, which are small to begin with, and more numerous centrally; the surrounding cells are normal. The sides of excrescences appear dark while their apex is bright.
- *Stage 2*: Size of the guttae becomes equal to that of endothelial cells.
- *Stage 3*: Guttae grow in size and become considerably larger than that of endothelial cells. The borders of the endothelial cell become blurred due to the presence of guttae.
- *Stage 4*: Guttae coalesce, blurring the adjacent boundaries; multiple apical bright spots can be seen (coalesce of adjacent guttae). In advanced disease,

TABLE 2.6.3: Different rates of endothelial loss following ocular surgeries.

Surgery	EC loss
Phacoemulsification	• 5–8% at 3 weeks and 6 months[10] • 10.5% at 1 year[6]
ECCE	9.1% at 1 year[6]
SICS	4.21% at 6 weeks (4.72% for ECCE and 5.41% for phacoemulsification)[7]
ICCE	15–50%[8]
PKP	11% ± 20% at 6 months and 20% ± 23% at 12 months[9]
DALK	14.2% ± 11.7% at 1 month (the loss was 8.6% at 1 year and 13.9% at 5 years compared to the 1 month endothelial cell density)[10]
DSAEK	34% ± 22% at 6 months 38% ± 22% at 1 year[9]
DMEK	35% at 6 months, 38% at 1 year, 43% at 2 years, 55% at 5 years[11]
PPV	9.0% ± 14.6% at 3 months[12]
Trabeculectomy	7% after penetrating surgery and 2.6% after nonpenetrating surgery at 3 months (noncombined surgeries)[13]

(DALK: deep anterior lamellar keratoplasty; DMEK: Descemet's membrane endothelial keratoplasty; DSAEK: Descemet stripping automated endothelial keratoplasty; ECCE: extracapsular cataract extraction; ICCE: intracapsular cataract extraction; PKP: penetrating keratoplasty; PPV: pars plana vitrectomy; SICS: small incision cataract surgery)

complete disorganization of the adjacent endothelial mosaic is seen (few authors call it stage 5).

8. What are the changes seen in specular microscopy in iridocorneal endothelial (ICE) syndrome?

Ans. Specular microscopy of FECD demonstrates the following changes:
- Rounding off of cell angles
- Loss of shape, many pentagonal cells are evident
- Cells appear more granular
- The appearance of central dark areas in endothelial cells
- In advanced cases, loss of endothelial mosaic
- The typical appearance of central black with bright borders is reversed, i.e., there will be black central areas and white borders (also known as ICE cells).

9. What are the changes seen in specular microscopy in diabetes?

Ans. The following changes can occur in diabetes:
- A rapid decrease in ECD with age
- Normal corneal thickness
- Increased polymegathism
- Increased pleomorphism
- Decreased percentage of hexagonality.

10. How do guttae appear in specular microscopy?

Ans. Corneal guttae are focal excrescences of collagenous basement membrane material, which have accumulated on Descemet's membrane, across the central cornea.[15]
- Corneal guttata are focal droplet-like accumulations of nonbanded collagen on the posterior surface of Descemet's membrane that appear as dark areas in between the bright endothelial cells.[16]

- These are commonly found in elderly people (9.6% of people older than 40 years and 3.3% of those between 20 and 40 years old had corneal guttata without edema).[16]
- Most common corneal disorder with gutta formation includes Fuchs' corneal endothelial dystrophy.

Other conditions where guttae are seen include trauma, congenital glaucoma, macular dystrophy, and corneal dystrophy resulting from Big-h3 R124H mutation (granular dystrophy, Reis–Bücklers dystrophy, lattice dystrophy, and Avellino dystrophy).[16]

11. What are pseudoguttae?

Ans. These are transient guttata-like features, usually found in cases of trauma, or intraocular inflammation. Pseudoguttae are considered to be formed due to endothelial edema or pigmentation.

12. How to void error in specular microscopy?

Ans. The following precautions may reduce the amount of error:
- By taking an average of multiple readings from the same reason using the same settings
- By keeping the image analysis method similar at every follow-up
- By measuring both density and morphology
- Regional variations must be kept in mind such as the ECD is higher in paracentral and peripheral areas compared to the central area.

REFERENCES

1. Hu V, Hughes EH, Patel N, Whitefield LA. The effect of aqualase and phacoemulsification on the corneal endothelium. Cornea. 2010; 29(3):247-50.
2. Maurice DM. Cellular membrane activity in the corneal endothelium of the intact eye. Experientia. 1968;24(11):1094-5.
3. Laing RA, Sandstrom MM, Leibowitz HM. Clinical specular microscopy. II. Qualitative evaluation of corneal endothelial photomicrographs. Arch Ophthalmol. 1979;97(9):1720-5.
4. Laing RA, Sandstrom MM, Leibowitz HM. Clinical specular microscopy. I. Optical principles. Arch Ophthalmol. 1979;97(9):1714-9.
5. Armitage WJ, Dick AD, Bourne WM. Predicting endothelial cell loss and long-term corneal graft survival. Invest Ophthalmol Vis Sci. 2003;44(8):3326-31.
6. Bourne RRA, Minassian DC, Dart JKG, Rosen P, Kaushal S, Wingate N. Effect of cataract surgery on the corneal endothelium: modern phacoemulsification compared with extracapsular cataract surgery. Ophthalmology. 2004;111(4):679-85.
7. George R, Rupauliha P, Sripriya AV, Rajesh PS, Vahan PV, Praveen S. Comparison of endothelial cell loss and surgically induced astigmatism following conventional extracapsular cataract surgery, manual small-incision surgery and phacoemulsification. Ophthalmic Epidemiol. 2005;12(5):293-7.
8. Neetens A, Dierens M, Delgadillo R. Endothelial Cell Damage after Intracapsular Cataract Extraction and Primary Anterior Chamber Pseudophakos Implantation. Ophthalmologica. 1983;187(2):114-7.
9. Price MO, Gorovoy M, Benetz BA, Price FW Jr, Menegay HJ, Debanne SM, et al. Descemet's Stripping Automated Endothelial Keratoplasty Outcomes Compared with Penetrating Keratoplasty from the Cornea Donor Study. Ophthalmology. 2010;117(3): 438-44.
10. Zhang Y, Wu S, Yao Y. Long-term comparison of full-bed deep anterior lamellar keratoplasty and penetrating keratoplasty in treating keratoconus. J Zhejiang Univ Sci B. 2013;14(5):438-50.
11. Baydoun L, Tong CM, Tse WW, Chi H, Parker J, Ham L, et al. Endothelial cell density after descemet membrane endothelial keratoplasty: 1 to 5-year follow-up. Am J Ophthalmol. 2012;154(4):762-3.

12. Koushan K, Mikhail M, Beattie A, Ahuja N, Liszauer A, Kobetz L, et al. Corneal endothelial cell loss after pars plana vitrectomy and combined phacoemulsification–vitrectomy surgeries. Can J Ophthalmol. 2017;52(1):4-8.
13. Arnavielle S, Lafontaine PO, Bidot S, Creuzot-Garcher C, D'Athis P, Bron AM. Corneal endothelial cell changes after trabeculectomy and deep sclerectomy. J Glaucoma. 2007;16(3):324-8.
14. Jackson AJ, Robinson FO, Frazer DG, Archer DB. Corneal guttata: a comparative clinical and specular micrographic study. Eye (Lond). 1999;13(Pt 6):737-43.
15. Vogt, A. Die Sichtbarkeit des lebenden Hornhautendothels. Graefes Arhiv für Ophthalmologie. 1920;101:123-44.
16. Akimune C, Watanabe H, Maeda N, Okada M, Yamamoto S, Kiritoshi A, et al. Corneal guttata associated with the corneal dystrophy resulting from a betaig-h3 R124H mutation. Br J Ophthalmol. 2000;84(1): 67-71.

2.7 ULTRASONIC PACHYMETER

Pranita Sahay, Mohamed Ibrahime Asif, Manasi Tripathi, Namrata Sharma

INTRODUCTION

Pachymetry is derived from the Greek word: *Pachos* meaning thick and *metry* meaning to measure. It refers to the measurement of corneal thickness. Central corneal thickness (CCT) is an indirect indicator of endothelial cell function. Pachymetry is used prior to refractive surgery, for screening ectatic corneal diseases and for glaucoma suspects.

Normal range: In healthy eyes, it ranges from 0.49 to 0.56 mm at the center, 0.52 mm to 0.57 mm in the paracentral region, and 0.7 mm to 0.9 mm at the limbus. Also, the thinnest quadrant is the temporal cornea followed by inferior. In general, a CCT of more than or equal to 0.7 mm suggests corneal endothelial cell dysfunction. Also, if the thickness of the center of the cornea is more than the midperipheral cornea, it points toward endothelial cell dysfunction.

PRINCIPLES

Broadly, pachymeters are based on either ultrasonic principles or optical principles. Most modern pachymeters are based on optical principle. The ultrasonic measurement is based on the reflection of ultrasonic waves from the anterior and posterior corneal surfaces. The time difference (transit time) between the echoes of the reflected ultrasonic signal from the anterior and posterior surface of the cornea to the transducer is used to measure the corneal thickness.

Corneal thickness is calculated by following the simple formula:

Corneal thickness
= (Transit time × Propagation velocity)/2

The speed of sound in the cornea is 1,640 m/s.

An ultrasonic pachymeter has the following important components **(Figs. 2.7.1 and 2.7.2)**:
- *Probe handle:* Which constitutes piezoelectric crystal that emits an ultrasonic beam of 20 MHz
- *Transducer:* Which sends ultrasonic waves and receives echoes from the corneal surface
- *Tip*: Having a diameter not >2 mm

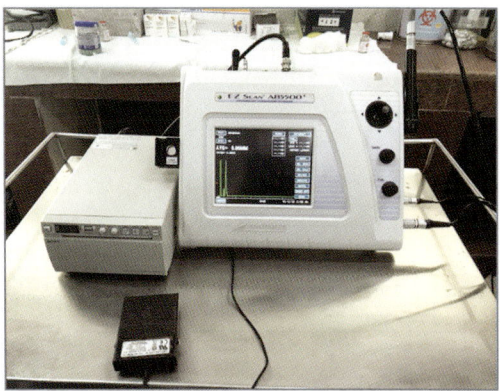

Fig. 2.7.1: A-scan pachymeter.

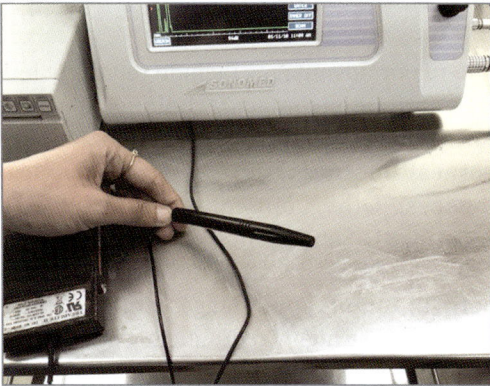

Fig. 2.7.2: Pachymeter probe.

TECHNIQUES OF PACHYMETRIC MEASUREMENTS

There are two types of pachymetric techniques:
1. *Spot measurements:* This technology is used in traditional optical pachymetry, specular microscopy, confocal microscopy, ultrasound pachymetry, and optical low-coherence reflectometry.
2. *Wide area mapping:* This technique provides the ability to map a wide area of the cornea and includes slit scanning optical pachymetry and very high-frequency (VHF) ultrasound imaging.

Pachymetric mapping provides several advantages over spot measurements:
- Mapping technique might help to reveal corneal abnormalities such as KC and PMD.
- It also allows preoperative planning for corneal surgeries that primarily do not concern just the center of the cornea, such as astigmatic keratotomy (AK), intracorneal ring segment (ICRS) implantation, DALK, and photo-therapeutic keratectomy.

Conventional ultrasound spot pachymetry is still the gold standard because of its reliability, ease of use, and relatively low cost.

OTHER TECHNIQUES OF PACHYMETRY

Methods of pachymetry **(Flowchart 2.7.1)** include the following:
- *Ultrasonic techniques:*
  - Conventional ultrasonic pachymetry
  - UBM
- *Optical techniques:*
  - Manual optical pachymetry
  - Specular microscopy
  - Scanning slit technology
  - OCT (ASOCT, IOLMaster 700)
  - Optical low coherence interferometry (OLCI) (Lenstar)
  - Confocal microscopy
  - Laser Doppler interferometry
  - Partial coherence interferometry (PCI)
- *Alternative measurements:*
  - Pentacam
  - Pachycam
  - Ocular response analyzer (ORA)

After being introduced by Henderson and Kremer introduced in 1980, ultrasonic pachymetry has been widely practiced and is regarded as the gold standard. Older units were more expensive and subject to alignment errors. With the improvement in ultrasound

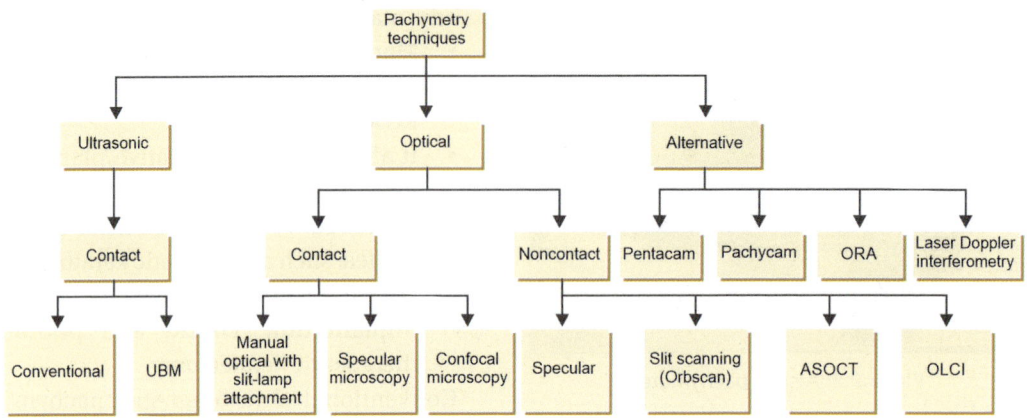

Flowchart 2.7.1: Pachymetry techniques.

(ASOCT: anterior segment optical coherence tomography; OLCI: optical low coherence interferometry; ORA: ocular response analyzer; UBM: ultrasound biomicroscopy)

technology, these instruments give less intersession and intraobserver variation with consistent and repeatable readings when compared to optical pachymetry.[1] They can be used intraoperatively and require no coupling medium. However, ultrasound pachymetry comes with a few disadvantages. Being a contact procedure; topical anesthesia is required, so is most undesirable in the early postoperative period. They have poor resolution and have limited accuracy, as the probe is handheld. For accurate measurements, it is essential to ensure that the probe is perpendicular. Reproducibility also relies on placing the probe at the center of the cornea. Indentation on the cornea can lead to underestimation of CCT. Modern ultrasound pachymeters are lightweight with good portability, have memory storage capability, IOP correction factor, high accuracy of ±5 microns, and resolution of 1 micron.

Maurice and Giardini first described optical methods of pachymetry as early as in 1951. These methods used various equations depending upon variables, such as corneal refractive index and anterior radius of curvature, to calculate corneal thickness and often had variable accuracy.

The major advantages include relatively low cost and a noncontact technique. Specular microscopes were later designed to measure corneal thickness using electromechanical devices. Other optical methods utilize rotating 3D Scheimpflug camera (available in Pentacam and Galilei devices) to obtain corneal tomography images noninvasively and provide a highly reproducible measure of CCT along with helping in the evaluation of regional changes in corneal thickness.

Anterior segment OCT is an easy and comfortable method for patients since it is a noncontact procedure and allows rapid image acquisition. It allows quantification of structures including corneal epithelium and images through corneal opacity. However, it may not always be used interchangeably with ultrasound pachymetry for CCT measurement.

The Orbscan device uses slit-scanning technology and measures the corneal thickness along with anterior and posterior corneal elevations. It, however, overestimates corneal thickness by almost 5%.

Optical low coherence interferometry methods use a diode laser beam and are attached to slit lamps. They measure only the CCT and have a precision of up to 1 micron.

Confocal microscopy is unique as it uses a computerized scanning system to provide total corneal thickness while evaluating cornea at high magnification (20× to 500×). It has moderate to good repeatability and has slower data acquisition as compared to other methods.

USES

- *Refractive surgeries:* CCT is used while planning refractive surgeries[2] as adequate preoperative thickness is critical in reducing the risk of developing postrefractive surgery ectasia. Residual stromal bed thickness of 250–300 μm is recommended before going for LASIK surgery. Patients with thinner corneas should be considered for surface ablation procedures.
- *Glaucoma suspects:* Corneal thickness influences IOP. Tonometry often overestimates or underestimates IOP in eyes with thicker and thinner corneas, respectively. Thin CCT is an independent risk factor for the development of glaucomatous optic neuropathy.[3] A correction factor of 0.7 must be used and deducted or added for every 10 μm above or below, respectively, from the average corneal thickness (530 μm for Indian population).
- *Congenital glaucoma:* CCT has been reported to be higher in cases of primary congenital glaucoma.[4] Pachymetry is essential for management of pediatric glaucoma.
- *Post-keratoplasty patients:* Pachymetry measurement tells about the health of a transplanted cornea. Serial measurement of CCT can be used for follow-up of post-keratoplasty patients to record the progress of corneal deturgescence. Besides, increase in CCT is an early indication of endothelial dysfunction or graft failure. Serial CCT measurement following an acute episode of graft rejection helps in detecting the response to pulse steroid therapy.
- *CL:* Prolonged CL wear can cause corneal edema and hypoxia. This is seen most commonly with daily wear, extended wear, and therapeutic lenses.
- *Corneal ectasia:* Pachymetry helps to determine and to monitor abnormalities of corneal structure or function. Corneal thinning is noted in disorders like KC and PMD while corneal thickening is seen in cases of endothelial dystrophy and other causes of endothelial dysfunction. Pachymetry is essential for patients undergoing corneal crosslinking (CXL). Corneal thickness <400 microns (without epithelium) is a contraindication for CXL due to potential risk of damage to corneal endothelium by the UV rays. Therefore, in such patients, certain modifications in CXL are essential such as transepithelial CXL, hypoosmolar riboflavin-assisted CXL, lenticule-assisted CXL, bandage CL-assisted CXL, customized epithelial debridement technique, and iontophoresis-assisted CXL (I-CXL).[6]
- *Corneal decompensation:* Corneal thickening is seen in endothelial dysfunction due to FECD and herpetic endotheliitis. In cases of FECD with corneal stromal swelling of 20% or CCT >640 μm, the risk of corneal decompensation after cataract surgery is significant.[5]
- *Decision making:* CT is an essential determinant for deciding upon the type of surgery, e.g., in cases of KC [to decide for corneal collagen crosslinking, ALTK, DALK or intracorneal ring segment (ICRS)]. Similarly, CCT is essential to decide whether to go for a triple procedure or only DSAEK in cases of FECD with cataract.

VIVA QUESTIONS

1. What is Artemis digital ultrasound?
Ans. Artemis is a VHF digital ultrasound that uses a 50 MHz VHF ultrasound transducer with immersion scanning technology. These waves are swept in an arc by a high-precision mechanism to acquire B-scans, which follow the surface contour of anterior or posterior segment structures. Artemis possesses an adjustment mechanism for the radius of curvature to enable maximum perpendicularity and enhanced signal to noise ratio. Digital signal processing significantly enhances the signal to noise ratio compared to analog processing by a factor of 3, thereby reducing the noise. Its axial resolution is 21 micron, and 3D-layered pachymetry (using multiple meridional scans) has precision <1.0 micron.

2. What is layered corneal pachymetry?
Ans. Layered corneal pachymetry is measuring the individual thickness of different components of the cornea like the epithelium, stroma, cornea, flap, and residual stromal bed. This can be done using Artemis VHF ultrasound, which has high repeatability.

3. What is normal corneal thickness?
Ans. Mean CCT is 515 microns (410–625 microns). In the paracentral region, the corneal thickness varies from 522 microns inferiorly to 574 microns superiorly while in the peripheral zone, thickness varies from 633 microns inferiorly to 673 microns superiorly.

4. Impact of CCT on IOP measurement.
Ans. Deviations from average CCT are a source of error in the measurement of IOP. In cases with corneal edema, IOP is often underestimated. Similarly, in patients with normal corneas, IOP is often overestimated in thicker corneas whereas, underestimated in thinner corneas. Ehler et al. have reported that the average error is 0.7 mm Hg per 10 microns of deviation from the mean 520 microns.

5. What are the modifications of corneal crosslinking in thin corneas?
Ans. These are transepithelial CXL, hypo-osmolar riboflavin-assisted CXL, lenticule-assisted CXL, bandage contact lens-assisted CXL (CA-CXL), customized epithelial debridement technique, and iontophoresis-assisted CXL (I-CXL).

REFERENCES

1. Salz JJ, Azen SP, Berstein J, Caroline P, Villasenor RA, Schanzlin DJ. Evaluation and comparison of sources of variability in the measurement of corneal thickness with ultrasonic and optical pachymeters. Ophthalmic Surg. 1983;14(9):750-4.
2. Marsich MW, Bullimore MA. The repeatability of corneal thickness measures. Cornea. 2000;19(6):792-5.
3. Kass MA, Heuer DK, Higginbotham EJ, Johnson CA, Keltner JL, Miller JP, et al. The Ocular Hypertension Treatment Study: a randomized trial determines that topical ocular hypotensive medication delays or prevents the onset of primary open-angle glaucoma. Arch Ophthalmol. 2002;120(6):701-13.
4. Lopes JE, Wilson RR, Alvim HS, Shields CL, Shields JA, Calhoun J, et al. Central corneal thickness in pediatric glaucoma. J Pediatr Ophthalmol Strabismus. 2007;44(2):112-7.
5. Seitzman GD, Gottsch JD, Stark WJ. Cataract surgery in patients with Fuchs' corneal dystrophy: expanding recommendations for cataract surgery without simultaneous keratoplasty. Ophthalmology. 2005;112(3):441-6.
6. Deshmukh R, Hafezi F, Kymionis GD, Kling S, Shah R, Padmanabhan P, et al. Current concepts in crosslinking thin corneas. Indian J Ophthalmol. 2019;67(1):8-15.

2.8 ORBSCAN

Alisha Kishore, Pranita Sahay, Ritu Nagpal

INTRODUCTION

A wide range of devices are available for performing corneal topography. Adequate knowledge is needed about the advanced computerized systems along with the normal ranges of various parameters for evaluation. "Orbscan" (Bausch and Lomb Inc, Rochester, NY, USA) and "Pentacam" (Oculus GmBH, Wetzlar, Germany) are the most common systems in use. Orbscan is scanning slit, noncontact tomography system.[1]

PRINCIPLE

Scanning Slit System

A series of slit-lamp beams are compiled across the cornea to create a profile of the cornea. The curvature of the anterior surface of the cornea along with posterior surface and anterior surface of the lens and iris can be assessed. The concept of "*slit scanning*" and "*triangulation*" is used to extrapolate the actual spatial location of multiple points on the surface.

The entire cornea is covered with 40 vertical slits, 20 from the right and 20 from the left **(Figs. 2.8.1A and B)**, normal to the surface at each point of acquisition capturing the backscattered light. Each of the slits has 240 points, so a total of 9,600 points and data for points in between is interpolated. The acquisition time is 1.5 seconds.

Orbscan II combines both a scanning slit and Placido disc system. Orbscan IIz is integrated with a Shack–Hartmann aberrometer in the Zyoptix workstation.

INTERPRETATION OF DIFFERENT MAPS

There are four different maps known as quad map. It includes the anterior elevation map, posterior elevation map, curvature map, and the pachymetry map.[2] The map should be read in the following order.

Details of the Patient

Check the *details* of the patient, which includes name, date, and eye. Check the scale range and step interval, which can be absolute or normalized.

Absolute scale (standardized): There is same dioptric power step on every map. The advantage is that it allows a direct comparison of two different maps and rapid pattern recognition of topographic maps is possible.

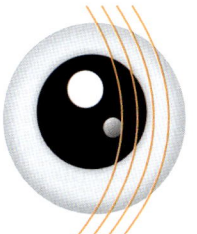 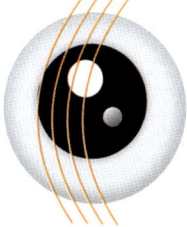 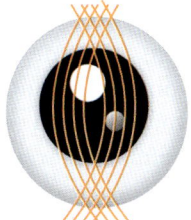

A 20 slits to the right and 20 slits to the left **B** Overlapping images (40 total)

Figs. 2.8.1A and B: Scanning slit imaging in Orbscan.

The disadvantage is that because of large steps it does not show subtle changes. It should be used for routine clinical analysis.

Normalized scale (relative): In this, the dioptric power step is based on the patient's cornea. The advantage is that since the dioptric power is smaller, therefore, it will show more detailed changes. However, the disadvantage is that the two maps cannot be compared directly. It is more sensitive and useful for research.[3]

Color scale: In all the four maps (i.e., power, curvature, elevation, and pachymetry) color scale is used using the concept of the BFS as explained below, where:
- *Red* is toward the higher side.
- *Blue* is toward the lower side for power, curvature, elevation, and pachymetry.
- *Green* denotes the reference surface.

Data Overview

Data overview includes **(Fig. 2.8.2):**[4]
- *Simulated keratometry (Sim K):* Maximum power of the surface along any axis and the power orthogonal to that axis (Sim K1 and Sim K2) in the central 3 mm area; the difference between Sim K1 and Sim K2 gives the value for astigmatism.
- *Irregularity index at 3 mm and 5 mm zone:* KC screening and HOAs
- *White-to-white diameter:* Measures the horizontal corneal diameter from limbus to limbus. The normal value is between 11 and 13 mm. It provides essential clinical information for diagnostic purposes (e.g., microcornea and relative anterior microphthalmos) as well as for surgical procedures:
  - Haptic size calculation in AC IOL and phakic IOL
  - Size of capsular tension ring (CTR)

```
Case, 10
N2 Y249984 M32
20.04.01 11:26:15
Screen

Sim K's: Astig:   –1.6°    @ 36°
Max:              44.9°    @ 126°
Min:              43.3°    @ 36°
3.0 MM Zone:  Irreg:       ± 1.9 D
Mean Pwr      44.0         ± 1.2 D
Astig Pwr     1.7          ± 1.4 D
Steep Axis    119          ± 38°
Flat Axis     16           ± 38°
5.0 MM Zone:  Irreg:       ± 2.5 D
Mean Pwr      43.0         ± 1.8 D
Astig Pwr     0.7          ± 1.7 D
Steep Axis    90           ± 44°
Flat Axis     21           ± 44°
White-to-white (mm): 11.3
Pupil diameter (mm): 4.5
Thinnest: 510 um @ (–0.7, –0.7)
ACD (Endo): 2.87 mm
Kappa: 6.75* @ 199.55*
Kappa intercept: –0.72, –0.04
```

Fig. 2.8.2: Data overview. (ACD: anterior chamber depth)

- IOL power calculation in cataract surgery using third-generation formulas
- *EK:* Corneal endothelial graft size should be 3 mm less than the smallest diameter of the recipient cornea as larger graft are more challenging to unfold
- *Corneal refractive surgeries:* Mesopic pupil diameter is closely related to horizontal white-to-white so more stringent approach in preoperative evaluation for ablation zone planning
- *Pupil diameter:* Photopic pupil size
- Thinnest point of the cornea
- *ACD:* From corneal endothelium to the lens; the normal value is between 2.5 and 3.5 mm.
- *Angle kappa:* It is the angle formed between the visual axis (line connecting fixation point with the fovea) and pupillary axis (the line that passes perpendicularly through the center of cornea and center of the pupil). It is crucial in refractive surgery

as proper centration is required for optimal results as a large angle kappa may lead to alignment errors during photoablation in laser refractive surgery as well lens decentration in intraocular refractive surgery. The decentration of ablation zones can lead to undercorrection and irregular astigmatism. Decentration of IOLs may cause photic phenomenon and decreased lens effectiveness. A positive angle kappa causes pseudoexotropia, and a negative angle kappa causes pseudoesotropia. The normal value is 5°.

Elevation Map

Elevation map uses the concept of the BFS **(Fig. 2.8.3)**.[5] In this a hypothetical sphere is calculated that resembles the shape of the cornea to be measured as close as possible and then compares the real surface to the hypothetical sphere. Areas above the surface of the sphere appear in warm colors (red) and areas below in cool colors (blue) in the color scale **(Fig. 2.8.4)**. Both anterior (top left of the quad map) and posterior elevation maps (top right of the quad map) are there, also known as the anterior and posterior float.

Anterior elevation map provides an overall diagnostic view of the cornea. Besides, it is important for CL trial.

Orbscan does not measure the posterior surface, but calculates it from the anterior surface and then produces a posterior elevation map. Relative elevation measures height difference in microns from a best fitting reference sphere. Posterior elevation map is vital for early diagnosis of cases of corneal ectasia. It is used for screening of cases of suspected or FFKC cases before any refractive surgery. A posterior float elevation of >40 µm is suggestive of posterior ectasia.

The normal cornea is *prolate*, which means that the meridional curvature decreases from the center to the periphery. It causes the normal cornea to rise centrally above the reference surface resulting in a central hill. Immediately surrounding the hill is an annular sea where cornea dips below the reference surface. In the far periphery, the prolate cornea again rises above the reference surface producing peripheral islands **(Fig. 2.8.5)**.

The regular astigmatic cornea is toric, which means that the meridional curvature has maximum and minimum directions, which are 90° apart. The steep part falls below the reference surface. The flat part rises above the reference surface resulting in central saddle topography **(Fig. 2.8.6)**.

The anterior elevation and posterior elevation map should be studied carefully and together to understand the shape of the cornea and look for any abnormal shape. Elevation patterns can be either "regular ridge, irregular ridge, incomplete ridge, island or unclassified". Among these patterns,

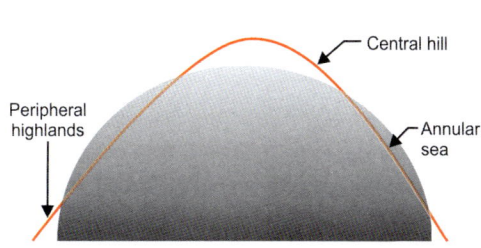

Fig. 2.8.3: The concept of best-fit sphere.

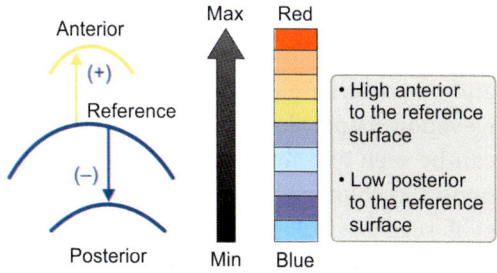

Fig. 2.8.4: The concept of color scale.

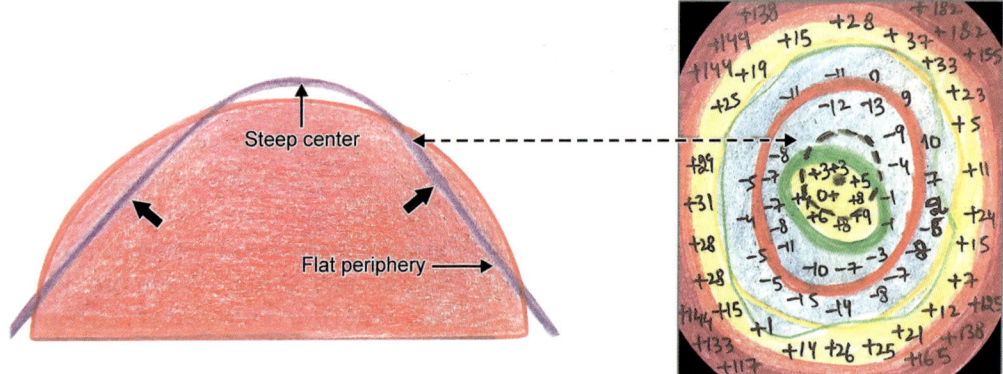

Fig. 2.8.5: Normal anterior elevation map of the cornea (prolate shape).

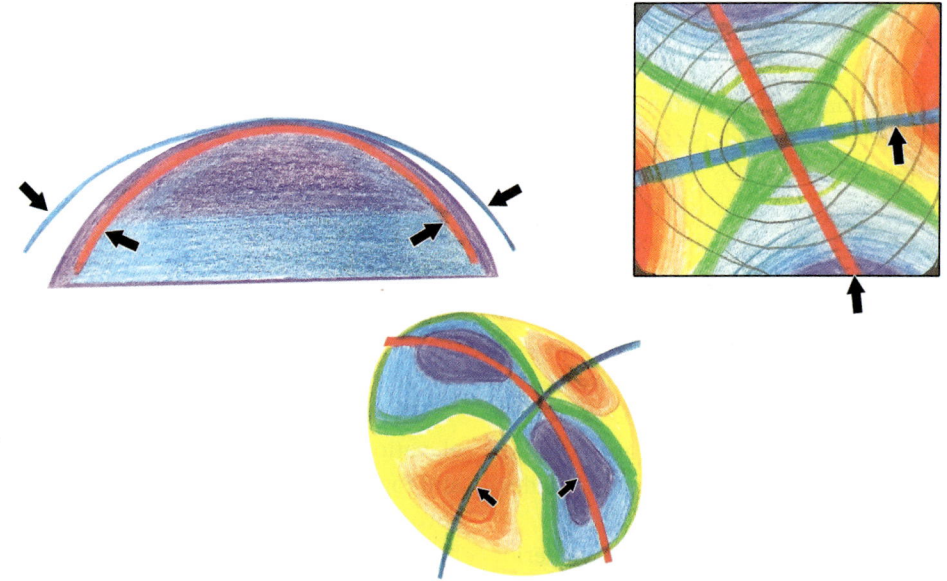

Fig. 2.8.6: Astigmatic elevation map.

the most commonly seen on anterior elevation map is incomplete ridge and island and on posterior elevation is island. On the elevation maps, abnormally elevated areas can be seen and further accuracy depends upon the color scale and step size. Tanabe et al. suggested 10 and 20 µm scale range on the anterior and posterior elevation maps, respectively. According to them, maps with three or more colors in the central zone (3 mm) were considered to be abnormal. Fam et al. reported that posterior elevation of 40 µm or more has a sensitivity of 57.7% and specificity of 89.9%. They have suggested anterior elevation ratio, which is anterior elevation/anterior BFS. If this is 0.5122 or less, it is more significant compared to posterior elevation alone.

Curvature Map

Axial keratometry map or sagittal curvature map, which is the bottom left map on the quad map **(Fig. 2.8.7)**; a fixed center of curvature is used for calculating the power at all points. The values are directly comparable to keratometry. The color scale as for the elevation map is also used for the keratometry map. This map is important for diagnosis and grading of ectatic corneal disorders such as KC and CL fitting.

Pachymetry Map

Pachymetry map is calculated by the distance between the anterior and posterior surface. It is the bottom right map on the quad map **(Fig. 2.8.7)**. The color scale is used to denote the pachymetry values.

It is important to note that the hot color represents increased thickness (or otherwise near normal thickness) while cool colors denote decreased corneal thickness (or otherwise ectatic cornea). These findings are just opposite to curvature map where hot colors denote ectatic cornea.

Pachymetry map is significant for treatment planning of cases of KC. Some of the crucial points to remember are as follows:

- ALTK—minimum thickness 400 microns
- DALK—increased risk of perforation if thinnest pachymetry is <250 microns
- Intacs—contraindicated if the thickness is <350 microns in mid-periphery
- LASIK—minimum thickness if >499 microns (for microkeratome, although it varies from surgeon to surgeon)

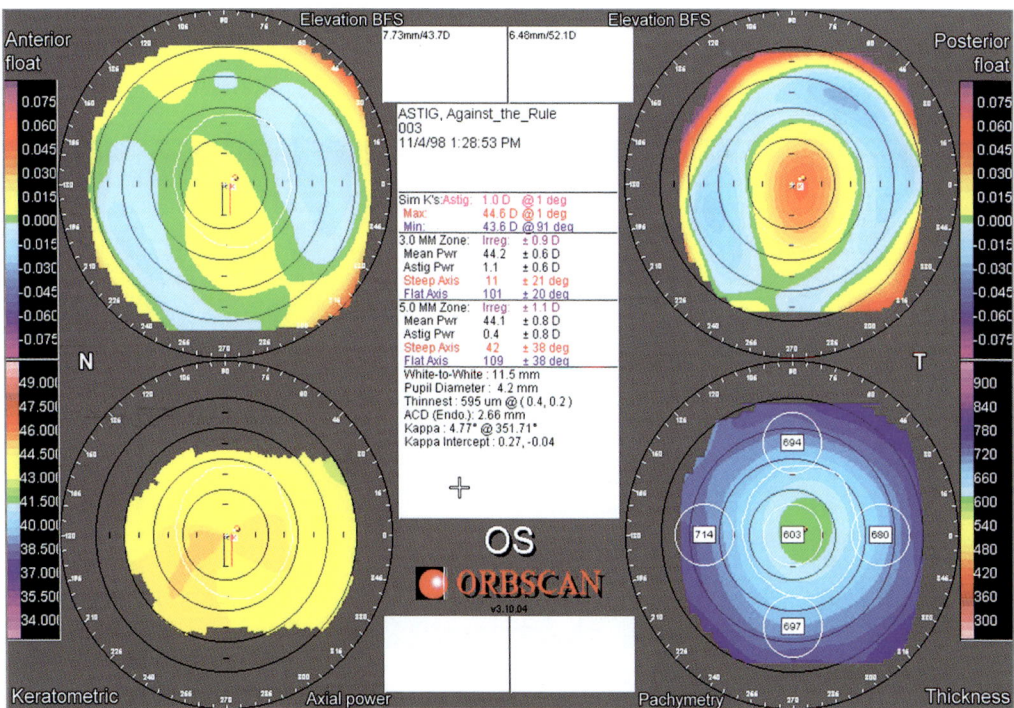

Fig. 2.8.7: Orbscan quad map (top left is the anterior elevation map, top right is the posterior elevation map, bottom left is the curvature map, and bottom right is the pachymetry map).

- Corneal corneal crosslinking—5% decrease in corneal thickness in 6 months suggests progression.

Compare

Always *compare* previous maps of the same eye and also compare with the other eye.

CLINICAL APPLICATIONS

Orbscan is used in the following conditions:
- *Detection of irregular corneal astigmatism in:*
  - KC
  - CL-induced corneal warpage
  - PMD
- *Preoperative evaluation:*
  - LASIK
  - AK
  - Intrastromal corneal ring segments (Intacs)
  - PKP
- *Applications to CL fitting:*
  - *Routine rigid gas permeable (RGP) fitting:* Preprogrammed protocol and simulated fitting.

HOW TO READ AN ORBSCAN MAP OF KERATOCONUS

Figure 2.8.8 shows is an Orbscan quad map of a patient X of the left eye with anterior elevation map at the top left and posterior elevation map at the top right side with color scale steps of 0.005 mm. The bottom left map is the axial curvature map with color steps of 1 D and the bottom right map is the pachymetry map with color steps of 20 µm. The Sim K maximum is 59.9 D at 149, and Sim K minimum is 54.7 D at 59° with astigmatism of 2.2 D at 149°. The irregularity index along the 3 and 5 mm zones is given. The white-to-white diameter is 11.9 mm with a pupil diameter of 3.9 mm. The thinnest pachymetry is 437 µm, which is located inferotemporally as shown by the plus mark position. The

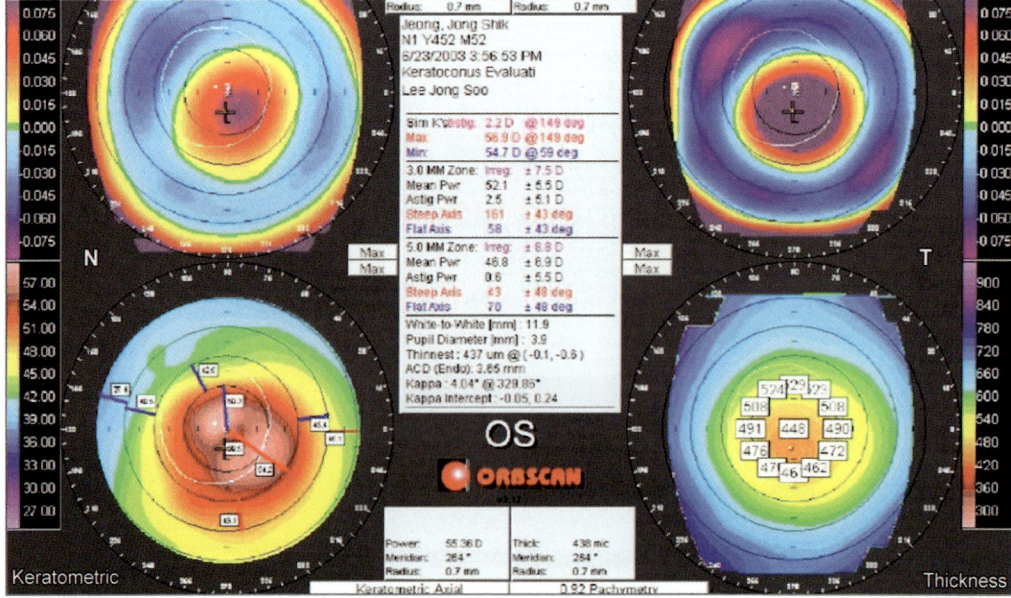

Fig. 2.8.8: Orbscan of a case of keratoconus.

ACD is 3.65 mm, and the angle kappa is 4.04° which is normal.

The anterior elevation map shows inferotemporal steeping as shown by the red color with corresponding steepening on the posterior elevation map. The axial curvature map shows asymmetric bowtie pattern with skewing of radial axis. The pachymetry map shows thinning along the corresponding area. On correlating it with the clinical picture this is most likely a case of KC. Also, it is important to compare with the fellow eye and any previous records if available for progression.

LIMITATIONS

- It lags in accuracy and reproducibility to the Scheimpflug devices and the readings were not interchangeable.
- It inaccurately identifies the postoperative posterior corneal surface and routinely locates the surface anteriorly.

VIVA QUESTIONS

1. Compare the different topography systems.

Ans. Different topography systems include:
- Placido disc (reflection)-based
- *Elevation-based:*
  - Slit scanning (Orbscan)
  - Scheimpflug imaging (Pentacam and Galilei)

Refer to **Tables 2.8.1** and **2.8.2** for details.

2. Describe the importance of white-to-white diameter in corneal surgery.

Ans. Refer to text.

3. Describe the importance of angle kappa.

Ans. Refer to text.

4. State the various cutoffs for diagnosis of KC in Orbscan.

Ans. Refer to **Table 2.8.3**.

5. What is the irregularity index and mention its clinical importance?

Ans. Irregularity index is proportional to the SD of the curvature of the surface. Orbscan calculates this index in the 3 mm and the 5 mm zone. Any further improvement of vision that cannot be corrected with refraction can be correlated with this index. The higher the value, the more the irregular astigmatism or HOA. The index is considered to be significant and suggestive of KC if it is >1.5 D in the central 3 mm zone or more than 2–3 D in the 5 mm zone. However, this should always be correlated clinically.

6. Describe the advantages of Orbscan pachymetry over ultrasonic pachymeter.

Ans. Advantages of Orbscan include:
- *Noncontact method:*
  - Less chance of infection
  - Error due to the eccentricity of the probe is minimized
- Measurement of several parts of the cornea

TABLE 2.8.1: Difference between Placido and slit scanning technologies.

	Placido-based	*Slit scanning-based*
Number of images scanned	One image, one surface	Multiple images, multiple surfaces
Mechanism	Angle-dependent specular reflection	Omni direction diffuse backscatter
Measures	Measures slope (as a function of distance between mires)	Measures triangular elevation
Data on the central cornea	Missed	Present
Accuracy	Able to acquire limited data points so less accurate	More number of data points and hence more accurate

TABLE 2.8.2: Difference between Pentacam and Orbscan.

	Pentacam	Orbscan
Principle	Scheimpflug	Scanning slit and Placido disc system
Number of measured data points per scan	>25,000	9,600
Effect of eye movement	Maintains the central point (thinnest point) of each meridian; thus can reregister these central points and eliminate eye movement	Takes a vertical image separate slice, which has no common point; thus cannot reregister for any eye movement
Accuracy	10 times more accurate	Less accurate
Lens details	Measures anterior and posterior lens shape, lens thickness, and lens densitometry	Measures only anterior lens shape

TABLE 2.8.3: Signs suggestive of early keratoconus on Orbscan.

Parameter	Criteria
Pachymetry	Thinnest point <470 µm
	A difference of >100 µm from the thinnest point to the values of the 7 mm optic zone implies a steep gradient of thinning from mid-periphery to the thinnest point
	Thinnest point on cornea should correspond with the highest point of elevation on the posterior corneal surface
Posterior elevation map	Posterior high point >50 µm above the best-fit sphere
	Best-fit sphere with a power >55 D on the posterior profile
	Roush criteria: Relative difference >100 µm between the highest and lowest point on the posterior elevation map
Power map	Keratometric mean power map >46 D
	Bow tie pattern or lazy C on the axial power map is suspect when astigmatism shifts >20° from a straight line
	Change within the central 3 mm optic zone of the cornea >3 D from superior to inferior can be correlated to the presence of vertical coma (most common aberration in keratoconus)
Composite integrated information	Highest point on the posterior elevation coincides with the highest point on the anterior elevation, the thinnest point on pachymetry, and point of steepest curvature on the power map
	Efkarpides criteria: Ratio of the radii of anterior and posterior best-fit sphere of the cornea should be >1.21. Between 1.23 and 1.27 would be suspect and >1.27 is diagnostic
	Astigmatic discrepancy of >1.5 D in 3 mm zone and discrepancy >2 D in the 5 mm zone

- Simultaneous analysis of anterior and posterior corneal surfaces and pachymetry
- Less technician dependent
- Repeatability

7. Describe the importance of BFS.
Ans. The posterior surface of the cornea is first to be involved in corneal ectasia. A value of 51 D or more is suggestive of primary posterior corneal elevation and 55 D or more for FFKC. The ratio of anterior to posterior BFS is also important. If it is >1.27, it is a contraindication for refractive surgery. Below 1.21 is acceptable and between 1.21 and 1.27 is considered as KC suspect.

REFERENCES

1. Marinez CE, Klyce SD. Keratometry and Topography. In: Krachmer (Ed). Cornea: Fundamentals, Diagnosis and Management, 3rd edition. Amsterdam: Mosby Elsevier; 2011. pp. 161-75.
2. DOS Times. (2014). Topography for the Refractive Surgeon. [online] Available from http://dos-times.org/pulsar9088/20140424040901240.pdf [Last accessed October, 2024].
3. Roberts C. Corneal topography: A review of terms and concepts. J Cataract Refract Surg. 1996;22(5):624-9.
4. Manudhane A, Arora R, Goyal JL, Jain P, Gaurav Goyal. (2013). Corneal Topography. [online] Available from http://dos-times.org/pulsar9088/20131113064559307.pdf [Last accessed October, 2024].
5. Dharwadkar S, Nayak BK. Corneal topography and tomography. J Clin Ophthalmol Res. 2015;3:45-62.

2.9 CORNEAL BIOMECHANICS

Ritu Nagpal, Chandradevi Shanmugam

INTRODUCTION

Corneal biomechanics refers to the study of the mechanical behavior of the corneal tissue, including its ability to maintain shape, respond to IOP, and recover from trauma or surgical intervention. These biomechanical properties are central to understanding disease progression, such as in KC, as well as optimizing refractive surgeries like LASIK and corneal crosslinking.

In this chapter, we will explore the structural composition of the cornea, its mechanical properties, the impact of diseases and surgical procedures on corneal biomechanics, and the latest innovations in measuring and analyzing these properties.

ANATOMY OF THE CORNEA: STRUCTURAL BASIS FOR BIOMECHANICS

The cornea consists of five primary layers, besides the proposed pre-Descemet layer, each contributing to its overall biomechanical integrity. The stroma comprising over 90% of corneal thickness, is composed of collagen fibers and proteoglycans arranged in a highly organized, lamellar structure. This organization is key to the cornea's mechanical strength and transparency.

The stroma's layered structure is the primary determinant of corneal biomechanics. The arrangement of collagen fibrils in parallel lamellae gives the cornea both tensile strength and elasticity, allowing it to withstand IOP while maintaining its shape.

BIOMECHANICAL PROPERTIES OF THE CORNEA

Elasticity and Stiffness

The cornea exhibits both elastic and viscoelastic properties. Its ability to return to its original shape after deformation is crucial for maintaining optical clarity and proper focus. Elasticity is largely dependent on the collagen fiber network in the stroma. Corneal stiffness, quantified by Young's modulus, describes the cornea's resistance to deformation under stress. A stiffer cornea is less likely to undergo significant shape changes, which is important for maintaining visual acuity.

Viscoelasticity

Unlike purely elastic materials, the cornea demonstrates viscoelasticity, meaning its deformation response to applied stress involves both immediate (elastic) and time-dependent (viscous) components. Viscoelasticity helps the cornea dissipate mechanical energy from external forces, such as rubbing or trauma, without permanent damage.

Hysteresis

Corneal hysteresis is a measure of the cornea's ability to absorb and dissipate energy. It reflects the difference between the deformation of the cornea during loading and unloading cycles, offering insights into its viscoelastic properties. Low corneal hysteresis is often associated with a greater risk of ectatic diseases like KC, as well as increased susceptibility to glaucoma.

MEASURING CORNEAL BIOMECHANICS

Advances in technology have enabled the measurement of corneal biomechanical properties in vivo. Key devices include the following.

Ocular Response Analyzer

The ORA measures corneal hysteresis and corneal resistance factor (CRF) by applying a rapid air puff to the cornea and analyzing the resultant deformation. It offers valuable data for glaucoma risk assessment, as well as for screening patients before refractive surgery.

Corvis ST

The Corvis ST uses a high-speed Scheimpflug camera to visualize the dynamic response of the cornea to an air puff. It provides information on corneal stiffness, deformation amplitude, and other biomechanical parameters. This technology is particularly useful for diagnosing ectatic diseases and planning surgical interventions.

Brillouin Microscopy

Brillouin microscopy emerging noncontact technique uses light-scattering to map the biomechanical properties of the cornea at a microscopic level. It offers the potential to detect early changes in corneal biomechanics, which may precede clinical signs of disease.

CORNEAL BIOMECHANICS IN HEALTH AND DISEASE

Keratoconus

Keratoconus is characterized by progressive thinning and weakening of the corneal structure, leading to irregular astigmatism and visual impairment. Biomechanically, the cornea becomes less stiff and more susceptible to deformation. Early detection of biomechanical changes can facilitate timely intervention with treatments like corneal crosslinking (CXL), which aims to stiffen the cornea and halt disease progression.

Post-Refractive Surgery Biomechanics

Refractive surgeries like LASIK, PRK, and SMILE reshape the cornea to correct refractive errors. However, these procedures also alter the biomechanical properties of the cornea, potentially increasing the risk of postoperative complications such as ectasia. Surgeons must carefully evaluate corneal thickness, shape, and biomechanical strength before performing these procedures to minimize risks.

Glaucoma

Corneal biomechanics also play a role in glaucoma management. Low corneal hysteresis is linked with a higher susceptibility to glaucoma, independent of IOP. Incorporating corneal biomechanical assessments into glaucoma diagnostics may help in identifying patients at higher risk and personalizing treatment plans.

THERAPEUTIC IMPLICATIONS OF CORNEAL BIOMECHANICS

Corneal Crosslinking

Corneal cross-linking is a widely used treatment for KC and other ectatic disorders. By applying riboflavin and UV light to the cornea, CXL induces the formation of new collagen cross-links, increasing corneal stiffness and stabilizing the disease. Understanding the biomechanical impact of CXL has allowed for refinements in the technique, such as accelerated protocols and customized treatments.

Impact on Intraocular Lens and Refractive Surgery Outcomes

Intraocular lenses and corneal refractive surgeries rely on accurate corneal measurements to optimize visual outcomes. A deeper understanding of corneal biomechanics has led to improvements in surgical planning and IOL power calculations, especially in patients with biomechanically compromised corneas due to previous surgeries or diseases.

Corvis ST

The *Corvis ST* is an advanced diagnostic tool designed to measure corneal biomechanical properties in vivo, revolutionizing the way we assess the cornea's response to mechanical stress. Utilizing high-speed Scheimpflug imaging and air-puff applanation technology, the Corvis ST provides critical insights into corneal stiffness, elasticity, and deformation dynamics.

Principles of Corvis ST Technology

The Corvis ST operates using two core components:

1. *Air-puff induced corneal deformation:* The device releases a controlled puff of air directed at the cornea. The force of this air causes the cornea to deform, flatten, and then return to its natural shape.
2. *Scheimpflug imaging:* During this deformation process, a high-speed Scheimpflug camera captures thousands of images per second (up to 4,300 frames/sec), documenting the entire dynamic response of the cornea to the air puff.

These images are then analyzed to extract important biomechanical parameters, including the amplitude of deformation, corneal applanation times, and corneal velocity during different phases of the air puff.

Key Parameters Measured by Corvis ST

The Corvis ST provides a range of data points that describe the mechanical response of the cornea. Key parameters include:

- *Deformation amplitude:* Deformation amplitude refers to the maximum amount of deformation (or "sinking") that the cornea experiences under the force of the air puff. A higher deformation amplitude indicates a more flexible or softer cornea, while a lower amplitude suggests a stiffer cornea. This parameter is vital in diagnosing ectatic conditions, such as KC, where the cornea becomes weaker and more prone to deformation.
- *Applanation times (A1 and A2):* Applanation refers to the moment when the cornea is flattened by the air puff. The Corvis ST measures two applanation events:
  - *A1 time:* The time taken for the cornea to reach its first flattening point
  - *A2 time:* The time taken for the cornea to return to its second flattening point during the recovery phase after maximum deformation

These applanation times provide insights into corneal stiffness. A stiffer cornea will have shorter applanation times, while a softer cornea will take longer to return to its normal shape.

- *Velocity of corneal deformation:* The velocity at which the cornea moves during the deformation and recovery phases is another important biomechanical marker. This data helps quantify the corneal tissue's resilience to external forces and its ability to return to baseline shape after mechanical stress.
- *Peak distance and deflection length:* The Corvis ST also measures the distance between the two highest points of corneal deflection (peak distance) and the total length of the deflected cornea. These parameters give insight into the distribution of stress and strain across the corneal tissue, which can help differentiate between normal and pathological corneas.
- *Stiffness parameter at first applanation (SP-A1):* SP-A1 is a parameter specifically developed to quantify corneal stiffness based on the speed of corneal deformation during the first applanation event. It is an essential tool for identifying patients with biomechanically weakened corneas, such as those with KC.
- *Integrated radius (IR):* The IR is a measure of the curvature of the cornea during its recovery phase. A stiffer cornea will have a higher radius of curvature, indicating a more rigid and less deformable tissue structure.

Clinical Applications of Corvis ST

The Corvis ST has become a crucial tool in several clinical areas, including corneal disease diagnosis, refractive surgery planning, and glaucoma risk assessment. Its ability to quantify corneal biomechanical properties has greatly improved decision-making in these fields.

- *Diagnosis and monitoring of KC:* KC is a progressive corneal disorder characterized by thinning and weakening of the corneal tissue, leading to irregular astigmatism and visual impairment. The Corvis ST's ability to detect subtle biomechanical changes in the cornea makes it a useful tool for early diagnosis and monitoring of KC.

Several specific biomechanical parameters from the Corvis ST are particularly useful for diagnosing KC:

Deformation amplitude: In KC, the cornea is softer and weaker, so it deforms more than a healthy cornea. A higher deformation amplitude is a hallmark of KC.

Applanation times (A1 and A2):
- *A1 time:* In KC, the cornea is more flexible, so this occurs later than in normal eyes.

- *A2 time:* Due to the weaker structural integrity in KC, this second applanation occurs earlier than in a healthy cornea.

Stiffness parameter at first applanation (SP-A1): In KC, the corneal stiffness is significantly reduced, leading to lower SP-A1 values. This parameter is particularly useful in distinguishing KC from healthy or borderline cases.

Deflection length: In KC, this deflection is more pronounced due to the weakened biomechanical properties of the cornea, leading to longer deflection lengths.

Ambrósio's relational thickness (ARTh): The ARTh is a calculated parameter that relates corneal thickness to biomechanical deformation. In KC, where the cornea is thinner and less stable, the ARTh value is lower, signaling an abnormal biomechanical response.

Biomechanical Index for Keratoconus [Corvis Biomechanical Index (CBI)]: One of the most significant innovations in the use of Corvis ST for KC diagnosis is the *CBI*. The CBI is a composite score that combines various biomechanical parameters, such as deformation amplitude, SP-A1, and applanation times, to create an objective risk profile for KC.

CBI score interpretation:
- A *CBI score of 0* typically indicates normal corneal biomechanics.
- A *CBI score close to 1* suggests a high likelihood of KC or biomechanical instability.

The CBI helps clinicians differentiate between healthy eyes, subclinical KC (where corneal shape may appear normal but biomechanical weakness exists), and advanced KC **(Fig. 2.9.1)**.
- *Diagnosis of subclinical (forme fruste) KC:* Subclinical KC, also known as forme fruste keratoconus, represents the earliest stage of the disease, often with no obvious topographical abnormalities. Corneal topography alone may miss these cases, but the Corvis ST's biomechanical measurements provide an early indication of biomechanical instability.

In these cases, a combination of increased deformation amplitude, abnormal applanation times, and a higher CBI score can suggest early KC, even if traditional imaging techniques show no signs of corneal thinning or distortion.
- *Early detection:* Biomechanical changes often occur before visible structural abnormalities in the cornea. The Corvis ST can detect early signs of KC by measuring increased deformation amplitudes, delayed applanation times, and reduced corneal stiffness, even when traditional topography shows a normal corneal surface.
- *Monitoring progression:* By periodically measuring corneal biomechanics, the Corvis ST can track disease progression, helping clinicians determine when interventions such as corneal collage crosslinking (CXL) may be necessary to halt further weakening.
- *Refractive surgery screening:* Refractive surgeries, such as LASIK, PRK, and SMILE, alter the corneal structure to correct visual errors. However, performing these surgeries on corneas with biomechanical instability can lead to postoperative complications, including corneal ectasia (a progressive thinning of the cornea after surgery). The Corvis ST is highly effective in identifying patients who may be at risk for ectasia by assessing corneal biomechanical strength.
- *Preoperative screening:* The Corvis ST provides critical data on corneal stiffness and deformation amplitude, allowing

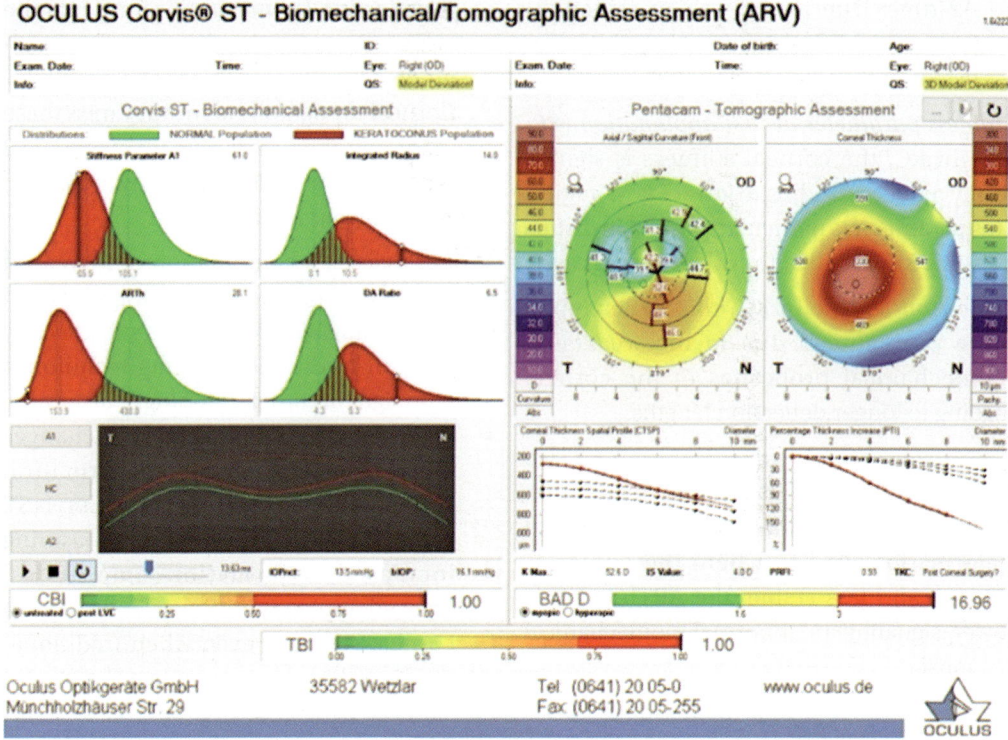

Fig. 2.9.1: Corvis-ST image of a patient with advanced keratoconus depicting altered Corvis Biomechanical Index (CBI) score.

surgeons to identify eyes with weaker biomechanical properties, which may disqualify them from refractive surgery.
- *Postoperative monitoring:* Postsurgery, the Corvis ST can monitor the biomechanical changes induced by the procedure, helping clinicians ensure that the cornea remains stable and does not develop ectasia.
- *Corneal crosslinking evaluation:* CXL is a treatment for KC that strengthens the cornea by increasing collagen cross-links in the stroma. The Corvis ST can be used to evaluate the biomechanical effects of CXL both before and after treatment.
- *Preoperative assessment:* By measuring the baseline biomechanical properties of the cornea, the Corvis ST helps determine the severity of the disease and the need for CXL.
- *Postoperative evaluation:* After CXL, the Corvis ST can measure the increase in corneal stiffness, providing objective evidence that the procedure has successfully stabilized the cornea.
- *Glaucoma risk assessment:* Recent studies have demonstrated a relationship between corneal biomechanics and glaucoma. Patients with low corneal hysteresis or reduced corneal stiffness are more prone to glaucomatous optic nerve damage, independent of IOP. The Corvis ST, in combination with other biomechanical tools, is increasingly used to assess glaucoma risk.
- *Glaucoma susceptibility:* The Corvis ST can identify biomechanically weaker

corneas, which may indicate a higher risk of developing glaucoma. This allows clinicians to adjust monitoring and treatment strategies, even in patients with normal IOP.
- *IOP compensation:* The Corvis ST measures IOP while taking into account the biomechanical properties of the cornea, offering a more accurate assessment of true IOP levels. This is particularly important for glaucoma patients with abnormal corneal biomechanics, where traditional tonometry may underestimate IOP.

Advantages of Corvis ST over traditional methods: The Corvis ST offers several advantages over traditional methods of assessing corneal biomechanics, such as tonometry or pachymetry:
- *Dynamic measurements:* Unlike static devices, the Corvis ST captures the dynamic behavior of the cornea during deformation, providing a more comprehensive view of its biomechanical properties.
- *In vivo, noninvasive assessment:* The Corvis ST allows for noninvasive, real-time measurement of corneal biomechanics in a clinical setting, without requiring any contact with the cornea beyond the air puff.
- *Comprehensive biomechanical profile:* The device provides a detailed biomechanical profile of the cornea, including stiffness, elasticity, and viscoelastic properties, which are invaluable for both diagnostic and surgical purposes.

Limitations and considerations: Despite its many advantages, there are some limitations to the Corvis ST:
- *Sensitivity to external factors:* Factors such as corneal hydration, patient cooperation, and ocular surface irregularities may influence the accuracy of the Corvis ST measurements.
- *Interpretation of data:* While the Corvis ST provides a wealth of data, proper interpretation requires expertise in biomechanics and corneal diseases. It is essential to integrate Corvis ST data with other clinical findings to make informed decisions.

FUTURE DIRECTIONS IN CORNEAL BIOMECHANICS

The field of corneal biomechanics is rapidly evolving. Advanced imaging techniques, such as Brillouin microscopy and optical coherence elastography, are poised to revolutionize our understanding of corneal tissue mechanics. Additionally, the integration of artificial intelligence in biomechanical analysis holds the promise of more precise and predictive models for disease diagnosis and treatment planning.

Research is also exploring the use of synthetic or bioengineered materials to replace or reinforce damaged corneal tissue, offering potential new treatment avenues for corneal ectasia and trauma.

CONCLUSION

Corneal biomechanics is an essential aspect of understanding the function, health, and diseases of the eye. By analyzing how the cornea responds to mechanical forces, we can better diagnose, manage, and treat a wide range of conditions, from KC to glaucoma. The continued advancement of biomechanical measurement technologies will further enhance our ability to provide tailored treatments that improve patient outcomes.

2.10 APPLIANCES AND INSTRUMENTS IN CORNEA

Pranita Sahay, Mohamed Ibrahime Asif, Devesh Kumawat, Namrata Sharma

KERATOPLASTY

Globe Fixation Rings

Flieringa Ring (Fig. 2.10.1)

Flieringa ring is made of stainless steel and is useful for maintaining the architecture of the globe once the host corneal button has been removed. They are available in 11 sizes from 12 to 22 mm.

Uses:
- Vitrectomized eyes
- Pediatric cases, as the eyeball has a tendency to collapse in these cases after trephination due to low sclera rigidity
- Aphakic eyes
- Ocular hypotony
- PKP combined with cataract surgery (optical triple procedure)

Disadvantages:
- It can distort the shape of the eyeball and causes an oval cut during trephination and subsequent high astigmatism.
- Very rarely, it can result in sclera perforation while passing sutures to fixate the ring.
- Subconjunctival hematoma

McNeill–Goldman Ring (Fig. 2.10.2)

McNeill–Goldman ring provides support at four strategically placed sutures. The ring features medial and temporal openings for greater access to the surgical field and two lid retractors to prevent eyelid closure by the patient. It is available in three sizes—small, medium, and large. The adult size has an inner diameter of 17 mm and outer diameter of 24 mm. It is made of stainless steel.

Corneal Marking Instruments

Radial keratotomy (RK) marker **(Fig. 2.10.3)**, Vajpayee corneal marker (20 radial arms), and Anis corneal marker (8 radial arms) are the various instruments that guide the optimal placement of sutures in keratoplasty.

Corneal Trephines

Different types of trephines are discussed in the following text.

Conventional Circular Cutting Trephines
- *Handheld* **(Fig. 2.10.4)**:
  - Ranging from 3 to 17 mm diameter

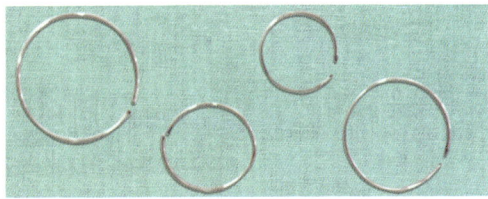

Fig. 2.10.1: Flieringa ring.

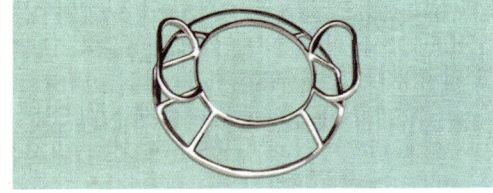

Fig. 2.10.2: McNeill–Goldman ring.

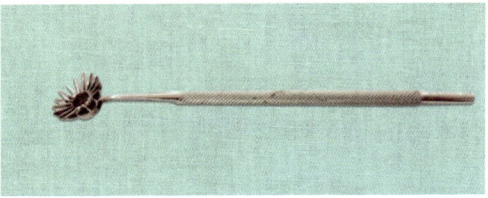

Fig. 2.10.3: Radial keratotomy (RK) marker.

- In some trephines, there is a central obturator, which can be adjusted to select the depth of the corneal cut and hence an inadvertent entry into the AC. However, the obturator obscures the view of central cornea, which may result in inaccurate centration during the trephination of the recipient's cornea.
- Examples of handheld trephines with obturator are the Castroviejo trephine **(Fig. 2.10.5)** and the Grieshaber–Franceschetti trephine.
- *Mechanized:* The disadvantages associated with motor driven trephines include corkscrew edge effect in the corneal stroma.
- *Suction-fixation type:* It is devised to obtain a perpendicular cut in the recipient cornea. These trephine systems essentially consist of an outer corneal suction ring for fixation and an inner circular cutting blade.
    - Hessburg–Barron trephine **(Fig. 2.10.6)** has a crosshair device for improved centration and an outer ring of corneal marks at equal intervals to assist in suture placement. It is available in diameters 6.0–9.0 in 0.5 mm increments as well as diameter of 7.75 mm. For each spoke (90°) turned, the blade is lowered or raised approximately 0.06 mm.
    - Barron vacuum punch **(Fig. 2.10.7)** features a solid stainless steel blade, which is permanently mounted in nylon housing. Four steel guide posts align with four corresponding holes in the cutting block base, automatically centering the blade over the donor cornea.
- *Special-purpose type: The Olson calibrated cornea trephine system* used to trephinate both the donor and recipient corneas. The system consists of an AC maintainer, reusable blade holder (with micrometer setting), and suction ring. One revolution of the micrometer is equivalent to 500 microns.
    - *Skin biopsy punches*: The skin biopsy punches, which have been used in dermatological practice, are especially useful in harvesting of small patch

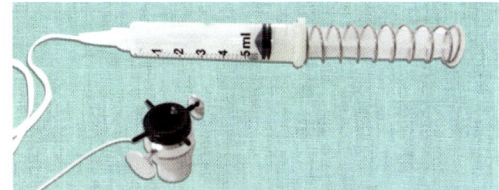

Fig. 2.10.6: Hessburg–Barron trephine.

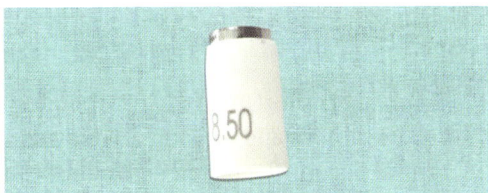

Fig. 2.10.4: Handheld.

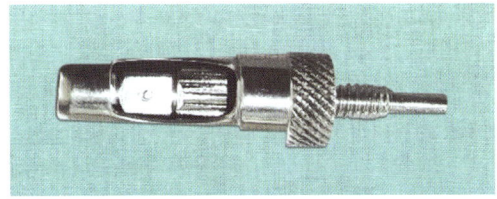

Fig. 2.10.5: Castroviejo trephine.

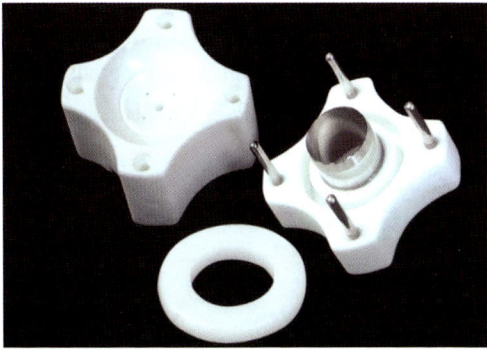

Fig. 2.10.7: Barron vacuum punch.

grafts used for tectonic purposes in cases of impending/frank perforation.

Single-Point Cutting Trephines

The single point cutter trephines were designed to decrease corneal torsion, e.g., *Leiberman single point cutter*.

Combination Trephines

Hanna trephine system has got a circular razor-cutting blade and incorporates many of the salient features of single point cutting trephines.

Noncontact Trephines (Lasers)

Laser noncontact trephination eliminates corneal topography distortion provides the visualization of the entire cornea and enhances centration.

Graft Holder (Paton Spatula) (Fig. 2.10.8)

The graft is placed over viscoelastic and is kept covered till the recipient dissection is complete.

Cutting Blocks

The various cutting blocks available for corneal grafting are Paraffin block, Teflon block **(Fig. 2.10.9)**, and Polycarbonate and nylon blocks.

- *The Kaufmann corneal cutting block*: This is the simplest design which consists of a Teflon block with metal cover.
- *The Brightbill polytef cutting block*: This modern, compound curved block approximates the central, midperipheral, and peripheral curvature of donor. The Brightbill polytef cutting block uses three wells, each with a different radius of curvature and diameter. Two concentric inlays of colored polytef are present. The outer black polytef zone has a chord length of 12.5 mm and corresponds to the limbus and a second white polytef inlay with an 8 mm chord length corresponds to the central zone of the donor cornea. Slippage of the moist donor cornea at the time of cutting can cause oval graft. This can be prevented by repeated drying of the well in which the donor is placed or by using a thin, slightly moistened layer of cotton in the well.

Corneal Endothelial Punches

To cut a donor button from endothelial side corneal punches are also available which use disposable trephine blades. The advantage of corneal punch is that they yield sharp vertical cuts without beveling.

- *Cottingham corneal punch:* It is a metal punch with a universal style handle. Additionally, it also has two replaceable base plugs.
- *Troutman corneal punch:* It incorporates a centered block and a piston carrier with a central piston. The piston accommodates blades of 7–9 mm. This relies on the surgeon's thumb to incise the cornea.

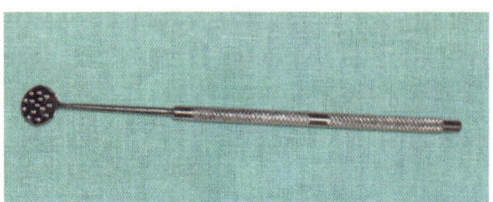

Fig. 2.10.8: Graft holder (Paton Spatula).

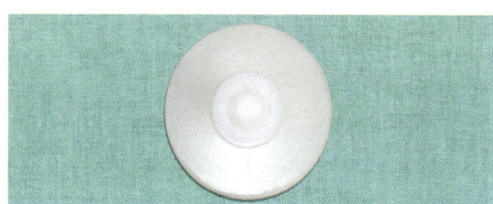

Fig. 2.10.9: Teflon block.

- *Iowa PK press corneal punch:* It incorporates a spring-loaded piston with an expandable edge to accommodate 6–9.5 mm trephines to harvest various sizes the donor graft from the endothelial side. It has a unique two color cutting block, which aids in centration of the donor tissue. The recessed base assumes that the block is held centrally under the trephine block.
- *Lieberman gravity-action punch:* It is a guillotine-style punch with a heavy head, which uses the force of gravity rather than the surgeon's hand to punch the cornea.
- *Rothman–Gilbard corneal punch:* It uses a piston which is not spring loaded. The suction block has eight evenly spaced suction holes which anchor the corneal button firmly so that there is minimal movement during trephination. The button has eight precisely placed marks and can be sutured into the host bed by suturing every mark on the button with the marks placed on the host bed.

There are four trephine assemblies, which use artificial anterior chamber (AAC). These include *Krumeich, Hanna, Olson,* and *Lieberman* systems. This involves cutting the donor corneas from the epithelial side rather than the endothelial side. Pressure in the AAC is adjusted to the IOP with the help of attachments of the infusion tubing.

Cutting Instruments

Blade Breaker (Fig. 2.10.10)

A disposable razor blade is broken and mounted on the tip of a metallic pencil handle. This is one of the best instruments available for cutting tissues in straight or curved lines. Blade breaker is used to enter

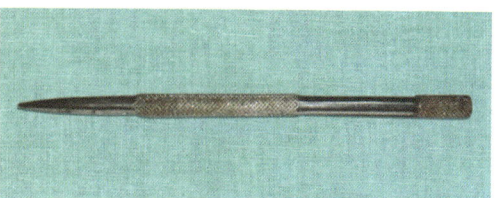

Fig. 2.10.10: Blade breaker.

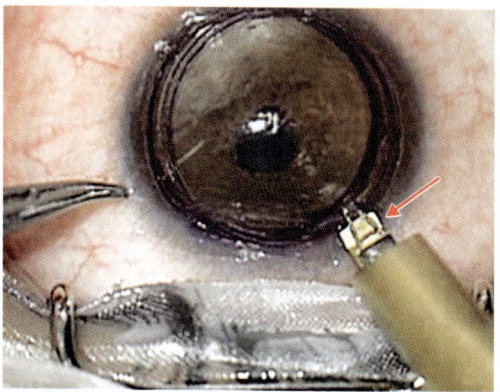

Fig. 2.10.11: Diamond knife.

the AC in a controlled manner after a deep cut has been created in the recipient's cornea by a trephine. Blunt side of the blade can sometimes be used for blunt dissection of adherent iris.

Diamond Knife (Fig. 2.10.11)

Diamond knife is the sharpest cutting instrument and is available in various sizes and shapes. It is the most durable instrument and useful for stab incisions as well as to complete the trephine cuts.

Corneal Scissors (Fig. 2.10.12)

Ideally, all corneal scissors should have an immobile lower blade. Troutman microscissor is the prototype, which has blades 5 mm in length and is curved on a radius of 5 mm. The lower handle, which controls the upper blade, has a flexible spring. This is a very light and fine scissors and mainly

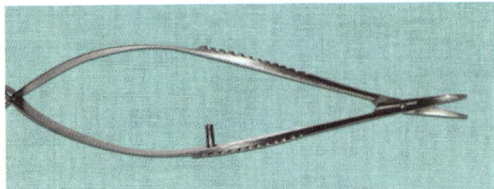

Fig. 2.10.12: Corneal scissors.

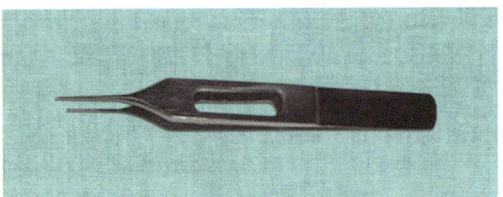

Fig. 2.10.14: Pierse–Hoskins forceps.

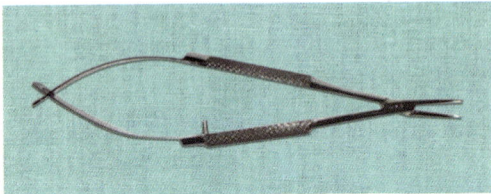

Fig. 2.10.13: Barraquer's curved needle holder.

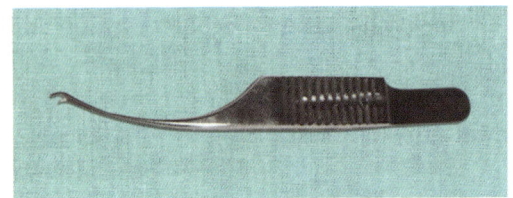

Fig. 2.10.15: Colibri forceps.

used to complete the cutting of the trephine incision. The blades should be kept vertical and must be curved to follow the curvature of the trephine, while cutting the host cornea. It is often used to remove the irregular tags from the wound margin. Corneal scissors are used to complete the trephination of the host cornea after creation of the circular cut following AC entry. Curved Vannas scissors can also be used for the same.

Holding Instruments

Needle holders used in ophthalmic microsurgery consists of two handles, which are supported between index finger and thumb. Needle holder, which is lightweight, with nonslip curved handle and curved jaws is preferred for PK. The curvature of the jaw varies from a uniform smooth to a hockey stick shape. The jaws should be atraumatic to the steel needles, but the grip should be firm. Barraquer's curved needle holder (**Fig. 2.10.13**) is an example.

Grasping Instruments

Varieties of forceps are used for PK. However, they can be broadly classified into toothed, nontoothed, or forceps used for special purposes.

Toothed Forceps

- *Pierse–Hoskins forceps* (**Fig. 2.10.14**): It is a fine toothed tissue-holding forceps used to hold the corneal tissue firmly. Pierse–Hoskin's forceps is the most frequently used tissue-holding forceps in corneal grafting surgery. It is a 2 × 1 fine toothed lightweight instrument and extensively used for suture tying.
- *Colibri forceps* (**Fig. 2.10.15**): This is another example of tissue holding forceps. The advantage of this instrument is that it is less likely to damage surrounding tissues due to its curved shape.

Nontoothed Forceps

The nontoothed forceps have flat edges that help in holding or picking up structures like 10-0 nylon suture. McPherson forceps (**Fig. 2.10.16**) is the prototype of this variety. It can be used for suture tying and for burying the suture knots.

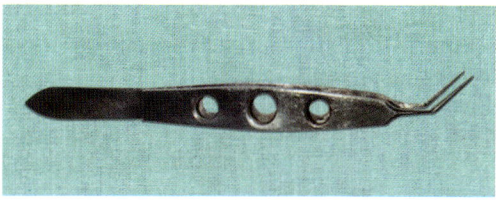

Fig. 2.10.16: McPherson forceps.

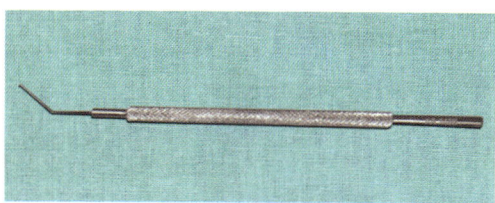

Fig. 2.10.19: Sinskey.

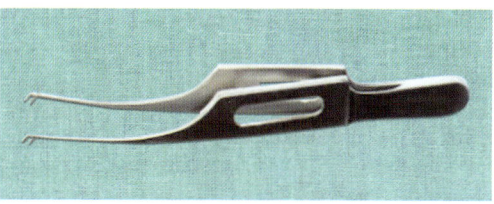

Fig. 2.10.17: Polack double corneal forceps.

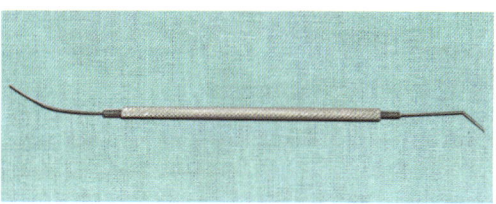

Fig. 2.10.18: Double-ended iris repositer.

iris and lens capsule, dissection of iris from retrocorneal membranes and iris-supported implants, lysis of broad-based anterior synechiae, and sweeping the donor tissue to undermine its edges below the host tissue. IOL manipulators such as Sinskey **(Fig. 2.10.19)** and Lester hooks are very useful for placing and stabilizing an AC lens.

Qualitative Keratometers

The keratometers are very helpful to assess the degree of corneal toricity at the end of the surgery. These can be of two types depending on whether they are attached to the microscope or they are handheld.

Keratometers with Microscopic Attachment

There are a number of surgical keratometers like *Smirmaul*, *Troutman*, and *Terry* that are physically attached to the microscope and work by reflecting projected light off the surface of the cornea. However, these are not portable and require a regular smooth refracting surface to reflect the image and are quite expensive.

Handheld Keratometers

Simpler, cost-effective, and portable methods as Mandel intraoperative keratometer and *Maloney* keratometer are available, which work by reflecting a circle from the corneal surface. Maloney keratometer is a titanium cone-shaped instrument, which is designed to reflect the microscope light in rings on the

Forceps with Special Functions

- *Double corneal forceps, Colibri style:* It has two 2.75 mm long tips separated 1 mm with 0.4 mm Pierse tips. It is 72 mm long and has a serrated handle.
- *Colibri style Polack double corneal forceps* **(Fig. 2.10.17)**: It is used for the first corneal suture. The cut edge of the graft is gently grasped at the junction of the epithelium and stroma with fine toothed forceps.

Spatulas and Hooks

Spatulas and hooks are mainly used in the reconstruction of the AC, the manipulation of the iris, and assistance in IOL placement. A double-ended iris repositor **(Fig. 2.10.18)** is useful for lysis of synechiae between the

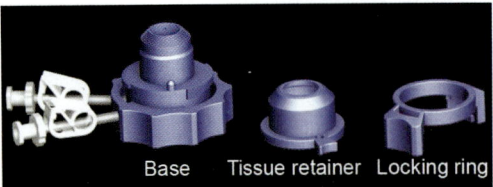

Fig. 2.10.20: Barron's.

cornea to detect astigmatism. In the absence of the expensive intraoperative surgical keratometers, a safety pin can also be used to monitor the intraoperative astigmatism. The circle of the safety pin is reflected off the corneal surface and any observed ovality implies excessive curvature in the axis of the shortest diameter of the oval. This is used for readjusting and replacement of the sutures and helps to reduce astigmatism intraoperatively and postoperatively.

Instruments for Donor Cornea Dissection in Lamellar Keratoplasty

- *Artificial anterior chamber and clamp [Barron's* **(Fig. 2.10.20)**, *Moria's* **(Fig. 2.10.21)**, *etc.]:* The chamber is used to mount the donor tissue and maintain adequate pressure while lamellar dissection or full thickness trephination is being performed. It is designed in a bright blue color to provide a high-contrast background for visualizing the cornea and aiding in the lamellar dissection of the cornea.
  The chamber is composed of three pieces: (1) Base with tissue pedestal, (2) tissue retainer, and (3) locking ring. The base has two ports with silicone tubing: (1) In-line pinch clamps and (2) Luer Lock connectors. Either port may be used to inject or aspirate viscoelastic material, balanced salt solution, preservation media, or air.
- King's clamp **(Fig. 2.10.22)**

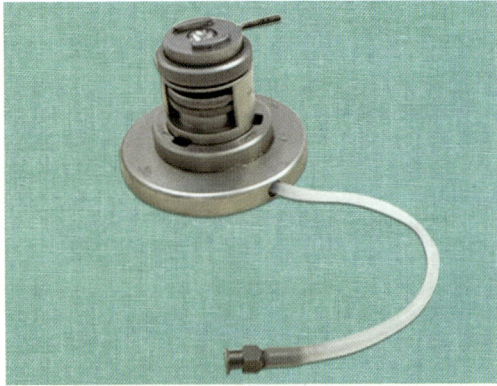

Fig. 2.10.21: Moria's.

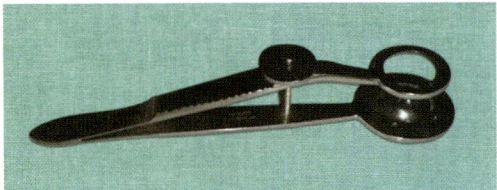

Fig. 2.10.22: King's clamp.

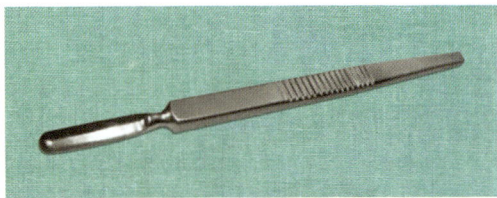

Fig. 2.10.23: Tooke's knife.

Lamellar Dissectors

- *Tooke's knife* **(Fig. 2.10.23)**: The pocket for the initiation of the lamellar dissection may be performed with a Tooke's knife. It has a smooth blade at one end, which can be inserted intralamellarly to create a pocket.
- *Paufique's knife* **(Fig. 2.10.24)**: It has a double-edged sharp-angled blade that helps in outlining the graft, making the pocket, and dissecting the lamellar plane.
- *Desmarre's lamellar dissector:* It is used in the open type of dissection, which has a

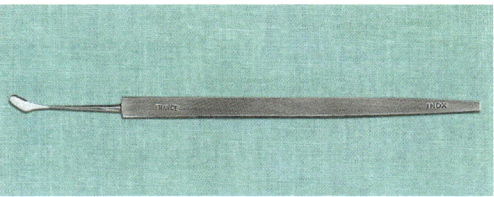

Fig. 2.10.24: Paufique's knife.

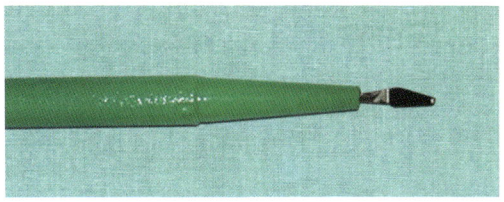

Fig. 2.10.25: Crescent knife.

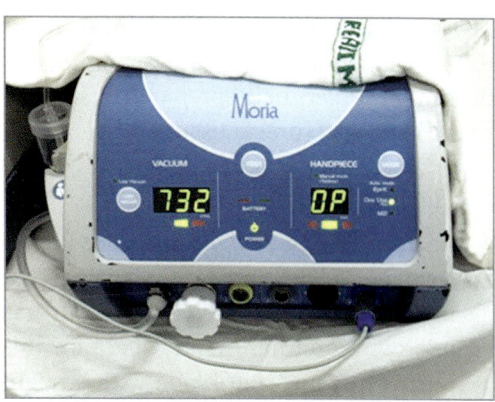

Fig. 2.10.26: Microkeratome.

curve in its vertical meridian and it is used to sweep across the fibers in a cutting and teasing motion. A duckbill-shaped lamellar dissector is used for closed type of dissection, which is curved in the horizontal dimension.
- *Gill's lamellar dissector:* It has a 3 mm wide blade, which can be either straight or curved.
- *Guarded diamond knife:* It is a micrometer-adjusted guarded diamond knife, useful for obtaining irregular-shaped lamellar grafts.
- *Crescent knife* **(Fig. 2.10.25)***:* This is another useful instrument for the lamellar dissection. It has a 2.0 mm blade. It is also used in pterygium surgery and small-incision cataract surgery (SICS).

Automated Lamellar Therapeutic Keratoplasty Machine

The Moria ALTK microkeratome system utilizes the Moria Carriazo-Barraquer (CBm) microkeratome **(Fig. 2.10.26)** and an artificial chamber, which is manually driven by the surgeon. Multiple microkeratome heads may be used to achieve dissection of various thicknesses ranging from 130 to 350 μm (130, 150, 250, 300, and 350 μm). The Moria ALTK AAC requires a donor scleral rim that is symmetrically greater than 16 mm (maximum 19 mm) in diameter to provide proper vacuum during the microkeratome pass. The surgical time is greatly reduced as compared to manual dissection technique.

Another machine available is the Amadeus II microkeratome with an AAC (Ziemer Group). The assembly unit comes equipped with four interchangeable suction units (with diameters of 8.5, 9.0, 9.5, and 10.0 mm) and a choice of five blade holders (for a flap thickness of 200, 250, 350, 400 or 450 μm).

Descemet Stripping Automated Endothelial Keratoplasty Instruments

For Donor Dissection

Donor tissue can be prepared manually as in Descemet stripping endothelial keratoplasty (DSEK), using an automated microkeratome as in DSAEK or with the aid of femtosecond laser. Irrespective of the mode of tissue dissection, an AAC is required to aid dissection. Donor tissue can be prepared at the time of surgery or preprepared by surgeon or eye bank staff (precut tissue).

For Recipient Preparation

- *Instruments for making incision:* Blades such as 15°, 30°, and 45° for inserting AC maintainer. Alternatively one can use microvitreoretinal (MVR) blade for this purpose. A crescent blade with straight sides and rounded tip is used for making scleral tunnel.
- *Instruments for Descemet scoring and scraping:*
  - Reverse Sinskey hook **(Fig. 2.10.27)**
  - Descemet's stripper such as Melles stripper, Steinert Descemet stripper, and Gorovoy irrigating stripper can be used instead of Sinskey hook.
  - DSAEK scraper **(Fig. 2.10.28)** such as Terry scraper, Rosenwasser scraper, Melles PLK scraper or Daya Descemet scraper have angled broad smooth tip with sharp edge and can be used to score as well as take out the host Descemet's membrane.

- Stripping forceps such as Snyder stripping forceps, tips of which are angled upward, often serrated to grasp the edge of Descemet's membrane to complete stripping technique.

For Graft Insertion

- *Forceps techniques:*
  - Taco folding technique (60:40 overfold/40:60 underfold/50:50) using compression forceps or non-appositional DSEK forceps
  - Trifold or burrito fold technique with forceps
- Needle-assisted technique
- Rosenwasser shovel
- Suture pull—through insertion technique
- Donor glides—Busin glide **(Fig. 2.10.29)**, TAN EndoGlide, and Sheets glide
- Donor inserters—EndoSerter, Neusidl corneal inserter, and EndoInjector (EndoShield)
- Others—Macaluso DSAEK endothelial lenticule inserter, Daya Endostar, IDEEL injector, Rieck Glide, and Al-Ghoul vacuum-assisted injector.

DSAEK Spatula (Stripper)

It is designed to strip the recipient's Descemet's membrane during the DSAEK procedure. The DSAEK strippers are available in 45° and 90° angled models, in both irrigating and nonirrigating versions. The angled tips facilitate the efficient dissection and removal of Descemet's membrane without

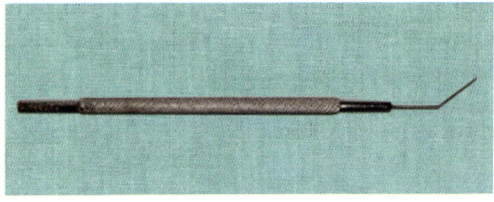

Fig. 2.10.27: Reverse Sinskey hook.

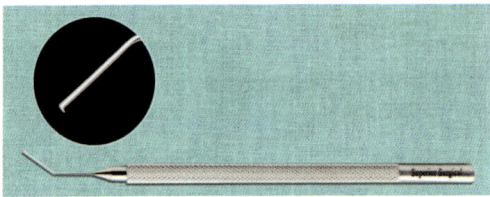

Fig. 2.10.28: DSAEK scraper.

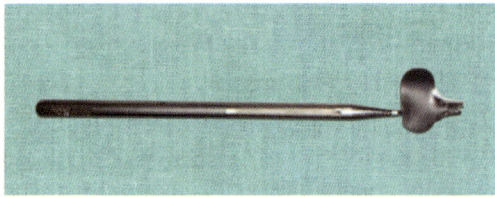

Fig. 2.10.29: Busin glide.

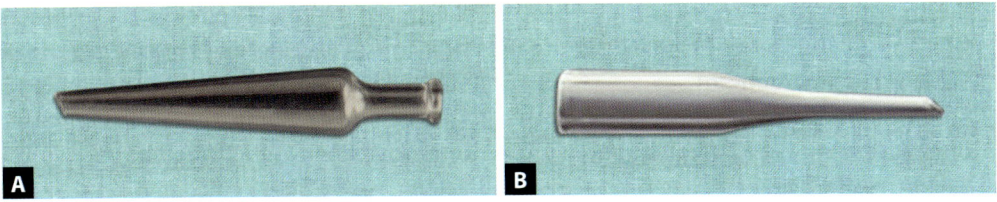

Figs. 2.10.30A and B: Glass injectors—DMEK Jones tube and Geuder glass injector.

inadvertent damage to the stroma. The strippers are made of surgical steel.

Busin Glide (Fig. 2.10.29)
Busin glide allows insertion of the taco by pull through technique through 3.2 mm incision. It facilitates the unfolding of the graft and simplifies centration of the donor button in the AC. It helps to minimize intraoperative manipulation of the graft and the possibility of endothelial loss.

DSAEK Busin Forceps
It is a microincision forceps with 20 G diameter and distal action. It is designed to position the graft in the glide and to pull it from the glide into the AC. Its tips have been designed specifically to contact the periphery of the graft such that the endothelial and the stromal surfaces remain untouched in the optical zone.

Descemet's Membrane Endothelial Keratoplasty Instruments

For Graft Insertion
- Modified IOL injection cartridges (Alcon B cartridge)
- Staar microinjector
- Viscoject IOL injector
- Modified AMO Emerald IOL injector and tip
- Glass injectors—DMEK Jones tube and Geuder glass injector **(Figs. 2.10.30A and B)**

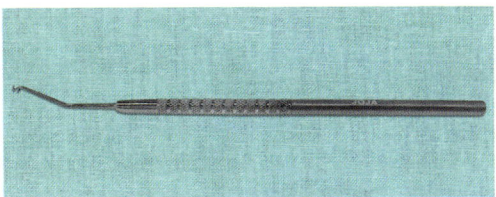

Fig. 2.10.31: S-stamp.

To Check Orientation of the Graft before Injection
- Staining the graft with 0.06% trypan blue
- Veldman Venn technique
- S-stamp on the stromal side **(Fig. 2.10.31)**

To Check Orientation after Insertion
- Moutsouris sign
- Handheld slit lamp—described by Bukhart et al.
- Endoilluminator or light probe—described by Agarwal et al.
- iOCT

■ VIVA QUESTIONS

1. What are the indications for use of Flieringa ring?
Ans. Refer to text.

2. Classify corneal trephines.
Ans. Refer to text.

3. What are the advantages of using suction trephine?
Ans. The following are the advantages of using suction trephine:

- Precise depth of trephination (250 microns for full rotation in Hessburg–Barron vacuum trephine)
- Better stabilization and less chance of slippage due to suction that is maintained during trephination
- Less endothelial cell loss compared with the posterior punch in donor tissue preparation.

4. What are the types of lamellar dissector?
Ans. Refer to text.

5. What are open and closed type of lamellar dissection?
Ans. In *closed method* of lamellar dissection the plane of dissection is not under direct visualization because the anterior lamellar flap is maintained in its original position close to the stromal bed and the dissector is advanced between the two layers. The advantage of this technique is it results in an even dissection plane with an increased likelihood that the dissection stays in the same plane throughout. However, the chances of corneal perforation are high when compared to open method. In *open method* of lamellar dissection, the plane of dissection is visualized by lifting the overlying corneal flap vertically. Slight traction of this flap caused tractional splitting of the stromal fibers at the leading edge of this dissection and the lamellar dissector is then applied in a pressing or sweeping motion at the base of the stromal fibers under traction.

6. What are different techniques of DALK?
Ans. Refer ophthalmology clinics (Part 1).

7. What are the different techniques of donor tissue insertion in DSAEK?
Ans. Refer to text.

8. Conditions where host Descemet's membrane scoring is not required.
Ans. There are two school of thoughts in this regard. However, most of the cornea surgeons believe that host Descemet's membrane peeling is not routinely indicated except in cases of scarred or wrinkled Descemet's membrane, Descemet folds, and prominent guttae that can impair the postoperative visual function. It should be absolutely avoided in cases of regraft following PK. In few cases the Descemet's membrane may be either absent or adherent to the underlying stroma making it extremely difficult to score under the hazy overlying corneal stroma.

9. What are the different techniques of donor tissue insertion in DMEK?
Ans. Refer to text.

CHAPTER 3

Cataract

3.1 INTRAOCULAR LENS MASTER

Deepali Singhal, Alisha Kishore, Arpit Sharma, Prafulla Kumar Maharana

■ INTRODUCTION

Method of optical biometry was introduced by Carl Zeiss Meditec in 1998. It is the gold standard in optical biometry and measures the distance from the corneal apex to the retinal pigment epithelium.

■ PRINCIPLE

IOLMaster 500 **(Fig. 3.1.1)** is based on the concept of partial coherence interferometry. It measures the time required for the infrared light to travel to the retina. The recently introduced IOLMaster 700 uses first swept-source optical coherence tomography (OCT)-based biometry.

■ USES

The following parameters can be measured:[1]
- Axial length (AL)—in the range from 14 to 38 mm with the interval scale of 0.01 mm
- Radius of curvature of cornea—in the range from 5 to 10 mm with the interval scale of 0.01 mm; it determines the value by measuring the relative position of six spots on the cornea. These are projected in hexagonal pattern with a diameter of 2.5 mm.
- Anterior chamber depth (ACD)—in the range from 1.5 to 6.5 mm with the interval scale of 0.01 mm
- White-to-white (WTW) diameter—in the range from 8 to 16 mm with the interval scale of 0.1 mm
- Intraocular lens (IOL) power calculation formulas—SRK II, SRK/T, Holladay 1 and 2, Hoffer Q, and Haigis formula are integrated **(Fig. 3.1.2)**. For calculating IOL power after laser in situ keratomileusis (LASIK)/photorefractive keratectomy (PRK)/laser epithelial keratomileusis (LASEK), Haigis-L formula is used. Phakic lens power calculation is also integrated.

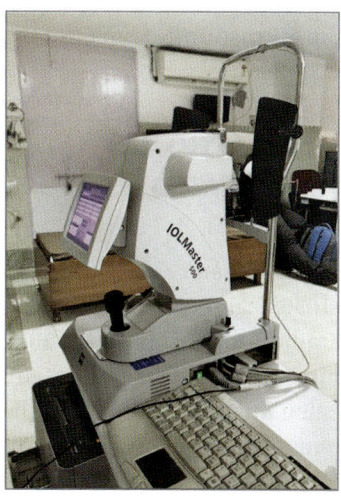

Fig. 3.1.1: IOLMaster 500.

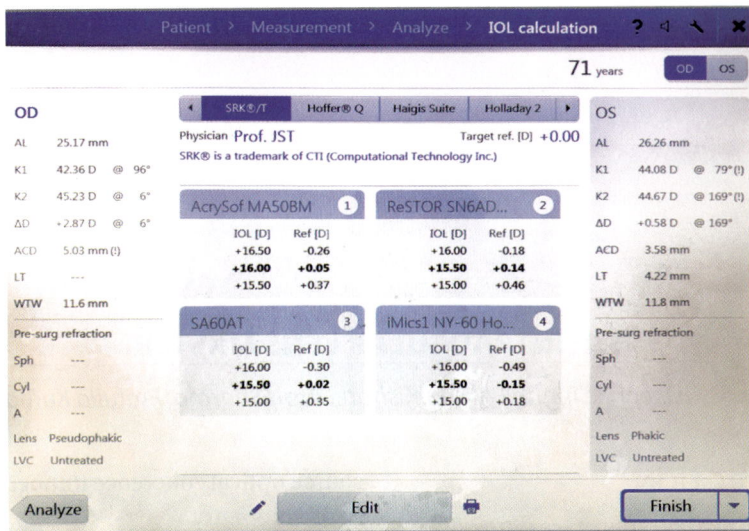

Fig. 3.1.2: IOLMaster 700 with different intraocular lens (IOL) power calculation formula.

Constants of various IOL are optimized. Also with the Holladay 2, only the postoperative refraction of the patient is needed. All the other information is filled automatically. There is no need for the data to be exported.

ADVANTAGES

- Integrated device, which measures AL, keratometry, and IOL power calculation with wide range of options for calculating power.
- All measurements are done along visual axis for accurate AL measurement. It is useful even in cases of staphyloma, pseudophakics, eyes filled with silicone oil, and patients with phakic lens.
- Faster acquisition time; both keratometry and AL can be measured simultaneously in the dual mode. Different modes can be changed automatically and is user-independent.
- Patient comfort since the measurements are distance-independent. It is, therefore, useful in patients with poor fixation.
- Higher success rate compared to other devices as there is better cataract penetration. The signals to noise values are also increased, thereby increasing the reliability. It should be >2.0.
- The IOLMaster can be integrated with CALLISTO eye for better management in the operating room. It helps in toric IOL alignment without marking the cornea. It can also be connected with A-scan ultrasound device for quick AL measurement.

INTERPRETATION OF INTRAOCULAR LENS MASTER (FIG. 3.1.3)

This is an IOLMaster of a patient named X with ID 163638 and date of birth 24/05/1968. The examination was done on 28/11/2017 under surgeon Y. The formula used for IOL power calculation is SRK/T with the target refraction as plano, which means emmetropic. The AL of the right eye is 22.66 mm and the left eye is 22.44 mm, which is within normal

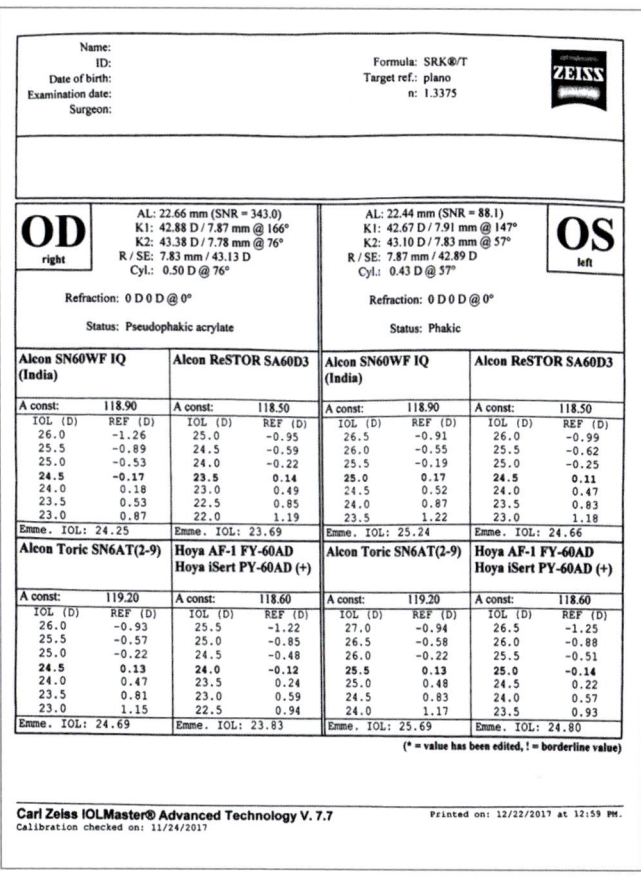

Fig. 3.1.3: IOLMaster of a right-eye pseudophakic patient for left-eye cataract surgery.

limit and the difference between the two eyes is <0.3 mm. The keratometry value of the right eye is 42.88/43.38 D @166°/76° with an astigmatism of 0.50 D at 76°. The right eye is pseudophakic. The keratometry value of the left eye is 42.67/43.10 D @147°/57° with an astigmatism of 0.43 D at 57°. The left eye is phakic. So, the patient is for left-eye cataract surgery. IOL calculations for Alcon IQ, ReSTOR, Toric, and Hoya have been calculated. The IOL, which has been used in the right eye, should be used in the left eye. For example, if Alcon IQ of 24.5 D was used in the right eye, then in the left eye, Alcon IQ of power 25.5 D should be used, which will give a refraction of –0.19, which will comparable to the right eye of –0.17 at 24.5 D. It is important to correlate the findings clinically.

■ VIVA QUESTIONS

1. **What is the difference between LenStar and IOLMaster?**

   Ans. Refer to **Table 3.1.1**.

2. **State the advantages of IOLMaster 700.**

   Ans. IOLMaster 700 **(Fig. 3.1.4)** has integrated swept source OCT and Barrett suite.[2] Its various advantages include:
   - Refractive surprises are less.
   - Repeatability

TABLE 3.1.1: Difference between LenStar and IOLMaster.

	LenStar	IOLMaster
Manufacturer	Haag-Streit	Zeiss
Principle	Optical low-coherence reflectometry	Partial coherence interferometry
FDA approved	October 2009	March 2000
Laser used	Superluminescent diode (820 nm)	Infrared diode laser (780 nm)
Measurement	Dual-zone keratometer with a total of 32 marker points on two concentric rings of 1.65 mm and 2.3 mm in diameter	It measures the relative position of six spots on the cornea. These are projected in hexagonal pattern with a diameter of 2.5 mm
Pupillometry	Can be measured	Cannot be measured
Lens thickness	Can be measured	Cannot be measured
Central corneal thickness	Can be measured	Cannot be measured

(FDA: Food and Drug Administration; IOL: intraocular lens)

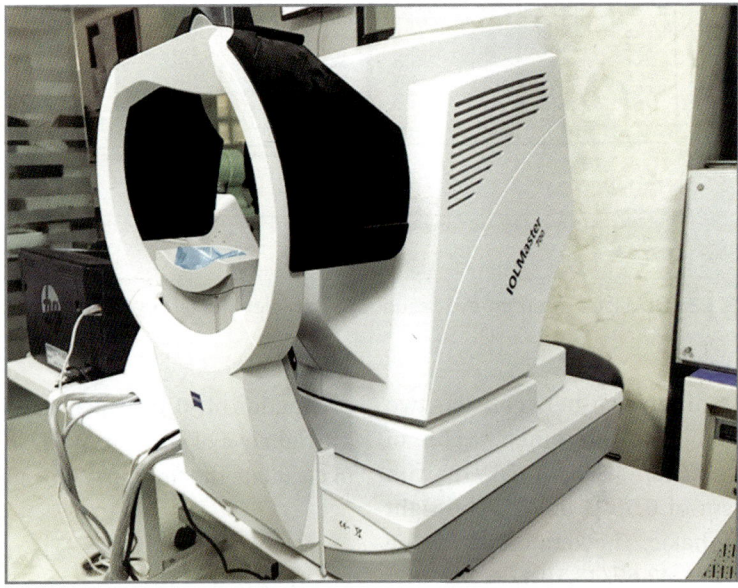

Fig. 3.1.4: IOLMaster 700.

- Integration of swept-source OCT provides measurement based on image. It provides a longitudinal section of the eye. It helps in identifying conditions such as lens tilt.
- Accurate measurement since image of the fovea **(Fig. 3.1.5)** tells about the fixation.
- Central corneal thickness and lens thickness can be measured additionally.
- More effective in cases of posterior subcapsular cataract (PSC) and dense nuclear cataract as compared to IOLMaster 500.

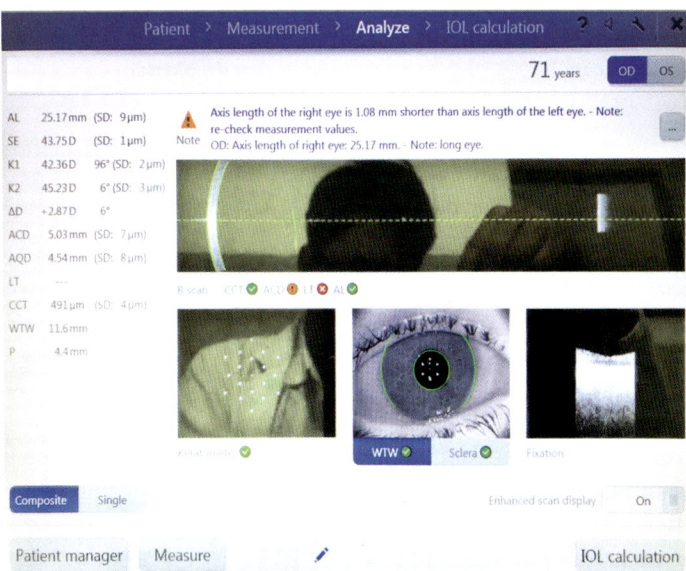

Fig. 3.1.5: IOLMaster 700 showing foveal image.

TABLE 3.1.2: IOLMaster 700 versus 500.		
Parameters	**500**	**700**
AL measurements	PCI	Swept-source OCT
LT and central corneal thickness (CCT)	Not available	Possible
ACD measurements	Optical section through the anterior chamber by means of a slit-illumination system	Swept source OCT images
	Not possible in pseudophakic eyes	Possible
	Prone to error	More accurate
Identify irregular eye geometries	Not possible	Possible
Dense PSC/dense cataracts	Inaccurate measurement	Accurate
Patients with poor fixation, irregular eye geometries	Inaccurate	Useful

(ACD: anterior chamber depth; AL: axial length; IOL: intraocular lens; LT: lens thickness; OCT: optical coherence tomography; PCI: partial coherence interferometry; PSC: posterior subcapsular cataract)

3. Give the difference between IOLMaster 500 and IOLMaster 700.
Ans. Refer to **Table 3.1.2**.[3]

4. State the difference between A-scan and IOLMaster for AL measurement.
Ans. Refer to **Table 3.1.3**.[4]

5. What is partial coherence interferometry?
Ans. Partial coherence interferometry uses a low coherence length infrared light of 780 nm and is split into two parts by an external Michelson interferometer. A coaxial dual beam is produced out of which one goes to

TABLE 3.1.3: Difference between AL measurement using A-scan and IOLMaster.

	A-scan	IOLMaster
Signal transmission	Ultrasound waves	Laser
Measurement	• From corneal apex to the internal limiting membrane • Measures along the anatomical axis	• From corneal apex to retinal pigment epithelium • Measures along the visual axis
Contact procedure	Contact	Noncontact
Accuracy	• Less resolution • Approximately 0.10–0.12 mm	• Better resolution and more accurate • Approximately 0.012 mm

(AL: axial length; IOL: intraocular lens)

a reference mirror and the other component is reflected at several intraocular interfaces that separate media of different refractive indices. For the measurement of AL, reflection sites are the anterior surface of the cornea and the retinal pigment epithelium. If the delay of these two components produced by the interferometer equals an intraocular distance within the coherence length of the light source, an interference signal (called partial coherence interferometry signal) is detected, similar to that of ultrasound A-scan, but with a very high resolution and precision.

6. What is swept-source OCT?

Ans. Swept-source OCT utilizes longer wavelength of 1,040 nm compared to 840 nm in spectral domain OCT. This overcomes the scattering of light by the retinal pigment epithelium. Also, there is deeper penetration into the choroid allowing more accurate imaging of vitreous, retina, and the choroid. The axial resolution is increased and there is faster acquisition time.

REFERENCES

1. Meditec CZ. (2016). IOLMaster 500 from ZEISS: Defining Biometry. [online] Available from https://applications.zeiss.com/C1257A290053AE30/0/6D036B2F9E9161C8C1257BF30033EF8F/$FILE/IOLMaster_500_Brochure_EN_32_010_0022II.pdf [Last accessed January, 2019].
2. Meditec CZ. (2017). ZEISS IOLMaster 700: Getting Fewer Refractive Surprises. [online] Available from https://zeiss.taimaz.com/wp-content/uploads/2018/06/TAIMAZ_iolmaster_700_brochure_en_32_010_0009v-.pdf. [Last accessed January, 2019].
3. Akman A, Asena L, Güngör SG. Evaluation and comparison of the new swept source OCT-based IOLMaster 700 with the IOLMaster 500. Br J Ophthalmol. 2016;100:1201-5.
4. Holladay JT. Ultrasound and optical biometry. Cataract Refract Surg Today Eur. 2009;26:18-9.

3.2 LENSTAR

Yogita Gupta, Deepali Singhal, Prafulla Kumar Maharana

■ INTRODUCTION

LenStar LS900 **(Fig. 3.2.1)** is a high-resolution, noncontact, and noninvasive optical biometry device. When it was first introduced in 2009[1] by Haag-Streit manufacturer, it became popular as the first optical biometry device, which could measure crystalline lens thickness.

■ PRINCIPLE

The LenStar is based on optical low-coherence reflectometry (OLCR).[2] Like the IOLMaster, it uses the effect of time domain interferometric or coherent superposition of light waves to measure ocular lengths of the eye in a similar technique to one-dimensional OCT. The IOLMaster uses a diode laser, whereas the LenStar uses 820 μm superluminescent diode[2] with a Gaussian-shaped spectrum, which allows a higher axial resolution; hence, the terminology OLCR, rather than partial coherence interferometry, has been coined.[1]

■ EQUIPMENT

LenStar obtains measurements after user focuses or aligns the image of the eye on the computer monitor while patient fixates on a flashing red light **(Fig. 3.2.2)**.

Central corneal topography is obtained using two rings of diameters 1.65 mm and 2.3 mm of 16 light spots each, reflected off the air/tear interface. These 32 closely spaced measurement points give a dual-zone keratometry system.

The retinal thickness can also be determined from the scans by subjective alignment of the cursor. The horizontal iris width (WTW) is measured as the horizontal diameter of a best fit circle to the iris boarder and the pupil diameter is measured as the diameter of a best fit circle to the pupil boarder.

■ USES

LS900 measures nine parameters: (1) AL, (2) keratometry, (3) lens thickness, (4) corneal thickness, (5) retinal thickness, (6) ACD, (7) WTW diameter, (8) pupil diameter, and (9) eccentricity of the visual axis with respect to the center of cornea **(Fig. 3.2.3)**. Besides it also gives aqueous depth, radii for flat and steep meridian, and axis of flat meridian.

■ ADVANTAGES

- The dense cataract measurement (DCM) mode allows penetration through dense cataract and allows biometry in aphakic, pseudophakic, or silicone oil-filled eyes.

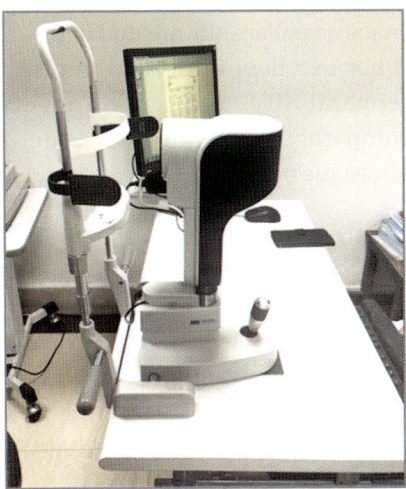

Fig. 3.2.1: LenStar LS900 device for optical biometry.

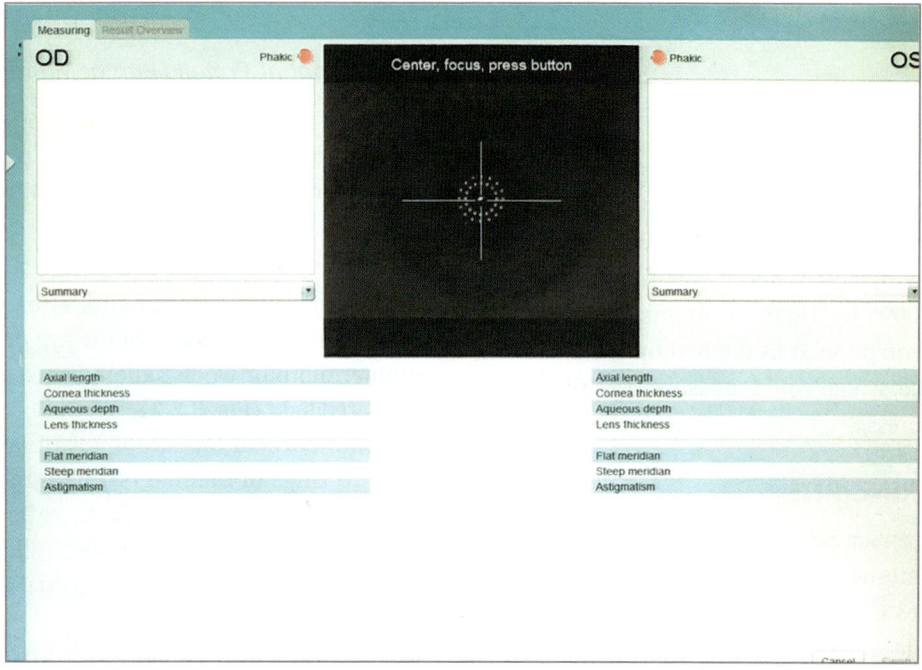

Fig. 3.2.2: Patient fixation in LS900.

- LenStar Pro version has automated positioning system (APS) that tracks eye movement to capture reliable measurements in one click.
- When planning for toric or premium IOLs, the Pro version of the LS900 can be used to measure 6-mm optical zone with the option of adding T-cone toric platform, a double-ring placido disc topographer, which improves refractive outcomes.
- It helps in determination of the appropriate IOLpower by including the modern IOL formulae like Barrett Universal II, Barrett True-K, Haigis, Hoffer Q, Holladay 1, SRK/T, SRK II, Masket, Modified Masket and Shammas No-history, and Hill RBF methods. The option of EyeSuite IOL toric planner software also includes the Barrett Toric Calculator.
- It is patient-friendly and high-speed device with each scan capturing all measurements in 30 seconds.[3]
- It uses a separate external PC, which allows good memory for storage and enables regular software updates.
- It has excellent intra- and intersession repeatability and good accuracy, comparable with the IOLMaster and ultrasonic biometry.

VIVA QUESTIONS

1. **What is the principle of LenStar?**
   Ans. Refer to text.

2. **What are the advantages of LenStar over IOLMaster?**
   Ans. Refer to text and also chapter on IOLMaster.

OD
Right eye
Phakic

LS900 16 Jul, 2019 - 1
- AL [mm] 25.42¹
- CCT [µm] 516
- AD [mm] 2.99
- ACD [mm] 3.51
- LT [mm] 4.09
- R1[mm/D/°] 8.08 / 41.75 @ 93
- R2[mm/D/°] 7.56 / 44.66 @ 3
- R [mm/D] 7.82 / 43.15
- +AST [D/°] 2.91 @ 3
- n 1.3375
- WTW [mm] 12.18

Warnings:
⊕ 1: Significant difference between OD and OS

Target Refraction: 0.00   Template: Room No. 279

SN60WF — Alcon
IOL [D]	Eye [D]
14.50	0.73
15.00	0.41
15.50	**0.08**
16.00	-0.25
16.50	-0.58

SRK/T A=119.00

AcrySof MA60AC — Alcon
IOL [D]	Eye [D]
15.00	0.51
15.50	0.19
16.00	**-0.13**
16.50	-0.46
17.00	-0.79

SRK/T A=119.20

Tecnis 1 ZCB00 — AMO
IOL [D]	Eye [D]
15.00	0.57
15.50	0.25
16.00	**-0.07**
16.50	-0.40
17.00	-0.73

SRK/T A=119.30

CT LUCIA 601P/PY — Zeiss
IOL [D]	Eye [D]
15.00	0.51
15.50	0.19
16.00	**-0.13**
16.50	-0.46
17.00	-0.79

SRK/T A=119.20

ReSTOR SN6AD1/3 — Alcon
IOL [D]	Eye [D]
14.50	0.73
15.00	0.41
15.50	**0.08**
16.00	-0.25
16.50	-0.58

SRK/T A=119.00

Symfony ZXR00 — AMO
IOL [D]	Eye [D]
15.00	0.57
15.50	0.25
16.00	**-0.07**
16.50	-0.40
17.00	-0.73

SRK/T A=119.30

OS
Left eye
Phakic

LS900 16 Jul, 2019 - 1
- AL [mm] 26.03¹
- CCT [µm] 519
- AD [mm] 3.03
- ACD [mm] 3.55
- LT [mm] 3.71
- R1[mm/D/°] 8.17 / 41.31 @ 88
- R2[mm/D/°] 7.54 / 44.75 @ 178
- R [mm/D] 7.86 / 42.96
- +AST [D/°] 3.43 @ 178
- n 1.3375
- WTW [mm] 11.92

Warnings:
⊕ 1: Significant difference between OD and OS

Target Refraction: 0.00   Template: Room No. 27

SN60WF — Alcon
IOL [D]	Eye [D]
13.00	0.66
13.50	0.34
14.00	**0.02**
14.50	-0.31
15.00	-0.64

SRK/T A=119.00

AcrySof MA60AC — Alcon
IOL [D]	Eye [D]
13.00	0.75
13.50	0.44
14.00	**0.12**
14.50	-0.21
15.00	-0.53

SRK/T A=119.20

Tecnis 1 ZCB00 — AMO
IOL [D]	Eye [D]
13.50	0.49
14.00	0.17
14.50	**-0.15**
15.00	-0.48
15.50	-0.81

SRK/T A=119.30

CT LUCIA 601P/PY — Zeiss
IOL [D]	Eye [D]
13.00	0.75
13.50	0.44
14.00	**0.12**
14.50	-0.21
15.00	-0.53

SRK/T A=119.20

ReSTOR SN6AD1/3 — Alcon
IOL [D]	Eye [D]
13.00	0.66
13.50	0.34
14.00	**0.02**
14.50	-0.31
15.00	-0.64

SRK/T A=119.00

Symfony ZXR00 — AMO
IOL [D]	Eye [D]
13.50	0.49
14.00	0.17
14.50	**-0.15**
15.00	-0.48
15.50	-0.81

SRK/T A=119.30

EyeSuite™ IOL, V4.3.2
SID: 1800

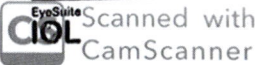
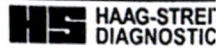

Fig. 3.2.3: A report of LS900.

REFERENCES

1. Buckhurst PJ, Wolffsohn JS, Shah S, Naroo SA, Davies LN, Berrow EJ. A new optical low coherence reflectometry device for ocular biometry in cataract patients. Br J Ophthalmol. 2009;93:949-53.
2. Haag-Streit Diagnostics. (2017). LENSTAR LS 900: Improving Outcomes. [online] Available from https://www.haag-streit.com/fileadmin/Haag-Streit_USA/Lenstar/Landing/papers/Brochure_Lenstar_eng.pdf [Last accessed January, 2019].
3. Haag Streit LENSTAR®. (2017). LENSTAR LS 900® The First Optical Biometer of the Entire Eye. [online] Available from https://www.doctor-hill.com/lenstar_haag_streit/lenstar_main.htm [Last accessed January, 2019].

3.3 A-SCAN

(Surg Capt) Srujana D, Mohamed Ibrahime Asif, Pranita Sahay, Ritu Nagpal

INTRODUCTION

A-scan ultrasound **(Fig. 3.3.1)** is a one-dimensional amplitude modulation scan, used commonly to determine the AL of the eye. Measurement of AL is an important component of any IOL calculation formula prior to cataract surgery. Besides, A-scan is also used in conjunction with B-scan imaging to measure the size and characterize the ultrasonic properties of any mass lesion located in the posterior segment or in orbit.

PRINCIPLE

A-scan ultrasonography is based on the principle of calculating the time required for the sound waves to go across the eye using a 10-MHz ultrasound transducer **(Fig. 3.3.2)** and conversion of it to a quantitative (linear) value through a velocity formula.

Using an estimated average velocity through the various ocular media: cornea (1,620 m/s), aqueous (1,532 m/s), lens (1,641 m/s), and vitreous (1,532 m/s), the biometric software calculates the AL. This value should be altered when velocities differ as in performing AL measurements in aphakia, pseudophakia, and silicon-filled eye. Special precaution must be taken in silicone oil-filled eyes. The refractive index of silicone oil is considerably less than vitreous humor; hence

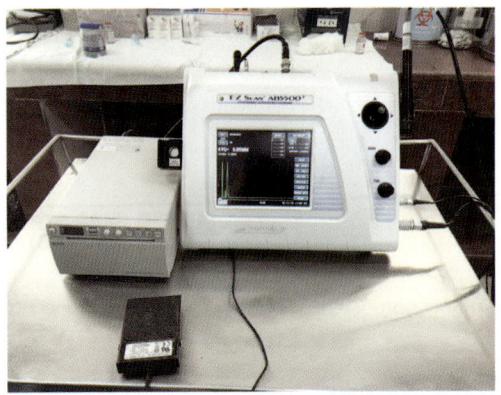

Fig. 3.3.1: A-scan.

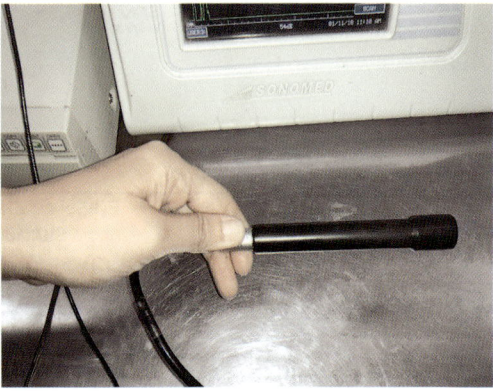

Fig. 3.3.2: Ultrasonic probe.

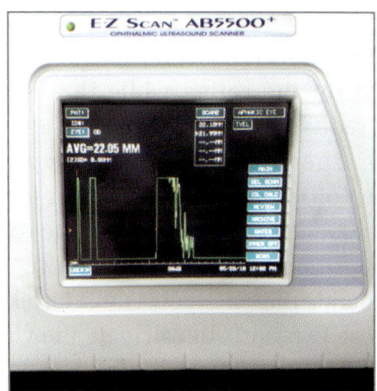

Fig. 3.3.3: Display of contact A-scan showing spikes at various ocular interfaces.

pathology, are less likely to fixate accurately, causing errors. To avoid any error, the average of 10, most reliable readings with 100% spike must be calculated.

In the manual mode when an acceptable scan is obtained, the operator has to freeze the scan with a foot pedal. The gates (corneal and retinal) should then be moved to the correct place and the reading taken. While doing this, it is advisable to keep the gain at the lowest level at which a high-quality reading is obtained.

In automatic mode, the machine freezes the image when the spikes fall in a certain range. However, prior to measurement, the machine must be calibrated, and the velocity settings must be appropriately chosen depending upon the condition of the eye. It is important not to apply too much pressure over the cornea, or else compression of the cornea could lead to an underestimation of the measured AL. For example, in the case of Sanders–Retzlaff–Kraff (SRK) formula, an error of 1.0 mm will result in approximately 2.50 D postoperative refractive surprise. This may further increase while measuring AL in short or long eyes. Thus, in case of an underestimation of AL, there will be a myopic surprise while in case of an overestimation, there will be a hyperopic surprise in the postoperative period. It is important to note that a greasy corneal surface due to prior application of ointment or lubricants can also lead to an error in IOL power calculation.

this must be taken into consideration along with the type of IOL while calculating the IOL power in silicone oil-filled eyes.

While performing A-scan, multiple spikes are seen in the display, each representing reflection of the waves from different parts such as the cornea, anterior surface of the lens, posterior surface of the lens, and the retina. The gap between the spikes from the corneal and retinal surface provides the AL of the eye **(Fig. 3.3.3)**.

■ METHOD

After instilling topical anesthetic, the ultrasound probe (6 mm in diameter) of A-scan is placed gently over the apex of the cornea. The patient is asked to fix a target light on the probe or is asked to fixate his thumb raised by the technician to keep the eye aligned along the pupil-macular axis. High spikes are obtained when the sound beam is perpendicular to the ocular interfaces. If the beam strikes the optic nerve instead of the macula, scleral and orbital fat spikes are absent. Hence, alignment of the probe is critical as incorrect alignment can give erroneous readings. Patients with poor vision, such as dense cataracts or due to other

Another source of error is not choosing the right IOL mode. The velocity of the sound wave is more in cases of polymethylmethacrylate (PMMA)/acrylic/silicon IOL than through the crystalline lens. Hence, in these eyes, pseudophakic mode has to be used.

Repeat scan: Repeat scan is indicated in the following situations:

- AL <22 mm or >25 mm; in short or long eyes, the indentation effect can lead to significant error; hence, it is better to repeat the measurement several times till reliable results are obtained.
- Eyes with posterior staphyloma
- If the difference is measured, AL between the two eyes is >0.3 mm.
- *If repeated measurements vary by >0.2 mm, discrepancy between patients refractive status and the measured AL*: It is always a good practice to compare the refractive error of the patient with the AL. For example, an AL of 30 mm having an error of +2.00 D, one should repeat measurements of A-scan.

A-SCAN IN SPECIAL SITUATIONS

- *Silicon oil-filled eye:* The speed of ultrasound wave in silicon oil is around 987 m/s (with a viscosity of 1,000 centistokes and 1,040 m/s for 5,000 centistokes) while in vitreous humor, it is 1,532 m/s; hence, the AL measured is usually falsely high in oil-filled eye. Theoretically, the correction factor comes out to be 0.64 mm. Murray et al. derived the conversion factor of 0.71 for silicon oil of viscosity 1,300 centistokes.[1]

  The second major challenge in oil-filled eyes is the difficulty in identifying the ocular interfaces accurately. The identification of the retinal interface is challenging in oil-filled eyes due to sound attenuation. Besides, the majority of oil-filled eyes are myopic and may be having posterior staphyloma, which further can amplify the error.

  The situation becomes worse when the eye is partially silicone oil-filled. The oil bubble moves with movement of the eye producing shifting retinal echoes. In the supine position, often the routinely followed technique, the oil bubble would rest on the retina while the liquefied vitreous will stay on top of it. If the measurements are taken in this position, then ultrasound wave will cross the layer of liquefied vitreous first, prior to crossing the silicone oil-filled portion. Thus, separate measurements must be taken for these two parts to calculate the vitreous cavity depth accurately. The best approach to deal with such cases is to perform the measurement with the patient in a seated position. The liquefied vitreous will shift superiorly leaving only the silicone oil in the optical axis through which the ultrasound beam would pass. Also, with contact A-mode, the echoes from the tip of the probe merge with the echoes from the cornea to become a single broad echo, leading to difficult identification of the anterior corneal spike. Further, lens opacities also generate additional echoes that interfere with the instrument's ability to detect the posterior capsule spike and to measure the proper lens thickness.
- *Posterior staphyloma:* In the presence of staphyloma, the anatomic AL (corneal apex to the most posterior portion of the globe) may not correspond to the refractive AL (corneal apex to the center of the macula). This could lead an erroneous AL measurement.
- *Others:* Several other factors can also produce errors in AL measurement on A-scan. The difficulty in delineating the anterior and posterior corneal surfaces can lead to an error in exact positioning of the anterior spike for AL measurement. Similarly for lenticular opacities, the presence of IOL can produce multiple echoes that can lead to errors in AL measurement.

IMMERSION SCAN

In this, the coupling fluid rather than the ultrasound probe comes into contact with the corneal apex. This excludes any compression of the cornea and hence avoids any errors in AL measurement **(Fig. 3.3.4)**. The coupling fluid requires a Prager Scleral Shell **(Fig. 3.3.5)**, or a set of Ossoinig or Hansen Scleral Shells to be placed within the palpebral aperture. A shell of size 20 mm usually fits most eyes, a larger cup may be required for the bigger eye with large palpebral fissure, and a smaller cup for eyes with a narrow palpebral fissure.

For performing the scan, the patient is asked to lie down supine, looking up at the ceiling. The Prager shell is placed between the eyelids. Normal saline or lubricant eye drop is used to fill the shell that acts as the coupling media. The ultrasound beam is then aligned with the macula by asking the patient to look at the fixation light, and the measurements are taken. Although both saline and a higher concentration of methylcellulose 1% can be used as coupling fluid, 1% methylcellulose is the best as saline is too thin and a higher concentration of methylcellulose is too thick.

Accuracy

The accuracy of immersion scan is within 0.12 mm. Thus, the use of this technique could lead to a refractive surprise of approximately 0.28 D. This error may be more in short or long eyes.

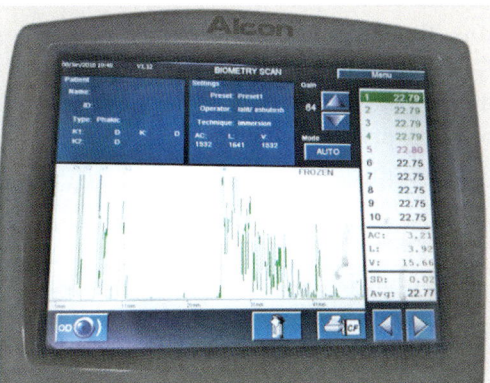

Fig. 3.3.4: Display of immersion A-scan showing spikes at various ocular interfaces.

Advantages

Immersion scan has following advantages:
- Better reproducibility and accuracy
- Avoids corneal compression thereby displaying true ACD and exact AL
- Possible to identify anterior corneal spike clearly (c.f. applanation A-scan)
- In posterior staphylomatous eyes, it is (immersion B-scan) extremely useful in identification of the macula in relation to staphyloma.
- Allows measurement of correct AL in oil-filled eyes by identifying retro silicon space accurately.
- Posterior staphyloma, recurrent retinal detachment (RD), epiretinal membranes, and retained perfluorocarbon (PFC) bubbles can be detected, and gates can be adjusted to give the exact AL.

VIVA QUESTIONS

1. **What is Artemis very high-frequency (VHF) digital ultrasound?**

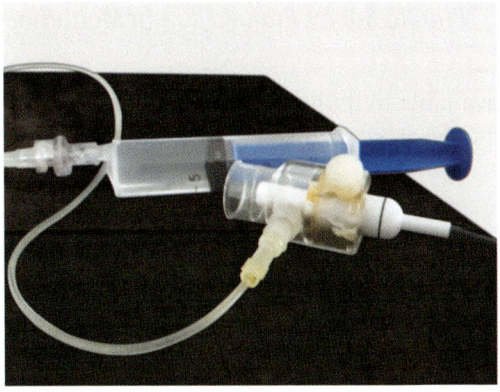

Fig. 3.3.5: Prager scleral shell.

Ans. Artemis uses a 50-MHz VHF ultrasound transducer with immersion scanning technology. It acquires high-precision B-scans that approximately represent the surface contour of anterior or posterior segment structures. The radius of the curvature adjustment mechanism to enable maximum perpendicularity and enhanced signal-to-noise ratio allows for excellent precision. Its axial resolution is 21 µ, and three-dimensional (3D) layered pachymetry (using multiple meridional scans) has precision <1.0 µ.

2. **What is the AL at birth?**
Ans. AL at birth is 14.5–15.5 mm.

3. **State the changes in AL with age.**
Ans. The change in the AL of the eye occurs in three phases:
1. *Phase 1 (birth to age 2 years):* This is a period of rapid growth. In the first 6 months, the AL increases by 4 mm while in the subsequent 6 months, it increases by 2 mm.
2. *Phase 2 (age 2–5 years):* The growth slows down and the AL increases by 1 mm.
3. *Phase 3 (age 5–13 years):* The growth further slows down and the AL increases by another 1 mm.

4. **What is the impact of cataract surgery on AL in congenital cataract?**
Ans. The impact of cataract surgery on AL change is controversial with few reports suggesting a reduction while few reporting increased axial elongation of the eye following cataract surgery. Unilateral cataract surgery, especially during infancy, has been reported to be associated with more axial elongation in the operated eye than bilateral cataract surgery.

5. **What is the advantage of A-scan over IOLMaster?**
Ans. Though IOLMaster is more precise than A-scan, it is disadvantageous in patients with dense cataract (media opacities), corneal opacity, dense vitreous hemorrhage, and if patients are not able to fix.

REFERENCE

1. Murray DC, Durrani OM, Good P, Benson MT, Kirkby GR. Biometry of the silicone oil-filled eye: II. Eye (Lond). 2002;16:727-30.

3.4 APPLIANCES AND INSTRUMENTS IN CATARACT SURGERY

Pranita Sahay, Prafulla Kumar Maharana

VON GRAEFE'S KNIFE (FIG. 3.4.1)

Von Graefe's knife is a long, narrow, and thin blade with a sharp tip with cutting edge on one side. It was used for making the corneoscleral entry in cataract surgery.

KERATOMES (FIG. 3.4.2)

This is a thin blade with a diamond-shaped apex and cutting edge on both sides. It is available in both straight and curved design as well as in various sizes (2.2, 2.8, 3, 3.5, and

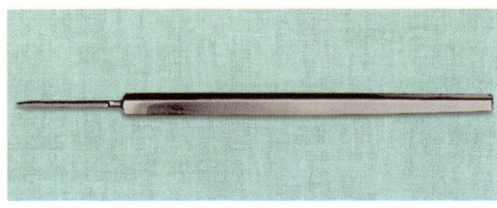

Fig. 3.4.1: von Graefe's knife.

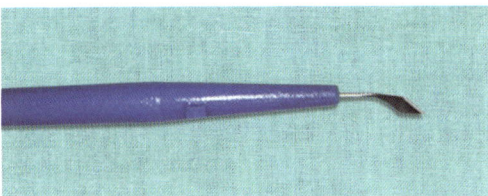

Fig. 3.4.2: Keratomes.

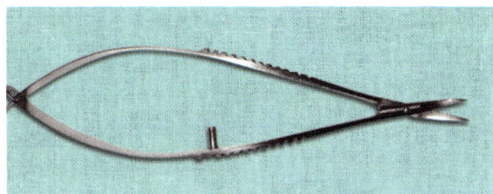

Fig. 3.4.4: Corneal scissors.

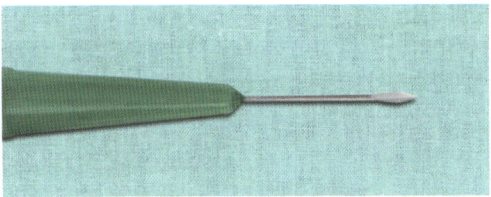

Fig. 3.4.3: Microvitreoretinal (MVR).

5.5 mm). It is used for making self-sealing corneal incisions in cataract surgery.

MICROVITREORETINAL OR V-LANCE BLADE (FIG. 3.4.3)

This is a fine straight instrument with triangular knife at its distal end having cutting edge on both the sides. It is used for making the side port entry at the limbus as well as sclerotomy for vitreoretinal surgery. The incision width with this blade is approximately 1.1 mm.

One special use of microvitreoretinal (MVR) is posterior-assisted levitation (PAL) technique, described by Charles Kelman to salvage a dropping nucleus during cataract surgery. In this technique, a pars plana sclerotomy is done at the 11 o'clock meridian, 3 mm behind the limbus using an MVR blade. A spatula is passed through the sclerotomy and placed behind the nucleus, which is then elevated forward into the anterior chamber (AC) and subsequently managed by phacoemulsification or manual removal. The other special uses of MVR include transcorneal venting incisions in Descemet stripping automated endothelial keratoplasty (DSAEK) to drain residual interface fluid and stab incisions to drain intrastromal fluid pockets in cases of corneal hydrops.

The limitation of MVR is similar to other sharp instruments, i.e., chances of inadvertent prick injuries to the operating surgeon. During cataract surgery, it can lead to Descemet's membrane detachment (DMD) and inadvertent damage to iris or lens capsule especially if the tip is bent or blunt.

CORNEAL SCISSORS (FIG. 3.4.4)

Corneal scissors is fine, curved scissors that works on spring action. The main differentiating feature of conjunctival scissors is that it is short and stout.

Uses

- To enlarge the corneal or corneoscleral incision for intracapsular cataract extraction (ICCE)/extracapsular cataract extraction (ECCE)
- To enlarge corneal incision in keratoplasty
- To cut the scleral tissue flap

The main advantage of enlarging the corneal incision with corneal scissors is that it enlarges the wound exactly along the limbus. The limitation is that it may lead to ragged margins of the cut edges especially if it is not sharp.

VANNAS SCISSORS (FIG. 3.4.5)

Vannas scissors are fine scissors that work on spring action. They have two wings to

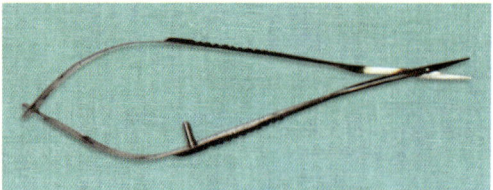

Fig. 3.4.5: Vannas scissors.

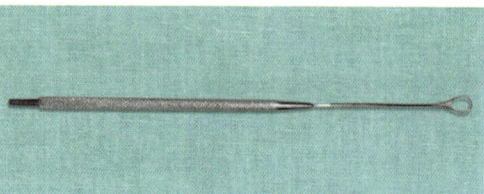

Fig. 3.4.7: Wire vectis.

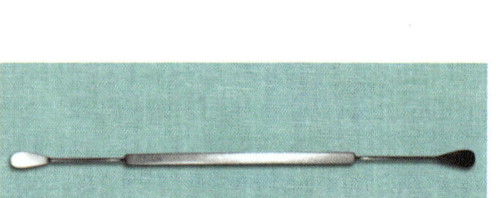

Fig. 3.4.6: Lens spatula.

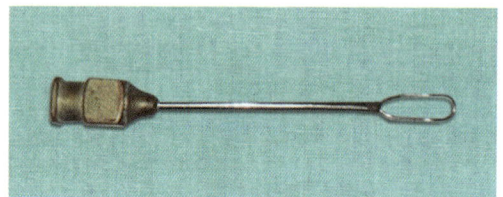

Fig. 3.4.8: Irrigating wire vectis.

operate—(1) one sharp and (2) one blunt. These can be curved, straight, or angulated.

Uses

- For cutting sutures
- For performing anterior capsulotomy in ECCE
- For cutting the vitreous strand while performing anterior vitrectomy
- For excising the host corneal ledge during keratoplasty

■ LENS SPATULA (FIG. 3.4.6)

Lens spatula has a metallic handle with spoon-shaped end, which is used to apply pressure at 12 o'clock position in Smith's technique and expression of nucleus in ECCE.

■ WIRE VECTIS (FIG. 3.4.7)

Wire vectis is a wire loop attached to metallic handle.

Uses

It is used to remove subluxated lens in ICCE and nucleus in ECCE.

While it is extremely useful in retrieving the nucleus pieces in the event of posterior capsular rent (PCR) during cataract surgery, it can lead to complications like iridodialysis and giant retinal tear if performed blindly or when a desperate attempt is made to retrieve an already sinking nucleus from anterior vitreous cavity.

■ IRRIGATING WIRE VECTIS (FIG. 3.4.8)

Irrigating wire vectis is a modification of the wire vectis and has a hollow rim with a 0.3 mm opening at the anterior end and a hollow handle at the posterior end, which is attached to a hub similar to that of a hypodermic needle through which fluid can be injected. The advantage of using irrigation is that there is less chance of pulling unaimed structures like iris during nucleus delivery.

Use

It is used for hydro-/viscoexpression of the nucleus in ECCE and small-incision cataract surgery (SICS).

SIMCOE'S IRRIGATION AND ASPIRATION CANNULA (FIG. 3.4.9)

It is available in the classical and reverse design with both right-handed and left-handed models available in each design. It has an irrigation system through the main port and aspiration system through the port on the side, which is attached to a syringe through a silicon tube.

Uses

- For irrigation and aspiration of cortical matter in ECCE and open sky cataract surgery in keratoplasty
- For aspiration of hyphema

Simcoe cannula is extremely useful in the setting of PCR with retained cortical matter. One modification to minimize vitreous loss is to remove the irrigation cannula and aspirating the retained lens matters after filling the AC with viscoelastics (dry IA). By removing the irrigating fluid, hydration of vitreous is prevented, thereby reducing further vitreous loss.

DASTOOR'S IRIS REPOSITOR (FIG. 3.4.10)

It is a flat and straight/bent blade with blunt edges.

Uses

- To reposit the iris in the AC
- To tuck the donor cornea underneath the host cornea in keratoplasty surgery

CYSTOTOME NEEDLE (FIG. 3.4.11)

Cystotome needle is prepared with a 26-gauge needle by bending the needle tip down while holding the bevel up. Then, while maintaining this needle orientation, bend the needle up near the hub. Experience will aid in determining the optimal preferred angles. Most commonly, bends near 90° are common at the tip and slightly less than this angle at the hub. However, authors recommend a bend that is >90° so that the tip of the needle and its contact point with the anterior capsule are clearly visible. This would prevent capsulotomy-related complications like

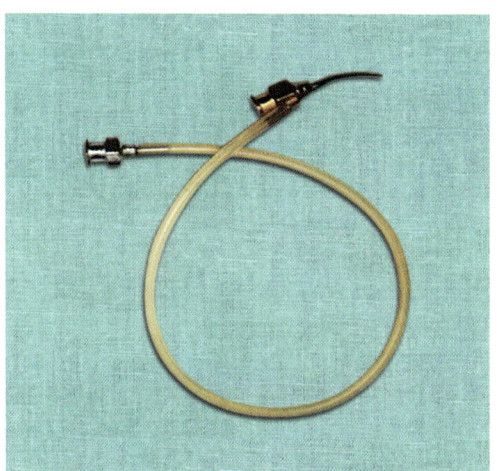

Fig. 3.4.9: Simcoe's irrigation and aspiration cannula.

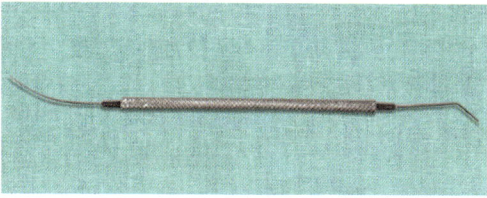

Fig. 3.4.10: Dastoor's iris repositor.

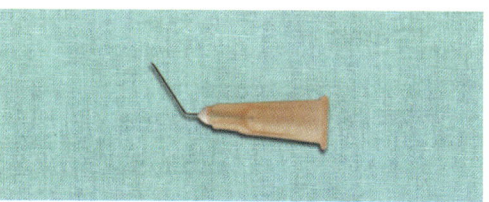

Fig. 3.4.11: Cystotome needle.

rhexis extension. Some surgeons introduce a third bend downward in the middle of the needle to get more vertical displacement of the tip to aid in reaching down into deep ACs.

The advantage of 26-gauge needle is that it is disposable (useful in camp/mass surgery setup), more controlled, and can be used through the sideport incision compared to utrata forceps. The limitation is that the torque generated is less compared to the utrata forceps hence, it is not preferred in cases like pediatric cataract where the capsule is extremely elastic and the chances of extension is high.

Uses

- It is used to make the anterior capsulotomy in ECCE as well as capsulorhexis in phacoemulsification.
- To initiate posterior capsulorhexis in pediatric cataract surgery

UTRATA CAPSULORHEXIS FORCEPS (FIG. 3.4.12)

The forceps have a fine precise tip with a sharp point that enables to initiate the capsular tear and then securely grasp the capsule to perform the capsulorhexis. It also has an "iris stop platform" to stop the shafts of the forceps from completely closing when tips are closed. This avoids inadvertent trauma to iris tissue. A 2.2 mm incision is required to insert this instrument into the AC. The force generated is much better compared to cystotome, hence preferred in pediatric cataract, intumescent lens, fibrosed capsule, lax capsule (subluxated lens), posterior capsulorhexis, and hypermature cataract. The limitation is that it needs a larger incision and chamber stability is often difficult in inexperienced hand.

McPHERSON'S FORCEPS (FIG. 3.4.13)

McPherson's forceps is a fine, sharp-tipped nontoothed forceps with angulation.

Uses

- Holding the IOL while implanting it
- Holding the suture while tying the knot
- Suture removal
- Removal of capsular tags/retained lens matters/foreign body (FB) from AC.

ARRUGA'S INTRACAPSULAR (CAPSULE HOLDING) FORCEPS (FIG. 3.4.14)

This forceps has a cup at inner side of the tip of each limb to create enough vacuum force for

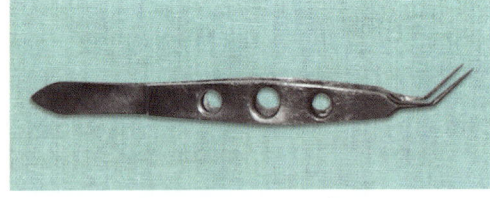

Fig. 3.4.13: McPherson's forceps.

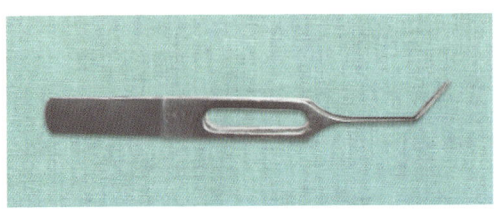

Fig. 3.4.12: Utrata capsulorhexis forceps.

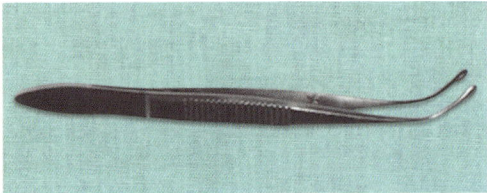

Fig. 3.4.14: Arruga's intracapsular (capsule-holding) forceps.

a tight grip. The edges of the cup are smooth and atraumatic to the lens capsule.

Uses

- It is used to remove the lens during forceps method of ICCE.
- It is also used to remove the lens capsule remnant after accidental ECCE.

INTRAOCULAR LENS HOLDING FORCEPS (FIG. 3.4.15)

Intraocular lens holding forceps are spring action forceps with short, blunt, and curved blades having smooth edges and tips.

Use

To hold the optic of nonfoldable PMMA IOL during implantation.

SINSKEY HOOK OR INTRAOCULAR LENS DIALER (FIG. 3.4.16)

This is a fine instrument with a bent blunt tip. The tip can engage the dialing holes of the IOL.

Uses

- Dialing of the nonfoldable PMMA IOL for proper positioning in the capsular bag or sulcus
- Also used in nucleus manipulation in phacoemulsification
- Useful to check for any vitreous strand by sweeping across the suspected area

CHOPPER (FIG. 3.4.17)

Chopper is similar in appearance to the Sinskey hook but the difference lies in the tip, which is sharp with cutting edges in a chopper. A sharp chopper is useful in cases of hard cataract.

Use

To split or chop the nucleus into smaller pieces during phacoemulsification

PHACO NEEDLE TIP (FIG. 3.4.18)

Phaco needle tip is made of titanium with a distal opening of 0.9 mm in diameter with a

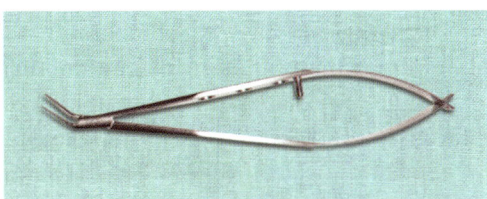

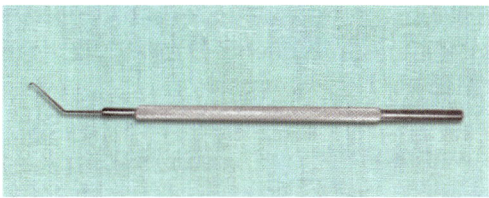

Fig. 3.4.17: Chopper.

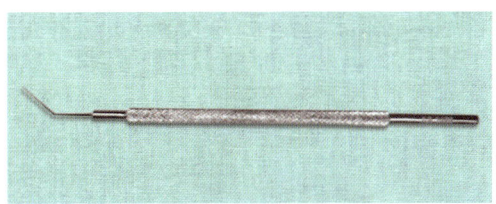

Fig. 3.4.15: Intraocular lens (IOL) holding forceps.

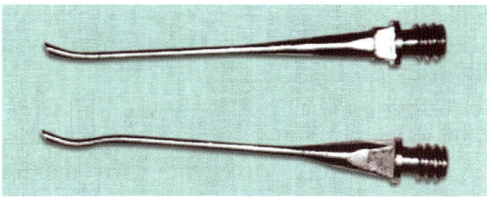

Fig. 3.4.16: Sinskey hook or intraocular lens (IOL) dialer.

Fig. 3.4.18: Phaco needle tip. The 45° conventional tip with a 22° bend (top) and the new 45° balanced tip (bottom). Note the single bend in the conventional tip and two bends in the new balanced tip.

silicon sleeve, which has two openings on the side 180° apart, through which the irrigation fluid flows. The phaco needle threads directly onto the phaco handpiece.

The tip can have bevel of 0°, 15°, 30°, 45°, or 60°. The greater is the angulation of the bevel tip, the better is the sculpting effect and visibility of the tip but leads to poor occlusion. The 30° bevel offers the best compromise and leads to better sculpting, visibility as well as occlusion. The silicon sleeve acts as an insulator and the fluid flowing through the sleeve keep the tip cool and prevents wound burn.

The Kelman tip has a 22° angulation of the shaft of 3.5 mm from the tip. This enhances the emulsification as well as allows the surgeon to use the phaco tip in manipulating the nucleus during surgery. Kelman tip makes phacoemulsification faster; however, the chances of PCR are higher.

The Flared tip has an outer diameter greater at the tip than 1–2 mm behind it. This helps to enhance the emulsification effect and reduce the postocclusion surge.

The Cobra tip is bell-shaped tip, which increases the surface producing the ultrasound to reduce the level of energy required.

Balanced Tip

It is a phaco tip that has especially been designed for torsional ultrasound. Its design though similar to Kelman tip but has two curves near the tip. There is increased lateral movement at its tip but decreased lateral movement at the incision site compared to conventional phaco tips. Therefore, it is especially useful in cases with hard cataract as it reduces the cumulative dissipated energy, total ultrasound time, torsion amplitude, aspiration time, fluid used, and wound burn.

■ VIVA QUESTIONS

1. What are the different types of surgical incisions in cataract surgery?

Ans. The different surgical incisions for cataract surgery are:
- *Scleral:* It induces less astigmatism and is self-sealing but has increased risk of conjunctival ballooning and subconjunctival hemorrhage. Peritomy, cauterizing of blood vessels that are inherent to this incision, can increase the surgical time although marginally. In addition, it is difficult to perform under topical anesthesia. Best suitable for cases where a PMMA IOL is planned or when corneal diameter is less (e.g., Iridofundal coloboma (IFC)) or when endothelium status is compromised.
- *Limbal:* It has advantages of both corneal and sclera incisions. It induces less astigmatism, has good wound apposition, and less patient discomfort. The risk of iatrogenic limbal stem cell deficiency is very rare but is a possibility with large limbal incisions. Similar to scleral incision, it is difficult to perform under topical anesthesia.
- *Corneal:* It is easy to construct with minimal manipulation of conjunctiva but the disadvantages are that it induces astigmatism and has poor wound apposition. These kind of incisions are free of any bleeding (preferred for patients on anticoagulants) and most suited for surgery under topical anesthesia. Corneal incisions are the most preferred incision for phacoemulsification.

2. What are the types of clear corneal incision?

Ans. The types of clear corneal incision are:
- *Uniplanar:* Easy to construct but poor self-sealing

- *Biplanar:* Relatively easy to construct with better self-sealing
- *Triplanar:* Relatively difficult to construct with better self-sealing but risk of DMD is more
- *Hinged:* Very difficult to construct but best self-sealing

3. What is hydrodissection and hydrodelineation?

Ans. Hydrodissection is separation of the cortex from lens capsule by injecting fluid while hydrodelineation is the separation of the epinucleus from the inner compact nucleus by injection of fluid.

4. What are soft-shell, ultimate soft-shell, and tri-soft shell techniques?

Ans.
- *Soft-shell technique:* A low-viscosity dispersive ophthalmic viscosurgical device (OVD) (Viscoat) is injected first onto the surface of the lens, followed by a viscous cohesive, which pushes the dispersive up into a smooth layer against the endothelium, providing a protective layer.
- *Ultimate soft-shell technique:* Uses viscoadaptive (Healon 5) and balanced salt solution (BSS) instead of dispersive OVD. The BSS layer allows ease in turning the capsulorhexis, provides an area to place capsular dye, and provides area for circulation of BSS, thus avoiding phaco handpiece overheating and possible corneal burns.
- *Tri-soft shell technique:* Uses layers of dispersive against the cornea, viscous cohesive centrally to establish stability, and BSS on the lenticular surface for a low-viscosity surgical space.

5. What is the ideal size of capsulorhexis?

Ans. Ideally the rhexis should cover 0.5 mm of the IOL all around. Therefore, the ideal size is around 5–5.5 mm. 0.5 mm overlap prevents the posterior migration of "A" cells, thereby reducing the chances of posterior capsular opacification (PCO).

6. Concept of continuous curvilinear capsulorhexis (CCC) was given by:

Ans. Howard Gimbel and Thomas Neuhann.

7. Name the various capsulotomy techniques that have been described in literature.

Ans. The different capsulotomy techniques are:
- *Vogt's technique:* Toothed forceps is used for grasping and ripping out a part of anterior capsule.
- *Kelman's "Christmas-tree" approach:* Cystitome is used to peel anterior capsule in a triangular or Christmas-tree morphology
- *"Can-opener" technique:* Cystitome is used for interconnecting perforations of anterior capsule to create a circular window. This technique provides precise control of size and shape of the capsular opening
- *Galand "letterbox" technique:* Two steps procedure in which the anterior capsular opening is completed after implantation of the IOL.

8. What are the causes of capsulorhexis run-out?

Ans.
- Shallow AC
- Inadequate viscoelastic injection
- Weak zonules [as in pseudoexfoliation (PXF) syndrome]
- High positive vitreous pressure (e.g., either due to excessive injection of anesthesia or inadequate anesthesia)
- Large CCC that may disrupt the anterior zonules
- Intumescent cataract
- Hypermature cataracts
- *Pediatric cataracts*—with elastic anterior capsules

9. What is capsulorhexis rescue technique?

Ans. In this technique, described by "Little et al.", a cohesive OVD is injected at the site of extending capsulorhexis to flatten the anterior capsule followed by grasping and pulling the extending edge of rhexis toward the center. After this maneuver, the rhexis can be continued regularly.

10. What are the various chopping techniques?

Ans. The classic "Nagahara technique" of *horizontal chopping* involves movement of both the phaco tip and chopper toward each other in the horizontal plane during the chop. The phaco tip is deeply buried in the center of the nucleus using high vacuum, with insertion of chopper under the anterior capsule engaging the endonucleus near the equator followed by inward movement of the chopper toward the phaco tip to crack the nucleus into two pieces.

Vertical chopping involves burying the phaco tip in the center of the nucleus using high vacuum. After ensuring that the center of the nucleus is adequately impaled with the phaco tip, a chopper with a sharp tip is buried within the nucleus adjacent to the phaco tip. The phaco tip is then lifted up while the chopper is depressed down, which results in cracking of the nucleus along the natural fault lines in the nucleus.

Stop-and-chop phaco involves creation of a central groove in the nucleus followed by division of the nucleus into two pieces through sculpting and cracking. This is followed by subsequent chopping of the two nucleus pieces.

11. Give the advantage of balanced phaco tip.

Ans. Refer to text.

12. What are the different techniques of performing ICCE?

Ans.

- Verhoeff and Kirby described the use of forceps to hold the upper anterior surface of the capsule to deliver the upper pole first.
- *Arruga's capsule forceps method/tumbling technique:* Arruga's capsule holding forceps is used to hold the anterior surface of the lens capsule at 6 o'clock position. The lens is then lifted slightly with gentle sideways movements to break the zonules. The lens is then delivered by gentle sliding movements by the forceps along with pressure at 6 o'clock position near the limbus by a lens expressor.
- Barraquer described the use of *suction cup* for holding the lens capsule and subsequent delivering of the lens.
- *Indian Smith method:* The lens is delivered with tumbling technique by applying pressure on limbus at 6 o'clock position with lens expressor and counterpressure at 12 o'clock with the lens spatula. In this technique, the lower pole of lens is delivered first.
- *Cryoextraction:* In this technique, the tip of cryoprobe is placed on the anterior surface of the lens in the upper quadrant. With a temperature of $-40°C$, an adhesion is created between the lens capsule and the cryoprobe. With gentle rotator movements, the zonules are broken and the lens is extracted out by sliding movements. The upper pole of the lens is delivered first.
- *Irisophake* method
- *Wire vectis method:* It is used in cases with subluxated or dislocated lens. In this technique, the loop of wire vectis is slid below the subluxated lens, which is then lifted and delivered.

- Alpha-chymotrypsin is used in cases where the zonules are found to be very resistant.

13. What are the different techniques for delivering the nucleus in SICS?
Ans.
- *Blumenthal's AC maintainer technique:* The nucleus is engaged into the corneoscleral tunnel followed by injection of ophthalmic viscosurgical device (OVD) both above and below the nucleus. A lens glide is then passed behind the nucleus and with the help of intermittent hydropressure generated by the AC maintainer, the nucleus is delivered out of the tunnel's mouth.
- *Wire vectis technique:* Wire vectis is used to deliver the nucleus.
- *Irrigating vectis technique/Microvectis technique:* Irrigating wire vectis is used to deliver the nucleus by either hydroexpression or viscoexpression. The irrigating wire vectis is 4 mm in width and 9 mm in length. The anterior surface is concave with three 0.3 mm openings at one end. The other end is continuous with the main body and can be attached to a syringe or infusion set.
- *Phacofracture technique:* After the nucleus is prolapsed at the iris pupillary plane, a wire vectis is insinuated under the nucleus followed by positioning of a nucleotome on the anterior surface of nucleus. The *two* instruments are then maneuvered toward each other leading to cleavage of the nuclear substance. Nuclear forceps, which have a 9.0 mm long jaw (each having a double row of teeth), are used to deliver the nucleus fragments.
- *Fish hook technique:* In this technique, initially only the superior pole of nucleus is brought into the AC. OVD is injected both in front and behind the nucleus. The tip of 30G needle is bent in the form of hook and is then maneuvered behind the nucleus to hook the undersurface of the nucleus. Once the nucleus is hooked, it is delivered by applying gentle pressure over the posterior lip of the tunnel.
- *Ruit's technique:* OVD is injected around the nucleus to prolapse it into AC. An irrigating Simcoe cannula is then inserted below it, which aids in delivering the nucleus with hydropressure.
- *Phacosandwich technique:* In this technique, the nucleus is prolapsed into AC and delivered by sandwiching the nucleus between a dialer and vectis.
- *Viscoexpression:* Viscoelastic is continuously injected into AC to deliver the nucleus.

CHAPTER 4

Retina and Uvea

4.1 OPHTHALMOSCOPE

Alisha Kishore, Hannah Shiny R, Suman Meena, Pranita Sahay

BINOCULAR INDIRECT OPHTHALMOSCOPE

Introduction

Ophthalmoscopy, also called Fundoscopy, is a test that allows viewing inside the fundus of the eye and other structures using an ophthalmoscope. Broadly, it can be categorized as direct and indirect. Marc Antonie Giracid Tenlon of France invented the first binocular indirect ophthalmoscope in 1861. Charles Schepens described the first binocular indirect ophthalmoscope in 1945 **(Fig. 4.1.1)**.

Principle

The parts of an indirect ophthalmoscope are a headset with binocular viewing box and a light source, which can be adjusted. The view box has prisms acting to optically reduce the interpupillary distance of the observer forming a binocular stereoscopic image. The light is brought to focus on an angled mirror, which is then reflected into the patient's eye. Light passes through the pupil and is reflected from the retinal surface. The reflected light is then brought to focus with a handheld convex lens **(Fig. 4.1.2)**. Indirect ophthalmoscope works on the principle that by placing a convex lens in front, the eye is made highly myopic.

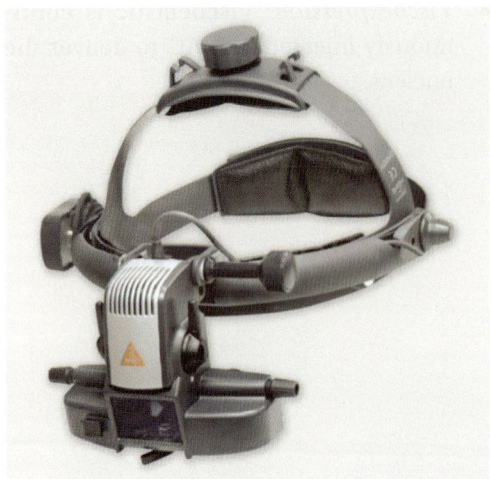

Fig. 4.1.1: Indirect ophthalmoscope.

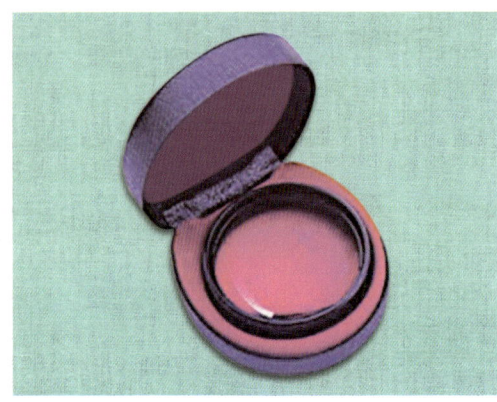

Fig. 4.1.2: 20 D lens.

The image is formed between the lens and the observer and is inverted and real.

In the emmetropic eyes, reflected light from the retina are parallel and is hence brought to focus by the condensing lens. An inverted image is therefore formed at the principal focus of the lens, which lies between the lens and the observer.[1]

In hypermetropia, the emerging rays will diverge and appear to come from an imaginary enlarged upright image situated behind the eye. The condensing lens, therefore, uses this as an object and forms an inverted image of it. Since the rays are divergent, the final image will be situated in front of its principal focus.[1]

In the myopic eye, the rays coming from the fundus are convergent and therefore an inverted image is formed in front of the eye. A second smaller image is then formed by the condensing lens at a point within its focal length.[1]

The most commonly used handheld lens is a 20 D aspheric lens. It has a field of view of 46°/60° and provides an image magnification of 3.13×. The working distance is 50 mm.[2] The magnification of various lenses is described in **Table 4.1.1**.

Technique

The prerequisites for an indirect ophthalmoscopic examination are a darkroom and fully dilated pupil of the patient. The procedure is explained to the patient, and he is made to lie in the supine position or sit comfortably. Adjust the headset of the ophthalmoscope to a comfortable position. Move the eyepiece to set the interpupillary distance. The examination is carried out at an outstretched arms distance. The light of the ophthalmoscope, the condensing lens, the patient's pupil, and the retina must fall on one line. A bright red reflex appears when the examiner aligns his viewing access with the patient's pupil. The handheld lens is then placed over the patient's eye and adjusted until an image is identified. The most convex surface of the lens must face the examiner. The opposite surface is marked on most lenses by an unpainted edge and this must face the patient. The periphery of the retina is examined first because it is the least light-sensitive part. The examiner has to stand opposite to the clock-hour position to be examined, e.g., to examine the inferior quadrant the examiner stands toward the patient's head.[2]

Scleral Indentation

The peripheral retina can be examined in detail, by performing scleral indentation. Schepens scleral indentor **(Fig. 4.1.3)**,

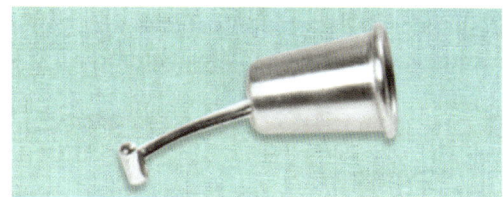

Fig. 4.1.3: Schepens scleral depressor.

TABLE 4.1.1: Field of view, magnification, and working distance of various lenses.

Lens	Field of view	Magnification	Working distance
14 D	36°/43°	4.30×	75 mm
20 D	46°/60°	3.13×	50 mm
28 D	53°/69°	2.27×	33 mm
2.2 Panretinal lens	56°/73°	2.68×	40 mm

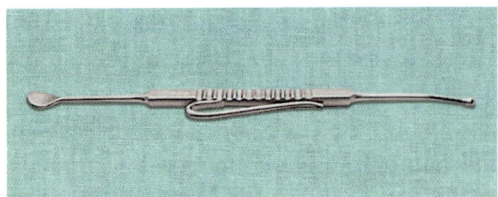

Fig. 4.1.4: Josephberg–Besser scleral depressor, double-ended.

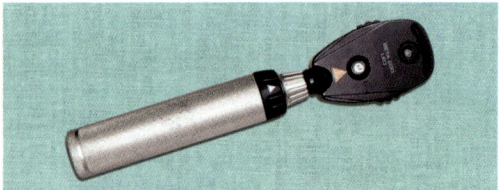

Fig. 4.1.5: Direct ophthalmoscope.

sockets indentor **(Fig. 4.1.4)**, or a cotton tip applicator can be used.[2]

Instillation of topical anesthesia reduces the pain during the procedure. In order to visualize the superior peripheral retina, the scleral depressor is positioned vertically at 12 o'clock while the patient looks down. The patient is then asked to look superiorly, allowing the visualization of the indent of the depressor with indirect ophthalmoscopy. If the indent is not visible, it indicates that the depressor is placed too anteriorly, or the indent is too less.

The nasal and temporal periphery of the retina is the most difficult to indent because of lesser fornix space and presence of canthal ligaments.[2]

Indentation must be done very gently in patients who have undergone filtering surgeries as it can cause bleb leakage. Scleral depression is deferred in patients with globe rupture and hyphema following trauma.

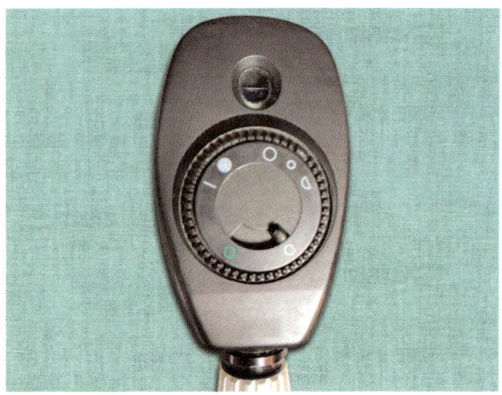

Fig. 4.1.6: Head of direct ophthalmoscope.

■ DIRECT OPHTHALMOSCOPE

Introduction

Scientists discovered that using a coaxial illumination observation system, with the light source kept close to the eye, visualization of the retina is possible. Charles Babbage made the first practical ophthalmoscope. Following which Von Helmholtz in 1851 described the direct ophthalmoscope.[3,4] As the name indicates, a direct image is formed on the retina in a direct ophthalmoscope, and there is no intermediate image formation, unlike in an indirect ophthalmoscope.[3]

Parts

It consists of a metallic optical tube containing a lamp, aperture dial assembly, mirror/prism, and objective and condensing lens **(Figs. 4.1.5 and 4.1.6)**.[4]

Illumination System

It consists of a halogen lamp powered by rechargeable battery, an aperture dial with different apertures including Linkz star, cobalt blue filter, medium and large spot, hemispot, slit and pinhole **(Fig. 4.1.7)**. It has two condensing lenses, one on each side of the aperture dial. It also has angled mirrors at 45°, which are nowadays replaced in a modern ophthalmoscope by prisms **(Table 4.1.2)**.[4]

Observation System

It has condensing lens of power +1 to +10, +15, +20, +40, and −1 to −10, −15, −20, −25, −35, a viewing window with antireflective coating

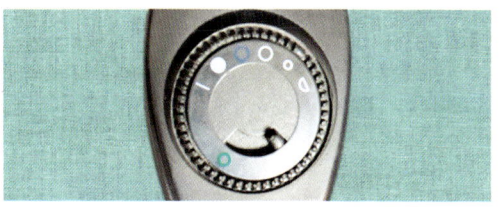

Fig. 4.1.7: Apertures of direct ophthalmoscope.

to avoid glare and a red-free filter to detect nerve fiber layer defects.[4]

Optical Principle

The image formed depends on the distance at which the ophthalmoscope is used. When used for distant direct ophthalmoscopy at a distance of 25 cm a real, inverted, unmagnified image is formed. When fundoscopy is done at a very near distance to the subject's eye, a virtual, erect image is formed.

The emergent rays of light from an emmetropic patient are parallel and are

TABLE 4.1.2: Uses of various apertures in a direct ophthalmoscope.

Aperture type		Use
Small spot		For seeing through small pupil, provides approximately a 5° cone
Large spot		For viewing in dilated pupil
Macular spot/pinhole		To observe only fovea, enables view through even 2 mm pupil
Hemispot or half-circle diaphragm		• Reduces corneal reflex and improved depth of perception; avoids fundus reflection while examining the fundus • It is also helpful in the observation of certain fine retinal details that are seen best in the transitional zone between illuminated and nonilluminated retina

Contd...

Contd...

Aperture type	Use
Slit	Accurate evaluation of retinal elevation and depression (diagnosis of retinal detachment, tumors, disc edema), anterior chamber depth
Cobalt blue	• For corneal abrasions • To enhance the visibility of fluorescein, for use in fluorescein angioscopy and as a handheld light source for fluorescein staining of the cornea
Linkz star/fixation star with polar coordinates	Graduated cross-hairs for measuring eccentric fixation or locating lesions
Red-free filter	• Better visualization of blood vessel, hemorrhage, and retinal nerve fiber layer (RNFL) • Differentiate between retinal and choroidal lesion • It also makes small macroaneurysms and small hemorrhage standout more clearly. • RNFL defect • Helpful in estimating cup-to-disc (C/D) ratio

Note: Not all filters are present in every ophthalmoscope.

brought to focus on the observer's retina. If the patient is hypermetropia, the emergent rays are divergent and will be brought to focus on the observer's retina only if the latter accommodates or if a convex lens is used. On the other hand, if the subject is myopic, the emergent rays are convergent and should be interposed by a concave lens to bring them to focus on the observer's retina.

When the accommodation of the subject and the observer is at rest, the refractive error of the observer is corrected fully, the mirror of the ophthalmoscope is held at the anterior focal point of the eye 15.7 mm in front of the cornea, and if the disc is seen, then the eye is emmetropic. If the image formed is not clear, the convex lenses of increasing power are turned in front of the observer's eye and the highest power, which produces a clear image give the measure of hypermetropia. If the image becomes progressively blurred with the convex lens, then the concave lens is turned on, and the highest power, which forms a clear image gives the myopic power of the patient. If astigmatism is present, then the blood vessels are blurred unequally in different directions, and when spherical lenses are presented in the ophthalmoscope, only the vessels that are perpendicular to that meridian will become clear.

The direct ophthalmoscope magnifies images to 15 times. The field of view is 5° and is directly proportional to the size of the subject's pupil, the axial length of the patient and inversely proportional to the distance between subject and observer.[3]

Technique

First examine the patient from a distance of 1 m to look for abnormality of the lid, orbit, and ocular deviation. Then, the examination is carried out at 25 cm from the subject. A red reflex or any media opacity can be seen. To identify the position of the opacity, the patient is asked to look in all four gazes, and movement of the opacity is noted. Opacity lying behind the lens moves against the ocular movements, whereas any opacity lying in the cornea or anterior chamber moves along with ocular gaze. Any squint can be seen as an unequal reflex (Brückner test). One should also look for relative afferent pupillary defect (RAPD). The retina should be brought to focus by moving closer to the patient. As the retina gets focused, look for the blood vessels and trace them backward to reach the optic disc. The macula is focused by asking the patient to focus into the light. The right eye should be examined using the right eye of the observer and vice versa.

Modifications of ophthalmoscope include a panoptic ophthalmoscope, which works on the principle of axial point-source optics. This enables a large field of view and reduces corneal reflexes.[4,5]

■ VIVA QUESTIONS

1. At what distance is the distant direct ophthalmoscopy performed?
Ans. At 25 cm.

2. How will you quantify disc edema using direct ophthalmoscope?
Ans. The direct ophthalmoscope is first focused on the surface of the disc. The dioptric power at which the disc is focused clearly is noted and then the ophthalmoscope is used to focus on the adjacent retina for which the dioptric power is noted again. The difference between the two dioptric powers gives the amount of elevation. Every addition of +3 D equals to 1 mm elevation in phakics and 2 mm in aphakics.

3. Mention the differences between direct and indirect ophthalmoscope.
Ans. Refer to **Table 4.1.3**.

4. Is there any light exposure hazard with the use of direct ophthalmoscope?
Ans. Prolonged exposure to intense light damages the retina. Hence, the minimum intensity of light, which allows clear visualization of structures should be used.

TABLE 4.1.3: Difference between direct and indirect ophthalmoscope.

	Direct ophthalmoscope	Indirect ophthalmoscope
Stereopsis	Absent	Present
Magnification	15 times	5 times
Static field of view	2-disc diameter	8-disc diameter
Dynamic field of view	Up to equator	Up to ora serrata
Retinal image	Virtual, erect	Real, inverted
Technique	Easy	Difficult
Illumination	Good	Excellent
Uses	Diagnostic mainly	Diagnostic and therapeutic (laser)

Persons at risk are:
- Infants
- Aphakes
- Persons with retinal disease
- Eye exposed to retinal photography, the same procedure repeated within of 24 hours.

During operating conditions at a maximum light intensity, the duration of exposure should not exceed the durations as described in **Table 4.1.4** (for HEINE direct ophthalmoscopes).

5. How will you optimize lamp life?
Ans. Keep on time <2 minutes with off time not <15 minutes.

REFERENCES

1. Abrams D. Duke-Elder's Practice of Refraction, 10th edition. London: J & A Churchill Ltd; 1954.

TABLE 4.1.4: Recommended exposure to light with direct ophthalmoscope when operated at maximum intensity.

Distance from instrument to patient (mm)	Duration (min)
10	≤8–10*
50	≤3–8*
100	≤1–3*

* The higher duration is for LED bulbs.

2. Wirthlin RS, Young TA. Pearls on indirect ophthalmoscopy. Tech Ophthalmoscopy. 2005;3(3):138-40.
3. Yanoff M, Duker JS. Ophthalmology, 3rd edition. St Louis: Elsevier Health Sciences; 2009.
4. Keeler CR. Babbage the unfortunate. Br J Ophthalmol. 2004;88:730-2.
5. Mark HH. On the evolution of binocular ophthalmoscopy. Arch Ophthalmol. 2007; 125(6):830-3.

4.2 FUNDUS FLUORESCEIN ANGIOGRAPHY

Nasiq Hasan, Priyanka, Brijesh Takkar, Rohan Chawla, Atul Kumar

INTRODUCTION

Fundus fluorescein angiography (FFA) was devised by two medical students (Novotny and Alvis) in 1959.[1] Blood flow through vessels of retina can be visualized using this technique, which allows sequential imaging with passage of time. It is a useful diagnostic modality that allows monitoring of posterior segment diseases and assesses the efficacy of retinal therapeutics.

The basic principle of FFA revolves around three phenomena:
1. *Luminescence* is the emission of light from any source not resulting due to high temperature.
2. *Fluorescence* is *luminescence* that is maintained by continuous excitation of electrons.
3. *Phosphorescence* continues to emit light even after the excitation is stopped.

There are earlier reports of performing FFA using oral fluorescein. However, in today's era, sodium fluorescein is injected intravenously. It is 80% protein-bound and the molecules fluoresce on excitation at a particular wavelength. In a fundus camera, a blue excitation filter permits only the blue light from a white source to enter the retina and absorbs all other light. This blue light excites the fluorescein in the bloodstream, which starts emitting green–yellow light at 520–530 nm. A barrier filter keeps out the blue excitation light (all wavelengths <520 nm) and allows only green–yellow light (all wavelengths >520 nm) to be captured electronically as a digital image.

Pseudofluorescence is a phenomenon that occurs when nonfluorescent light cannot be filtered by the entire filter system as seen in the case of old worn-out filters.

■ SODIUM FLUORESCEIN

Properties

Sodium fluorescein has the following properties:
- It is a water-soluble orange–red crystalline hydrocarbon, also known as *resorcinol phthalein sodium* ($C_{20}H_{10}Na_2O_5$) or uranine ($C_{20}H_{12}O_5Na$).
- It has a molecular weight of 376.27 Da.
- It is excited by blue light (465–490 nm) and emits green light (520–530 nm).
- *80% of the dye is protein-bound*, and this fraction does not fluoresce, only the unbound 20% fluoresces.
- The commercial concentration of solutions available is 10 mL of 5% fluorescein, 5 mL of 10% fluorescein, and 3 mL of 25% fluorescein.
- The fluorescein diffuses through the choriocapillaris, but cannot diffuse through the inner or outer blood-retinal barriers.
- It is usually eliminated by the kidney within 24 hours, although can be found in the body for a few weeks.

Side Effects

Side effects include the following:[2]
- Transient nausea and vomiting
- Vasovagal attacks
- Pain due to extravasation of dye
- Inadvertent arterial injection
- Thrombophlebitis
- Anaphylaxis
- Seizures
- Cardiorespiratory arrest

Contraindications

Contraindications include the following:
- *Absolute contraindications:*
  - Known history of allergy to the dye
  - Previous anaphylaxis to fluorescein angiography (FA)
- *Relative contraindications:*
  - The first trimester of pregnancy (although there are no reported complications)
  - Severe renal impairment
  - Recent cerebrovascular accident (CVA), myocardial infarction (MI), and unstable angina
  - History of heart disease, arrhythmia, and pacemakers are no contraindications.

■ FUNDUS CAMERA

The following systems have been used to acquire fluorescein images:
- Film-based fundus camera
- Digital fundus camera **(Fig. 4.2.1)**
- Confocal scanning laser ophthalmoscope (cSLO).

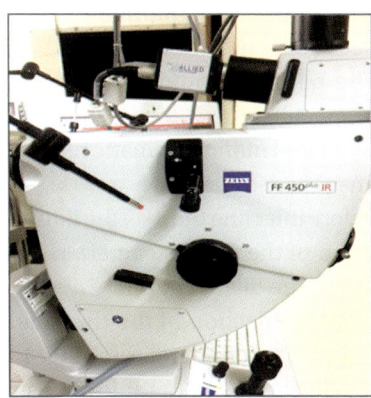

Fig. 4.2.1: Digital fundus camera.

Confocal scanning laser ophthalmoscope uses a near-infrared laser beam instead of the flash bulb used in digital and film-based systems.[3] This helps in the quick scanning of the retina and producing *high-resolution and high-contrast images in a very short span of time.* They use longer wavelength lasers and hence can be used to obtain fundus autofluorescence (FAF) and indocyanine green (ICG) images too.

Fundus cameras range from *30° to 50° field of view*; however, there are machines which can provide widefield and ultra-widefield images *up to 200°*. Montage system is used to capture peripheral angiograms with conventional cameras; however simultaneous imaging of each fundus field is not possible.

The exciter filter transmits blue light at 465–490 nm, which is the absorption peak of fluorescein excitation and the barrier filter transmits light at 525–530 nm, which is the fluorescent or emitted peak of fluorescein.

TECHNIQUE

Following are the steps of FFA:
1. Explain about the procedure to the patient and take informed consent.
2. The patient should ideally be *fasting* while performing FFA given the high likelihood of nausea and vomiting during the procedure.
3. The patient sits comfortably with a loose neck collar in front of the camera.
4. The patient should be positioned for proper alignment, focus, and comfort.
5. Color and monochromatic red-free filter images are obtained.
6. Before injecting the dye, the illuminating beam of the fundus camera is centered within the dilated pupil.
7. A bolus injection of the dye is administered in a peripheral vein **(Fig. 4.2.2)**.
8. Images are usually rapidly taken very second up till maximal fluorescence.
9. After early phase, images of the fellow eye and retinal periphery may be clicked.
10. When photography is done, the patient should be reassured about the discoloration of urine.

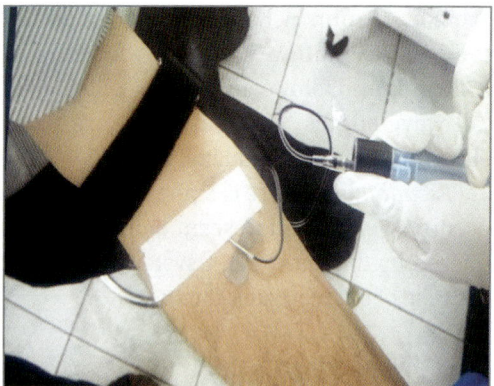

Fig. 4.2.2: Intravenous injection of fluorescein dye via the antecubital vein using a 24 G scalp vein attached to the 10-cc syringe.

PHASES OF FUNDUS FLUORESCEIN ANGIOGRAPHY

- *Arm-to-retina circulation time:* 10–12 seconds
- *Posterior ciliary arteries*: 9.5 seconds
- *Choroidal flush (or prearterial phase):* 10 seconds
- *Retinal arterial phase:* 0–12 seconds
- *Arteriovenous phase (laminar stage or early venous stage):* 14–15 seconds
- *Venous phase:* 16–17 seconds
- *Late phase:* 5 minutes

The foveal avascular zone (FAZ) is relatively hypofluorescent due to the presence of dense xanthophyll pigments, taller and more retinal pigment epithelium (RPE) cells, and absence of retinal capillaries in the center of fovea.

Choroidal Phase

Choroidal phase is due to the permeability of choriocapillaris to dye, causing a widespread area of hyperfluorescence.

A cilioretinal artery, if present, will fill during this phase as it is derived from posterior ciliary circulation.

Arterial Phase

Arterial phase is seen 2 seconds later when dye enters into retinal arterioles.

Arteriovenous Phase

Next the retinal capillaries fill followed by the laminar flow in veins seen as thin columns of dye along their walls.

Venous Phase

The arteriovenous phase is followed by a venous phase where the venous columns become broader as the dye fills up the venous lumen.

Mid Phase

About 2-4 minutes after injection, the veins and arteries remain roughly equal in brightness.

Late Phase

Gradual removal of dye can be seen at ~10 minutes postinjection. Disc margin remains hyperfluorescent due to staining **(Figs. 4.2.3A to C)**.

ABNORMAL FLUORESCEIN PATTERNS

Hypofluorescence: Reduced or absent normal fluorescence; it can be categorized to:
- *Blocked fluorescence—masking of fluorescence* **(Fig. 4.2.4A)**:
  - Any opacity anterior to the fluorescence like blood or media opacification
  - Additionally, choroidal fluorescence can be blocked by occurrence of abnormal pigment in RPE cells.
- Vascular filling defects—absence of vascular circulation **(Fig. 4.2.4B)**

Hyperfluorescence: Increased fluorescence
- *Leakage:* The area of fluorescence increases in both size and intensity with time **(Fig. 4.2.5A)**, e.g., neovascularization and macular edema.
- *Pooling:* The area of fluorescence is the same, but the intensity increases with time in a confined anatomical space **(Fig. 4.2.5B)**, e.g., focal serous retinal detachment and pigment epithelial detachment (PED).
- *Staining:* Increase in intensity over time in the late frame, but margins are irregular **(Fig. 4.2.5C)**, e.g., macular scars, drusen, and laser mark.

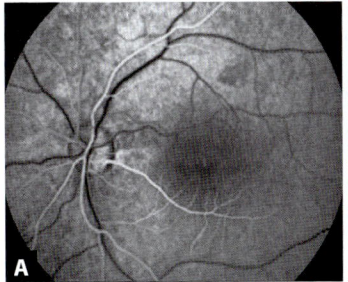 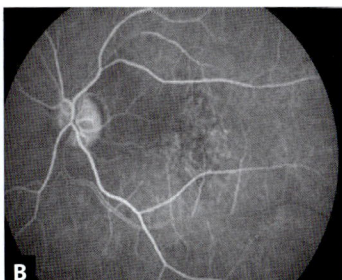 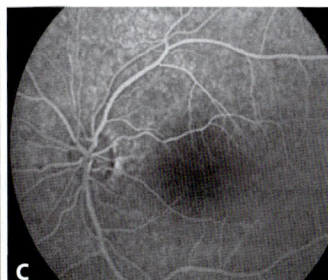

Figs. 4.2.3A to C: Normal fluorescein angiogram. (A) Arterial phase in which only the artery is filled with the dye; (B) Arteriovenous phase showing laminar flow along the walls of the veins; (C) Venous phase showing filling of veins also.

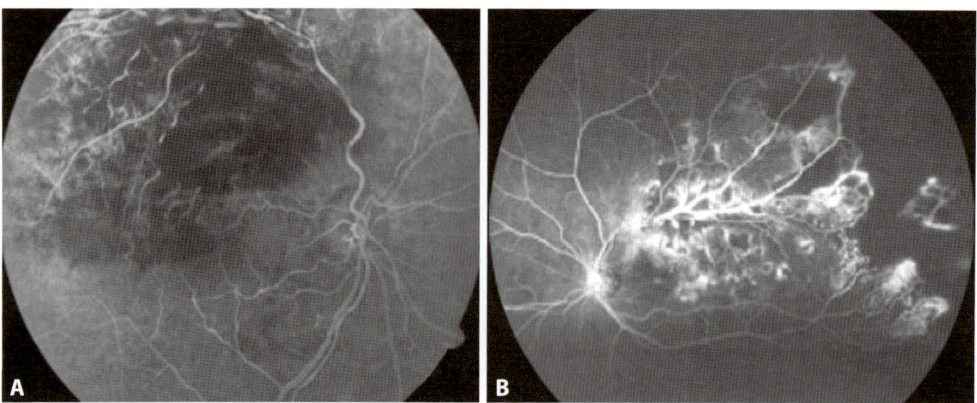

Figs. 4.2.4A and B: Hypofluorescence. (A) Blocked fluorescence where the underlying retinal vessels are obscured; (B) Vascular filling defects showing peripheral capillary nonperfusion areas in the temporal retina.

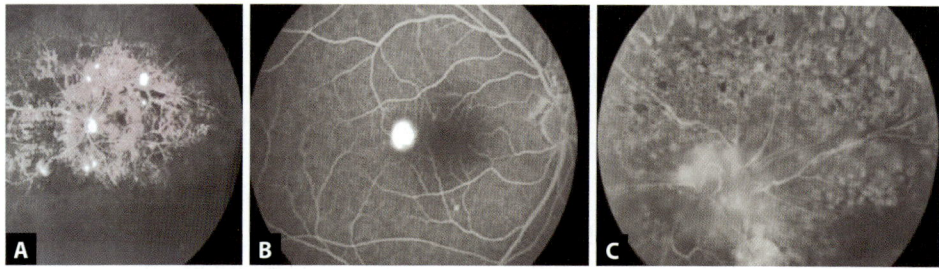

Figs. 4.2.5A to C: Hyperfluorescence. (A) Leak; (B) Pooling; (C) Stain.

- *Transmitted fluorescence (window defect):* Increased fluorescence from the underlying choroidal vasculature due to the absence of overlying pigment **(Fig. 4.2.6)**, e.g., geographical atrophy
- *Autofluorescence:* Continuous emission of fluorescent light from ocular structures in the absence of fluorescein dye, e.g., optic nerve head drusen, astrocytic hamartoma, and lipofuscin

CHARACTERISTIC FFA FEATURES OF CERTAIN CONDITIONS

- *Central serous choroidopathy*: Two types of leakage patterns are seen on FFA:
  1. Smock stack pattern **(Fig. 4.2.7)**
  2. Inkblot pattern **(Fig. 4.2.8)**

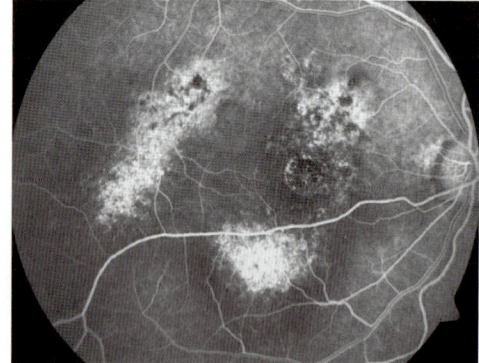

Fig. 4.2.6: Window defect is seen as hyperfluorescence as the overlying retinal pigment epithelium (RPE) shows atrophy.

- *Diabetic retinopathy (DR)*: Different stages of DR can have the following presentation:

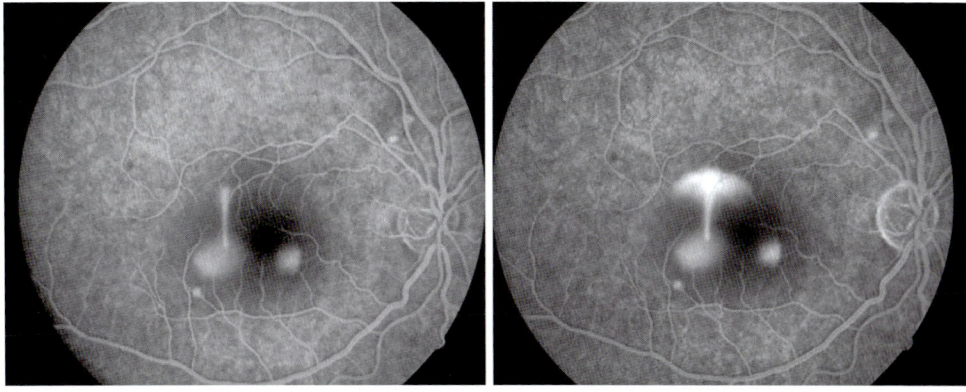

Fig. 4.2.7: Smokestack pattern of central serous chorioretinopathy (CSC) leak showing increasing hyperfluorescence in terms of area and intensity with time.

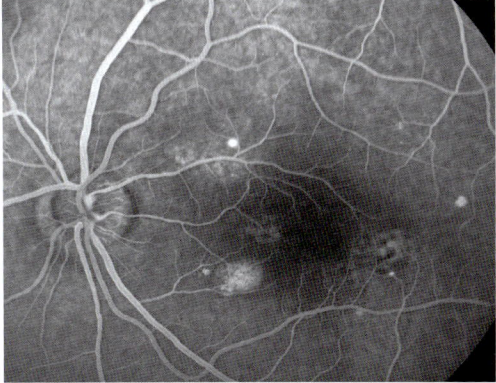

Fig. 4.2.8: A well-defined inkblot leak is seen superonasal to the fovea. A pigment epithelial detachment is seen temporal to the fovea. Additional areas of stippled hyperfluorescence are also visible.

- *Nonproliferative diabetic retinopathy (NPDR):*
  - *Mild NPDR:*
    - *Microaneurysms*: Appear as hyperfluorescent dots, which may leak in later phases **(Fig. 4.2.9A)**.
  - *Moderate NPDR:*
    - *Microaneurysms*: Appear as hyperfluorescent dots, which may leak in later phases.
    - Superficial and deep retinal hemorrhages cause blocked choroidal fluorescence.
    - Hard exudates **(Fig. 4.2.9B)**
  - *Severe NPDR:*
    - All features as in mild NPDR.
    - *Capillary nonperfusion (CNP) areas*: Appear as areas of hypofluorescence and usually outlined by dilated capillaries **(Fig. 4.2.9C)**.
    - Intraretinal microvascular abnormalities (IRMAs) are segmental and irregular dilatation of capillary bed lying within CNP areas. They may slightly leak in later phases at their growing tips.
    - Soft exudates cause blockage of choroidal fluorescence.
- *Proliferative diabetic retinopathy (PDR):*
  - Neovascularization of the disc (NVD) or neovascularization elsewhere (NVE) **(Fig. 4.2.9D)** on the retinal surface. These cause leakage of dye profusely, which increases in the late phase.
  - Preretinal (subhyaloid) hemorrhages block both retinal and choroidal fluorescence.

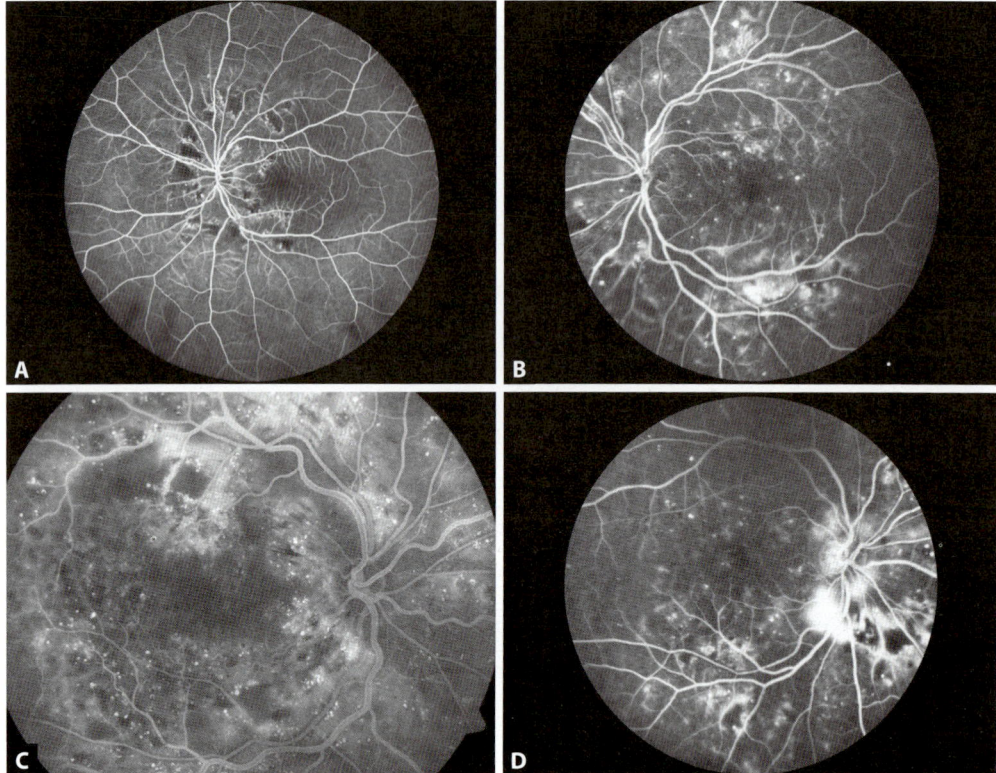

Figs. 4.2.9A to D: (A) Fluorescein angiogram of a diabetic patient showing focal hyperfluorescent microaneurysms; (B) Fluorescein angiogram of a diabetic patient showing multiple hard exudates, focal hyperfluorescent microaneurysms, and few areas of flame-shaped hemorrhages; and (C) This is a late phase fluorescein angiogram of a diabetic patient showing diffuse leak at the macula. Hypofluorescent capillary nonperfusion areas are also visible. Focal hyperfluorescent microaneurysms are also seen. Neovascularization of the disc (NVD) or neovascularization elsewhere (NVE) is not seen; (D) Fluorescein angiogram of a diabetic patient showing multiple areas of leaking NVE and NVD along with other features of severe nonproliferative diabetic retinopathy (NPDR).

- *Diabetic macular edema (DME)* **(Figs. 4.2.10A and B)**:
  - *Focal diabetic maculopathy:*
    - Focal leaks from microaneurysms in the macular area
    - Hard exudates cause blocked choroidal fluorescence, may also show staining.
  - *Diffuse diabetic maculopathy (cystoid):*
    - Dilated retinal capillaries leak diffusely into the macular area.
    - Typical petaloid or honeycomb pattern of cystoid macular edema (CME) may also be seen **(Fig. 4.2.10A)**.
  - *Ischemic diabetic maculopathy:* FAZ appears broken, i.e., CNP areas merge into FAZ.
- *Age-related macular degeneration (ARMD):*
  - Dry ARMD:
    - Geographical atrophy is usually seen as window defects with transmitted fluorescence from underlying choroid.

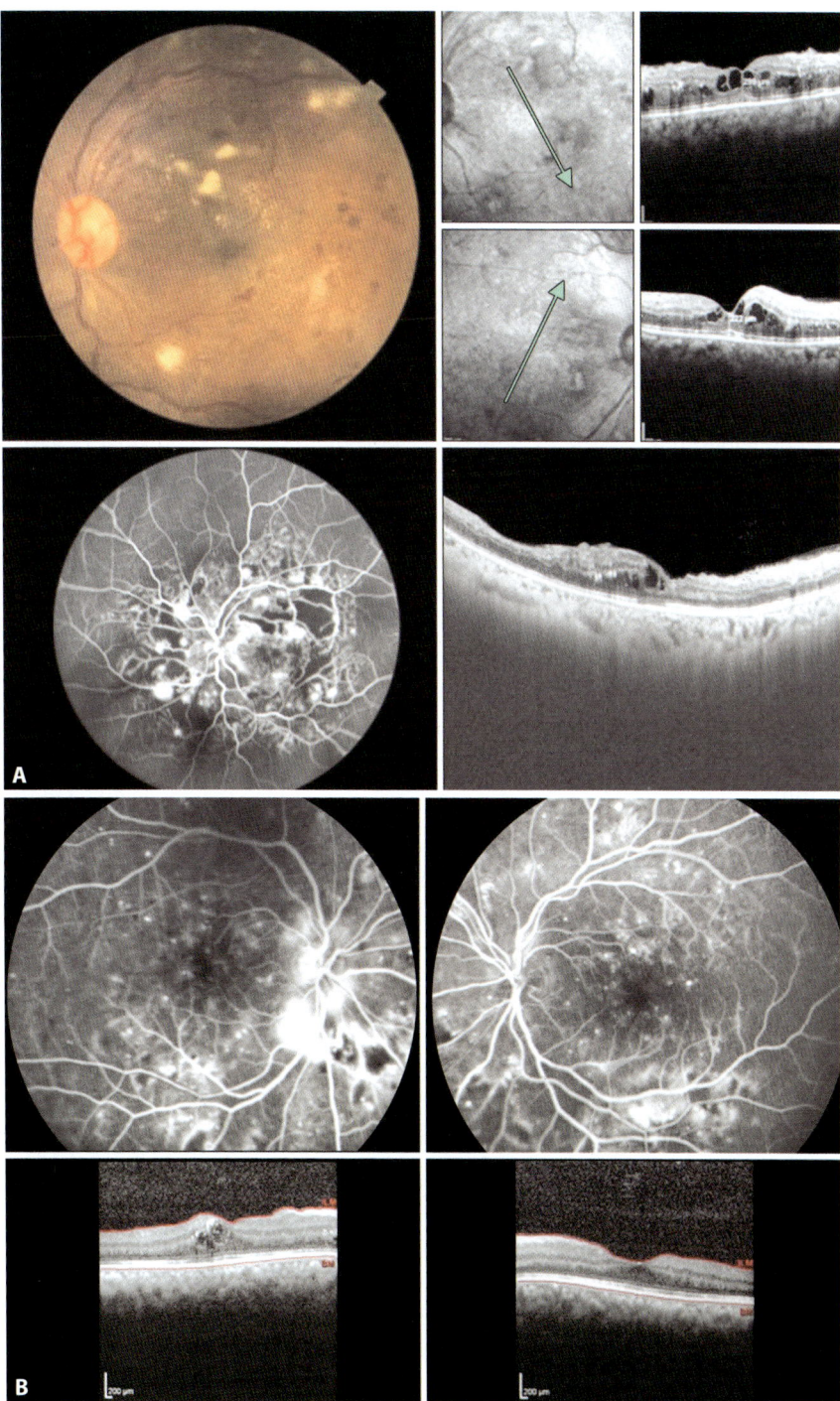

Figs. 4.2.10A and B: Diabetic macular edema corroborated with optical coherence tomography (OCT) findings.

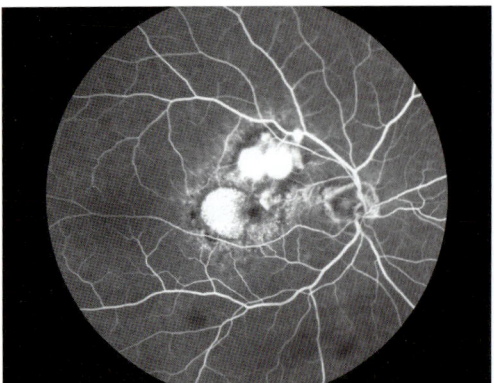
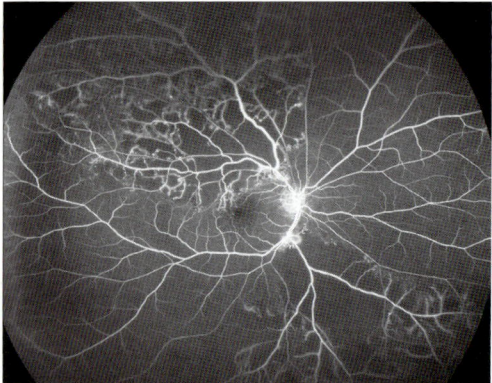

Fig. 4.2.11: Venous phase angiogram showing areas of well-defined hyperfluorescence, extrafoveal, and increasing with time. At the fovea, there is an area of pooling of fluorescein with an adjacent diamond-shaped area of leak. Associated stippled hyperfluorescence is also seen. Findings are suggestive of a combined type 1 and 2 choroidal neovascular membrane.

Fig. 4.2.12: This is a widefield (Optos) fluorescein angiogram showing two areas of vascular block (venous) one in the superotemporal quadrant and the other in the inferonasal quadrant. Both these areas show areas of capillary nonperfusion and few microaneurysms. Few focal leaking microaneurysms are also visible superior to the fovea. Neovascularization is not evident.

- Drusen can be hyperfluorescent (staining in late phase) or hypofluorescent depending on the concentration of lipid material.
- *Wet ARMD:*
  - Choroidal neovascular membrane (CNVM) can be seen as areas of the leak, serous PED as pooling and subretinal fibrosis/disciform scar as staining. Further submacular and intraretinal hemorrhage are seen as blocked hypofluorescence.
  - "Classic" choroidal neovascularization (CNV) is typically seen as a leak, in the early phase, which intensifies throughout the transit phase. It is uniform, with "lacy" margins **(Fig. 4.2.11)**.
  - "Occult" lesions are typically seen in the late phase of FA. It consists of two described forms on FA: (1) Fibrovascular PED (FVPED) and (2) late leakage of undetermined source (LLUS).
  - FVPED is seen as an irregular elevation of the RPE with stippled or granular irregular fluorescence. LLUS is seen as areas of hyperfluorescence at the level of RPE seen in late phases.
- *Vascular occlusion:* The characteristic findings are:
  - Delayed filling of the occluded retinal veins with areas of CNP **(Figs. 4.2.12 and 4.2.13)**
  - Blocked fluorescence from intraretinal or preretinal hemorrhages
  - Leak from neovascularization or macular edema **(Fig. 4.2.14)**
  - Macular ischemia, which is seen as an increase in FAZ area **(Fig. 4.2.15)**

Note: Fluorescein angiography is recommended *only* after the intraretinal hemorrhages have adequately cleared out from the retina. It is not advised in acute cases as dense intraretinal hemorrhages may make interpretation difficult due to blockage of fluorescence.

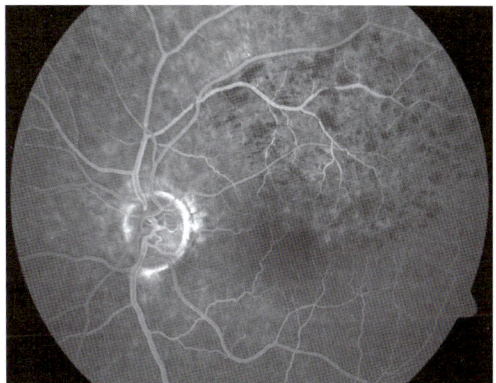

Fig. 4.2.13: Fresh superior-temporal branch retinal vein occlusion (BRVO) depicting scattered hemorrhages in the area of drainage of the major vein and macular hemorrhages. Late fundus fluorescein angiography (FFA) image showing blocked fluorescence in the area of the hemorrhages along with minimal leakage of the capillary bed.

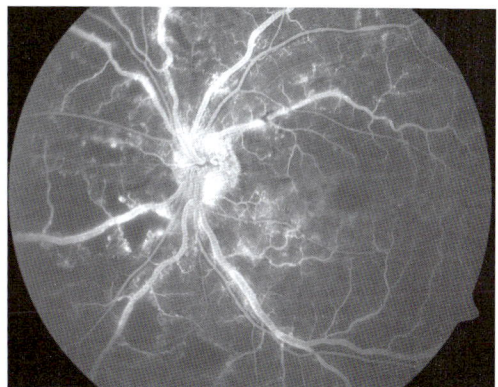

Fig. 4.2.15: Central retinal vein occlusion (CRVO) showing dilated veins with capillary nonperfusion areas involving the entire retina.

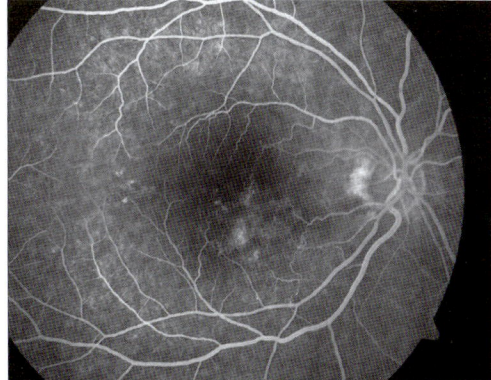

Fig. 4.2.14: Fundus image showing macular branch retinal vein occlusion, corresponding venous phase angiogram showing focal leakage at macula, and collateral formation.

Ultra-widefield FA (UWFA)[4] has been recommended in vascular occlusion to look at the peripheral vascular status and presence of CNP areas and to mark the areas for targeted retinal photocoagulation or sectoral laser photocoagulation.

- *Neuro-ophthalmology:* FFA has been used to study diseases like nonarteritic anterior ischemic optic neuropathy (NAION) extensively, and also helps in determining telangiectasia over the optic disc that is considered typical of diseases like Leber hereditary optic neuropathy (LHON).
- *CME:* CME shows the petaloid appearance of fluorescence.

ADVANCES IN FUNDUS FLUORESCEIN ANGIOGRAPHY

Advances in FFA include following:
- *Confocal scanning laser ophthalmoscope:* Uses low-power laser beam to sweep through the retina and the reflected beam is recorded by a detector. The standard size is a field of 30° × 30°, but may be increased using attachments. Advantages include better resolution, reduction of noise, patient comfort through less bright light, and imaging in small pupil sizes.
- Ultra-widefield FFA is done using a camera, which gives a *200° field* of view, which equates to 82.5% of the total retinal surface area. It uses a wide ellipsoid mirror to image retina through an undilated pupil. It can even be used in nondilating pupils that is typically

difficult with older cameras. Pediatric sedation is less imaging for diseases like retinopathy of prematurity (ROP), familial exudative vitreoretinopathy (FEVR), and Coats' disease may also be done.[5] More importantly, it allows simultaneous imaging of near-total retina that was not possible with conventional FFA. Newer studies document its role in targeted laser photocoagulation of CNP areas in diseases like retinal vein occlusion (RVO), PDR, etc. Evaluations for retinal vasculitis have found it advantageous in determining the true extent and laterality of the disease. It also allows autofluorescence analysis and magnified central imaging.

- Retcam with FFA to look for vascular loops and adequacy of the laser in ROP babies; widefield system is considered gold standard for pediatric imaging.

REFERENCES

1. Novotny HR, Alvis DL. A method of photographing fluorescence in circulating blood in the human retina. Circulation. 1961;24:82-6.
2. Lipson BK, Yannuzzi LA. Complications of intravenous fluorescein injections. Int Ophthalmol Clin. 1989;29(3):200-5.
3. Webb RH, Hughes GW, Delori FC. Confocal scanning laser ophthalmoscope. Appl Opt. 1987;26(8):1492-9.
4. Atkinson A, Mazo C. Imaged Area of the Retina. Dunfermline, UK: Optos PLC; 2015.
5. Friberg TR, Gupta A, Yu J, Huang L, Suner I, Puliafito CA, et al. Ultrawide angle fluorescein angiographic imaging: a comparison to conventional digital acquisition systems. Ophthalmic Surg Lasers Imaging. 2008;39:304-11.

4.3 OPTICAL COHERENCE TOMOGRAPHY

Priyanka Ramesh, Nawazish Shaikh, Nasiq Hasan, Aayush Majumdar, Atul Kumar

INTRODUCTION

Optical coherence tomography (OCT) is a noninvasive technique of imaging the retina and optic nerve. It gives high-resolution images of the retina and optic nerve head. It is being used extensively in the diagnosis and management of many retinal and choroidal pathologies. It is also used in the diagnosis as well as follow-up of glaucoma.

The principle of "Michelson interferometry" or low-coherence interferometry is used in OCT. A ray of light is divided into a reference and a sample beam. The sample beam falls on the retina and is backscattered and interferes with the reference beam to form interference patterns. These interference patterns are used to reconstruct axial A-scans. Multiple A-scans are constructed at each point of the retina, and these are together reconstructed to give a two-dimensional cross-sectional image.[1,2]

TYPES OF OPTICAL COHERENCE TOMOGRAPHY (TABLE 4.3.1)

- *Time-domain OCT:* It used a single-photon detector and moving mirror. This caused limitation in the speed of imaging. It had an axial resolution of 10 μm and a transverse resolution of 20 μm. The OCT could take 400 A-scans per second and used 820 nm wavelength light. For example, Stratus OCT (Carl Zeiss Meditec, Inc, Dublin, California).
- *Spectral-domain OCT:* It uses 840 nm wavelength of light. Also called Fourier-

TABLE 4.3.1: Types of optical coherence tomography.

OCT	Time-Domain	Spectral-Domain	Swept-Source
Image acquisition	• Super luminescent diode (810 nm) • Single photon detector • Moving reference mirror	• Broadband super luminescent diode – 840 nm • Array of detectors • Fixed reference mirror	• Swept source tunable laser (1,050 nm) • Single detector
Scanning speed (A scans/sec)	400	27,000	100,000–400,000
Axial resolution	10 micron	5–7 micron	5 micron
Transverse resolution	20 micron	14–20 micron	20 micron
Range of imaging	VR interface to RPE	Cortical vitreous to choroid; up to sclera using EDI mode	Cortical vitreous to sclera

(EDI: enhanced depth of imaging; OCT: optical coherence tomography; RPE: retinal pigment epithelium; VR: virtual reality)

domain OCT or high-definition OCT (HD-OCT). It uses an array of detectors to acquire all the A-scans and hence it is faster than the time-domain OCT. A-scan rate is 27,000 Hz and has an axial resolution of 5–7 µm. For example, Cirrus HD-OCT (Carl Zeiss Meditec, Inc, Dublin, California).

- *Swept-source OCT:* This is a newer type of OCT, which uses a broadband super-luminescent diode light source of 1,050 nm wavelength. The longer wavelength has better penetration and therefore has better visualization of structures deep to the retinal pigment epithelium (RPE). The A-scan rate is 100,000 Hz. The axial resolution is 3–5 µm.[3]

INTERPRETATION OF OPTICAL COHERENCE TOMOGRAPHY

First identify the name, age, type of OCT scan, and the date of acquisition. The OCT is read from inner layers to the outer layers.
- The vitreous has to be commented as well as the vitreoretinal interface.
- The different layers of the retina have to be seen.
- The retinal pigmented epithelium (RPE)–Bruch's membrane complex integrity has to be commented on.
- The choroid has to be seen for the thickness and normal pattern.
- The sclera-choroidal junction has to be seen.

The layers of retina seen in an OCT image are as follows **(Fig. 4.3.1)**:
- Precortical vitreous
- Internal limiting membrane (ILM)
- Nerve fiber layer
- Ganglion cell layer
- Inner plexiform layer
- Inner nuclear layer
- Outer plexiform layer
- Outer nuclear layer (Henle's layer in the macula)
- External limiting membrane
- Myoid zone
- Ellipsoid zone
- The outer segment of photoreceptors
- Interdigitation zone
- RPE–Bruch's complex
- Sattler's layer
- Haller's layer
- Choroid-sclera junction

Causes of change in reflectivity in OCT are summarized in **Table 4.3.2**.

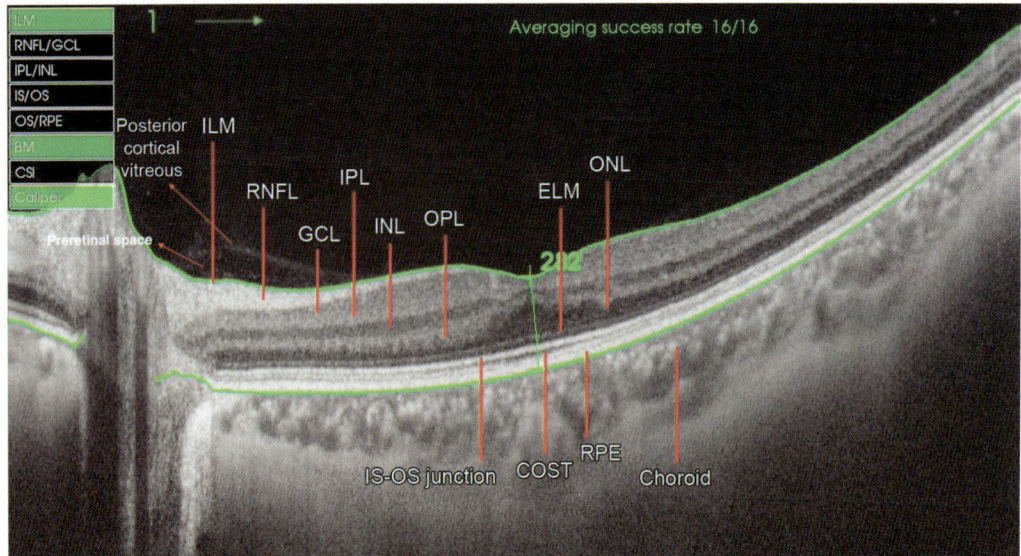

Fig. 4.3.1: Normal layers in OCT.[4-6] (COST: cone outer segment tips also known as interdigitation zone; ELM: external limiting membrane; GCL: ganglion cell layer; ILM: internal limiting membrane; INL: inner nuclear layer; IPL: inner plexiform layer; IS-OS junction: inner segment-outer segment junction; OCT: optical coherence tomography; ONL: outer nuclear layer; RNFL: retinal nerve fiber layer; RPE: retinal pigmented epithelium)

TABLE 4.3.2: Causes of hyporeflectivity and hyper-reflectivity in OCT.	
Hyporeflectivity	**Hyper-reflectivity**
Fluid (DME, CME, NSD, serous PED)	Exudation
Anatomical gaps in tissues: • Retinoschisis • Traction • Dystrophy	Vitreous opacities: • Vitreous cells • Asteroid hyalosis
Shadowing	Blood
Lumen of blood vessels	Calcification
(CME: cystoid macular edema; DME: diabetic macular edema; optical coherence tomography)	

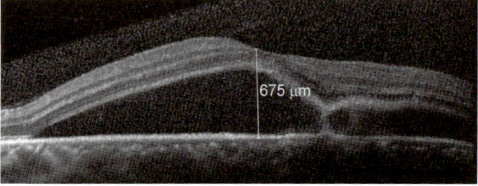

Fig. 4.3.2: Central serous chorioretinopathy (CSC).

CLINICAL CASES/EXAMPLES

- *Central serous chorioretinopathy (CSC)/central serous retinopathy* **(Fig. 4.3.2)**:
  - An elevation of the inner layers of the retina, which is suggestive of a neurosensory detachment.
  - There is also an elevation of the RPE and Bruch's complex, which is suggestive of a pigment epithelium detachment, which is suggestive of CSC.
  - Acute CSC in which there is neurosensory detachment whereas the other retinal layers are not distorted.
  - Chronic CSC in which there are large cystic spaces in the retinal layers with RPE disruption.
- *Cystoid macular edema (CME)* **(Figs. 4.3.3A to C)**: There is the presence of cystic spaces in the retina corresponding to the outer plexiform layer.
- *Diabetic macular edema (DME)* **(Figs. 4.3.4A to C)**: There is the presence of

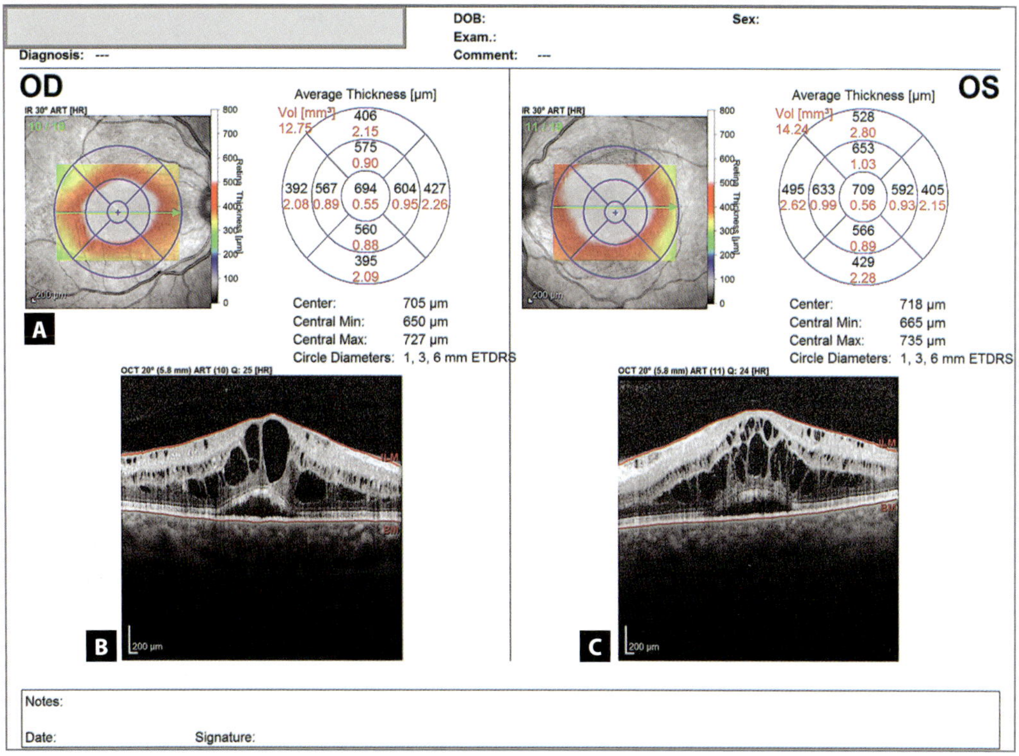

Figs. 4.3.3A to C: (A) *Retinal thickness map:* Top left image shows the color-coded macular thickness map showing thickening at the macular region and macular thickness values are seen in 1, 3, and 6 mm circles in the top right image. (B and C) The corresponding spectral domain optical coherence tomography image of right eye and left eye, respectively, depicting cystoid macular edema.

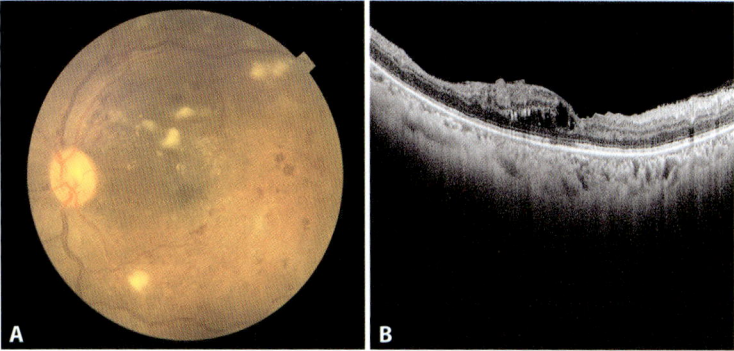

Figs. 4.3.4A and B

cystic spaces in the inner retina. There is the presence of hyper-reflective dot-like lesions, which could either be hard exudates (with back shadowing), or hyper-reflective foci (without back shadowing). There may be associated thickening of the posterior hyaloid, which is seen as a hyper-reflective band called "thick taut posterior

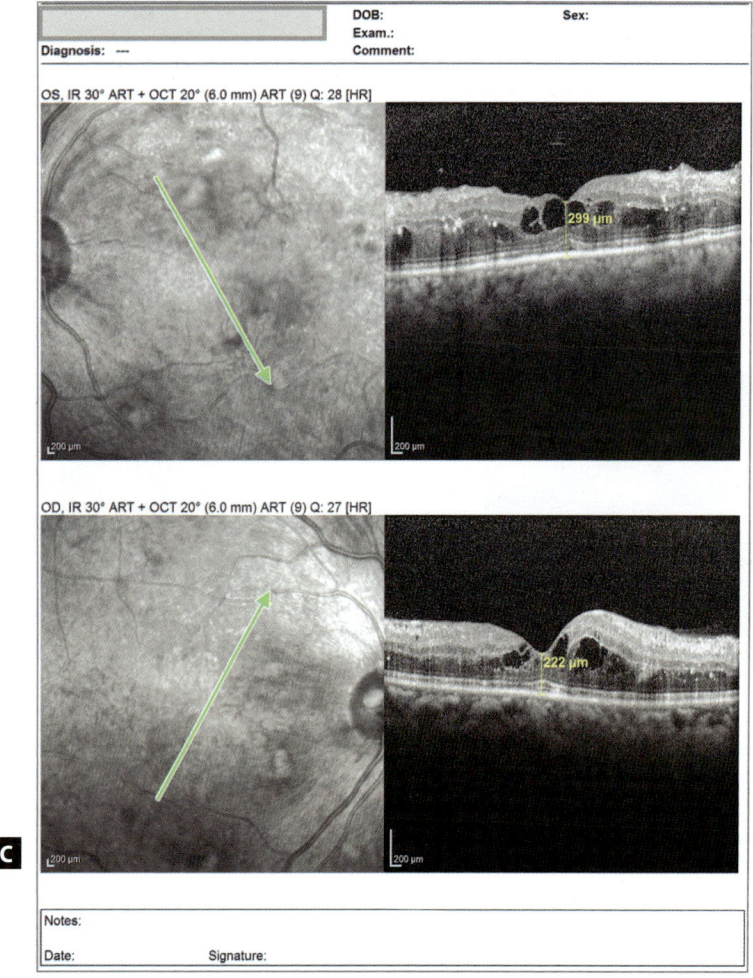

Fig. 4.3.4C

Figs. 4.3.4A to C: Diabetic macular edema.

hyaloid". OCT may be used in patients with DME to predict visual outcomes by use of biomarkers such as disorganization of retinal inner layers (DRIL), outer retinal tabulation (ORT), hyper-reflective foci (HRF), neurosensory detachment and subfoveal choroidal thickness.
- *Macular hole (Figs. 4.3.5A and B):*
  - OCT is showing a macular hole extending full thickness in the retina with cystic spaces in between the retinal layers.
  - Colloidal bodies may be seen as hyper-reflective structures at the base of the macular hole.
  - The different dimensions of the hole can be calculated like minimum diameter, height, basal diameter, and also the different indices like diameter hole index, hole forming factor, tractional hole index, and macular hole index. (MHI). MHI >0.5 is a good prognostic marker for anatomical closure.

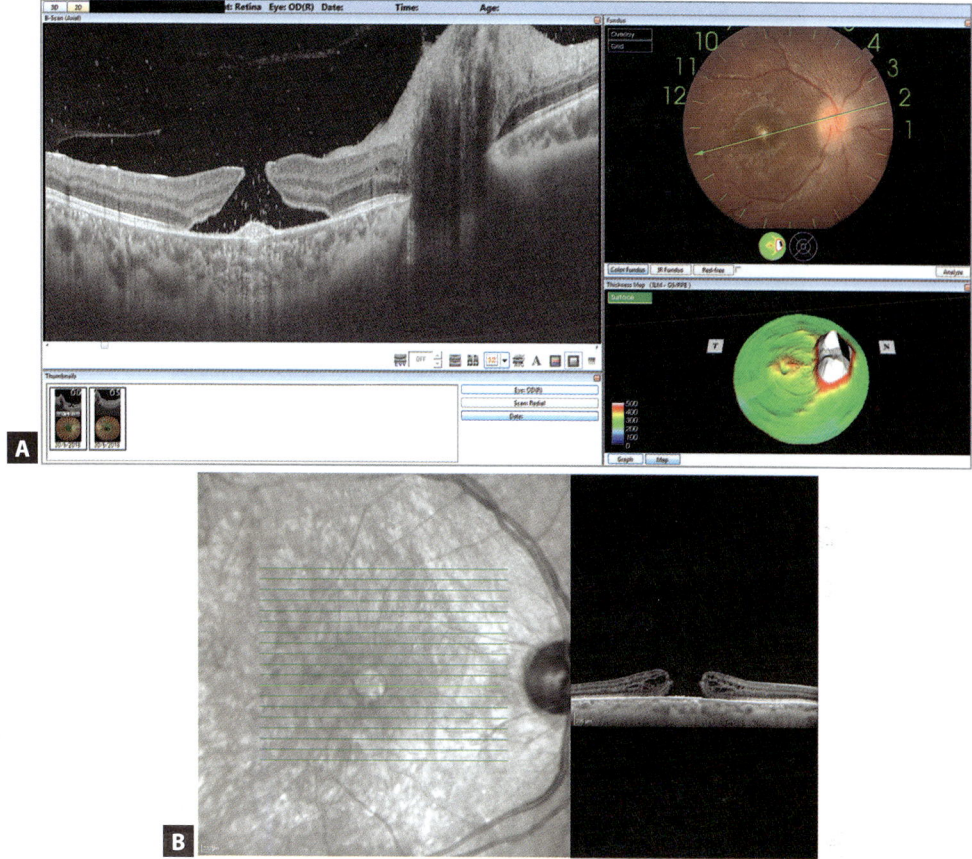

Figs. 4.3.5A and B: (A) Macular hole with choroidal neovascular membrane (CNVM); (B) Macular hole with cystoid changes.

- *Epiretinal membrane (ERM) (Fig. 4.3.6)*: There is the presence of a hyper-reflective membrane on the surface of inner retina with associated distortion of the retinal architecture. OCT based classification of ERM includes presence of ectopic inner foveal layers (EIFL) described by Govetto et al.
- *Vitreomacular traction (Figs. 4.3.7A and B)*:
  - OCT showing focal attachment of the posterior hyaloid in the perifoveal area with separation in the macular area
  - Vitreomacular adhesion (focal) in which the posterior vitreous cortex is attached only at the fovea and the foveal counter is normal.
  - Vitreoretinal traction may be classified as focal (<1,500 µm) or broad based (>1,500 µm).
- *Choroidal neovascular membrane (CNVM) (Fig. 4.3.8)*: There is the presence of a discontinuity in the RPE–Bruch's membrane complex and hyper-reflective structure extending beneath the RPE–Bruch's complex. Also a small area of neurosensory detachment. OCT can be used to differentiate between sub-RPE (type 1) or sub-retinal (type 2) CNVM.

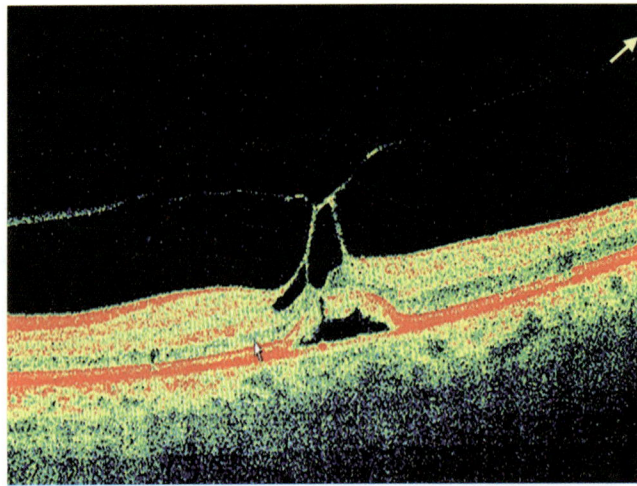

Fig. 4.3.6: Epiretinal membrane with vitreomacular traction (VMT).

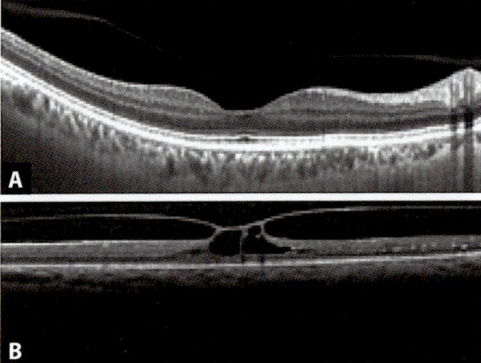

Figs. 4.3.7A and B: Vitreomacular traction.

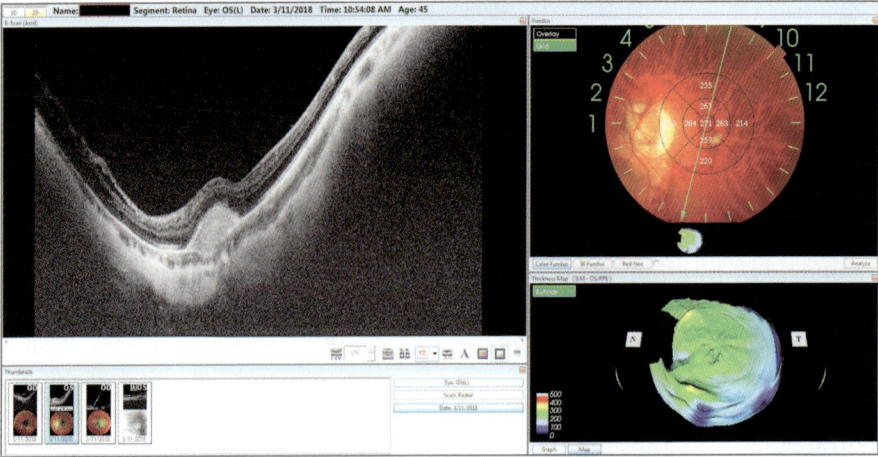

Fig. 4.3.8: Choroidal neovascular membrane.

- *Polypoidal CNV (Fig. 4.3.9)*:
  - Polypoidal choroidal vasculopathy (PCV) is characterized by the presence of PEDs, which are steep and called "thumb-like polyps" (star).
  - There is the presence of characteristic "double-layer sign" (arrow), which is because of the split of the RPE and Bruch's membrane due to the branching vascular network (BVN).
    - Enhanced depth of imaging (EDI) in SD-OCT or SS-OCT may be used to quantify the choroidal thickness in patients with pachychoroid spectrum.
- Inherited retinal dystrophies:
  - Stargardt's disease shows characteristic foveal thinning of outer retinal layers, with the flecks appearing as subretinal and intraretinal hyper-reflective deposits **(Fig. 4.3.10)**.

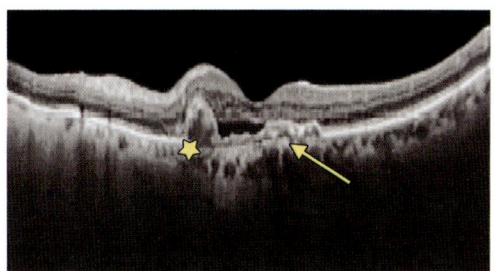

Fig. 4.3.9: Polypoidal choroidal neovascularization.

- Best vitelliform dystrophy shows the presence of a hypo-reflective space with thickening of the interdigitation zone which may be fuzzy appearing photoreceptors. This hypo-reflective space may be confused with sub-retinal fluid/NSD and may be differentiated by the clinical features as well as fundus autofluorescence imaging **(Fig. 4.3.11)**.

RECENT ADVANCES IN OPTICAL COHERENCE TOMOGRAPHY

- *Enhanced depth imaging:* This involves setting the zero-delay line from the ILM to the RPE to enhance imaging of the choroid and the choroid-scleral junction **(Figs. 4.3.12A and B)**.
- *Optical coherence tomography angiography:* It is a noninvasive method of visualizing the retinal microvasculature. It does not require dye injection. In simple words, in a stationary eye the only moving structures are red blood cells (RBCs) and a contrast is created between the retina and the blood vessels by assessing the signal changes in the moving RBCs in the blood vessels.
- *Ultra-widefield OCT (UWF-OCT):* Available in the Optos Silverstone (Optos

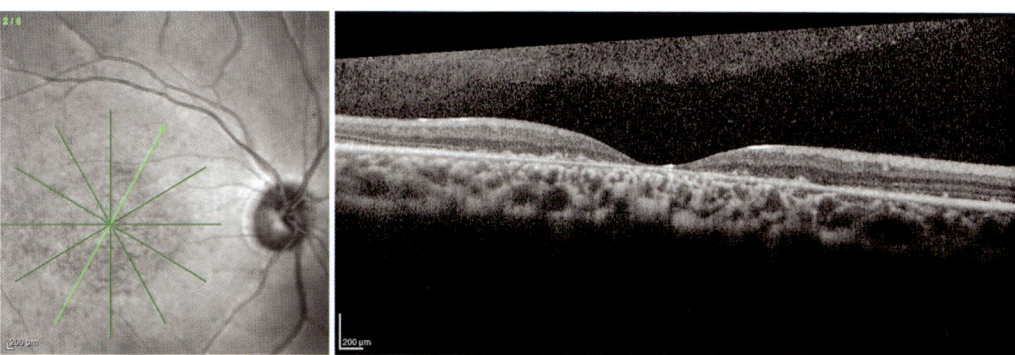

Fig. 4.3.10: Stargardt's disease.

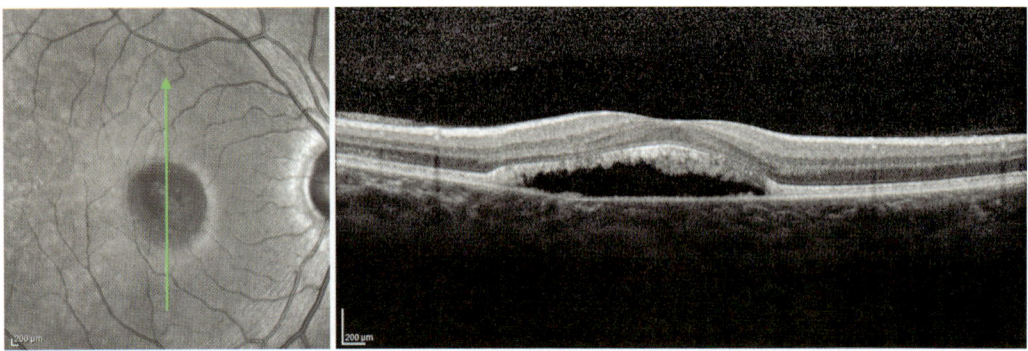

Fig. 4.3.11: Best's vitelliform macular dystrophy.

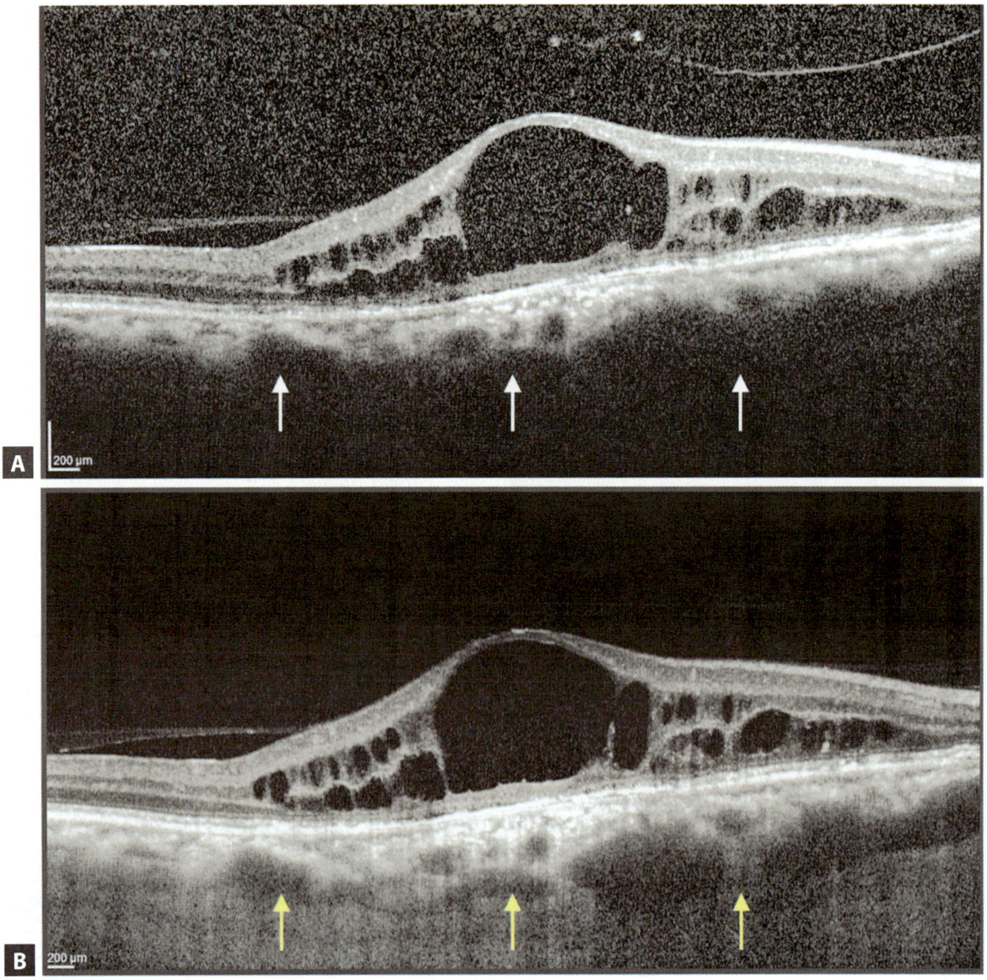

Figs. 4.3.12A and B: Enhanced depth imaging (EDI) on SD-OCT.

PLC Edinburgh) and now also present across various other platforms, the capability of capturing the far periphery of the retina with OCT has expanded its utility in various conditions like retinal detachment, retinoschisis, peripheral retinal degenerations, and ocular oncology.
- *Polarization sensitive OCT (PS-OCT):* It extends the concept of OCT, utilizing the information that is carried by polarized light to obtain additional information about ocular tissue. Several ocular structures alter the polarization state of the light (e.g., cornea, retinal nerve fiber layer, retinal pigment epithelium), showing a tissue specific contrast in PS-OCT images. Automated segmentation of the RPE and other pigmented structures (e.g., hard exudates) based on the polarization scrambling effect is one amongst many clinical applications of this modality.
- *Intraoperative OCT:* Evolving from initial handheld OCT to microscope mounted OCT, to the recent microscope integrated OCT platforms, incorporation of OCT scanning beam into microscope optics allows seamless, real time OCT feedback with parfocality. Clinical trials like PIONEER and DISCOVERY have concluded that iOCT significantly impacted surgical decision making in both anterior and posterior segment surgeries. Clinical utility is wide ranging, including:
  - *Anterior segment procedures:*
    - *DALK:* Real time evaluation of depth of dissection
    - *DSAEK/DMEK:* Graft orientation and graft-host apposition
    - *Cataract:* Posterior capsule status, IOL positioning
    - *Phakic IOL:* Vault measurement
    - *Glaucoma surgeries:* Scleral dissection depth, GDD tube positioning
  - *Posterior segment procedures:*
    - Membrane peeling procedures
    - Chorioretinopathy biopsies
    - Subretinal injections
    - Guided identification of tissue planes and occult breaks

REFERENCES

1. Gao SS, Jia Y, Zhang M, Su JP, Liu G, Hwang TS, et al. Optical coherence tomography angiography. Invest Ophthalmol Vis Sci. 2016;57(9):27-36.
2. Ryan SJ. Retinal reattachment: general surgical principles and techniques. In: Ryan SJ (Ed). Retina, 5th edition. Philadelphia: Elsevier Saunders; 2013. p. 1713.
3. Bhende M, Shetty S, Parthasarathy MK, Ramya S. Optical coherence tomography: A guide to interpretation of common macular diseases. Indian J Ophthalmol. 2018;66(1):20-35.
4. Staurenghi G, Sadda S, Chakravarthy U, Spaide RF. Proposed lexicon for anatomic landmarks in normal posterior segment spectral-domain optical coherence tomography: the IN OCT consensus. Ophthalmology. 2014;121(8):1572-8.
5. Govetto A, Lalane RA 3rd, Sarraf D, Figueroa MS, Hubschman JP. Insights Into Epiretinal Membranes: Presence of Ectopic Inner Foveal Layers and a New Optical Coherence Tomography Staging Scheme. Am J Ophthalmol. 2017;175:99-113.
6. Markan A, Agarwal A, Arora A, Bazgain K, Rana V, Gupta V. Novel imaging biomarkers in diabetic retinopathy and diabetic macular edema. Ther Adv Ophthalmol. 2020; 12: 2515841420950513.

4.4 INDOCYANINE GREEN ANGIOGRAPHY

Anusha Sachan, Nasiq Hasan, Atul Kumar

INTRODUCTION

Indocyanine green is a water-soluble, tricarbocyanine anionic dye. Its first application was used in measuring cardiac output. Flower and Hochheimer performed the first intravenous ICGA to image the human choroid in 1972. Hayashi and coworkers worked on improved filter combinations in 1980. The dye has a molecular weight of 774.96 Da and has maximum absorption at 790 nm and emission at 835 nm in the near-infrared wavelength. This allows penetration through macular pigment, blood, melanin, and pigments, thereby better angiography under challenging situations.[1-3]

Indocyanine green is 98% protein-bound compared to 80% of that of sodium fluorescein. This allows the dye to stay within the larger choroidal circulation resulting in its enhanced definition. The dye is eliminated through the bile without metabolism. ICG is known to have more side effects than sodium fluorescein. Nausea, vomiting, and pruritis are the most common side effects. Urticaria and difficulty breathing can occur, hypotensive shock and anaphylactic shock can also occur rarely. It is usually contraindicated in patients with iodine and seafood allergy, liver disease, end-stage renal failure, and uremia. It is a category-C drug in pregnancy. Differences between FFA and ICG have been summarized in **Table 4.4.1**.

ADMINISTRATION OF INDOCYANINE GREEN

Indocyanine green is used in the standard concentration of 25 mg/mL. Rapid intravenous (IV) injection is done with 5 mL saline flush and images are captured serially.

PHASES OF INDOCYANINE GREEN

- *Early phase*—first 1-minute postinjection—shows choroidal arteries.
- *Early mid-phase (1–3 minutes)*: Choroidal veins and retinal vessels
- *Late mid-phase (3–15 minutes)*: Choroidal vessels fading but retinal vessels are still visible.

TABLE 4.4.1: Differences between fundus fluorescein angiography (FFA) and indocyanine green (ICG) dye.

Features	*Fluorescein dye*	*ICG dye*
Molecular weight (kD, kilodalton)	375	775
Absorption wavelength (nm)	494	800
Emission wavelength (nm)	521	830
$t_{1/2}$ (minutes)	23	2.5
Excretion	Renal	Biliary
Waiting time after injection (minutes)	15	2
Side effects	++	+

- *Late phase (15–45 minutes)*: Hypofluorescent choroidal vessels and gradual fading of retinal vessels

The "hyper" lesions are described as hotspots.

The two technologies used for imaging ICG are the standard digital camera-based systems and SLO-based systems. The newer techniques of ICGA are real-time ICGA (30 frames/s), wide-angle ICGA (160° field), and digital subtraction ICGA. It has also been incorporated in ultra-widefield imaging (Optos) in the latest Optos California machines. Simultaneous FFA with ICG can also be done.[1-3]

ADVANTAGES OVER FUNDUS FLUORESCEIN ANGIOGRAPHY

- More useful in the presence of optical media opacification
- More useful for the understanding of choroidal pathologies due to its ability to penetrate melanin; example: CSCR, PCV, etc.
- Very useful in identifying feeder vessels of tumors and CNVMs
- It was an excellent guide for the treatment of age-related macular degeneration (ARMD) when anti-VEGF (anti-vascular endothelial growth factor) therapy was unavailable.
- In cases where background fluorescence is high or in cases with PEDs, differentiating pathologies may be difficult. In such cases, ICG was considered advantageous. However, with the advent of OCT angiography, this advantage is now lost.

DISADVANTAGES OF INDOCYANINE GREEN

Side effects are much more common than FFA, and severe too. It cannot be used in patients with specific allergies and those with hepatic dysfunction.

CLINICAL APPLICATIONS

Age-related macular degeneration: CNV has been classified depending on size and delineation into "focal hotspots" and "plaques". Plaques are further classified into well-defined, poorly defined, and a combination of both. The most common type was plaques (61% of the cases) and had a poor visual prognosis, compared to focal spots or "hotspots" (29%), which had a better prognosis, and they were considered to be potentially treatable by ICG-guided laser photocoagulation. ICGA also shows feeder vessels in its early phase.

Polypoidal choroidal vasculopathy: ICGA is very useful in detecting and characterizing polyps, which are seen as small hypercyanescent spots in early and late phase. ICGA helps in measuring the total size of the lesion, which includes polyps and BVN **(Fig. 4.4.1)** and allows us to select the spot size when considering photodynamic therapy (PDT).

Central serous chorioretinopathy: ICGA helps to assess the location of areas of

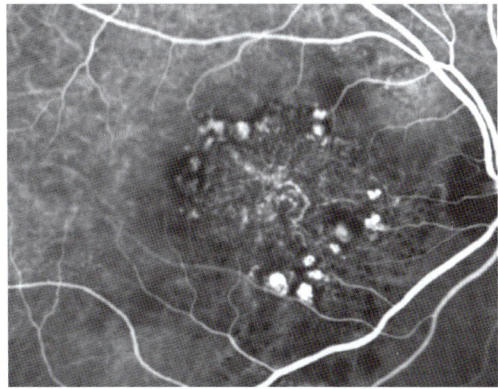

Fig. 4.4.1: Indocyanine green (ICG) frame reveals multiple polyps with branching vascular network (BVN) in an eye with polypoidal choroidal vasculopathy.

hyperpermeability, which can be useful when considering treatment with verteporfin PDT.

Choroidal inflammatory disease: ICGA helps in staging and determining the activity of the disease. Active lesion show areas of hypocyanescence or cold spots with poorly defined margins whereas healed lesions show well-defined margins. Aggressive lesions show areas of late hypercyanescence or hotspots.

Choroidal tumors: Indocyanine green angiography is useful to diagnose choroidal tumors that cannot be diagnosed with FA. It shows the intrinsic vascular pattern of the tumors.

REFERENCES

1. Agrawal RV, Biswas J, Gunasekaran D. Indocyanine green angiography in posterior uveitis. Indian J Ophthalmol. 2013;61(4): 148-59.
2. Ryan SJ. Retina, 4th edition. Philadelphia: Elsevier;2006.
3. Regillo CD. The present role of indocyanine green angiography in ophthalmology. Curr Opin Ophthalmol. 1999;10:189-96.

4.5 ELECTRORETINOGRAM

Sourabh Verma, Lohith Rambarki, Divya Agarwal

INTRODUCTION

Electroretinogram (ERG) **(Fig. 4.5.1)** is a record of change in electric potential of the eye in response to light stimuli. Holmgren first described it in 1865, and first recording in humans was done by Dewar.[1] Riggs and Karpe made corneal electrodes mounted on contact lens with which clinical recording of ERG became possible.[1] Pattern ERG (PERG) and standard full-field ERG (referred to as ERG) have found widespread use in diagnosis and prognostication of retinal and macular diseases. They provide objective data, which can be interpreted according to set norms. However, as its findings may be similar for many conditions, a precise correlation with clinical context and history is necessary. International Society of Clinical Electrophysiology of Vision (ISCEV) has established guidelines to record and interpret its results.[2]

PHYSIOLOGY

A potential difference of 1 mV exists between cornea and retina, cornea having a relative positive charge, called corneoretinal potential. Stimulation of retina by light leads to a generation of a cascade of electrical changes in the retina, which is recorded with the help of electrodes. ERG is a record of electrical activity from radially arranged retinal components, i.e., photoreceptors,

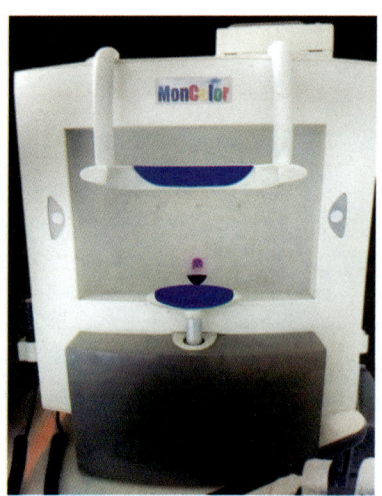

Fig. 4.5.1: Electroretinogram (ERG) machine.

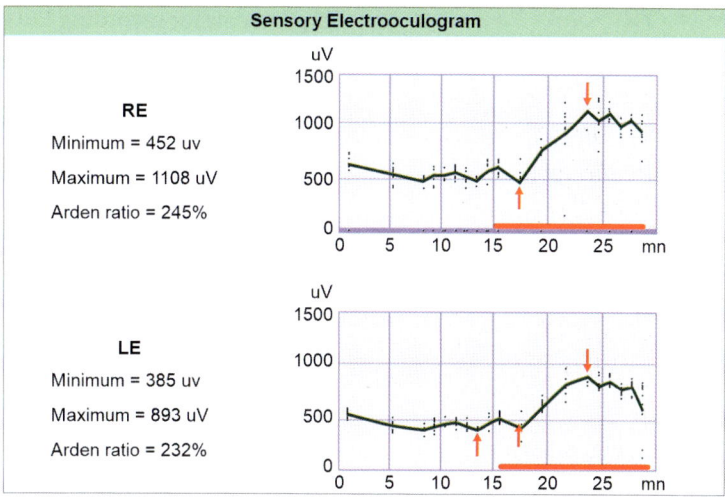

Fig. 4.5.2: Normal electroretinogram (ERG) wave. (LE: left eye; RE: right eye)

bipolar cells, Müller cells, and RPE. Horizontally arranged cells such as amacrine cell and ganglion cell have minimal effect on it.

The ERG waveform **(Fig. 4.5.2)** is composed of following parts:

- *A-wave:* It is the initial negative wave, which arises from *photoreceptors*. When recorded in isolation it is called Granit's P-III or late receptor potential.[3] Both rods and cones contribute to it after light-induced hyperpolarization and using specific stimuli can separate their individual responses.
- *B-wave (P-II component of Granit):* It is a positive wave after a wave. It arises due to *Müller cell membrane* potential change in response to potassium released from photoreceptors during hyperpolarization. It represents the activity of *the bipolar cell layer*. Small wavelets are found on the ascending limb of the b-wave, which represents a negative feedback circuit in the inner retina between amacrine cells, ganglion cells, and bipolar cells. They are recorded in the light-adapted retina using a bright flash of light and using filters to filter out low-frequency b-wave responses. Their frequency varies from 100 to 150 Hz.
- *C-wave (AKA P-I) component of Granit:* It is a small positive wave after b-wave arising from RPE. Since predominantly rods are in contact with RPE cells in interdigitation zone, cones are believed to have no contribution to it.

There is no contribution of retinal components proximal to ganglion cells and optic nerve.

DEFINITION OF PARAMETERS

- *Amplitude:*
  - A-wave amplitude—measured from baseline to tip of a-wave
  - B-wave amplitude—measured from trough of a wave to peak of b-wave
- *Latency:* The time between stimulus and initiation of the wave. It is approximately 2 ms for a-wave.
- *Implicit time:* The time period between stimulus and peak of a- or b-wave.

TYPES

- **On the basis of stimulus zone:**
  - Full-field ERG
  - Multifocal ERG (mfERG)
- **On the basis of stimulus type:**
  - Single flash ERG
  - Red flash ERG
  - Flicker ERG
  - Blue filter ERG
  - PERG
- **On the basis of the state of retinal adaptation:**
  - Photopic ERG **(Fig. 4.5.3)**
  - Scotopic ERG **(Fig. 4.5.4)**
  - Mesopic ERG

Full-field Electroretinogram

International Society of Clinical Electrophysiology of Vision has given revised guidelines for recording ERG, which are based on strength of stimuli (flash strength in $cd/s/m^{-2}$) and state of adaptation.[2]

Six protocols for recording ERG are as follows:
1. Dark-adapted 0.01 ERG—gives the rod-driven response of bipolar cells.
2. Dark-adapted 3 ERG—represents the combined response from both rod- and cone-driven bipolar cells; the rod response is more predominant.
3. Dark-adapted 10 ERG—represents combined response from rods and cones; prominent a-wave is seen.
4. Dark-adapted oscillator potentials—it represents amacrine cell activity.
5. Light-adapted 3 ERG—represents cone response; a-wave from cones and cone off bipolar cells; b-wave from on and off cone bipolar cells.
6. Light-adapted flicker ERG (30 Hz)—it is cone-driven response.

Patient Preparation

The pupil should be dilated. Before recording, a period of 20 minutes' dark adaptation

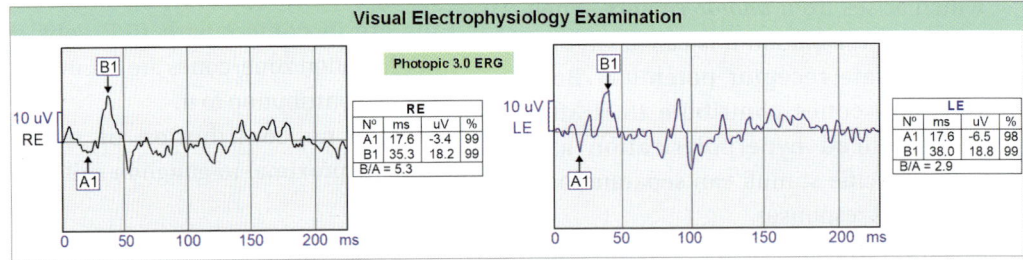

Fig. 4.5.3: Photopic electroretinogram (ERG). (LE: left eye; RE: right eye)

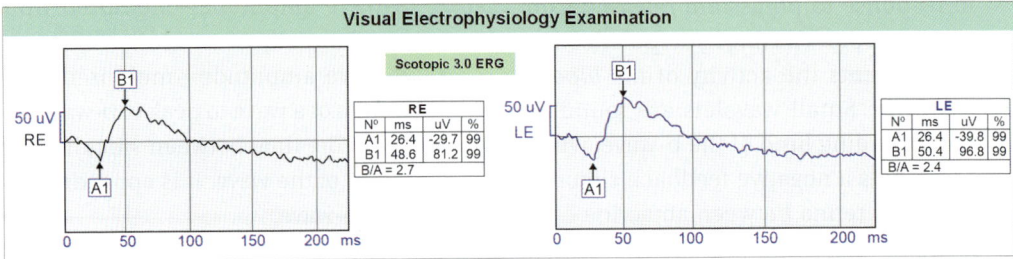

Fig. 4.5.4: Scotopic electroretinogram (ERG). (LE: left eye; RE: right eye)

for scotopic ERG and 10 minutes' light adaptation for photopic ERG is required. Any investigation using bright light should be avoided before it; if done, a 30-minute recovery period is required before recording. The patient is instructed to look at a fixation point. Scotopic ERG should be recorded before photopic ERG.

Electrodes

Active electrode: Different types are available, which can be placed on the cornea, conjunctiva or skin of lower lid **(Fig. 4.5.5)**. Most commonly used ones are embedded in the contact lens and placed on the cornea as they provide the most stable and reproducible recordings.

Reference electrodes: They serve as the negative pole. They can be placed on cornea conjunctiva or skin. Mostly they are placed on the lateral orbital rim. They should not be placed over muscle masses.

Ground electrodes/common electrodes: They are placed on forehead, mastoid or earlobe.

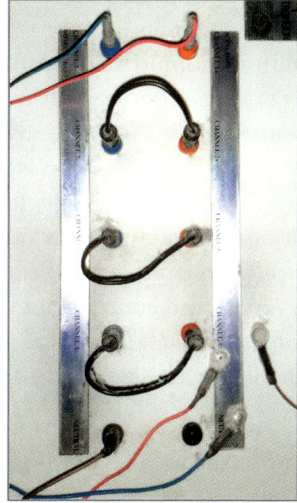

Fig. 4.5.5: Electroretinogram (ERG) leads.

Stimulus

A Ganzfeld field in the shape of a dome or integrating sphere to stimulate entire retina provides background illumination of about 17–34 cd/m^2. A fixation spot is provided. Duration of flash stimulus should be <5 ms, which is shorter than the integration time of photoreceptors. Different wavelengths can be used to stimulate rods and cones separately or in a combined fashion. Standard strength of stimulus is 3 $cd/s/m^{-2}$.

Factors Affecting Electroretinogram

- Area of retina illuminated
- Duration of stimulus
- Strength of stimulus
- Interval between stimulus
- Size of pupil

Abnormal Electroretinogram Responses and Associated Conditions

- Accentuated/supernormal response—characterized by the amplitude of a- and b-waves being greater than two standard deviations from the mean. It is seen in conditions such as early stages of siderosis bulbi, subtotal circulatory disturbance of retina, and albinism.[4,5]
- Subnormal response—characterized by a- and b-wave amplitude <2 standard deviations of the mean. As ERG gives an estimate of total retinal function, a subnormal response is seen only when a large area of the retina is not functioning. It is seen in retinal detachment, chloroquine and quinine toxicity, and early cases of retinitis pigmentosa. It can also found in systemic conditions such as vitamin A deficiency, anemia, and mucopolysaccharidosis.
- Extinguished response—a- and b-waves are not seen, and a flat ERG waveform is

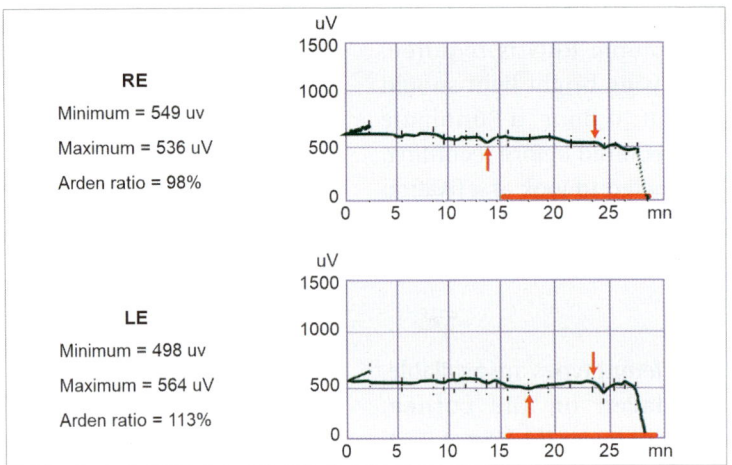

Fig. 4.5.6: Extinguishing electroretinogram (ERG). (LE: left eye; RE: right eye)

recorded **(Fig. 4.5.6)**. It is seen in advanced cases of siderosis bulbi, old retinal detachment, and retinitis pigmentosa. An extinguished response at birth characterizes Leber's congenital amaurosis. It can also be found in progressive conditions such as choroideremia, cancer-associated retinopathy, and chorioretinitis in later stages. Presence of an extinguished response signifies a poor visual outcome.

- Negative response—it is characterized by a large a-wave and absent b-wave (b/a <1) and signifies gross retinal dysfunction. It is seen in central retinal artery occlusion (CRAO), X-linked retinoschisis, melanocyte-associated retinopathy, Goldmann–Favre syndrome, etc.[1]
- Absent oscillatory potentials—they are absent in patients of DR and may point toward the conversion of NPDR to PDR. They are also abolished in other ischemic conditions of the retina such as CRAO.

Pattern Electroretinogram

Pattern ERG is a retinal response evoked by a contrast-reversing pattern, predominantly generated from ganglion cells driven by photoreceptors. Most commonly a black and white checkerboard pattern is used. The width of individual checks is 0.8° (±0.2°). Their shape should be square. In patients with abnormal visually evoked potentials (VEPs), PERG can help differentiate between an optic nerve retinal dysfunction.[6]

Pattern ERG recording is difficult as signal strength is only 2–8 µV. The standard PERG response is called transient response, as it is almost complete before the next reversal of contrast pattern. This allows clear separation of the wave components.

The patient should be given a proper refractive correction during testing, which is not necessary for ERG. Also, no mydriasis is required here. Rest of the setup is the same as standard ERG. During testing, luminance of lit area should be 80 cd/m^2 and mean luminance of screen remains constant during pattern reversal. The contrast between light and dark areas should be not <80%. A reversal rate of 4.0 ± 0.8 reversals per second (rps) is standard.[6]

The waveform consists of following parts:
- *N35:* Negative wave; peak time at approximately 35 ms

- *P50:* Positive wave; peak time at approximately 45–60 ms; the amplitude of P50 is measured from the trough of N35 to peak P50.
- *N95:* Large amplitude negative wave; peak time at approximately 90–100 ms; the amplitude of N95 is measured from the peak of P50 to trough of N95.
- P50 and N95 amplitude and peak time are important parameters to be reported. Implicit time is defined as the time between onset of contrast reversal and peak of the wave.

Uses of Pattern Electroretinogram
- A measure of central retinal function
- Differentiation between the optic nerve and macular dysfunction
- Evaluation of ganglion cell function and early diagnosis of glaucoma[7]
- Approximate determination of visual acuity

Multifocal Electroretinogram

Multifocal ERG is first developed by Eric Sutter in 1992. It is a topographical record of the local retinal electrophysiological response. It gives the cone-driven response, recorded under light-adapted condition. ISCEV (2007) has given clear guidelines to record and describe it.

Patient Preparation
Pupils should be fully dilated and 15 minutes of light adaptation under ordinary room light is required. Good central fixation is necessary and optimal refractive correction is provided. Rest of the precautions is the same as for recording ERG. Electrode placement is the same as for ERG. Recording can be done both monocularly and binocularly.

Stimulus
It consists of a display containing 61 or 103 hexagonal elements subtending an angle of 40°–50° with a central fixation point. Each hexagonal element has a 50% chance of illumination every time the frame changes in a pseudorandom pattern. Also, the size of elements increases from center to periphery to compensate for reducing the concentration of cones from center to periphery. Most commonly used frame frequency is 75 Hz. Background luminance and luminance of stimulus are 30 cd/m^2 and 100 cd/m^2, respectively. There should be a contrast of 90% or greater between lighted and darkened areas of the stimulus pattern. Test duration is 4 minutes for 61-element and 8 minutes for 103-element display.[8]

Response and Interpretation
Multifocal ERG test results are represented as:
- *Trace array:* It is the basic mfERG display. It should always be taken into account while reporting. It can be displayed with a retinal or field view, which should be specified along with the breadth of trace array. A trace length of 100 ms or more is used. Trace arrays are examined for any delayed signal and abnormal waveform. They show topographic variations and quality of records.
- *Topographic 3D response density plots:* It shows an overall signal strength per unit area of the retina. A normal plot in presence of central and steady fixation has a peak corresponding to the fovea, due to high cone density in this area and an evident depression corresponding to the blind spot. They give a quick, easy to understand representation of retinal function but should never be used in isolation to trace arrays. This is because an abnormal and delayed response can also produce a normal-looking 3D plot.
- *Ring and other regional averages:* A group of trace arrays from an area of interest

can be averaged to compare normal and abnormal areas. This comparison can be done between quadrants, hemiretinal areas, or successive rings from center to periphery. Latter is advantageous in diagnosing diseases, which produce retinal dysfunction with approximate radial symmetry.

First-order kernel: It is thought to represent the activity of outer retina, i.e., photoreceptors and Müller cells, and is obtained by subtracting the average of all responses from when a hexagon dark from the average of responses from when it is lit. The typical waveform is biphasic, consisting of an initial negative followed by a positive deflection. A third negative deflection is usually found and the three peaks obtained are designated as N1, P1, and N2, respectively.

Second-order kernel: It is thought to arise from the inner retina, especially ganglion cells and is a measure of mfERG responses to adaptation by successive flash. Its waveform consists of an initial positive (P1) followed by a negative (N1) peak.

Advantages of Multifocal Electroretinogram

- It gives a topographic representation of retinal function and help in identifying the site of disease
- Helpful in monitoring progression of the disease
- Distinguishing between inner and outer retinal disease

Affected By

- The decrease in amplitude and increase in implicit time is seen with increasing age.
- The amplitude of N1 and P1 are reduced in patients with cataract.
- Reduced first- and second-order kernel responses with increasing refractive error and axial length

Uses

- Toxic retinopathy—mfERG can be used in early detection of drug-induced retinopathy, e.g., in chloroquine, hydroxychloroquine, vigabatrin, and sildenafil.
- Differentiate diseases affecting inner (predominantly effects second-order kernel) and outer retinal layers (effects first-order kernel).
- Age-related macular degeneration (ARMD)—mfERG has been used to evaluate the extent of retinal involvement in ARMD. Significant reduction in P1 amplitude and N1 implicit time has been seen in the early foveal disease.
- DR—implicit time has been shown to be better than amplitude in detecting early DR.
- Central serous retinopathy—decreased amplitudes and increased implicit time is seen.
- Macular hole—decrease in response density in the foveal region
- ERM—decreased response density is seen, which improves after ERM removal.
- Vascular occlusions—decreased amplitudes and increased implicit time is seen.
- It has been useful in evaluating other acquired retinopathies such as multiple evanescent white dot syndrome (MEWDS), multifocal choroiditis (MFC), acute macular neuropathy (AMN), acute zonal occult outer retinopathy (AZOOR), acute idiopathic blind spot enlargement (AIBSE), Purtscher-like retinopathy, melanoma-associated retinopathy (MAR), cancer-associated retinopathy (CAR), etc.[9]

ELECTROOCULOGRAM

Electrooculogram is the measurement of the resting potential of the eye, between the cornea (positively charged) and retina (negatively charged). Like ERG, it is also a mass response and cannot be used for localized retinal conditions. Active electrodes are placed on both lateral and medial canthi, and a grounding electrode is placed on the forehead. There are three fixation lights and the right and left lights are lit alternatively to produce a saccadic movement in the eye. First baseline amplitude is recorded with stimulus lights on. A recording in dark-adapted state follows this with stimulus light off, and a recording in the light-adapted state with stimulus light on.

In dark-adapted state, resting potential decreases progressively reaching to a "dark trough" in approximately 10 minutes. The dark trough has contributions from RPE, photoreceptors and inner nuclear layer. The amplitude increases in light-adapted state and reaches a "light peak" in approximately 5 minutes. Light peak is affected by photoreceptors.

Arden ratio is calculated as the amplitude of light peak divided by the amplitude of dark trough. Its normal value is more than or equal to 180 and is considered abnormal below 165.

Clinically, it has found application only in diagnosing Best vitelliform dystrophy in which Ardens ratio is <165, but ERG is normal. In other retinal diseases, it usually does not provide any additional information over ERG.[10]

REFERENCES

1. Vincent A, Robson AG, Holder GE. Pathognomonic (Diagnostic) ERGs: a review and update. Retina. 2013;33(1):5-12.
2. McCulloch DL, Marmor MF, Brigell MG, Hamilton R, Holder GE, Tzekov R, et al. ISCEV Standard for full-field clinical electroretinography (2015 update). Doc Ophthalmol. 2015;130(1):1-12.
3. Perlman I. The Electroretinogram: ERG. 2001. In: Kolb H, Fernandez E, Jones B, et al. (Eds). Webvision: The Organization of the Retina and Visual System [Internet]. Salt Lake City (UT): University of Utah Health Sciences Center; 1995.
4. Wack MA, Peachey NS, Fishman GA. Electroretinographic findings in human oculocutaneous albinism. Ophthalmology. 1989;96(12):1778-85.
5. Wachtmeister L. Oscillatory potentials in the retina: what do they reveal. Prog Retin Eye Res. 1998;17(4):485-521.
6. Bach M, Brigell MG, Hawlina M, Holder GE, Johnson MA, McCulloch DL, et al. ISCEV standard for clinical pattern electroretinography (PERG): 2012 update. Doc Ophthalmol. 2013;126(1):1-7.
7. Tafreshi A, Racette L, Weinreb RN, Sample PA, Zangwill LM, Medeiros FA, et al. Pattern electroretinogram and psychophysical tests of visual function for discriminating between healthy and glaucoma eyes. Am J Ophthalmol. 2010;149(3):488-95.
8. Hood DC, Bach M, Brigell M, Keating D, Kondo M, Lyons JS, et al.; International Society For Clinical Electrophysiology of Vision. ISCEV standard for clinical multifocal electroretinography (mfERG) (2011 edition). Doc Ophthalmol. 2012;124(1): 1-13.
9. Lai TYY, Chan WM, Lai RY, Ngai JW, Li H, Lam DS. The clinical applications of multifocal electroretinography: a systematic review. Surv Ophthalmol. 2007;52(1):61-96.
10. Arden GB, Constable PA. The electrooculogram. Prog Retin Eye Res. 2006;25(2): 207-48.

4.6 MULTISPOT LASER SYSTEM

Anusha Sachan, Brijesh Takkar, Amber Bhayana

INTRODUCTION

The laser was first used in ophthalmology by Meyer-Schwickerath.[1] Laser photocoagulation is one of the most commonly performed ocular procedures.[2] It is aimed at the destruction of outer retina, especially photoreceptors which have high oxygen consumption. This results in decreased retinal oxygen demand along with increased diffusion of oxygen from choroid to inner retina, which improves the inner retinal homeostasis. This leads to a decrease in the production of angiogenic factors such VEGF and platelet-derived growth factor (PDGF) resulting in regression of neovascularization.[3]

Common indications include PDR, arterial and venous occlusions, and sealing breaks. Multiple types of lasers have been employed for this, including double-frequency neodymium-doped yttrium aluminum garnet (Nd:YAG) laser, argon laser, and diode laser. A relatively recently developed platform for quick delivery of laser spots is the multispot laser (MSL), and a commercially available form of the same is the pattern scanning laser (PASCAL). It was Food and Drug Administration (FDA) approved in 2005. Systems for scanning beam technology in retinal photocoagulation were first developed at Stanford University by Blumenkranz et al. around 2006. Other similar laser systems are also now available commercially.

MULTISPOT LASER NEODYMIUM-DOPED YTTRIUM ALUMINUM GARNET

It is a semiautomatic device, which delivers ultrashort pulses of double-frequency Nd:YAG laser in selected patterns.

With the PASCAL system, a maximum of 56 spots can be delivered together in 0.6 seconds. Each pulse has a duration of 10–20 ms compared with 100–200 ms of conventional laser delivery systems. Space between spots can be varied from 0.25 to 2 spot diameters. The short duration of pulses results in decreased thermal damage to surrounding structures, though laser power required may be higher. Spots can be delivered in different patterns such as square, arc or grid[4] selected by the physician by using control screen **(Fig. 4.6.1)**.[2,4]

Fluence is defined as (power × time)/area. If the spot size remains unchanged with a burn duration of 20 ms as in MSL, the fluence is less than with a 100-ms burn typically delivered with single-spot laser. Hence, reduced diffusion of heat and subsequent collateral damage occur. Multiple studies have shown better "qualitative visual aspects" with MSL in comparison to traditional laser systems. Another reason for the same is the inconsistent laser delivery typical of single-spot laser systems in real-world situations.

Advantages over conventional single spot systems:
- Decreased duration of the procedure
- Decreased thermal damage
- Increased precision and uniformity **(Figs. 4.6.2 to 4.6.4)**
- Less pain
- Less scarring (creep phenomenon) and collateral damage
- Customized patterns for different conditions such as the macular laser, laser around holes and breaks

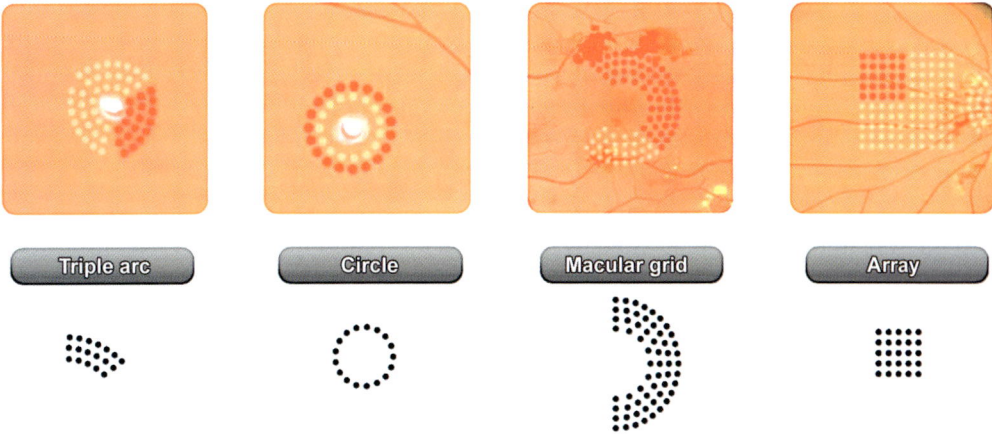

Fig. 4.6.1: Patterns of laser.

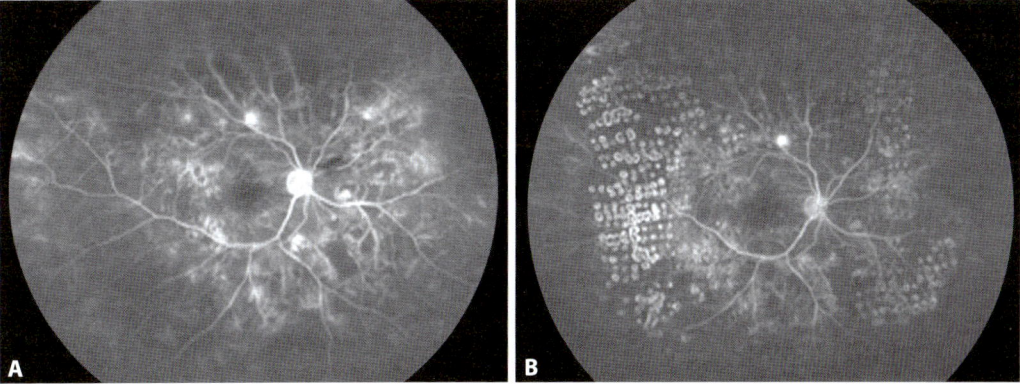

Figs. 4.6.2A and B: (A) A case of proliferative diabetic retinopathy (PDR) and (B) 3 months after pattern scanning laser (PASCAL).

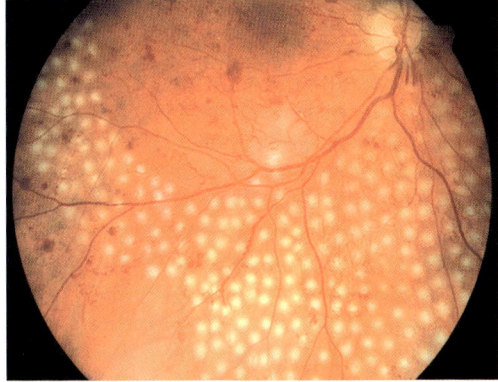

Fig. 4.6.3: Fundus image showing PASCAL laser spots in inferior retina of right eye.

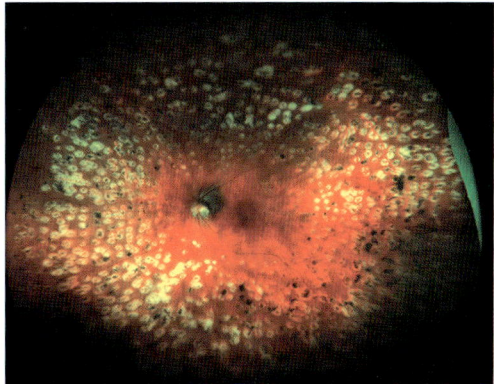

Fig. 4.6.4: Optos image depicting PASCAL laser panretinal photocoagulation in PDR.

A major practical utility is the ability to perform panretinal photocoagulation (PRP) for indications like PDR in a single sitting, rather than the traditional technique of 2–3 sittings. Even more useful may be the use in ROP that is considered a tedious laser, which is anecdotal as of now. A comparison between MSL and conventional systems has been drawn in.

Optical coherence tomography-based studies have shown that damage from burns in PASCAL is confined to outer retina. More precisely, maximum damage and healing response are seen at the level of inner segment/outer segment (IS/OS) junction and apical RPE. Also, burn marks, which may not always be visible on fundus biomicroscopy are seen more clearly on FAF as hypofluorescent spots.[5] Newer MSLs offer macular photocoagulation also, along with different color modes. However, the surgeon must titrate the desired laser burn before shooting in continuity as multiple burns will be delivered in a very short interval. Titration may be done with single spots that are also available with the MSL systems.

Examples of MSL available with the PASCAL system:
- *PASCAL 577 nm laser:* Subthreshold 577 nm yellow PASCAL laser has been used to treat DME with excellent results.
- *PASCAL red laser:* Useful when photocoagulation is to be done in the presence vitreous hemorrhage.

PATTERN SCANNING LASER TRABECULOPLASTY

It makes use of 633 nm aiming and 532 or 577 nm therapeutic lasers. A gonioscopic (PSLT gonioscopic lens) lens is used to project a laser pattern on trabecular meshwork. Half or the full length of trabecular meshwork can be treated. It is applied to 180° in 16 steps and 360° in 32 steps, respectively.[6] 13 spots are present in each row. Laser power is first titrated by using 10 ms pulse on the inferior segment of the eye to produce a visible blanching reaction. Once appropriate power is selected, using the same power and 5 ms pulse duration does the rest of the treatment. No visible reaction is seen. Studies have shown 20–30% reduction in intraocular pressure (IOP) at a mean follow-up of 1 month.

REFERENCES

1. Meyer-Schwickerath RE, Schott K. Diabetic retinopathy and photocoagulation. Am J Ophthalmol. 1968;66(4):597-603.
2. Salman AG. Pascal laser versus conventional laser for treatment of diabetic retinopathy. Saudi J Ophthalmol. 2011;25(2):175-9.
3. Funatsu H, Hori S, Yamashita H, Kitano S. Effective mechanisms of laser photocoagulation for neovascularization in diabetic retinopathy. Nippon Ganka Gakkai Zasshi. 1996;100(5):339-49.
4. TOPCON. (2018). Eye Care: Pattern Scanning Laser PASCAL Series. [online] Available from https://www.topcon.co.jp/en/eyecare/products/product/surgical/pascal/PASCAL_s_E.html [Last accessed January, 2019].
5. Joan W Miller, Szilárd Kiss. The Pattern Scanning Laser (PASCAL®) Photocoagulator for Diabetic Retinopathy. US Ophthalmic Rev. 2011;4(1):94-5.
6. IOVS. (2013). Patterned Laser Trabeculoplasty with PASCAL streamline 577. [online] Available from http://iovs.arvojournals.org/article.aspx?articleid=2146511 [Last accessed October, 2024].

4.7 ADAPTIVE OPTICS

Anusha Sachan, Divya Agarwal, Rohan Chawla

■ INTRODUCTION

Adaptive optics (AO) is a novel technology, which compensates for the eye's optical aberrations, allowing exceptional visualization of retinal structures in the eye, including individual photoreceptors, the microvasculature, retinal nerve fiber bundles, the RPE, and the lamina cribrosa (LC).[1,2] Junzhong Liang, David Williams, and Donald Miller at the University of Rochester (NY) developed the first AO fundus camera, which was able to image individual cones at multiple retinal eccentricities.[2] Retinal imaging modalities depend on the optical elements of the eye mainly the cornea and lens to produce retinal images and are therefore affected by the specific arrangement and curvatural imperfections of these optical elements known as wavefront aberrations. It can be a lower order aberration (defocus, astigmatism), which can be easily managed in imaging devices and higher order aberration (coma, trefoil), which are unstable aberrations and require complex corrections to allow excellent resolution.[3] The highest possible transverse resolution of retinal imaging is affected by the optical properties, which produces wavefront aberrations of the imaging light and degrade the quality of the image. In order to compensate or correct these wavefront aberrations and improve the image quality, a novel technology of AO has been tried. Initially, it was used for astronomy in the ground-based telescope, but now it has been integrated with many ophthalmic imaging devices like fundus photography, scanning laser ophthalmoscopy (SLO), and OCT for retinal imaging.[4]

■ PRINCIPLE

Adaptive optics retinal imaging system consists of three main components:
1. Wavefront sensor (typically Hartmann–Shack aberrometer)
2. Corrective element or adaptive optical element
3. Control system or software system.

A beam of light enters the eye, and a small part of it is reflected back into the optical system of the eye. This reflected beam of light forms a wavefront, which is detected by the wavefront sensor. The deformable mirror alters reflected light for optical aberrations based on the measurements of the wavefront sensor. This integration between the sensor and deformable mirror is controlled by the control system, which is a software to process information from the sensor and provide the feedback to the deformable mirror to reduce the optical aberrations of the imaging light and provide good quality of images **(Fig. 4.7.1)**.[1,3] By compensating for the wavefront aberrations of the eye, transverse (lateral) resolution up to 2 µm can be achieved, thereby allowing visualization of the cone mosaic and individual cone photoreceptors.

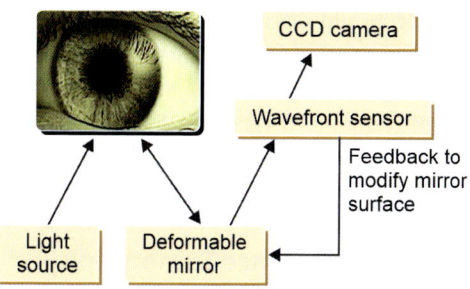

Fig. 4.7.1: Working principle of adaptive optics. (CCD: charge-coupled device)

Adaptive optics integrated with optical-retinal imaging modalities provides noninvasive histology of the retinal tissue. It allows in vivo visualization of cone photoreceptors, RPE, red and white blood cells, LC, and retinal blood vessels.[4] Imaging of rod photoreceptors is difficult due to its small diameter (<2 µm) and reduced waveguiding properties as compared to cones.[5,6]

ADAPTIVE OPTICS RETINAL IMAGING SYSTEMS

Fundus Camera

- Retina illuminated by krypton arc flash lamp, Xinetics deformable mirror
- Visualize cone mosaic (cone spacing, cone bidirectionality, temporal fluctuations in cone reflectance) and loss of fixation
- Advantage—incoherent light source to reduce speckle, brief imaging exposure
- Disadvantage—effective frame rate slow, images collected one at a time

Scanning Laser Ophthalmoscopy

- Greatly enhanced image quality through the use of a confocal pinhole to eliminate out-of-focus light
- Continuous, high resolution, raster scanning at a faster rate than AO fundus camera
- Eye tracking, laser modulation for stimulus delivery, multichannel imaging, and stabilized stimulus delivery for psychophysics and electrophysiology
- Advantage—confocality increases the contrast of the final image, axial sectioning of retina, and visualization of its various layers like nerve fiber layer, blood vessels, photoreceptors, and RPE.

Optical Coherence Tomography

Three-dimensional (3D) visualization of the nerve fiber layer, ganglion cells, and LC as well as the RPE mosaic and choriocapillaris was demonstrated using high-speed AO-OCT (120,000 scans/s).

INTERPRETATION

Adaptive optics image data from a normal individual is essential for establishing the baseline for the cone characteristics, in order to detect early pathological changes. In one of the AO prototype (rtx1, imagine eye, Orsay, France) 750 nm wavelength light is used to visualize different retinal layers. 850 nm wavelength light source capture sequential images of a 4 × 4 picture with frame rate 9.5 frames/s (total 40 frames). The final image is formed using image J software and region of interest is analyzed for three main parameters: (1) Cone packing density; (2) Cone spacing; and (3) Voronoi analysis (to access the regularity of photoreceptors and hexagonal polygons percentage) **(Figs. 4.7.2 and 4.7.3)**.

APPLICATIONS

- Functional AO imaging—high-speed AO fundus camera and adaptive optics scanning laser ophthalmoscopy (AOSLO) can be used to study temporal fluctuation in cone reflectance. Two hypotheses are there for temporal fluctuations. Firstly, it is caused due to molecular changes within

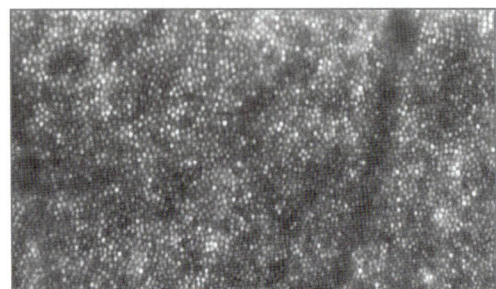

Fig. 4.7.2: White dots correspond to cone photoreceptors.

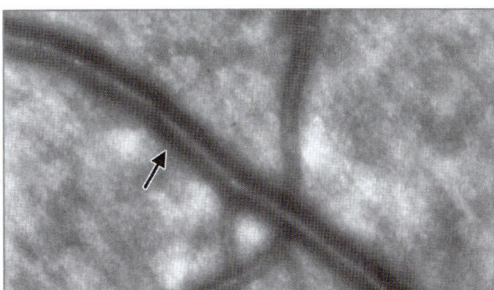

Fig. 4.7.3: The black arrow points to the vessel wall. Lumen is bright as compared to the vessel wall. The defocused retinal nerve fiber layer is in the background.

the photoreceptor during transduction; secondly, it is due to changes in the cone outer segment related to disc shedding. AO can be helpful in measuring this reflectance and providing the functional status of the normal and diseased retina. It is used in conditions like opsin mutations, acute macular neuropathy (AMN), and closed globe blunt trauma.[7]
- Photoreceptor density and structure in retinal diseases, e.g., Stargardt disease—abnormal cone morphology and packing
- *To assess the prognosis of disease:* In conditions of achromatopsia, patients with some amount of retained cone structure benefit more from gene therapy than those with a complete absence of cones.
- *Monitoring treatment outcomes:* Talcott et al. tried CNTF encapsulated implants in patients with retinal degenerations and monitoring was done with AOSLO. They concluded that AOSLO provided early information on progression or treatment than conventional modalities.[8]
- *Vascular analysis:* Vascular system gives an insight into the health of the retinal tissue. Diseases like diabetes, hypertension, and dyslipidemia can cause changes in the vessel architecture and lumen size. Preclinical abnormalities can be seen in retinal vasculatures like capillary dropout areas, abnormal AV tortuosity, and subclinical FAZ enlargement.[9]

LIMITATIONS

- Difficult to perform in patients with unstable fixation, dense cataract, and opaque media; imaging sessions are prolonged and demand excellent subject fixation, as the field of view studied is between 1° and 4°.[2]
- The system is very sensitive to media opacities, higher refractive error, and tear film deficiencies.
- Image processing and analysis are time-consuming processes that lack automated techniques.[2]
- High cost and expertise to interpret the images.

REFERENCES

1. Godara P, Dubis AM, Roorda A, Duncan JL, Carroll J. Adaptive optics retinal imaging: emerging clinical applications. Optom Vis Sci. 2010;87(12):930-41.
2. Retinal Physician. (2016). Adaptive Optics Retinal Imaging: applications and clinical implications. [online] Available from https://www.retinalphysician.com/issues/2016/may-2016/adaptive-optics-retinal-imaging-applications-and [Last accessed January, 2019].
3. Lombardo M, Lombardo G. Wave aberration of human eyes and new descriptors of image optical quality and visual performance. J Cataract Refract Surg. 2010;36(2):313-31.
4. Babcock HW. Adaptive optics revisited. Science. 1990;249(4966):253-7.
5. Lombardo M, Serrao S, Ducoli P, Lombardo G. Eccentricity dependent changes of density, spacing and packing arrangement of parafoveal cones. Ophthalmic Physiol Opt. 2013;33(4):516-26.
6. Alpern M, Ching CC, Kitahara K. The directional sensitivity of retinal rods. J Physiol. 1983;343:577-92.

7. Cooper RF, Dubis AM, Pavaskar A, Rha J, Dubra A, Carroll J. Spatial and temporal variation of rod photoreceptor reflectance in the human retina. Biomed Opt Express. 2011;2(9):2577-89.
8. Talcott KE, Ratnam K, Sundquist SM, Lucero AS, Lujan BJ, Tao W, et al. Longitudinal study of cone photoreceptors during retinal degeneration and in response to ciliary neurotrophic factor treatment. Invest Ophthalmol Vis Sci. 2011;52(5):2219-26.
9. Lombardo M, Parravano M, Serrao S, Ducoli P, Stirpe M, Lombardo G. Analysis of retinal capillaries in patients with type 1 diabetes and nonproliferative diabetic retinopathy using adaptive optics imaging. Retina. 2013;33(8):1630-9.

4.8 AMSLER GRID

Ankit Singh Tomar, Saurabh Verma, Atul Kumar

■ INTRODUCTION

In today's ever-changing healthcare environment, the best defense against disease is self-detection and monitoring. Many disease states such as diabetes and age-related macular degeneration can have long-term effects on the eyesight. Early detection of deteriorating vision is key to preventing permanent vision damage.

Marc Amsler, a Swiss ophthalmologist in 1945, developed Amsler grid. It evaluates the 20° of the visual field centered on fixation. It is principally useful in screening for and monitoring macular disease but will also demonstrate central visual field defects originating elsewhere. Patients with a substantial risk of CNV should be provided with an Amsler grid for regular use at home.

■ TECHNIQUE

The pupils should be undilated and slit-lamp examination should be avoided in order to avoid the photostress effect on the eyes. A presbyopic refractive correction should be worn if appropriate. The chart should be well illuminated and held at a comfortable reading distance, optimally around 33 cm.[1]

The following steps are followed:
- One eye is covered.
- The patient is asked to look directly at the central dot with the uncovered eye, to keep looking at this, and to report any distortion, broken lines, blurred area, dark area or waviness of the lines on the grid.
- Remind the patient to maintain fixation on the central dot.
- The patient may be provided with a recording sheet and pen and asked to draw any anomalies.[2]

■ TYPES

There are seven charts, each consisting of a 10 cm outer square. The charts and the relevant points are described in **Table 4.8.1**.

■ INTERPRETATION

Questions asked of the patient: A set of questions, as given in **Table 4.8.2**, is asked to the patient to interpret the results.

Uses: The various clinical conditions and their interpretations are given in **Table 4.8.3**. Amsler chart is extremely helpful in following diseases:[3]

TABLE 4.8.1: Types of Amsler charts and their salient features.[1]

Charts	Characteristics
Chart 1	• Most often used chart • It consists of a high-contrast white grid on a black background • The outer grid enclosing 400 smaller 5 mm squares • When viewed at about one-third of a meter, each small square subtends an angle of 1° • Absolute scotoma appears as not seen at all or black area • Relative scotoma appears as blur
Chart 2	• Similar to *Chart 1* but has diagonal lines that aid fixation for patients with a central scotoma • If the patient still is unable to achieve or maintain fixation, a larger white central spot may be applied to center of the grid
Chart 3	• Similar to *Chart 1* but has red squares • Red-on-black design stimulates the long wavelength foveal cones • Useful to detect subtle color scotoma and desaturation in cases such as toxic maculopathy, nutritional amblyopia, optic neuropathy, and optic tract lesions • Can be used to detect patients with functional vision loss in conjunction with red–green glasses (grid will not be seen when viewed through green lens)
Chart 4	• It has only white random dots distributed like stars in sky • It is useful in differentiating scotoma from metamorphopsia (no form to be distorted)
Chart 5	• It has horizontal lines and is useful in detecting metamorphopsia along specific meridians • It can be rotated to any meridian to check for irregularities in a particular area • It is of particular use in the evaluation of patients describing difficulty reading
Chart 6	• Similar to *Chart 5* but has a white background and the central lines 1° above and below fixation point are closer together • Enables evaluation that is more detailed
Chart 7	• It has a fine central grid of area 6° × 8° in the central area • Each square subtends an angle of a half degree • It is highly sensitive to early macular diseases and mild visual disturbance

TABLE 4.8.2: Questions asked to the patient while interpreting Amsler chart.

1.	Can you see the central dot?	To rule out central scotoma
2.	While looking at the central dot, can you see all four quadrants of chart simultaneously?	To rule out arcuate, altitudinal, quadratic or hemianopic field defect as well as field constrictions
3.	Does the grid appear to have any missing or distorted area?	To rule out paracentral, cecocentral, or altitudinal scotomas
4.	Any area of grid having an unusual appearance (lines appear wavy)?	To rule out metamorphopsia
5.	Any square shimmering or colored?	To rule out scintillating scotomas

- Dry age-related macular degeneration (ARMD)
- DR
- Macular degenerations
- ERM and other vitreomacular traction disorders
- Macular hole
- Toxic maculopathy

TABLE 4.8.3: Clinical conditions and their impact on Amsler chart interpretation.

Type of disease	Character	Example
Progressive disease	Which develop significant alterations over time	Toxic maculopathy/atypical retinitis pigmentosa (RP)
Active disease	May improve or worsen in short span of time	Optic neuritis or macular neuroretinopathy
Recurrent disease	Already suffering vision loss but at a risk of reactivation of disease process	Central serous choroidopathy, toxoplasma retinochoroiditis

- Optic neuropathy[3]
- Chiasmal lesion

VIVA QUESTIONS

1. What part of the visual field is evaluated by Amsler grid?
Ans. 20°

2. What are the indications of using the Amsler grid?
Ans. Refer to text.

3. How many types of Amsler grid are there?
Ans. Seven types **(Figs. 4.8.1 to 4.8.7)**

4. What instructions need to be given to the patients?
Ans. Refer to text.

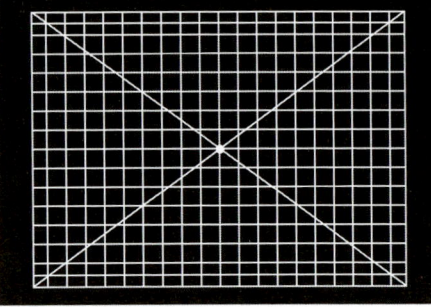

Fig. 4.8.2: Chart 2.

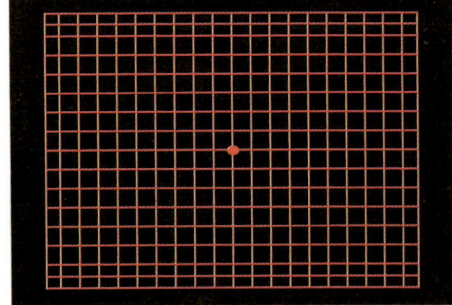

Fig. 4.8.3: Chart 3.

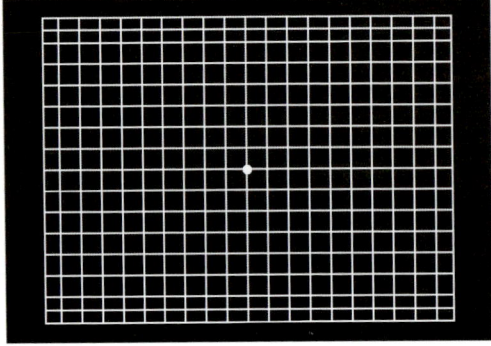

Fig. 4.8.1: Chart 1.

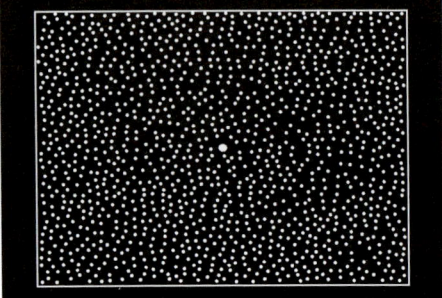

Fig. 4.8.4: Chart 4.

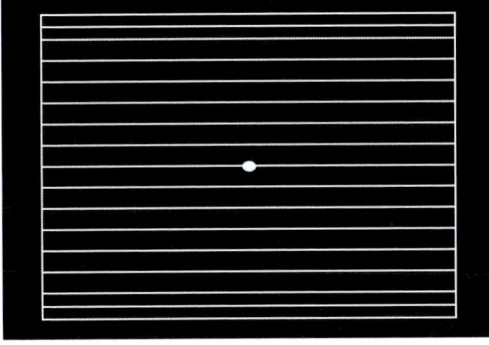

Fig. 4.8.5: Chart 5.

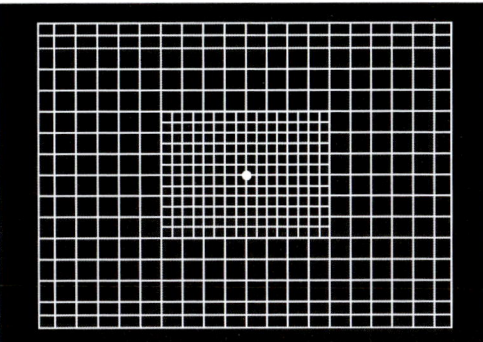

Fig. 4.8.7: Chart 7.

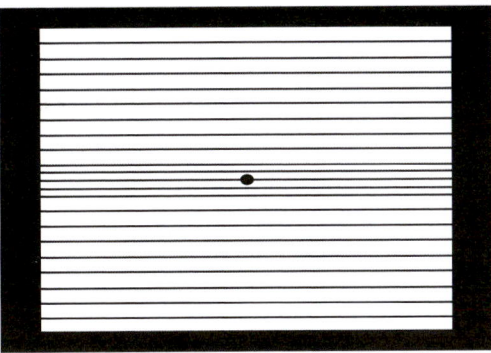

Fig. 4.8.6: Chart 6.

REFERENCES

1. Mattice E, Wolfe CP. Using the Amsler grid. J Ophthalmic Nurs Technol. 1986;5(1):34.
2. Lederman ME. Demonstration of scotoma on an Amsler grid examination. Am J Ophthalmol. 1985;100(5):740.
3. Easterbrook M. The sensitivity of Amsler grid testing in early chloroquine retinopathy. Trans Ophthalmol Soc UK. 1985;104 (Pt 2):204-7.

4.9 VITREORETINAL INSTRUMENTS

Devesh Kumawat, Pranita Sahay, Anusha Sachan, Atul Kumar

TROCAR AND CANNULA

- Trocars **(Fig. 4.9.1)** are used to make pars plana sclerotomy entries. Trocar needle can be 20G/23G/25G/27G.
- Microcannulas made up of polyimide and are already loaded over the needle trocars.
- Microcannula can be valved or non-valved.
- Plugs usage and instrument exchanges for its removal and placement are eliminated in valved cannulas.
- Trocar needle, microcannula, and trocar handle together constitute the trocar/cannula assembly. This system helps in instrument access from outside within eye without any obstruction and maintains entry hole between conjunctiva and sclera aligned.

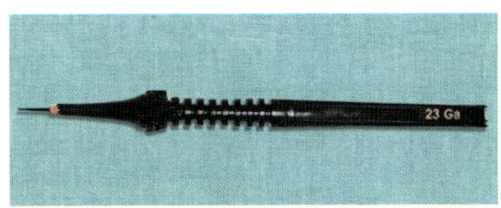

Fig. 4.9.1: Trocar.

INFUSION CANNULA

Self-retaining infusion cannulas **(Fig. 4.9.2)** of different sizes according to microcannula (20G/23G/25G/27G) are used to introduce irrigating solutions into the vitreous cavity.

VITRECTOMY CUTTER

- Vitreous cutters **(Fig. 4.9.3)** utilize suction and inclusive shearing force to cut vitreous.
- These can be of two broad types:
  1. Electrodynamic cutters are heavy and become hot on prolonged use. It can cause fatigue and aggravate tremors.
  2. Pneumatic cutters are lighter than the electrodynamic cutters and so they cause fewer tremors. They are cheaper and of higher efficiency.
- Vitrectomy cutters are of three types based on the cutting mechanism:
  1. Cutters using rotating mechanism.
  2. *Cutter using oscillating mechanism or Peyman type:* This type of cutter is more efficient and superior than rotating cutter as it produces less shearing effect on retina.
  3. *The Guillotine type cutters:* Most frequently used vitrectomy cutter; it has an outer tube, which has an opening through, which vitreous is aspirated. The inner tube slides across the port thus cutting the vitreous with minimal traction over retina.
- *Vitrectomy mode:* A standard high-speed vitrectomy cutter has a cutting frequency of up to 5,000 cpm and can be increased up to 7,500. High-speed cutting reduces traction on retina hence increases stability while cutting vitreous close to the retina. The vitrectomy machine supports both pneumatic and electric drive for pneumatic and electric vitrectomies when needed. It should be used in a single cut, fixed, and linear cutting control. Horizontal cutting probes have a new concept of radial reciprocating action, which minimizes the traction, turbulence, or fluttering of tissues (cutting blade moves from left to right across the port). Latest vitrectomy machine by Alcon "the Constellation" can cut vitreous up to a frequency of 7,000 cpm. Three different vitrectomy modes exists in the machine, i.e., proportional vacuum, 3D (dual dynamic drive), and momentary mode. Usually proportional vacuum mode vitrectomy is done.
- *3D technology:* This allows the surgeon to change the parameters of cut rate and vacuum simultaneously as needed throughout the surgery. Vacuum can be set to start at low level and rise to max at full foot pedal depression while cutting rate can be set to start at its max setting and decreased with foot pedal is depression. It allows more cutting of

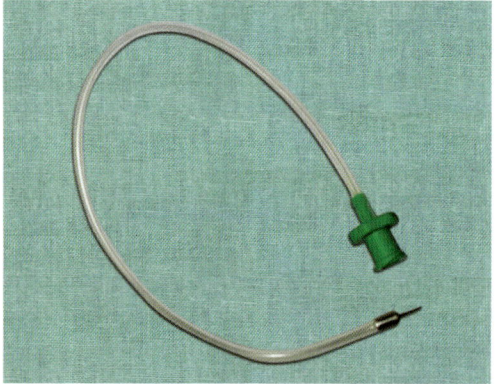

Fig. 4.9.2: Infusion cannula.

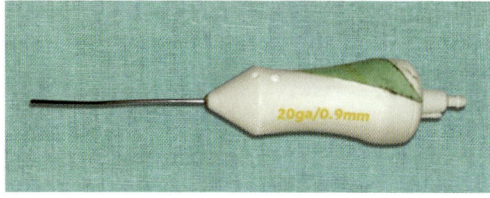

Fig. 4.9.3: Vitrectomy cutter.

vitreous while doing core vitrectomy and fine cutting without much traction when cutting near the retinal surface.

END GRASPING FORCEPS
- These forceps have jaws at the tip to hold tissues at the edge only **(Fig. 4.9.4)**.
- The tips are fine and allow visualization of the tissue while grasping.
- These are used for epiretinal membrane peeling.

INTERNAL LIMITING MEMBRANE FORCEPS
- These have fine tips with smaller jaws, which help in picking up of delicate tissues like ILM **(Fig. 4.9.5)**.
- These are used for ILM peeling in macular hole surgery.

SERRATED FORCEPS
- Serrated forceps have large flat grasping blades without jaws **(Fig. 4.9.6)**, which help in strong grip over tissues while managing proliferative vitreoretinopathy.

- These are used in tough epiretinal membrane peeling and retinal pucker release.

FOREIGN BODY FORCEPS
- Foreign body forceps are large-gauge forceps with serrated or diamond-dusted tips for removal of intraocular foreign bodies **(Fig. 4.9.7)**.
- These have stout jaws, which help in the firm holding of the foreign body.

EXTRUSION INSTRUMENTS
- *Charles flute needle:* It consists of a blunt needle attached to a detachable handle **(Fig. 4.9.8)**.
  - It is used for controlled passive extrusion of fluid during internal

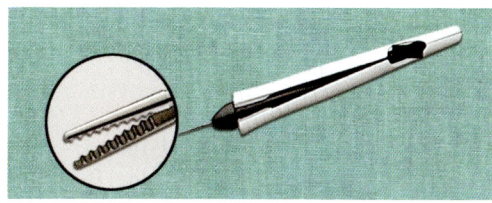

Fig. 4.9.6: Serrated forceps.

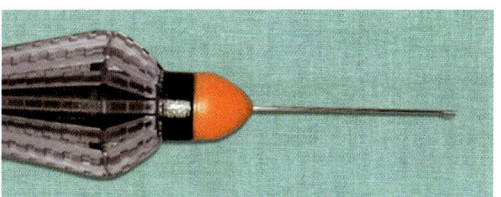

Fig. 4.9.4: End grasping forceps.

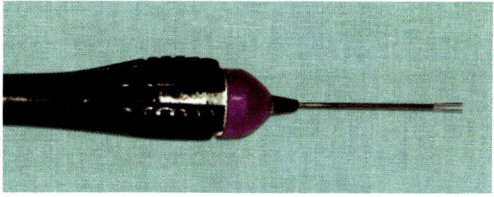

Fig. 4.9.7: Foreign body forceps.

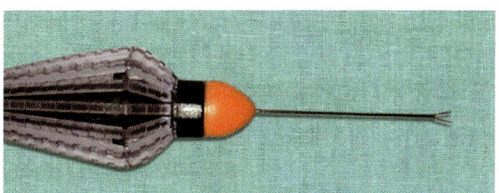

Fig. 4.9.5: Internal limiting membrane (ILM) forceps.

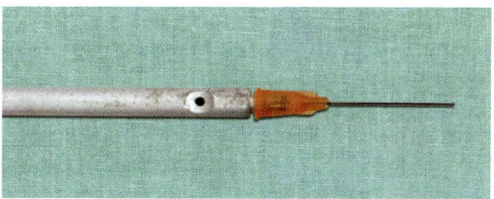

Fig. 4.9.8: Charles flute needle.

drainage of subretinal fluid, removal of preretinal blood, and fluid–air exchange.
- The internal channel leads to an exit port on the side of the handle. Egress of fluid occurs when cannula tip is in fluid, and exit port is open, driven by infusion pressure, which is above the atmospheric pressure.
- The blunt tip can be replaced with a soft silicone tip needle as well with decreased risk of iatrogenic retinal damage.

■ *Backflush* **(Fig. 4.9.9)** is a modified flute handle with large silicone reservoir. Pressure on this reservoir leads to retrograde flushing of the fluid or accidentally aspirated/incarcerated tissues. It can also be used to disperse sedimented preretinal bleed. It can be used with either blunt or soft-tip needle.

■ CANNULA

Cannula tips can be of several types:
- *Silicone brush tip cannula*: It has a soft silicon brush tip **(Fig. 4.9.10)**, which is used for gentle brushing and manipulation of the retina. These are excellent for removing blood from the retina surface.
- *Diamond-dusted soft silicone tip cannula*: These are used for the removal of triamcinolone particles from the retinal surface.
- *Charles flute cannula*: Smooth, finished tip provides atraumatic entry, reduces the risk of trauma to surrounding tissue, and helps to aspirate blood and debris.
- *Soft silicone tip cannula*: The soft, flexible tip on the cannula provides nontraumatic entry through retinal or macular tears or holes. These are used for fluid–fluid or fluid–air exchange in vitrectomy surgery.
- *Dual bore cannula*: Simultaneous infusion of heavy liquids like perfluorocarbon liquid (PFCL) and aspiration of intraocular fluids with dual-bore cannula helps to control and maintain a constant IOP during the procedure.

The cannula can be connected to flute handle or backflush handle or active extrusion handle.

■ DIAMOND-DUSTED MEMBRANE SCRAPER

Tano diamond-dusted membrane scraper (DDMS) **(Fig. 4.9.11)** helps to find the edge of the epiretinal membranes. It is made of tongue-shaped soft silicone with inert diamond dust. It is very helpful in ILM and epiretinal membrane removal; the

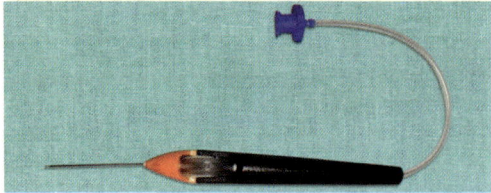

Fig. 4.9.9: Backflush.

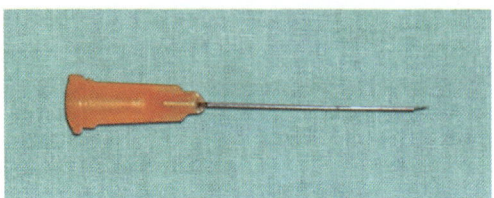

Fig. 4.9.10: Soft silicone tip cannula.

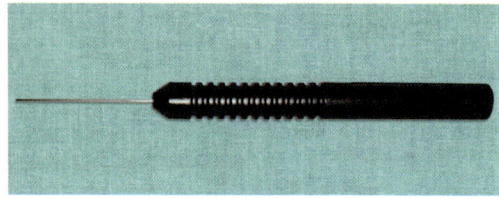

Fig. 4.9.11: Diamond-dusted membrane scraper (DDMS).

diamond-dusted soft silicone tip is grazed over the retinal surface to find the edge of membrane. The edge is then grasped with the ILM forceps to complete the membrane removal.

VITREORETINAL SCISSORS (FIG. 4.9.12)

- *Horizontal scissors* are used for delamination during epiretinal membrane removal. Their cutting edge moves conformal to the retinal surface. Their blades can have a gentle curve or can be straight, with an angle of 30° or 45° to the shaft.
- *Vertical scissors* have vertical blades with pointed tips that move along the axis of the shaft. Proximal blade moves down toward the fixed distal blade to cut the tissue vertically. These are used for epiretinal membrane segmentation.

GASS RETINAL DETACHMENT HOOK

Gass retinal detachment hook is used for localization of retinal breaks onto the sclera in retinal detachment surgery **(Fig. 4.9.13)**.

MAGNETS

Magnets are used to remove magnetic intraocular foreign bodies **(Fig. 4.9.14)**.

Electromagnets are more powerful than rare earth magnets (REMs) and their magnetic force can be varied, but they are used only as external magnets. REMs are available for both intraocular and extraocular uses.

SCHOCKET SCLERAL DEPRESSOR

Schocket scleral depressor has a rounded end used for depressing sclera and curved marking end for indenting posteriorly by reaching behind the globe **(Fig. 4.9.15)**.

VIVA QUESTIONS

1. What is the full form of MIVS?
Ans. Microincision vitrectomy surgery (MIVS) [initially known as transconjunctival sutureless vitrectomy (TSV)].

2. What is the dimension, color coding, and inventor of various trocar cannula?
Ans. Refer to **Table 4.9.1**.

3. Who is the father of vitreoretinal surgery?

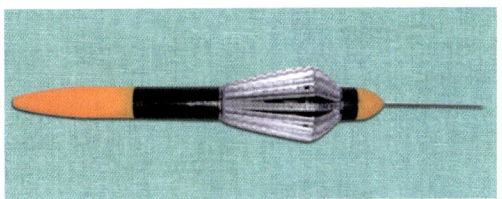

Fig. 4.9.12: Vitreoretinal scissors.

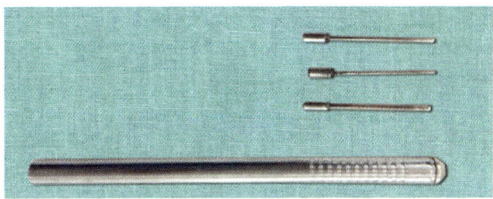

Fig. 4.9.14: Magnets.

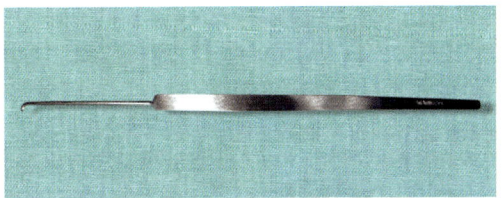

Fig. 4.9.13: Gass retinal detachment hook.

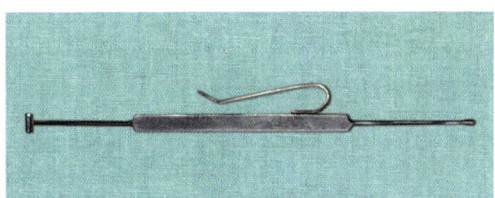

Fig. 4.9.15: Schocket scleral depressor.

TABLE 4.9.1: Dimension, color coding, and inventor of various trocar cannula.

Trocar cannula	Dimension (outer diameter in mm)	Color	Scientist
17	2.3		
19	1.1		
20	0.9	Yellow	O'Malley and Heintz
23	0.7	Orange	Eckardt
25	0.5	Blue–green	Fujji
27	0.4	Purple	Oshima

Ans. Robert Machemer in 1971 did first 17G single port closed pars plana vitrectomy in an egg by making a small opening in eggshell to remove its albumin.

4. What are the advantages of MIVS?

Ans. Following are the advantages of MIVS:
- Beveled incisions made with the help of these instruments are sutureless or require only a single 7-0 vicryl suture to close.
- Prevent herniation of retina and vitreous from port site
- Less chances of port site dialysis or retinal detachment
- Enhanced postoperative comfort and reduces healing time
- Port being closer to the distal tip of the vitrectomy cutter in smaller gauge system enhances the ability to go close to the retina (0.23 mm in 25G cutters and 0.43 in 20G cutters)
- Small cutters can be easily navigated through the gaps between the fibrovascular membranes and to create cleavage planes for easy dissection.

5. What are the disadvantages of MIVS?

Ans. Following are the disadvantages of MIVS:
- *Intraoperative:* Increased surgical time (due to the reduction in flow and aspiration), IOP rise, cannula retraction, retinal break formation, hypotony, jamming of vitrectomy cutters, and breakage of cutter or microcannula
- *Postoperative:* Postoperative hypotony and endophthalmitis

6. State the use of 41G instrument system.

Ans. It is a 0.1 mm diameter port cannula system, which is used to create small retinotomy to create perimacular subretinal blebs for submacular surgeries and in introducing tissue plasminogen activator (tPA) in patients with submacular bleed. These retinotomies do not require laser delimitation.

7. What is the benefit of valved small-gauge cannulas?

Ans. Valved cannulas help to reduce the turbulence and IOP variation in the vitreous cavity during insertion and removal of instruments through the ports during surgery.

8. How to reduce the malleability of 25G instruments?

Ans. As we are heading toward the smaller gauge instrument systems, reducing the thickness of the probe reduces its stiffness, which results in bending and difficulty to direct the instrument in the required direction. Addition of a stiffening sleeve is done to small-gauge instruments to reduce its malleability to promote good maneuverability.

9. What is bimanual vitreoretinal surgery?

Ans. When vitrectomy is done under chandelier light, then it is called bimanual vitreoretinal surgery. It provides a good opportunity to the surgeon to use his both

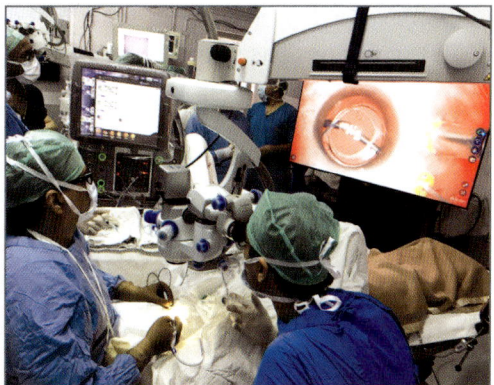

Fig. 4.9.16: "NGENUITY" 3D visualization system.

hands to dissect membranes with minimal damage in cases like DR.

10. What is digitally-assisted vitreoretinal surgery (DAVS)?

Ans. It is a novel concept of Novartis "NGENUITY" 3D visualization system, a platform for DAVS **(Fig. 4.9.16)**. It allows the surgeon to operate looking at a high-definition 3D screen, instead of bending their necks to look through the eyepiece of the microscope (heads-up viewing system). This microscope-free design is engineered to improve the surgeon's posture and help to reduce the fatigue during the surgery.

11. What are the various modes of vitrectomy?

Ans. These are:
- Momentary
- 3D
- Proportional

12. What is the duty cycle in vitrectomy?

Ans. The duty cycle of a vitrectomy probe is the percentage of time the port is open measured against the entire cycle of the cutter.

13. What are the various steps of a diabetic vitrectomy surgery?

Ans. The following are the critical maneuvers while doing a diabetic vitrectomy:
- *Segmentation:* Vertical cutting of epiretinal membranes into smaller segments to release circumferential traction
- *Delamination:* Finding the correct plane and horizontal cutting of individual neovascular frond from the retinal surface
- *En bloc:* Enables complete removal of all the fibrovascular tissue over the retinal surface; a small window is created in partially detached posterior hyaloid such that horizontally cutting scissor can create a plane between the epiretinal membranes and underlying retina.

14. What is the speed of vitrectomy cutters?

Ans. 750–7,500 cpm.

15. What is interface vitrectomy?

Ans. It describes the use of vitreous cutters, scissors, forceps, and other instruments at the interface between silicon oil, air, or PFCL and residual vitreous, epiretinal membrane, and retina.

4.10 OPTICAL COHERENCE TOMOGRAPHY ANGIOGRAPHY

Aayush Majumdar, Nawazish Shaikh, Saurabh Verma

■ INTRODUCTION

Optical coherence tomography angiography (OCTA) is a novel imaging modality for noninvasive evaluation of retinal and choroidal vasculature. By leveraging the principles of OCT technology, OCTA provides the means to noninvasive imaging of the vascular structures of the eye. In essence, it detects the motion of red blood cells (RBCs), in a stationary eye without the need of intravenous contrast. It is rapidly evolving as a critical alternative to conventional dye-based angiography for the diagnosis and management of various vascular disorders of retina and choroid.

PRINCIPLE

As described in the preceding chapter, OCT works on the principle of *"Michelson interferometry"*, in which a ray of low-coherence near-infrared light is divided into a reference and a sample beam. The sample beam falls on the retina and is backscattered and interferes with the reference beam to form interference patterns, which are used to reconstruct axial A-scans. Multiple A-scans are constructed at each point of the retina, and these are together reconstructed to give a two-dimensional cross-sectional B-scan. Sequential acquisition of spatially displaced B-scans generates volumetric data of the retina, while *sequential B-scans at the same location over a period will be unchanged, except for the motion of RBCs at this tissue level*. Comparing these sequential B-scans, on a pixel-by-pixel basis, generates a decorrelation signal, which helps in depth resolved motion contrast imaging of the retinal vasculature.

OCTA Algorithms

The OCT interferogram signal data consists of two attributes: (1) Phase and (2) intensity. Both can be analyzed for detection of decorrelation.

Phase-based Techniques

Used in the first-generation OCTA systems, these were *more sensitive* than intensity-based algorithms, but *more susceptible to effects of bulk eye motion*. These include:

- *Doppler OCT:* It measures retinal blood flow velocities based on the phase shift of reflected light using Fourier-domain OCT strategies. It could not detect microcirculation, and could only visualize major arteries and veins.
- *Phase-variance OCT:* It generates phase-based decorrelation signal without dependence on the Doppler angle, providing increased dynamic range with sensitivity to lower flow rates found in the microcirculation.

Intensity-based Techniques

Compared to phase-based techniques, these are *not as adversely affected by bulk eye motion*, but may be *less sensitive to slow blood flow*, requiring more OCT scans or split-spectrum imaging to generate increased signal-to-noise ratios. These include:

- *Speckle variance:* It can generate OCTA images approaching histologic specimens without additional motion compensation algorithms or optical modules.
- *Correlation mapping:* Stationary structures show high correlation between adjacent B-scans, whereas areas of blood flow exhibit lower correlation. Rather than assessing temporal changes in OCT signal, by comparing the signal intensity from a grid around a single pixel versus a grid around an adjacent pixel, areas of low correlation can be elucidated and subsequently presented as blood flow.

Complex or Mixed Signal-based Techniques

These utilize both intensity and phase decorrelation to use all available information and decrease the effect of bulk motion. These include proprietary algorithms like:

- Optical microangiography (OMAG) (Carl Zeiss Meditech)

- Split-spectrum amplitude decorrelation angiography (SSADA) (Optovue)
- OCTA ratio analysis (OCTARA) (Topcon)
- Full-spectrum amplitude decorrelation angiography (FSADA) with probabilistic algorithm (Heidelberg).

Imaging Attributes

- OCTA provides *depth-resolved, three-dimensional data* of the retina, often presented in two dimensions via an en face projection, conventionally segmented into four zones: (1) The superficial retinal plexus, (2) the deep retinal plexus, (3) the outer retina, and (4) the choriocapillaris (CC).
- *En face presentation* leads to loss of depth information but provides a simple representation of vascular flow much like the familiar fluorescein angiography images.
- En face imaging requires accurate *retinal layer segmentation*, which can be difficult in eyes with retinal pathology.
- OCTA data *can also be presented as cross-sectional B-scans analogous to traditional OCT, with overlay of flow information over structural OCT information.* This allows evaluation of both OCTA signals and co-registered structural data with its inherent depth information, helps in avoiding segmentation error, and illustrates projection artifacts in the form of "decorrelation tails" deep to the superficial vessels.
- *Volume rendering of OCTA data* is being used to visualize human retinal vasculature, maximizing the benefit of its three-dimensional nature. This technique eliminates segmentation errors and allows better recognition of projection artifacts but requires high-density volume data sets.

Quantitative Parameters

The OCTA utilizes morphological features of retinal vasculature to generate quantitative metrics, based on detection of flow signals above a specific background threshold. It requires additional image processing (binarization and skeletonization). It includes:

- *Perfusion density (PD):* It quantifies total area of blood flow in an imaging area. It is affected by vessel diameter, with false impression of increased perfusion in areas having large vessels/microaneurysms.
- *Vessel length density (VLD):* It minimizes the effects of vessel diameter and yields a more accurate representation of the capillary networks by creating a uniform width of all vessels in the imaged area
- *Vessel Diameter Index*
- *Fractal dimension:* It describes secondary branching of the microvasculature.
- *Foveal avascular zone (FAZ) size*

OCTA Imaging Artifacts

- *Motion artifact:* Aberrant decorrelation signals due to bulk eye motion, blinking, nystagmus, saccades or ocular drift can lead to degradation of the image quality. These artifacts include *vertical and horizontal white/dark lines*, and *blood vessel discontinuity* due to interrupted scanning **(Fig. 4.10.1)**. Strategies to reduce motion artifacts include:
    - Faster scanning speeds to reduce scan acquisition time
    - Hardware based eye-tracking strategies
    - Software-based motion correction algorithms (can themselves lead to stretch artifacts and vascular doubling artifacts when motion is severe).
- *Projection artifact:* False-positive decorrelation signal from deeper hyperreflective tissue due to overlying superficial

vasculature appear as *mirror images of superficial vascular plexus* **(Figs. 4.10.2A and B)**. Strategies to reduce projection artifacts include:
- *Slab subtraction method:* En face images from inner retinal slabs are subtracted from en face images of the avascular outer retina, resulting in the replacement of false-positive signals with dark vessel artifacts.
- *Projection-resolved OCTA algorithms:* Projected flow signals being weaker than actual flow signals, can easily be identified and removed without the need for predefined retinal segmentation.
- *Segmentation artifact:* Segmentation errors due to pathology disrupting normal retinal anatomy can lead to misinterpretation of OCTA images. This can be avoided by manual segmentation of OCT B-scans.
- *Shadow artifact:* Focal or general media opacities anterior to retina can lead to signal attenuation due to light scattering or absorption. Discrete hyperreflective structures within the retina (e.g., hard exudates, drusen) can also cause focal signal attenuation in retinal layers posterior to the hyperreflective structure **(Figs. 4.10.3A to C)**.
- *Suspended scattering particles in motion:* Brownian motion of small hyperreflective

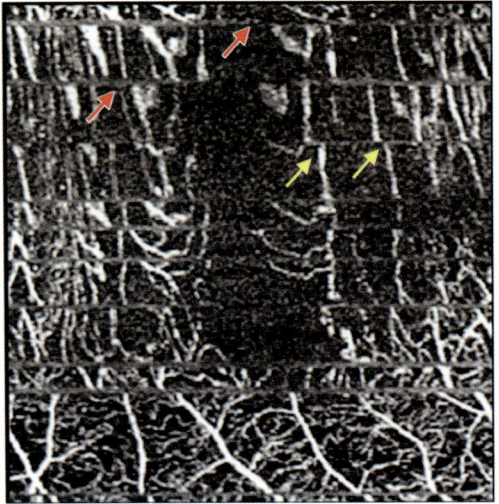

Fig. 4.10.1: *Motion artifacts:* Seen as horizontal white lines (red arrows) and areas of vessel discontinuity (yellow arrows).

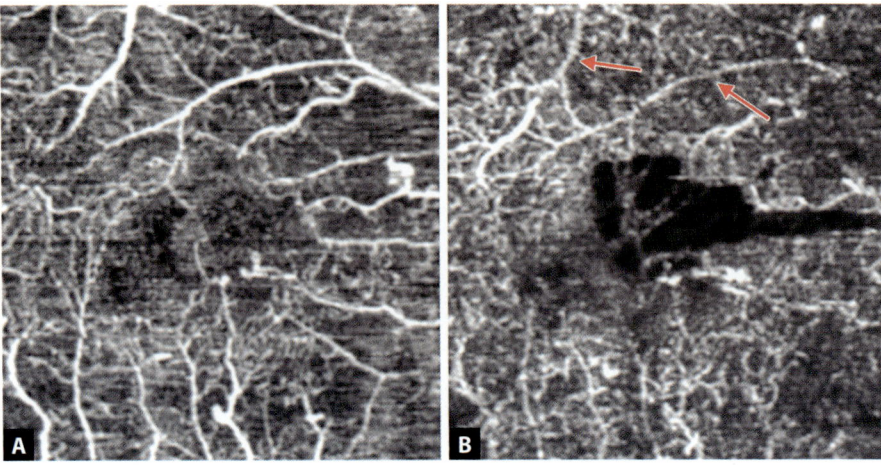

Figs. 4.10.2A and B: *Projection artifacts:* En face OCTA of the superficial retinal capillary plexus (SCP) (A) and deep retinal capillary plexus (DCP) (B) in the same patient demonstrates projection of mirror images of the large superficial vessels into the deeper retinal layers (red arrows).

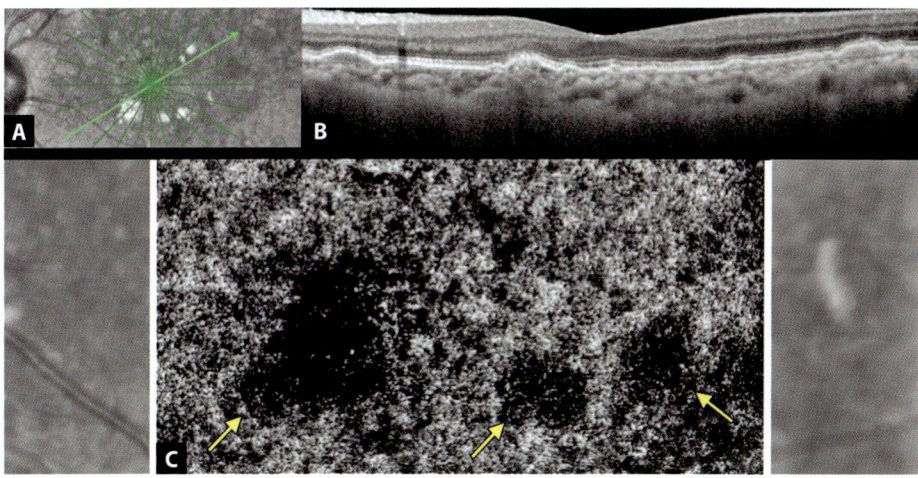

Figs. 4.10.3A to C: *Shadow artifacts:* Case of non-neovascular age-related macular degeneration with drusen seen on B-scan (A and B), leading to hyperreflective areas in OCTA imaging (yellow arrows) due to focal signal attenuation, mimicking flow deficits in the choriocapillaris (C).

particles (including large lipoproteins) in fluid-filled retinal spaces can lead to aberrant false-positive OCTA signals.

Advantages of OCTA

- Rapid and noninvasive imaging of retinal vasculature
- *No intravenous contrast required*: No dye-related complications especially useful in patients with history of allergy/anaphylaxis
- Provides detailed, depth-resolved microvascular resolution of all the vascular plexuses.

Limitations of OCTA

- Due to the need for dense A-scans and repeated imaging, achievable field of view with OCTA is limited to ~15 × 15 mm^2; thus it is mainly employed for localized imaging of macula and peripapillary area.
- It does not provide dynamic time-resolved information, such as arteriovenous transit time and leakage.
- It may miss low-flow structures like microaneurysms and polyps.

Interpretation of OCTA Findings

Unlike fluorescein angiography, which is a two-dimensional imaging system that illustrates the superficial vascular plexus with little contribution from the deep retinal capillary plexus, OCTA is capable of imaging the vascular anatomy at all levels of the retina and choroid.

The inner two-thirds of the retina is supplied by the central retinal artery, which branches into smaller arterioles, which further form four parallel capillary networks: (1) The *nerve fiber layer capillary plexus (NFLCP)* **(Fig. 4.10.4A)**, (2) the *superficial retinal capillary plexus (SCP)* **(Fig. 4.10.4B)**, (3) the *intermediate retinal capillary plexus (ICP)* **(Fig. 4.10.4C)**, and (4) the *deep retinal capillary plexus (DCP)* **(Fig. 40.10.4D)**. The NFLCP and SCP comprise the *superficial vascular complex (SVC)* **(Fig. 4.10.4E)**, and the ICP and DCP comprise the *deep vascular complex (DVC)* **(Fig. 4.10.4F)**. Flow between

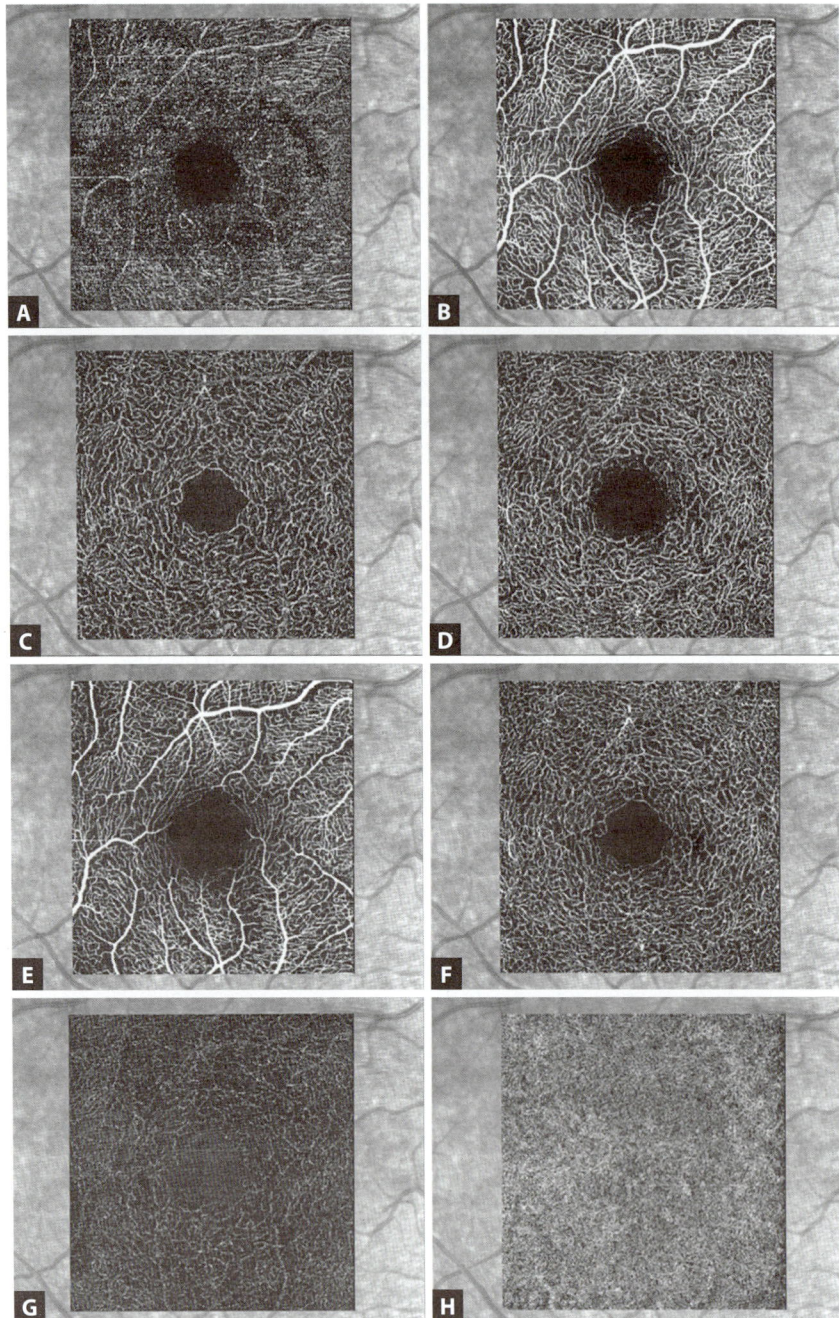

Figs. 4.10.4A to H: *OCTA segmentation in a healthy retina:* (A) Nerve fiber layer capillary plexus (NFLCP); (B) SCP; (C) Intermediate retinal capillary plexus (ICP); (D) DCP; (E) Superficial vascular complex (SVC = NFLCP + SCP); (F) Deep vascular complex (DVC = ICP + DCP); (G) Avascular outer retina; (H) Choriocapillaris. (DCP: deep retinal capillary plexus; DVC: deep vascular complex; SCP: superficial retinal capillary plexus; SVC: superficial vascular complex)

the capillary networks has been inferred from anatomic and pathologic studies, which suggest that the three capillary plexuses are predominantly organized in a serial fashion, with blood flow entering the SCP and traveling through the ICP and out the DCP **(Fig. 4.10.4G)**.

Outer one-third of the retina is supplied by the choroidal vasculature, comprising the short posterior ciliary arteries and long posterior ciliary arteries, which terminate as lobules of *CC* **(Fig. 4.10.4H)**. Imaging of CC is challenging in OCTA, as the individual capillary diameter approaches resolution limit of OCT, besides being more prone to segmentation defects and artifacts. CC imaging on SS-OCTA demonstrates a granular pattern, where bright spaces are thought to represent capillary flow, and the dark spaces are thought to represent intercapillary spaces with flow deficits.[1,2]

Clinical Applications of OCTA

- *Retinal vein occlusions:* In the acute phase, OCTA findings include vascular tortuosity, with venous dilation, microaneurysms, and nonperfusion, which is more prominent in the deep capillary plexus, as it is the site of major venous outflow **(Fig. 4.10.5)**. In chronic retinal vascular occlusions (RVOs), OCTA findings consist of collateralization, which tracks through the DCP, and neovascularization in the superficial retina, often near the border of nonperfused region. Besides these findings, OCTA may be utilized to assess the size and circularity of the FAZ as a sign of macular ischemia, especially in patients with unexplainable vision loss. Unlike fundus fluorescein angiography (FFA), due to absence of leakage, the FAZ is clearly outlined through the OCTA.
- *Retinal artery occlusions:* OCTA shows capillary dropout and a decrease in the flow of the superficial, intermediate, and deep capillary plexuses. "Ischemic cascade" refers to the progression of ischemia from the middle to the inner retina, since ischemia initially develop at the venular pole (DCP) and then progress anteriorly toward the arteriole pole (SCP).
- *Diabetic retinopathy (DR)*: OCTA may detect microvascular abnormalities before the onset of clinically evident retinopathy, providing an early biomarker of retinal disease in diabetic patients. These include microaneurysms, venous beading, enlargement of the FAZ, and capillary nonperfusion (CNP) **(Figs. 4.10.6A and B)**. However, up to 40% of microaneurysms may be missed by OCTA, as the slow flow of blood inside microaneurysms may be below the detection threshold. Neovascularization in proliferative diabetic retinopathy (PDR) can be easily identified with OCTA.
- *Diabetic macular edema (DME):* OCTA is also helpful in assessing the FAZ in

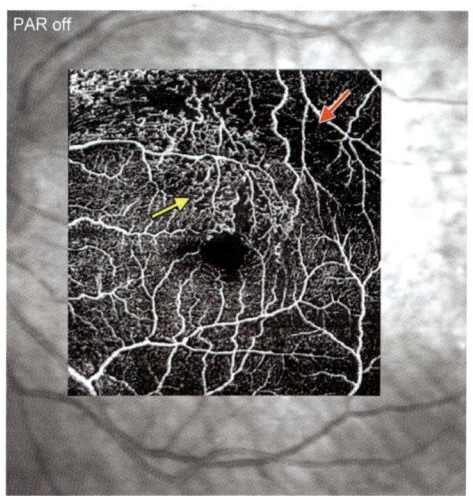

Fig. 4.10.5: OCTA in a case of branch retinal vein occlusion (BRVO) showing vascular tortuosity and venous dilation (yellow arrow), microaneurysms, and capillary nonperfusion areas (red arrow).

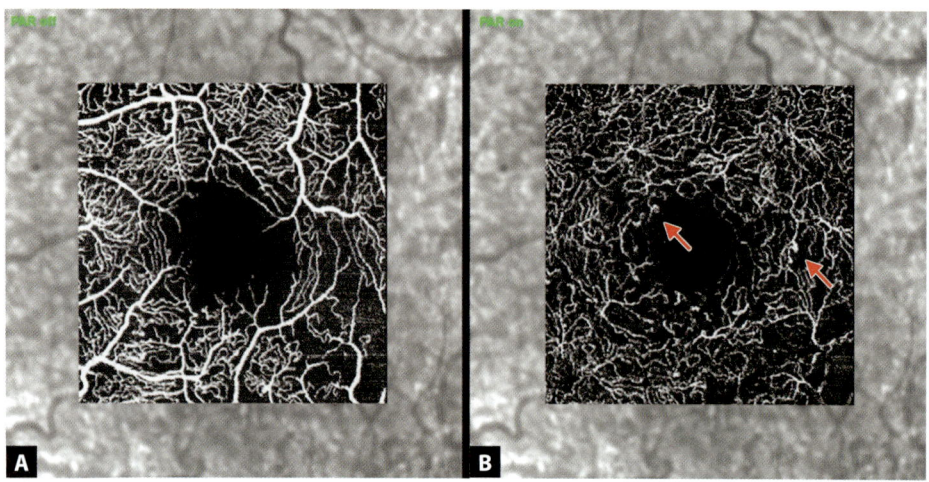

Figs. 4.10.6A and B: OCTA in a case of DR showing (A) enlargement of FAZ in SCP and (B) microaneurysms (red arrows) in DCP. (DCP: deep retinal capillary plexus; DR: diabetic retinopathy; FAZ: foveal avascular zone; SCP: superficial retinal capillary plexus)

patients with vision loss not attributable to DME. These patients may present with persistent reduction in visual acuity despite DME resolution with anti-VEGF (antivascular endothelial growth factor) therapy (evidenced by enlargement of FAZ, or DCP flow deficits) that can easily be identified with OCTA analysis.

- *Non-neovascular age-related macular degeneration (ARMD):* OCTA analysis has shown an inverse relationship between age and the density of SCP, ICP and DCP, and CC in the macula. OCTA imaging has revealed flow deficits in the CC of eyes with early and intermediate non-neovascular ARMD, immediately beneath and surrounding drusen. Further, CC flow impairment in areas of GA and to a lesser degree outside the GA lesions were significantly increased in eyes with ARMD compared with age-matched controls.
- *Neovascular age-related macular degeneration:* OCTA helps in qualitative and quantitative analysis of macular neovascularization (MNV). Various OCTA morphologies of type 1 and type 2 MNV have been described, including" "sea-fan", "medusa" **(Fig. 4.10.7)** and "dead tree" **(Fig. 4.10.8)** patterns. These patterns have been recently redefined into three principal stages of progression: Immature, mature, and hypermature. Type 3 MNV presents as a focal neovascular tuft that originates from the DCP and can be associated with a feeder vessel from SCP. Moreover, OCTA is a critical modality to detect nonexudative MNV, present in up to 27% of fellow eyes of exudative MNV, with high risk of future exudation and requiring close monitoring.
- *Macular telangiectasia (MacTel):* On OCTA, classical findings of MacTel include tortuous, dilated, or nonperfused capillaries with increased intervascular spaces and decreased foveal vessel density, primarily within the DCP **(Fig. 4.10.9)**. Often, MacTel may be confused with MNV and caution is advised in these patients. Multimodal imaging utilizing OCT, FFA, and OCTA in

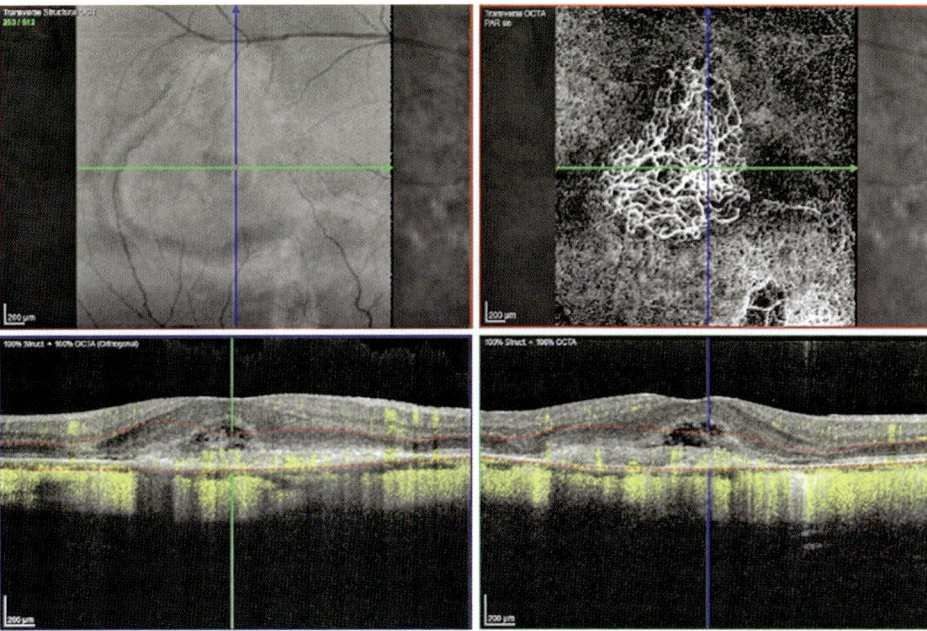

Fig. 4.10.7: OCTA in a case of neovascular age-related macular degeneration showing "medusa" appearance of macular neovascularization in the avascular outer retina (top right panel), corresponding to the Type-1 macular neovascularization seen in B-scans (bottom).

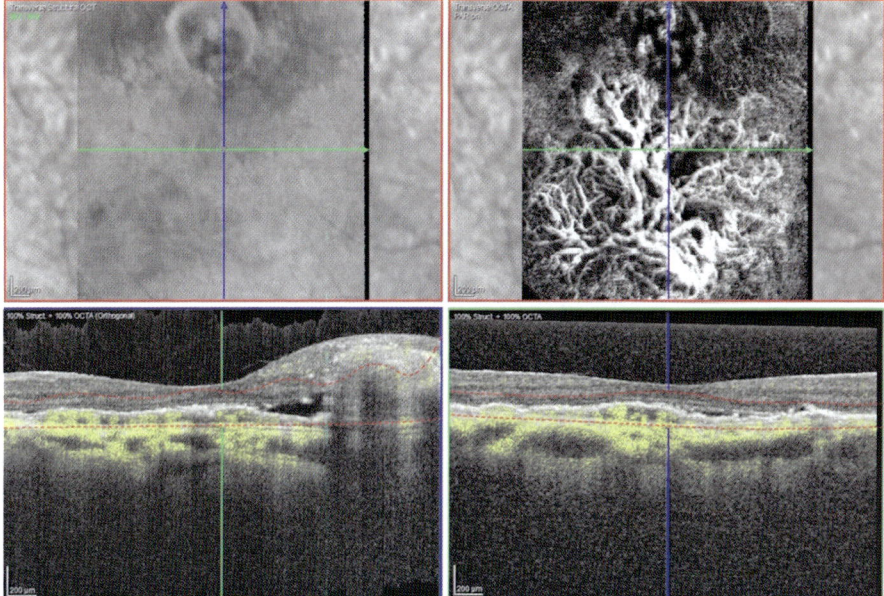

Fig. 4.10.8: OCTA in a case of neovascular age-related macular degeneration showing "dead tree" appearance of macular neovascularization in the avascular outer retina (top right panel), corresponding to the Type-1 macular neovascularization seen in B-scans (bottom).

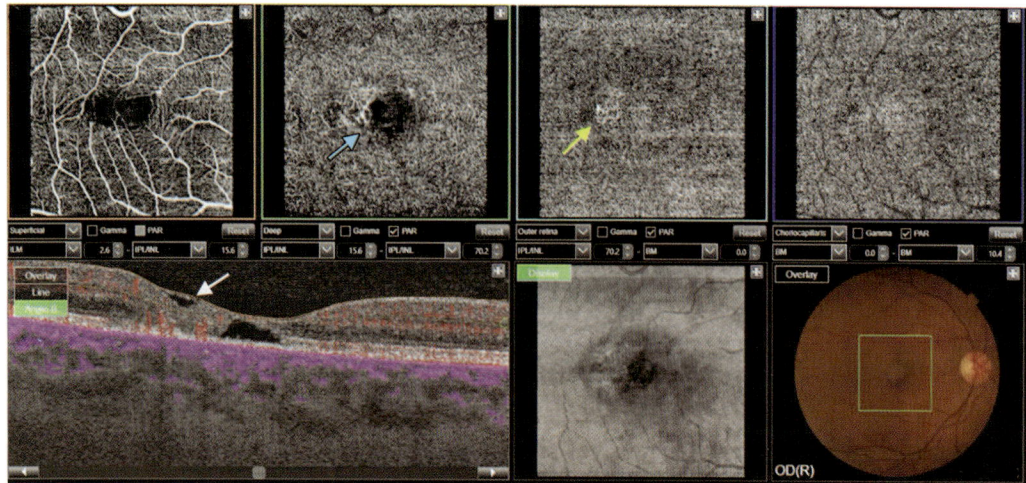

Fig. 4.10.9: OCTA in a case of MacTel showing telangiectatic vessels in the deep vascular complex (blue arrow), and projection artifact in the avascular outer retina (yellow arrow). Corresponding B-scan image shows characteristic temporal thinning (white arrow) with internal limiting membrane drape sign.

these patients provide the best diagnostic capability. It is also useful in identifying subretinal neovascularization, a sight threatening complication of MacTel.

- *MNV due to other disorders:* Disease processes like pathological myopia and chronic central serous chorioretinopathy can also be complicated by MNV. Identification of MNV and monitoring the response to anti-VEGF therapy are essential in disease management. It is imperative to highlight that in myopic patients, spontaneous coin-shaped hemorrhages may occur at the fovea, which can be due to myopic MNV or secondary to Bruch's membrane rupture. In such patients, OCTA may be done to localize the vascular network. However, when in doubt, multimodal imaging with FFA and OCTA provide the best opportunity to diagnose subtle MNV.

REFERENCES

1. Hou KK, Au A, Corradetti G, Sadda SR, Sarraf D. Optical Coherence Tomography Angiography. In: Sadda SR, Wilkinson CP, Wiedemann P, Schachat AP (Eds). Ryan's Retina, volume 3, 7th edition. Elsevier; 2023. pp. 115-44.
2. Shaikh NF, Vohra R, Balaji A, Azad SV, Chawla R, Kumar V, et al. Role of optical coherence tomography-angiography in diabetes mellitus: Utility in diabetic retinopathy and a comparison v/s fluorescein angiography in vision threatening diabetic retinopathy. Indian J Ophthalmol 2021.

4.11 ULTRA-WIDEFIELD IMAGING

Aayush Majumdar, Nawazish Shaikh, Saurabh Verma

■ INTRODUCTION

Retinal imaging is evolving with rapid technological advancement. The *Diabetic Retinopathy Clinical Research Network (DRCR.net)* originally defined ultra-widefield (UWF) images as image acquisitions with at least a 100° view of the fundus. Later, the *International Widefield Imaging Study Group* provided definitions of the various terms used to categorize the fundus fields of view **(Table 4.11.1)**. As widefield imaging becomes widely available, its role in clinical practice as well as research keeps expanding. The biggest advantage that it offers is idetection, analysis and documentation of ocular pathologies that may first present in the periphery, which may otherwise go undetected using traditional fundus photography.

■ HISTORICAL PERSPECTIVE

Panoret-1000: Based on Pomerantzeff's system, it was a handheld device with 100° field of view through undilated pupil

1926: Carl Zeiss Company develops first fundus camera with 20° field of view (later expanded to 30° and 50° fields of view)

1975: Pomerantzeff developed Equator-plus fundus camera-contact-lens based system with fiber optic-based transpupillary and transscleral illumination, with up to 148° field of view
Limitation: Limited resolution

1977: Lotmar describes Montage technique with traditional fundus camera—acquiring up your 19 images with a fixation lamp, rotatable mirror and mechanical steering of the camera, creating a 96° montage
Limitations:
- Requires patient cooperation
- Requires pupillary dilation
- Cannot acquire simultaneous images for dynamic studies like FA

1997: RetCam—contact-based digital imaging system with external fiber optic light source and interchangeable lenses providing up to 130° field of view
- *Advantages:* Primarily used to image neonatal and pediatric patients, especially useful in ROP telescreening programs
- *Limitations:* Lenticular opacities can produce scatter and glare, degrading image quality

2005: Staurenghi developed a confocal scanning laser ophthalmoscopy (SLO)-based imaging system using a contact-lens, with up to 150° field of view
Limitations:
- Need for topical anesthesia
- Lenticular opacities leads to poor image quality
- Difficult image acquisition

■ OPTOS

- Optos (Optos PLC, Dunfermline, United Kingdom) is a confocal scanning laser

TABLE 4.11.1: Nomenclature by International Widefield Imaging Study Group.

Nomenclature	Anatomical location	Field of view
Widefield	Imaging of mid-periphery of the retina up to posterior edge of ampulla of vortex veins	Up to 100°
Ultra-widefield	Imaging of far-periphery of the retina, including the anterior edge of the vortex vein ampulla up to pars plana	>200°
Panretinal	Imaging of entire retina	360°

ophthalmoscopy (SLO)-based UWF imaging system.
- *Provides largest single-frame view of the posterior pole:* It uses an ellipsoid mirror to image up to 200° (~82% of fundus).
- Red and green imaging channels are combined to create a pseudocolor image.

Advantages:
- Capable of imaging through undilated pupil
- Does not require any special CL
- No topical anesthesia required
- *Rapid image acquisition (~0.25s):* Quick 2D scanning with two galvanometer mirrors
- Guided eye steering allows images that extend beyond 200°
- Images are available instantly, and saved digitally for future comparison or telemedicine purposes.
- Provides a large depth of field, which can maintain the entire ocular fundus in focus
- Confocal optics capable of fundus photography, green-light fundus autofluorescence (UWF-FAF), fluorescein angiography (UWF-FA), indocyanine green angiography (UWF-ICGA) and OCT (UWF-OCT).
- *Optos Silverstone swept source OCT:* UWF imaging device with integrated, UWF-guided swept source OCT, capable of capturing specific peripheral pathology as far as 200°.

Limitations:
- Pseudocolor imaging can lead to misinterpretation of specific lesions.
- Although imaging beyond 200° is possible by eye steering, currently there is no inbuilt system for montage creation.
- *Map distortion*: Mapping three-dimensional fundus onto two-dimensional image leads to disproportionate imaging of peripheral regions, with horizontal warping and stretching (can be reduced by stereographic correction).
- Lower resolution imaging of the posterior pole as compared to other SLO systems like Heidelberg Spectralis (can be improved with recent ResMax™ feature)
- Large depth of focus leads to lash and lid artifacts.

By incorporating confocal scanning with green (red-free) laser light at 532 nm and also red light at 633 nm, Optos allows for additional diagnostic ability not found in most standard fundus camera systems. Using the Blend function, the images may be viewed together, providing a pseudocolor image of the fundus. Further, a "white-balance" mode can be used to more closely approximate the true colors of posterior segment pathology **(Table 4.11.2)**. The different SLO channels may be viewed separately. The shorter wavelength green (red-free) laser highlights the retinal vasculature and anterior retinal structures, whereas the longer wavelength red channel accentuates deeper retinal structures and the choroidal vasculature. When viewing in the green laser separation, retinal vessel detail and retinal hemorrhages are readily seen and often can enhance the discovery of hemorrhagic retinopathies—for example, diabetes and systemic hypertension.[1,2]

Clinical Applications

- *Diabetic retinopathy:* In the Early Treatment of Diabetic Retinopathy Study (ETDRS), seven standard field (7 SF) 30° fields of view were combined to create a 75° montage, and its assessment was the early standard for DR clinical trials. UWF imaging has shown sensitivity and specificity for the detection of DR, and has revealed potentially important clinical findings in the peripheral retina of

TABLE 4.11.2: Comparison between available imaging systems for widefield imaging.

	Optos	*Spectralis*	*Clarus*
Manufacturer	Optos PLC, Dunfermline, United Kingdom	Heidelberg Engineering, Inc., Heidelberg, Germany	Carl Zeiss Meditec Inc., California, USA
Optics	Confocal scanning laser ophthalmoscopy (cSLO) using a red (635 nm) and a green (532 nm) laser to scan the retina and reproduce a pseudocolor image	Noncontact lens/Staurenghi contact lens attached to the existing Heidelberg Spectralis or HRA2 cSLO platform	White LED flash consisting of red (585–640 nm), green (500–585 nm), and blue (435–500 nm) LED and an infrared laser diode (785 nm) creating a "true color" fundus image as seen during funduscopy
Field of view	200° (~82% of fundus) with single image, can be montaged up to 220° (~97% of fundus)	• 105° (noncontact lens) • 150° (Staurenghi contact lens)	Two horizontal images of 133° combined to image up to 200°
Advantages	• Noncontact imaging through undilated pupil • No contact lens (thus no topical anesthesia) needed	• Higher resolution imaging of posterior pole • Less lash artifact and therefore improved imaging of the superior and inferior periphery	• Partially confocal optics reduces eyelash and eyelid artifacts • Image formed by the combination of red, green, and blue provides a true color fundus image
Limitations	• Pseudocolor imaging can lead to misinterpretation of lesions • *Map distortion*: Mapping 3D fundus onto 2D image leads to disproportionate imaging of peripheral regions, with horizontal warping and stretching • Large depth of focus leads to lash and lid artifacts • Lower resolution imaging of the posterior pole as compared to other SLO systems like Heidelberg Spectralis	• Contact procedure (using Staurenghi contact lens for larger field of view) • Requires topical anesthesia • Limited view of superior and inferior periphery	Relatively longer image acquisition time

diabetic patients beyond the 7 SF ETDRS fields, including peripheral nonperfusion and neovascularization not evident with review of 7 SF photographs in 10% of cases. The use of UWF imaging detects a more severe stage of DR compared to 7 SF in 10% to 19% eyes. Up to 32% eyes were found to have neovascularization

elsewhere (NVE) and 75% had CNP areas outside the ETDRS 7 SF in one study. UWF imaging also has a critical role in telescreening programs, with real-time, point-of-care non-mydriatic UWF image acquisition and interpretation by nonphysician readers for identification of referable DR.
- *RVOs:* Peripheral neovascularization and nonperfusion areas can be documented.
- *Peripheral exudative hemorrhagic chorioretinopathy (PEHCR):* UWF imaging provides the capability to assess and monitor peripheral findings in both ARMD, such as the detection of peripheral choroidal neovascularization (CNV), PCV, and PEHCR. Recent studies have identified new findings, and are proposing new classifications for ARMD-like changes in the far periphery, even in those without macular involvement.
- *Retinal detachments:* Though clinical examination with binocular indirect ophthalmoscopy remains the gold standard for the diagnosis of retinal detachments and visualization of pathology in the far periphery, UWF imaging is becoming increasingly popular as a useful adjunct for preoperative documentation of retinal detachments, assisting in preoperative planning, and postoperative monitoring.
- *Pediatric retina:* UWF imaging is increasingly being used to diagnose and monitor a variety of pediatric retinal conditions in the outpatient clinic, without the need for examination under anesthesia, such as retinopathy of prematurity (ROP), pediatric uveitis, Coats' disease, familial exudative vitreoretinopathy (FEVR), hereditary dystrophies, juvenile X-linked retinoschisis, colobomas, etc. Although the RetCam is the most commonly used UWF imaging modality for ROP screening, the Optos system can be used with a special "flying baby" position to obtain higher resolution UWF images in ROP babies.
- *Oncology:* UWF imaging is useful for the diagnosis, monitoring, and progression of various tumors, such as choroidal nevus, uveal melanoma, choroidal metastasis, choroidal hemangioma, retinoblastoma, etc., which may be situated in the retinal periphery, or exhibit secondary effects such as exudation and inferior serous retinal detachment.
- Ultra-widefield imaging for retinal evaluation through undilated pupils is especially useful in cases of poorly dilating pupils, nondilating pupils with posterior synechiae, and patients unwilling for pupillary dilation.

Ultra-Widefield Fluorescein Angiography

Traditional FA is able to visualize 30°–50° of the retina at once. However, visualization of peripheral retina is essential in order to assess nonperfused areas, vascular leakage, microvascular abnormalities, and neovascularizations (NVs).[3,4]

Diabetic retinopathy: Comparison of UWF-FA with 7 SF revealed that UWF-FA detected 3.9 times more nonperfusion and 1.9 times more neovascularization, and resulted in the performance of 3.8 times more panretinal photocoagulation (PRP) laser sessions. Analysis of UWF–FA also identified peripheral nonperfusion and neovascularization not evident with review of 7 SF photographs in 10% of cases.
- Peripheral vessel leakage (PVL), seen as late hyperfluorescence extending beyond vessel wall in the setting of active retinopathy, has been linked to peripheral nonperfusion and neovascularization.

- Peripheral ischemia is an independent risk factor for DME development, quantified by "Ischemic Index", which is estimated by calculating pixels contained in nonperfused areas and dividing it by the number of pixels of the whole retina surface, thus generating a percentage of ischemia over the total retina area.
- UWF–FA has also been utilized for guided therapy, including targeted laser photocoagulation (TRP), in which laser energy is directed specifically into areas of retinal CNP, thus decreasing peripheral visual field loss and incidence of post-laser macular edema as compared to PRP.

Retinal vascular occlusions: UWF-FA is useful for the diagnosis of central retinal vein occlusion (CRVO) with peripheral nonperfusion. UWF-guided TRP reduced the anti-VEGF load, with decreased central subfoveal thickness and improved visual outcomes.

Pediatric retina: Several studies have elucidated the role of UWF-FA in the diagnosis and management of ROP, because FA may enhance detection of certain subtypes of ROP, and may better guide disease requiring treatment. Optos UWF imaging and FA have also led to improved classification systems and new insights into the pathophysiology and spectrum of phenotypes of disorders such as FEVR.

Uveitis: Early reports have shown the utility of UWF-FA for assessing the extent, severity, and progression of retinal disease and response to treatment in intermediate and posterior uveitis. There is increasing evidence that the assessment of PVL (i.e., angiographic leakage outside the ETDRS 7SF) may have importance in the grading of disease activity and management of disease. Prospective studies are warranted to incorporate PVL into the diagnosis and management of uveitis patients.

Ultra-Widefield Optical Coherence Tomography

Until recently, capturing the far periphery of the retina with OCT was not possible. However, UWF-OCT capabilities have been introduced in the Optos Silverstone (Optos PLC Edinburgh), the Heidelberg Spectralis HRA-OCT (Heidelberg Engineering USA) (using a steering technique), the Plex Elite 9000 (Zeiss, Oberkochen, Germany), and the Xephilio OCT-S1 (Canon Medical Systems, Japan), expanding the utility of UWF imaging in various conditions as follows:

Retinal detachment: UWF-OCT provides microstructural retinal details such as photoreceptor integrity and resolution of subretinal fluid in cases of retinal detachment. Sequential findings captured by the Optos Silverstone have provided illuminating insights into the response of the retina to treatments including laser retinopexy (coagulative necrosis and retinal splitting) and cryopexy (retinal layer destruction and RPE separation) **(Fig. 4.11.1)**.

Peripheral retinoschisis: UWF-OCT also helps in differentiating degenerative retinoschisis from retinal detachments. The management for these two conditions differs significantly, with retinoschisis often being a benign condition requiring no intervention, unless

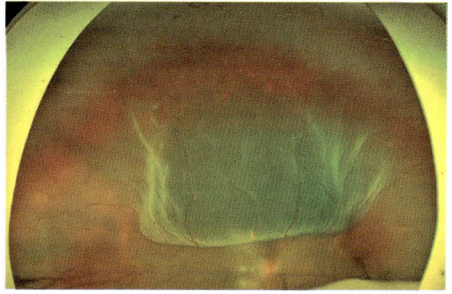

Fig. 4.11.1: Ultra-widefield image showing retinal detachment with multiple horse shoe tears in superior periphery.

retinoschisis is associated with retinal holes, a finding, which can also be visualized on peripheral OCT **(Figs. 4.11.2A to C)**.

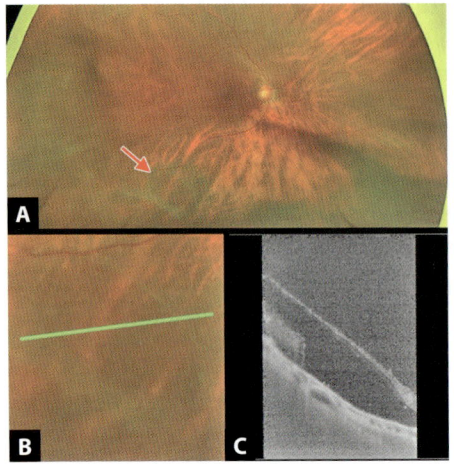

Figs. 4.11.2A to C: Ultra-widefield image showing (A) peripheral retinoschisis; (B) linear optical coherence tomography through the cyst reveals; and (C) splitting of retinal layers.

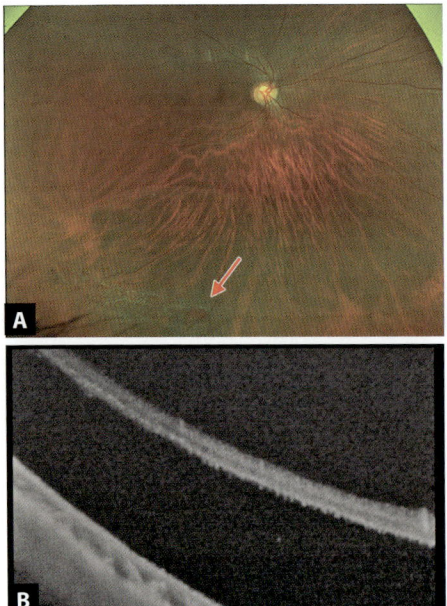

Figs. 4.11.3A and B: Ultra-widefield image showing (A) peripheral lattice degeneration with holes and (B) optical coherence tomography through the region revealed a shallow retinal detachment.

Peripheral retinal degenerations: UWF-OCT has been utilized for the characterization and documentation of peripheral retinal degenerations, including lattice degeneration, retinal tufts, retinal tears, retinal holes, and paving-stone degeneration. Apart from the microstructural details of peripheral retina, UWF-OCT also provides critical information about the vitreoretinal interface, the presence or absence of traction in lattice degeneration, and rules out tears and holes in cases of vitreoretinal tufts **(Figs. 4.11.3A and B)**.

Oncology: UWF-OCT is helpful in differentiating between choroidal naevi and choroidal melanoma in the retinal periphery. Presence of subretinal fluid on OCT is an important

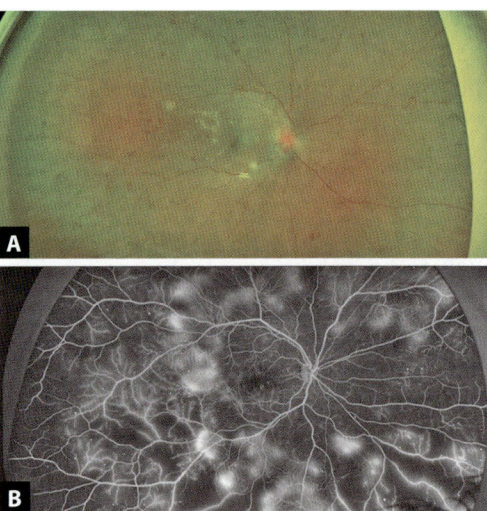

Figs. 4.11.4A and B: Ultra-widefield (UWF) image showing (A) diabetic retinopathy changes including microaneurysms, intraretinal hemorrhages and neovascularization seen throughout the retina including the periphery, which would have been missed by conventional fundus cameras; (B) Another case of PDR with UWF-FA showing leakage from peripheral NVEs and extensive peripheral CNP areas, especially in the inferonasal quadrant. (CNP: capillary nonperfusion; NVE: neovascularization elsewhere; PDR: proliferative diabetic retinopathy)

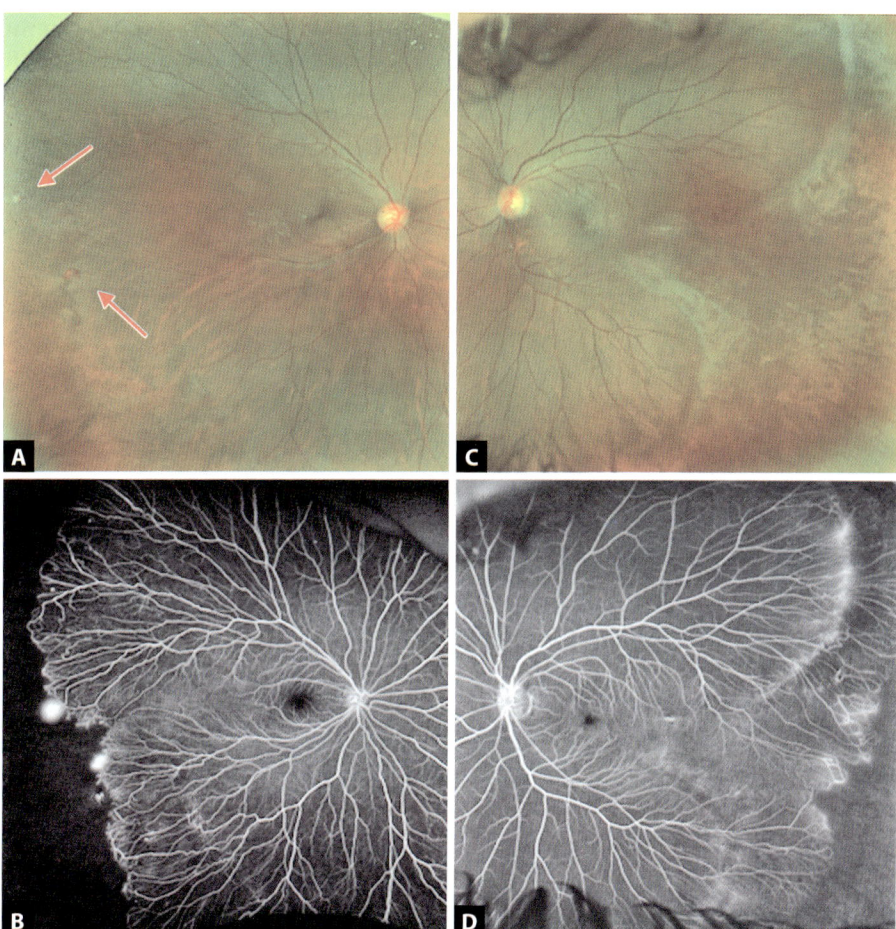

Figs. 4.11.5A to D: Ultra-widefield (UWF) images showing characteristic FEVR changes with (A) showing peripheral NVEs (red arrows) requiring photocoagulation, which are highlighted as late hyperfluorescent leaks in (B); another case with (C) fundus showing tongue-shaped areas of temporal peripheral avascularity; UWF-FA of the same eye (D) shows straightening of vessels, aneurysmal dilatations along with absence of neovascularization in the temporal periphery, thus not requiring photocoagulation. (FEVR: familial exudative vitreoretinopathy; NVE: neovascularization elsewhere)

risk factor for transformation of nevi into melanoma. UWF-OCT can be extremely valuable in cases of retinoblastoma, as subclinical tumors can be detected in the retinal periphery. It can also help in early detection of recurrences. Moreover, PEHCR lesions, usually found in the retinal periphery, can mimic choroidal melanomas, and are thus need to be properly characterized. They can be differentiated from melanomas by the presence of retinal exudation and RPE atrophy **(Figs. 4.11.4 and 4.11.5)**.

Pathological myopia: UWF-OCT can help in visualizing features of high myopia.

REFERENCES

1. Hou KK, Au A, Corradetti G, Sadda SR, Sarraf D. Optical Coherence Tomography

Angiography. In: Sadda SR, Wilkinson CP, Wiedemann P, Schachat AP (Eds). Ryan's Retina, volume 3, 7th edition. London: Elsevier; 2023. pp. 115-44.
2. Choudhry N, Duker JS, Freund KB, Kiss S, Querques G, Rosen R, et al. Classification and guidelines for widefield imaging: recommendations from the International Widefield Imaging Study Group. Ophthalmol Retina. 2019;3(10):843-9.
3. Rabiolo A, Parravano M, Querques L, Cicinelli MV, Carnevali A, Sacconi R, et al. Ultra-wide-field fluorescein angiography in diabetic retinopathy: a narrative review. Clin Ophthalmol. 2017;11:803-7.
4. Nidhi V, Verma S, Shaikh N, Azad SV, Chawla R, Venkatesh P, et al. Topographic distribution of retinal neovascularization in proliferative diabetic retinopathy using ultra-wide field angiography. Indian J Ophthalmol. 2023;71(8):3080-4.

CHAPTER 5

Glaucoma

5.1 GONIOSCOPY

Talvir Sidhu, Tanuj Dada

■ INTRODUCTION

The term "gonioscopy" is derived from the Greek words gonia – (angle) and Skopein – (view). It is a clinical biomicroscopic technique of examining the angle of the anterior chamber of the eye with the use of a special contact lens known as the gonioscope.

Alexios Tarantas first viewed the angle in a living keratoglobus eye during indentation by finger when trying to view the ciliary body. He coined the term gonioscopy and viewed the anterior chamber angle by indenting the limbus and using high plus lenses. Maximilian Salzmann is rightly called "*the father of gonioscopy*" as he recognized total internal reflection and introduced the goniolens and described angle pathology in detail.

■ PRINCIPLE

The anterior chamber angle situated at the attachment of iris-ciliary body complex to the sclera-corneal junction is called the irido-corneal angle. The angle structures are not visible due to *total internal reflection* of the light originating from angle at the corneal surface. *Total internal reflection* is an optical phenomenon that occurs when a ray of light traveling from denser to rarer medium (such as cornea to air) strikes the interface between two media at an angle larger than the "critical

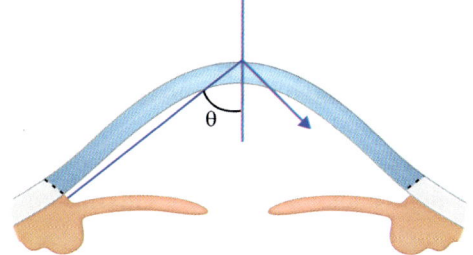

Fig. 5.1.1: Total internal reflection occurs at the cornea-air interface for light traveling from angle due to angle more than critical angle.

angle" for that pair of media. In this situation the light beam is completely reflected back to the denser medium. The critical angle for cornea-air interface is 46° **(Fig. 5.1.1)**. Hence, the light coming from angle structures strikes the cornea at an angle higher than the critical angle gets reflected internally. When a goniolens is applied over the cornea, the cornea-air interface is obliterated and the light is able to exit the eye and gets reflected from the gonio mirror and angle structures become visible **(Fig. 5.1.2)**.

■ INDICATIONS

- To identify open versus closed angle.
- To assess for risk of angle closure by identifying iris apposition to trabecular meshwork (TM)

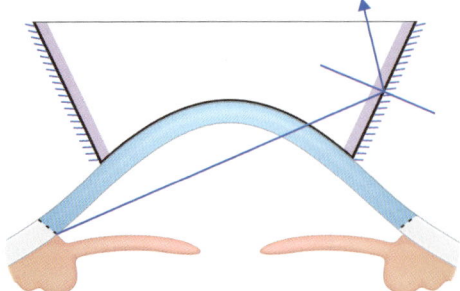

Fig. 5.1.2: A goniolens obliterates the cornea-air interface and light coming from angle can be seen as reflected from gonio mirror.

- To grade angle closure and distinguish between apposition and synechiae.
- To identify angle pathologies such as abnormal angle pigmentation, angle recession, foreign body in angle, developmental anomalies, neovascularization of angle, and grade them.
- Post-trabeculectomy patency of fistula/scleral opening.
- Laser procedures like selective laser trabeculoplasty (SLT)/argon laser trabeculoplasty (ALT).
- Intraoperatively to insert minimally invasive glaucoma surgery (MIGS) like iStent or perform surgery like goniosynechiolysis.

■ TYPES

Direct Goniolenses

A steeply convex domed lens obliterates the total internal reflection and allows the angle visualization. It is placed over the eye with patient lying in supine position for direct visualization of the angle by a handheld slit lamp or operating microscope. They are mostly used for surgical procedures or examination under anesthesia in children or in bed ridden patients.

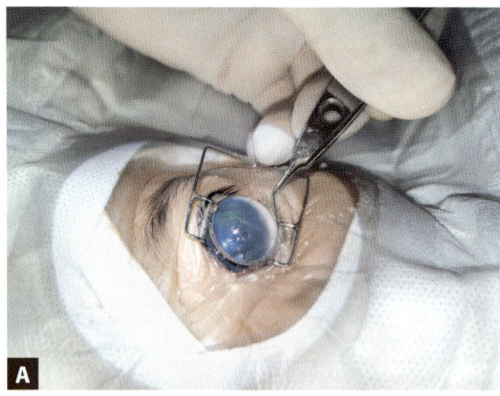
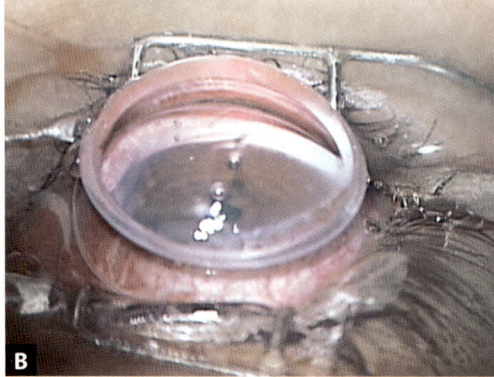

Figs. 5.1.3A and B: Koeppe lens—dome-shaped lens placed over eye for direct gonioscopy.

Examples: Koeppe lens (+50 D lens made of barium crown glass or plastic; prototype direct goniolens) **(Figs. 5.1.3A and B)**; Richardson–Shaffer (Small Koeppe lens for infants); Swan–Jacob (Surgical goniolens for children) **(Figs. 5.1.4A and B)**; Hoskins–Barkan (Prototype surgical lens); Thorpe (Surgical and diagnostic lens); Worst lens (Surgical goniolens for children).

Indirect Goniolenses

A corneal contact lens with mirrors is used to reflect the light coming from angle to obtain an inverted angle image. The lenses may have a large-sized corneal contact well which fit onto the sclera—*the scleral type lenses*, e.g., Goldmann one/two/three mirror lens

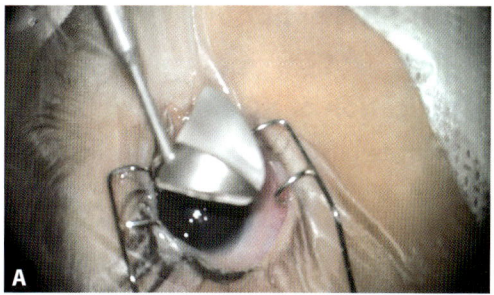
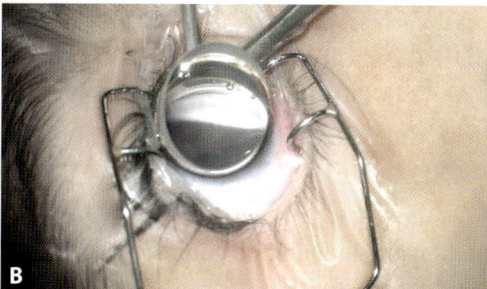

Figs. 5.1.4A and B: Swan–Jacob lens used intraoperatively to see the angle.

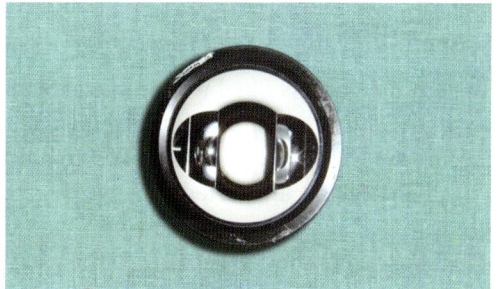

Fig. 5.1.5: Goldmann two mirror lens.

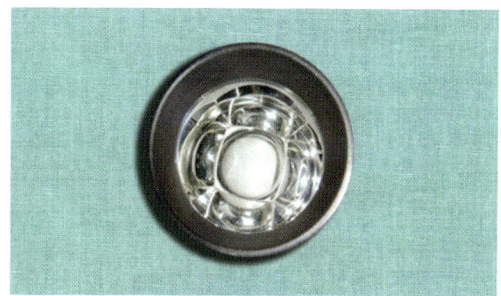

Fig. 5.1.6: Zeiss four mirror lens.

(Fig. 5.1.5) or a smaller lens contact surface which gently rests over the cornea—*the corneal type lenses*, e.g., Zeiss/Posner four mirror lenses **(Fig. 5.1.6)**.

The scleral type contact lenses have a large area of contact with eye and they fit over the sclera adjacent to the limbus. They are used for *manipulation gonioscopy* in case of closed angle due to convexity of iris, where the patient is asked to look toward the mirror the observer is viewing to open the angle being viewed. Manipulation helps to visualize the angle structures hidden behind a convex iris by allowing user to get an "over the hill" view. If too much pressure is applied, they falsely close the angle because the pressure directly goes to the limbus and folds may be visible at the limbal area in gonioscope mirror. Their curvature is steeper than the cornea, therefore a coupling fluid like methyl cellulose is required to obliterate the space left between contact lens and cornea while using a two mirror gonioscope.

The corneal type goniolens have a contact lens curvature similar to cornea and therefore they do not need coupling fluid. The well diameter is smaller than cornea therefore the contact lens rests on the cornea. Any pressure applied while doing gonioscopy leads to displacement of fluid into the angle, falsely opening the angle. These lenses are used for *indentation gonioscopy*, where pressure is applied with a corneal type goniolens to push the aqueous into the angle in a convex iris to visualize the angle structures. Indentation gonioscopy can help to differentiate between appositional and synechial angle closure. Sometimes, indentation gonioscopy is also used to abort the acute angle closure attack by pushing fluid into the angle as a therapeutic procedure (only in expert hands).

ADVANTAGES AND DISADVANTAGES OF DIRECT AND INDIRECT GONIOSCOPY (MANIPULATION AND INDENTATION)

Flowchart 5.1.1 shows the direct, manipulation and indentation gonioscopy.

Features of Indirect Goniolenses

Table 5.1.1 shows the features of indirect goniolenses.

Flowchart 5.1.1: Direct, manipulation and indentation gonioscopy.

- **Direct gonioscopy**
  - Erect and panoramic view
  - Minimal distortion of chamber and angle
  - Both eyes can be visualized simultaneously
  - Less magnification

- **Manipulation gonioscopy**
  - Small learning curve
  - Details are better visible
  - Excellent for documentation and imaging
  - Coupling fluid needed
  - Can underestimate the angle if rim of lens indents at the limbus

- **Indentation gonioscopy**
  - Differentiates between appositional and synechial angle closure
  - Coupling fluid not needed
  - Higher learning curve
  - Tendency to overestimate the angle if indentation on center of cornea

HOW TO PERFORM INDIRECT GONIOSCOPY

Application of a Goniolens

Patient is positioned at the slit lamp in a dim lit room as bright light can cause miosis and open up an "occludable angle." The gonioscope surface is cleaned and disinfected. Topical anesthetic is instilled in both the eyes (4% xylocaine or 0.5% proparacaine eye drops).

Scleral Type Lens

The concave well is filled with artificial tears or viscoelastic. Air bubbles should be avoided in the solution. The patient is asked to look up and the eyelids are parted with two fingers or the lower lid may be retracted with a swab stick. The gonioscope is placed near the lower limbus and quickly rotated into the eye to avoid spillage of the coupling fluid. The patient is asked to look straight and gonioscope is stabilized with the left hand and right hand is used to move the slit lamp into position to visualize the angle. The thumb, index, and middle fingers hold the lens, while the other two fingers stabilize the head of the patient.

Corneal Type Lens

The patient is asked to look straight and the lens is gently placed over the center of the

TABLE 5.1.1: Features of indirect goniolenses.

Type of the lens	Goldmann 1/2 mirror	Goldmann 3 mirror	Zeiss 4 mirror
Diameter of contact	12 mm	12 mm	9 mm
Overall diameter	15 mm	18 mm	9 mm
Mirror angulation	62°	59°	64°
Mirror height	17 mm	12 mm	12 mm
Radius of curvature	7.4 mm	7.4 mm	7.8 mm
Coupling fluid	Required	Required	Not required
Dynamic gonioscopy	Manipulation	Manipulation	Indentation

cornea. Two fingers hold the lens and others take support on the patient's forehead or cheek. The mirrors should be placed in the 12, 6, 3, and 9'o clock positions.

Minimal contact is maintained just to eliminate the air underneath the lens surface and avoid formation of Descemet's folds, which indicate too much pressure. If air bubbles form underneath lens surface, they can be easily removed by gently rocking the lens.

Angle Viewing

The patient is asked to look straight. The slit-lamp beam height should be adjusted to 2–3 mm in height and it should be a thin beam. The slit lamp should be put on while the beam is directed only into the angle without crossing the pupil. It is important to remember that image formed in the gonio mirror is of the opposite angle but it is not laterally inverted. The inferior angle is usually the widest and pigmented, and should be viewed first, followed by superior angle. The beam can be turned horizontal for viewing the temporal and nasal angle. In an open angle, usually all the angle structures are visible. However, in a closed angle, the posterior pigmented TM is not visible in at least 180° of the angle, known as occludable angle.

For manipulation, the patient is asked to look toward the examining mirror and angle is viewed over a steep iris. Indentation (or compression) gonioscopy can be performed by pressing a corneal type lens to push the aqueous into angle in eyes with primary angle closure glaucoma to differentiate an appositional from synechial angle closure. Examine each quadrant and note the findings.

GONIOSCOPY GRADING SYSTEMS

Shaffer's System

Shaffer's system describes the angle between trabecular meshwork and iris **(Table 5.1.2)**. Angles >20° are considered to be wide open and incapable of closure. The angle is not actually measured in degree, it is only a rough estimation of the angle width **(Fig. 5.1.7)**.

Spaeth System

The *Spaeth* system grades four aspects of angle anatomy **(Table 5.1.3)**:
1. Level of iris insertion

TABLE 5.1.2: Shaffer's system.

Grade number	Angle width	Comments
4	35–45°	Wide open—closure impossible
3	20–35°	Wide open—closure impossible
2	20°	Narrow—closure possible
1	≤10°	Extremely narrow—closure probable
Slit	Slit	Narrowed to slit—closure probable
0	0°	Closed

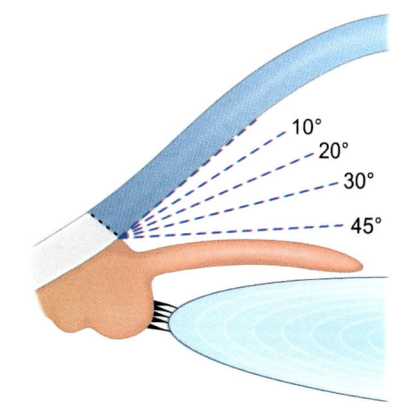

Fig. 5.1.7: Shaffer angle width determination.

SECTION 1: Appliances and Instruments

TABLE 5.1.3: The *Spaeth* system.

Insertion of iris root **(Fig. 5.1.8)**	• *Anterior:* Iris inserts anterior to the Schwalbe's line • *Behind Schwalbe's line:* Anterior to posterior limit of trabecular meshwork • *Centered on Sclera:* On the scleral spur • *Deep to scleral spur:* Behind the scleral spur • *Extremely deep:* On the ciliary band
Angular width slit **(Fig. 5.1.9)**	10° Narrow 20° 30° Wide 40°
Configuration of the peripheral iris **(Fig. 5.1.10)**	s = steep, anteriorly convex r = regular or flat q = queer, anteriorly concave
Angle pigmentation **(Fig. 5.1.11)**	*0:* None *1:* Minimal *2:* Mild *3:* Moderate *4:* Intense

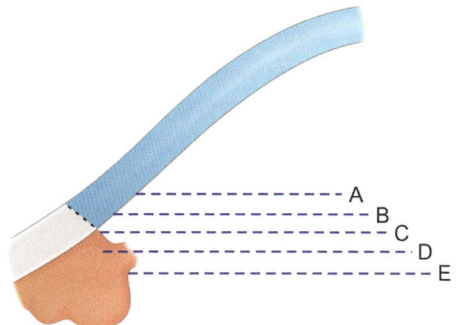

Fig. 5.1.8: Spaeth grading of site of iris insertion.

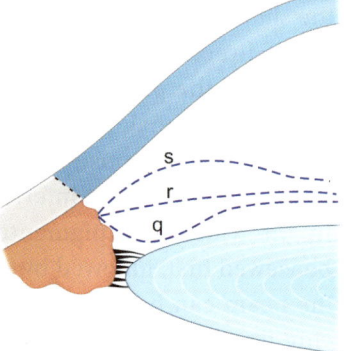

Fig. 5.1.10: Spaeth grading of peripheral iris curvature.

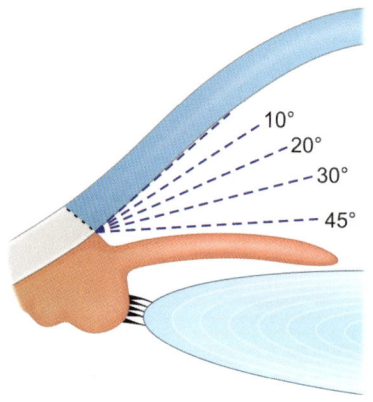

Fig. 5.1.9: Spaeth grading of angle width.

2. Angular width of angle recess
3. Iris configuration
4. Angle pigmentation.

■ RPC CLASSIFICATION

This is the classification routinely used at our Rajendra Prasad Centre for Ophthalmic Sciences, AIIMS, New Delhi for grading the angle with the patient in primary position.
- Grade 3 or less is considered as a narrow angle.
- *Grade 0:* Closed, no dipping of the slit lamp beam.

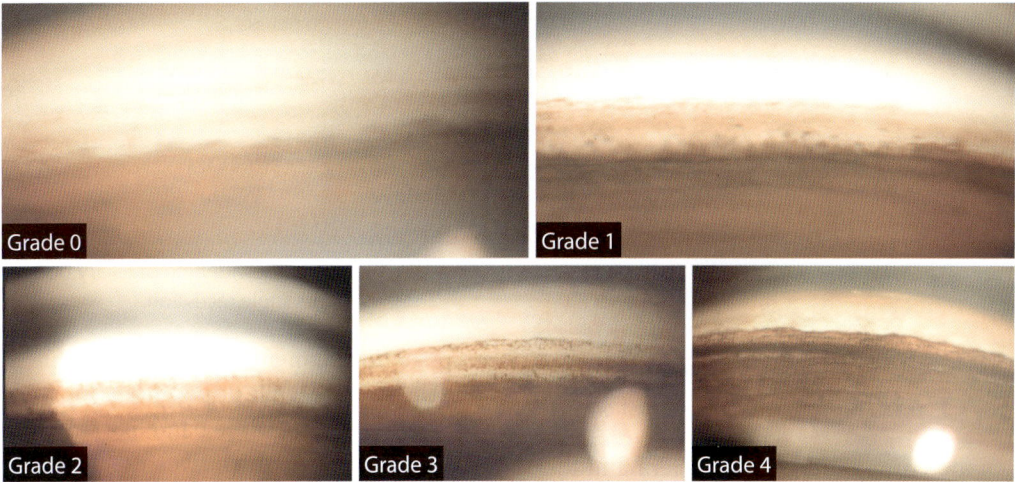

Fig. 5.1.11: Spaeth grading of angle pigmentation.

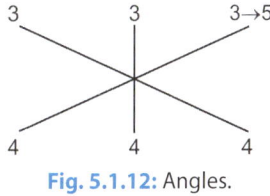

Fig. 5.1.12: Angles.

- *Grade 1:* Dipping of the beam.
- *Grade 2:* Schwalbe's line and anterior third of TM seen.
- *Grade 3:* Posterior two-thirds of TM is seen.
- *Grade 4:* Scleral spur is seen.
- *Grade 5:* Ciliary body band is seen.
- *Grade 6:* Last roll of iris seen.

The angle is written as shown in **Figure 5.1.12**.

This denotes the superior and inferior angle and the most posterior structure seen (3 = posterior TM visible in superior angle, 4 = scleral spur visible in inferior angle). The arrow 3→5 indicates the actual angle structure visible in primary gaze (in this case the TM = 3) and the structure which becomes visible after doing manipulative gonioscopy (in this case the ciliary body band = 5).

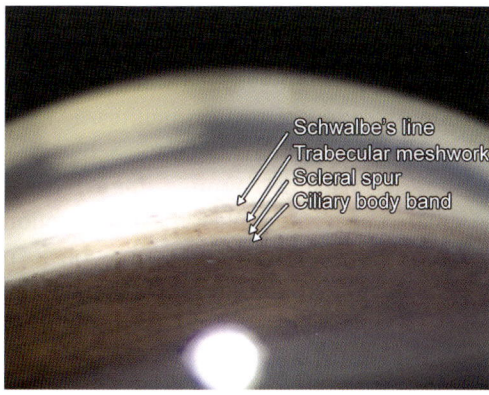

Fig. 5.1.13: Angle structures in a normal eye—Open.

NORMAL ANGLE STRUCTURES VISIBLE ON GONIOSCOPY

Gonioscopy helps us to determine the angle anatomy of a patient based on recognition of landmarks **(Fig. 5.1.13)**.

- *Schwalbe's line and corneal wedge:* Corneal wedge is used to locate the Schwalbe's line **(Figs. 5.1.13 and 5.1.14)**. It is formed by the meeting of the reflections of light from internal and external surface of cornea into one single light beam at the point where

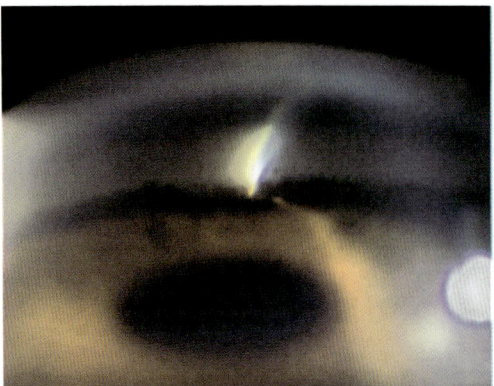

Fig. 5.1.14: Corneal wedge formation.

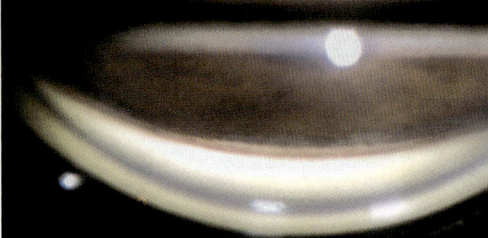

Fig. 5.1.15: Abnormal widening of ciliary body band-angle recession.

the cornea merges into sclera and loses its transparency. This is the point where the Descemet's membrane terminates. It marks the starting of angle structures. Sometimes pigmentation may lie anterior to the Schwalbe's line leading to confusion with TM, where corneal wedge helps in identification of angle structures. TM lies behind the corneal wedge and Schwalbe's line. It is visualized by projecting a thin and sharp beam at the angle. The pigmentation anterior to Schwalbe's line may be seen in pseudoexfoliation (PXF) called the Sampaolesi line, may be confused with TM. Corneal wedge is used to identify its location. A prominent Schwalbe's line may be seen in Axenfeld anomaly called a posterior embryotoxon.

- *Trabecular meshwork:* It starts right behind the Schwalbe's line. It is divided into anterior nonpigmented nonfunctional part and posterior functional pigmented part. The pigmentation of TM may vary from none to dark and is graded accordingly. Inferior TM tends to be more pigmented due to gravity and aqueous currents. The pigmentation may become especially heavy in pigment dispersion syndrome, PXF, and uveitis. Occludable angle is referred to an angle where 180° of posterior pigmented TM is not visible in primary gaze while doing gonioscopy.
- Scleral spur is a white band like structure behind the TM, which gives attachment to the ciliary body. Visibility of scleral spur in primary position denotes an open angle.
- *Ciliary body band:* The grayish portion of ciliary body visible behind the scleral spur is the ciliary body band. It may get abnormally widened after trauma—angle recession (see **Figure 5.1.15**) which is a sign of significant trauma to the eye. Ciliary body band may be wide in myopes and narrower in hyperopes.
- *Normal blood vessels:* They are usually visible in thin/blue-gray eyes and rarely in brown or black eyes. They can be seen as loops of vessels near root of iris that radially run toward the center of pupil. They never cross the scleral spur. Any vessel crossing the scleral spur is abnormal.
- Iris processes are finger like extensions arising from the iris and attaching in the angle at variable positions generally not crossing the TM. They follow the concavity of the iris and allow free movement of iris posterior during indentation. They may be confused with synechiae **(Fig. 5.1.16)**.

ABNORMAL ANGLES ON GONIOSCOPY

- *Primary angle closure disease (PACD):* Presence of an occludable angle (due to relative pupillary block or thick lens or increased lens vault) suggests PACD. Occludable angle is referred to an angle where 180° of posterior pigmented TM is not visible in primary gaze while doing gonioscopy. Manipulation or indentation gonioscopy is performed to look for blotchy pigments or goniosynechiae or permanent angle closure. Primary angle closure suspect (first stage of PACD) is defined as presence of an occludable angle, without goniosynechiae or raised intraocular pressure (IOP) or optic disc changes of glaucoma. Primary angle closure (second stage of PACD) is defined as presence of occludable angle with blotchy pigments or goniosynechiae, normal or raised IOP; without optic disc changes of glaucoma. Primary angle closure glaucoma is defined as presence of occludable angle with blotchy pigments or goniosynechiae, raised IOP, and optic disc changes suggestive of glaucoma **(Figs. 5.1.17A to D)**.

- *Traumatic glaucoma:* Irregular widening of ciliary body band may occur due to a

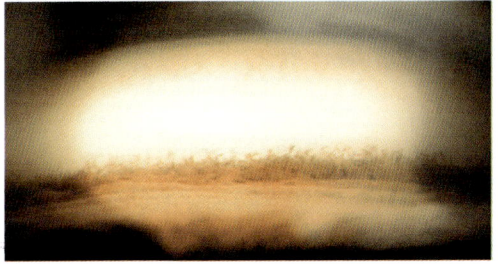

Fig. 5.1.16: Iris processes.

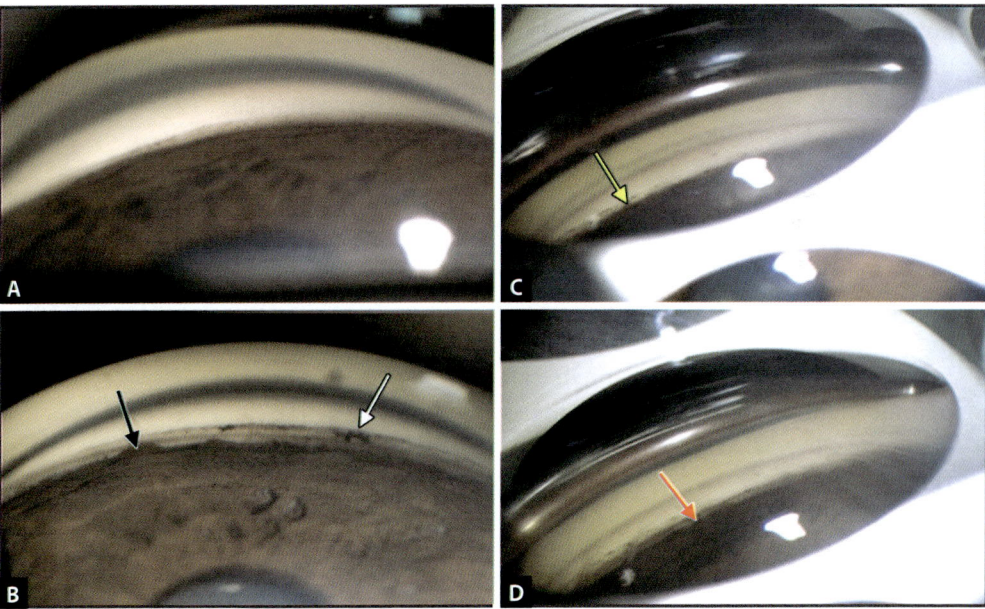

Figs. 5.1.17A to D: (A) Gonioscopy in primary gaze shows 180° angle where trabecular meshwork is not visible—suggestive occludable angle; (B) Goniosynechia—Tent like adhesion of iris (black arrow) to the trabecular meshwork is seen on manipulation gonioscopy using Goldmann lens and blotchy pigments seen in angle due to repeated adhesion of iris to trabecular meshwork (white arrow); (C) Zeiss type indentation goniolens applied over cornea shows occludable angle with pigmentation at the Schwalbe's line (yellow arrow); (D) Indentation goniosopy performed using the Zeiss type goniolens shows opening of angle showing the scleral spur and trabecular meshwork (red arrow).

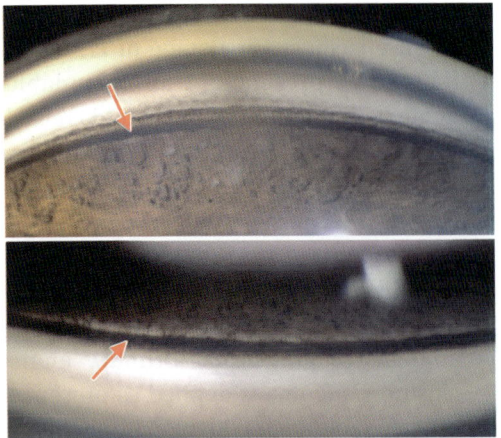

Fig. 5.1.18: Densely pigmented trabecular meshwork in both superior and inferior angles in pigment dispersion syndrome (red arrows).

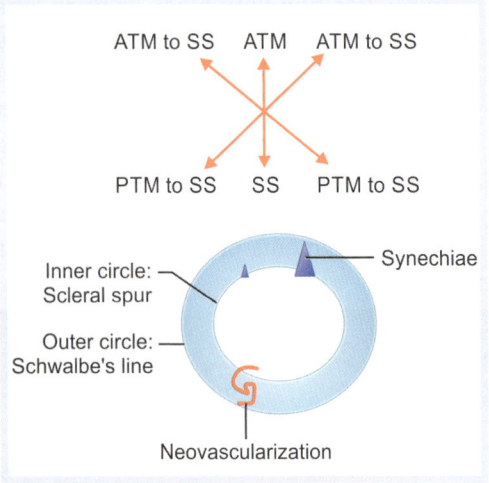

Fig. 5.1.19: Goniogram for easy recording of angle configuration. (ATM: anterior trabecular meshwork; PTM: posterior trabecular meshwork; SS: scleral spur)

split in the longitudinal and circular fibers of the ciliary muscle, also known as angle recession. It is suggestive of significant trauma to angle structures and increased lifetime risk of traumatic glaucoma **(Fig. 5.1.15)**.

- *Pigmentary glaucoma:* Pigment dispersion syndrome may result from posterior bowing of the midperipheral iris and rubbing with lens zonules, resulting in the release of iris pigment. This fine pigment deposits in the TM form a dense pigmentary band in both superior and inferior angle. PXF may result in salt pepper pigment deposition anterior to Schwalbe's line called the Sampaolesi line **(Fig. 5.1.18)**.

DOCUMENTATION OF GONIOSCOPY/ RECORDING—GONIOGRAM

- Posterior most structure visible in primary gaze with thin short slit beam.
- Posterior most structure on indentation or manipulation.
- Angle recess—degree
- Iris configuration—concave, regular, or steep
- Any specific angle abnormality:
  - Goniosynechiae
  - Pigmentation
  - Angle recession
  - Anterior insertion of iris
  - Iridodialysis/cyclodialysis
- Record any anomalies in the appropriate quadrant in a goniogram **(Fig. 5.1.19)**.

STERILIZATION OF GONIOSCOPES

Gonioscopy being an invasive procedure, infections can spread through infected gonioscopes. Hence, sterilization and disinfection of gonioscopes between uses is imperative.

A goniolens should be immediately rinsed with clean cold water with mild soap or detergent, after removing the lens from the patient's eye. After cleaning, the lens is disinfected. Disinfection may be done using either glutaraldehyde or bleaching powder.

The lens is soaked in 2% glutaraldehyde for at least 20 minutes or a 10% bleach solution (sodium hypochlorite) at 1 part bleach to 9 parts water for 10 minutes. The lens is then thoroughly rinsed with clean water and air dried. The gonioscope can also be wiped for 10 seconds with a sterile swab soaked in 70% isopropyl alcohol or cleaned with 1:1,000 merthiolate solution. Sterilization follows disinfection which is achieved by ethylene oxide (ETO) exposure. The sterilization of direct gonioscopes (Koeppe, Swan Jacob, etc.) used during surgery can be done with ETO gas sterilization. ETO is achieved by exposure at 56°C (130°F) for 1 hour.

Steam autoclave or soaking in alcohol should not be done.

VIVA QUESTIONS

1. What are the indications of doing gonioscopy?
Ans: Refer to text.

2. What are the different types of gonioscopes and their uses?
Ans: Refer to text.

3. What is the difference between manipulation and indentation gonioscopy?
Ans: Refer to text.

4. What is the benefit of doing indentation gonioscopy over manipulation gonioscopy?
Ans: Indentation gonioscopy can differentiate between appositional versus synechial angle closure, while manipulation gonioscopy cannot.

5. What are the structures seen in an open angle?
Ans: From the root of iris, the structures seen in an open angle are ciliary body band, scleral spur, posterior pigmented trabecular meshwork, anterior nonpigmented trabecular meshwork, and Schwalbe's line.

6. How do you differentiate between iris processes and goniosynechiae?
Ans: Iris processes are physiological whereas goniosynechiae are pathological attachment of iris to the trabecular meshwork. Iris processes are finger like projections whereas goniosynechiae are tent shaped. Iris processes follow the angle contour, move posteriorly, and may break while doing indentation gonioscopy whereas goniosynechiae do not move or break on indentation gonioscopy.

7. How do you differentiate between an open angle and a closed angle on gonioscopy?
Ans: The angle is visualized on gonioscopy with a thin light beam from a slit lamp, directed at the angle, not touching the pupil. If posterior pigmented trabecular meshwork is not visualized in at least 180° of the angle, it is deemed as a closed or occludable angle. In an open angle, the trabecular meshwork and the scleral spur are usually visualized in entire angle.

5.2 TONOMETRY

Jyoti Shakrawal, Talvir Sidhu, Shahnaz Anjum

■ INTRODUCTION

Intraocular pressure is the only modifiable risk factor in glaucoma. The regular monitoring of IOP is an important parameter in follow-up cases of glaucoma.

Therefore, the knowledge of practical application of IOP measurement is essential for every general ophthalmologist. The accuracy and precision in IOP measurement are of clinical significance.

■ TYPES

Flowchart 5.2.1 shows the types of tonometry.

■ PROTOTYPES

- Schiotz tonometer (indentation tonometer)
- Goldmann applanation tonometer (GAT) (introduced by Hans Goldmann and Theo Schmidt).

Schiotz Tonometer

Principles

- *Imbert–Fick's law:* This law states that the force (W) required to deform a perfectly dry, thin, and flexible sphere is equals to

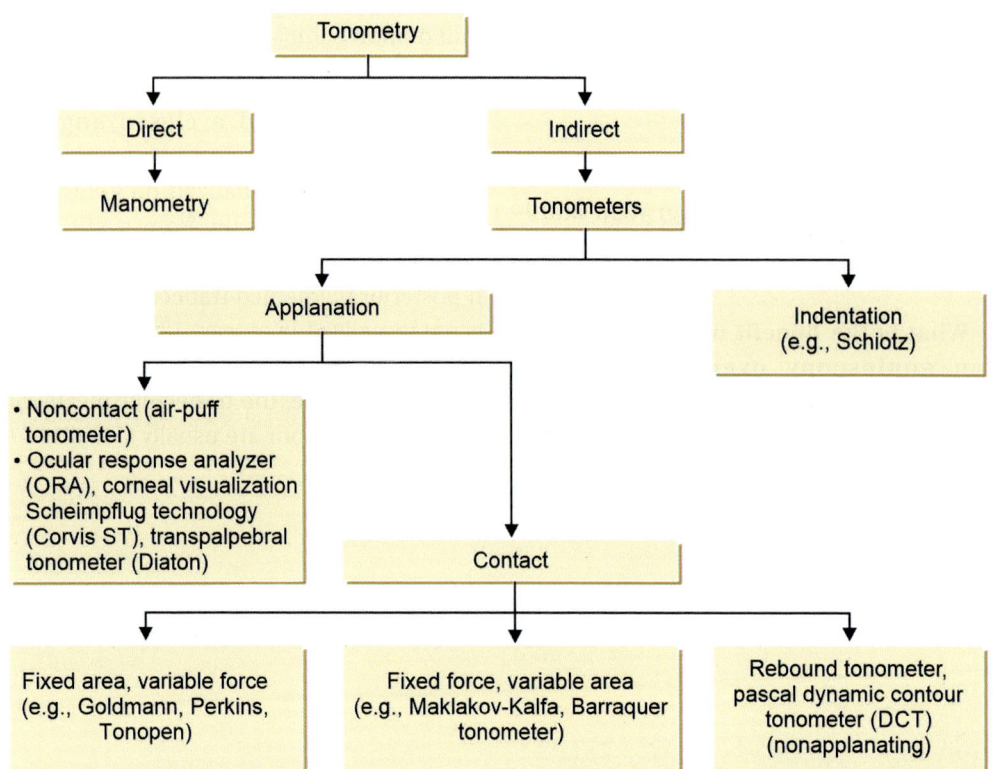

Flowchart 5.2.1: Types of tonometry.

product of area (A) deformed and pressure (P_t) inside that sphere **(Fig. 5.2.1)**:

$$W = P_t \times A$$

- *Modified Imbert–Fick's law:* As the cornea is neither perfect sphere nor absolutely dry, above equation needs some modification. The new equation considered surface tension due to tear meniscus and corneal resistance to applanation into account **(Fig. 5.2.2)**:

$$W + S = (P_t \times A_1) + B$$

Where, W is force of tonometer, P_t is intraocular pressure, and A_1 is applanation area.

The surface tension (S) and force required to bend the cornea (B) balance each other, whenever, the internal area of applanation is 7.35 mm², i.e., diameter of external applanated surface is 3.06 mm.

Goldmann Applanation Tonometer

Parts

The different parts of GAT are as follows **(Fig. 5.2.3)**:
- Measuring prism
- Feeler arm
- Weight insert
- Housing
- Revolving knob with measuring drum

Calibration

Following points are important for calibration of GAT:
- Ideally, should be done every month for verification of accuracy.
- It is done at dial positions 0, 2, and 6, which is equivalent to 0, 20, and 60 mm Hg.

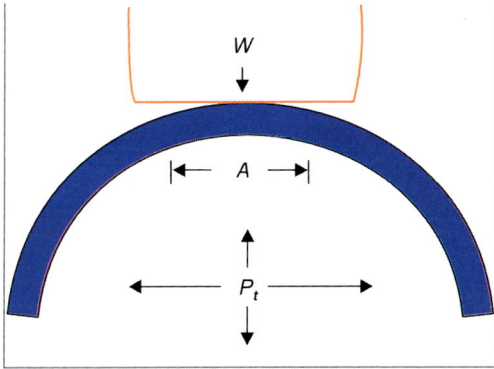

Fig. 5.2.1: The Imbert–Fick's law for the cornea ($W = P_t \times A$).

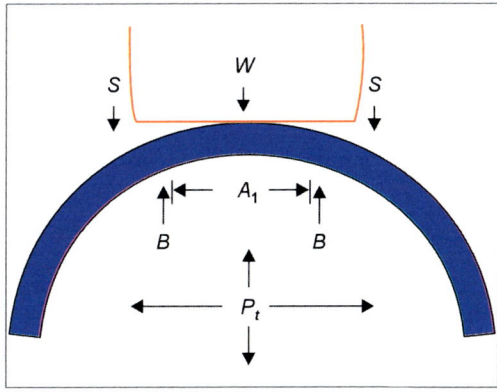

Fig. 5.2.2: Modification of Imbert–Fick's law for the cornea [$W + S = (P_t \times A_1) + B$].

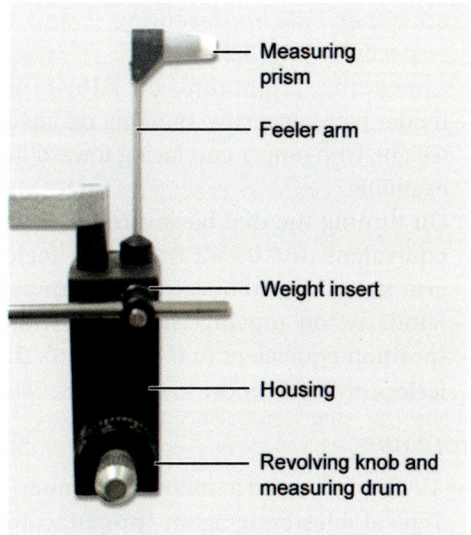

Fig. 5.2.3: Basic parts of Goldmann-type applanation tonometer.

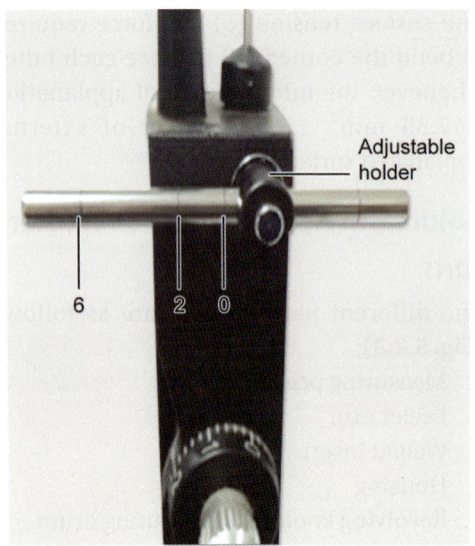

Fig. 5.2.4: Housing of Goldmann applanation tonometer with a bar-shaped check weight with five markings engraved on it (6, 2, 0, 2, 6).

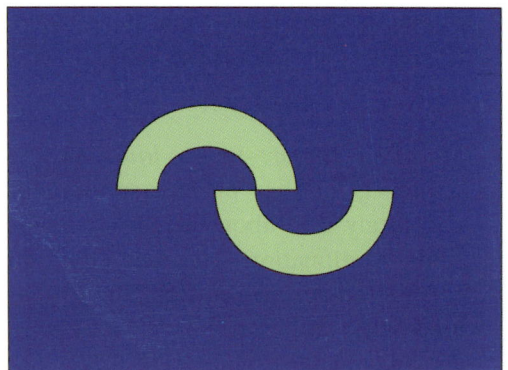

Fig. 5.2.5: Slit-lamp view of correct alignment of Goldmann mires.

- The dial positions 2 and 6 are checked by using check weight. While, dial position 0 is checked without check weight.
- The check weight is a bar-shaped rod with five markings engraved on it. The middle one represents 0, with two markings on either side representing 2 and 6, respectively **(Fig. 5.2.4)**.
- Check the alignment of adjustable holder with respective marking on check weight, with longer end facing toward the examiner.
- On turning the dial backward (position equivalent to 0.05 <2 or 6), the feeler arm should move toward the examiner. Similarly, on moving the dial forward (position equivalent to 0.05 >2 or 6), the feeler arm should move toward the patient.

Procedure

The GAT is performed in following manner:
- Topical anesthetic agent (proparacaine 0.5%) and fluorescein into conjunctival sac.
- 60° angle between illumination beam and viewing beam, and place cobalt blue filter.
- Prism with tonometer should fix in the notch.
- Keep the dial at low settings; approximately 1 (10 mm Hg).
- Obtain contact, observe cornea via viewing beam.
- Two semicircular, green color mires should be seen. When overlapping contact between inner edges of two semicircles visible, end point is reached **(Fig. 5.2.5)**.
- Regular pulsations of two semi-circular rings of equal size confirmed correct position of tonometer (mire thickness should be one-tenth of total diameter of applanated area).
- Doubling prism is used to applanate the cornea which optically splits circular area of contact with cornea into two horizontal semicircles by inducing horizontal shift.

Sources of Error

The different sources of error have been summarized in **Table 5.2.1**.[1,2]

TABLE 5.2.1: Sources of error in Goldmann applanation tonometer.

Central corneal thickness (CCT) and corneal curvature	• Thicker cornea—overestimation • Thinner cornea—underestimation • (For every 10 microns, change of 0.7 mm Hg) • Steeper cornea—overestimation
Corneal edema	Underestimation
Width of mires	• Thick mires—overestimation • Thin mires—underestimation
Astigmatism	• With-the-rule astigmatism—underestimation. Against-the-rule astigmatism—overestimation • (If >3 diopters, take average reading of two perpendicular axis, or align the minus cylindrical axis to red indicator of tonometer housing)
Repeated readings in short duration	Slight underestimation due to massaging effect on the globe
Incorrect calibration	Should be checked at least once in a month

Cleaning of Prism

- Sodium hypochlorite (1:10 household bleach)
- Isopropyl alcohol 70%
- Hydrogen peroxide 3%
- Soap and water wash

Contraindications to Goldmann Applanation Tonometer

- Globe rupture
- Ocular infection—corneal ulcers
- Allergy to fluorescein dye or topical anesthetic

Limitation

- Irregular corneal surface
- Over bandage contact lens

OTHER TYPES OF TONOMETER

- *Perkins applanation tonometer (Clement Clarke, Haag-Streit, UK)* **(Fig. 5.2.6):**
  - Handheld device and portable
  - Similar to GAT
  - Used in sitting or supine position, both, therefore helpful in children or bedridden patients.

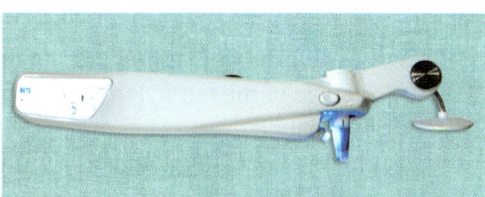

Fig. 5.2.6: Perkins applanation tonometer.

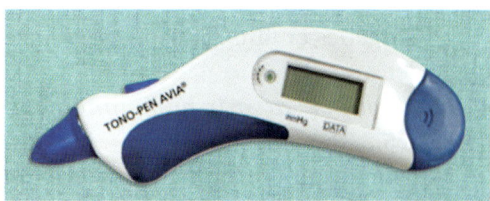

Fig. 5.2.7: Tonopen.

- *Tonopen (Reichert Technologies, Depew, NY, USA)* **(Fig. 5.2.7):**
  - Based on Mackay–Marg principle
  - A central plunger of diameter 1.02 mm is surrounded by a footplate. The moveable tip of the plunger is pressed against the cornea to generate a force, which is detected by a strain gauge. IOP readings are derived from the change in force detected by the instrument

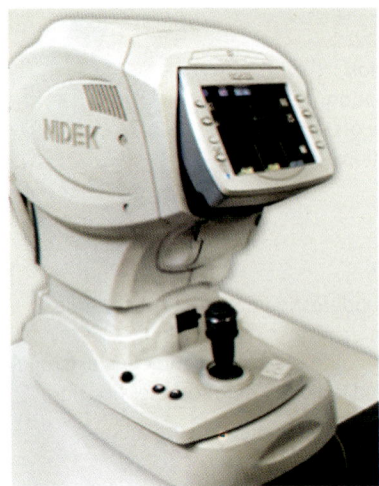

Fig. 5.2.8: Noncontact tonometer.

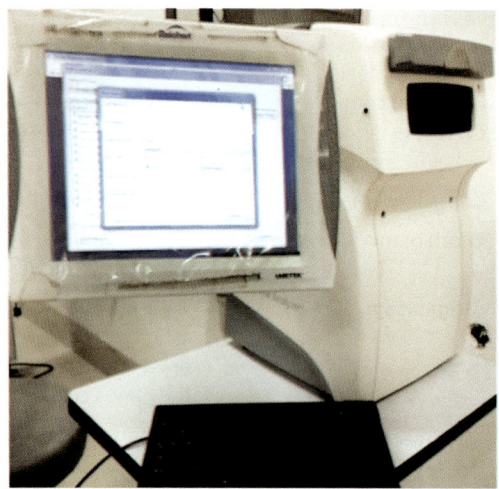

Fig. 5.2.9: Ocular response analyzer (Reichert, Depew, NY, USA).

in a waveform. This tonometer gives an average of the ten IOP readings of <85% variability.
- It underestimates IOP above 17 mm Hg and overestimates IOP below 17 mm Hg.
- Can be used in children, irregular corneal surface, after photorefractive surgeries or through bandage contact lens.

▪ *Noncontact or Air-puff tonometer* **(Fig. 5.2.8)**:
- The air puff records the intensity of rapid air pulse required to applanate or deform the central 3.6 mm of the cornea. The deformation is detected by reflected light from the cornea, which is aligned by an electro-optical system to get IOP reading. Minimum three readings must be taken to get average IOP reading.
- Fair agreement with GAT (± 3 mm Hg)
- Overestimate the IOP for pressures <10 mm Hg
- Underestimate the IOP for pressures >19 mm Hg
- Limited role in poor corneal surface or poor fixation

▪ *Pascal dynamic contour tonometer:*[3]
- Nonapplanating type, slit lamp mounted contact tonometer tip matching the corneal contour.
- The IOP is measured in real time as a pulsed curve according to systolic and diastolic cardiac cycle.
- The difference between the maximum (systolic) IOP and minimum (diastolic) IOP is the ocular pulse amplitude.
- IOP measurement is not affected by central corneal thickness (CCT), corneal edema, or rigidity.
- Overestimate IOP by 2.3–3.4 mm Hg approximately.
- Good agreement between dynamic contour tonometer (DCT) and GAT when CCT is 540–545 mm.[4]
- Difference between tonometers also increase, as CCT and IOP increases.

▪ *Ocular response analyzer (ORA) (Reichert, Depew, NY, USA)* **(Fig. 5.2.9)**:
- Measures the biomechanical properties (corneal hydration or

bioelasticity) of cornea, which influences IOP readings.[5]
- A continuous air jet is used to deform the anterior corneal surface until the desired applanation is achieved. It also measures the recovery of cornea from applanated state to normal state.
- Parameters measured are: Goldmann-correlated IOP, corneal-compensated IOP (IOPcc), corneal resistance factor (CRF), and corneal hysteresis (CH).
- Goldmann-correlated IOP (IOPg) is the average of the inward (P1) and outward (P2) applanation pressures and closely corresponds to Goldmann IOP. IOPcc is derived by using both IOP and corneal biomechanical factors.
- Corneal hysteresis measures corneal elasticity which is the cornea's capability to buffer the negative effects of pressure fluctuations in the eye. The second applanation pressure is usually lower than the first applanation pressure because cornea absorbs air pressure energy the first time. The difference between the two pressures denoted CH (P1-P2). Glaucoma patients have low CH. CRF is a measurement of corneal resistance.
- Important for taking IOP in various conditions of cornea like after refractive surgeries or keratoconus.

- *Rebound tonometer (I-care Finland, Helsinki)*[6] **(Fig. 5.2.10)**:
  - A very light weight, mushroom-shaped plastic probe which covers a central magnetic steel probe is used, which make momentary contact and rebounds back from the cornea. The strike of probe with cornea induces a voltage with is sensed as IOP.
  - No need for anesthesia.

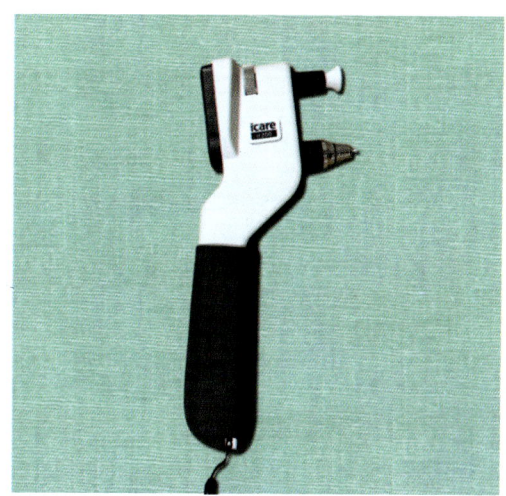

Fig. 5.2.10: Rebound tonometer (I-care Finland, Helsinki).

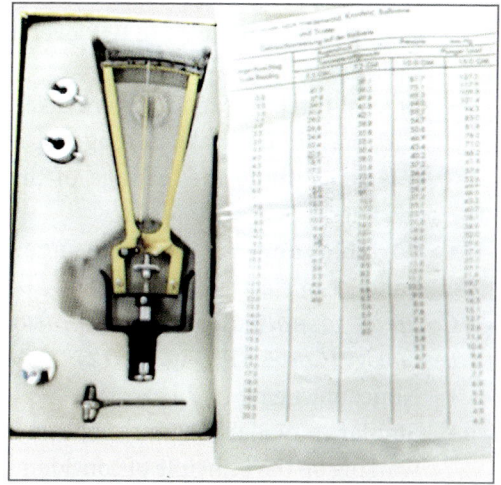

Fig. 5.2.11: Schiotz indentation tonometer.

  - Less discomfort to patient, can be used for home tonometry.
- *Indentation tonometer (Schiotz)* **(Fig. 5.2.11)**:
  - Indentation-based tonometer has a weighted metal plunger that is attached to a curved footplate, which matches the corneal curvature and

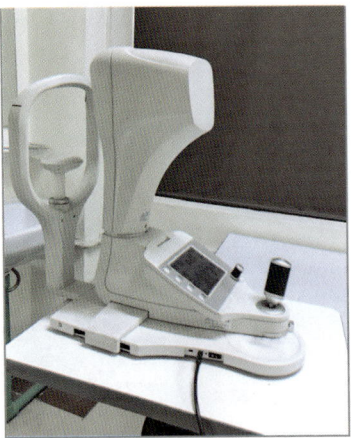

Fig. 5.2.12: Corneal visualization Scheimpflug technology (Corvis ST).

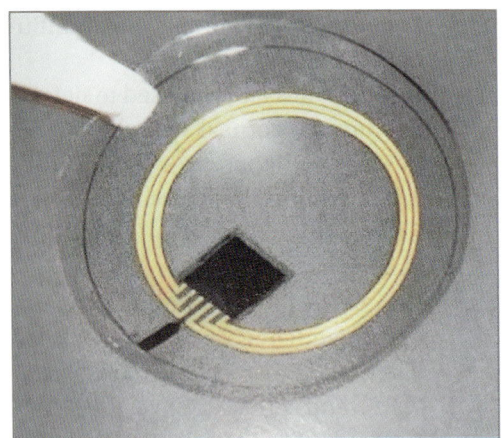

Fig. 5.2.13: Contact lens sensor (Sensimed, Lausanne, Switzerland).

rests over the cornea while measuring IOP. The plunger weighs 5.5 g and additional weights of 7.5 g/10 g/15 g can be added to measure IOP over a varied range.
- At least three IOP readings are taken and the Friedenwald nomogram is referred to note the average of the readings.
- Portable device, does not need batteries or electricity.

■ *Corneal visualization Scheimpflug technology (Corvis ST)* **(Fig. 5.2.12)**:
- Noncontact type
- Similar to ocular response analyzer, working on the principle of consideration of biomechanical properties of cornea.

■ *Transpalpebral tonometer (Diaton)*:
- Measures IOP through the eyelid
- Moderate correlation with applanation tonometry
- Can be used in presence of allergic conditions, viral infections

■ *Contact lens sensor (Sensimed, Lausanne, Switzerland)* **(Fig. 5.2.13)**

DIURNAL PHASING

Intraocular pressure is subject to cyclic fluctuations in whole day. Therefore, increase chances of missing peak IOP with one single reading. Normal variation is 3–6 mm Hg in normal eyes, which can increase up to 10 mm Hg in glaucoma patients before starting treatment. The *World Glaucoma Association (WGA)* guidelines advocate a minimum of IOP measurements at 8 AM, 12 PM, 4 PM, and 8 PM to assess its diurnal variation.

Indications:
- Normal tension glaucoma
- Ocular hypertension
- Progression despite adequate IOP during day time
- Advanced glaucoma patients at high-risk of progression
- After doing a peripheral iridotomy

CONCLUSION

- Both, indentation and applanation tonometry measure the IOP indirectly by some degree of globe deformation and converting it into the ocular pressure.
- IOP is affected by diurnal, environmental, and physiological factors.

- Establish a target IOP according to grade of glaucomatous damage, with minimal fluctuation during 24 hours IOP measurement.

VIVA QUESTIONS

1. Summarize different types of tonometers.
Ans. Refer to text.

2. What is the principle of applanation tonometry?
Ans. Refer to text.

3. How to calibrate a Goldmann applanation tonometer?
Ans. Refer to text.

4. What are the different ways of cleaning a Goldmann applanation prism?
Ans. Refer to text.

5. What are the factors related in establishing a target IOP?
Ans. Refer to text.

6. What is the best method to record IOP in following circumstances: corneal opacity; corneal edema; postlasik eyes; postkeratoplasty?
Ans. No single tonometer or method works best to gauge IOP across various corneal configurations; however, clinicians often prefer one type of device to another, depending on the circumstances. Goldmann applanation tonometry remains the gold standard, but it is susceptible to error due to variations in corneal biomechanics. However, in general, tonometry based on the principle of Mackay–Marg is considered the best.
- *Corneal opacity:* Tono-Pen may be useful to take the measurement in an area of the cornea that is clear.
- *Corneal edema:* Tono-Pen in the peripheral part of the cornea.
- *Postlasik eyes:* Both GAT and Tono-Pen are suitable for these eyes, but underestimation to be kept in mind.
- *Postkeratoplasty:* In eyes that have undergone penetrating keratoplasty, GAT pressure measurements are significantly lower than those obtained with the Tono-Pen. However, not proven which tonometer more accurately reflects the true IOP in such eyes.

7. What is scleral tonometry?
Ans. Measuring the IOP on the sclera can be an alternative to conventional corneal measurement in eyes with scarred corneas/keratoprosthesis. Tono-Pen is used to measure IOP at limbal and scleral area.

8. How to record IOP in GAT in presence of astigmatism?
Ans. In eyes with high astigmatism, two GAT readings should be obtained: one with the prism-oriented horizontally and the other with the prism-oriented vertically. "The mean of those two measurements is a better estimate of true IOP." Tono-Pen can also be used, as it is not influenced by the shape of the cornea in high astigmatism.

It is important to remember following facts:
- If the patient has <3.00 D of astigmatism, the prism is placed so that the patient's minus cylinder axis is aligned with the white line on the prism holder.
- If the patient has >3.00 D of astigmatism the prism is placed in the prism holder so that the patient's minus cylinder axis is aligned with the red line on the prism holder.
- It is important to remember that, as the prism is rotated according to the cylinder axis the mires will tilt with the direction of axis and the alignment has to be dome accordingly.

9. What is the normal range of IOP in infants, children, and adults?

Ans. In Indian eyes approximately
- Infants 8–10 mm Hg
- Children 10–14 mm Hg
- Adults 16–18 mm Hg

10. What is the time period for IOP spike following cataract surgery?

Ans. Most of the patients may experience an IOP >26–30 mm Hg following phacoemulsification, but most pressures will return to normal by 24 hours postoperatively. The peaks most commonly occur 8–12 hours after surgery.

11. What is the time period for IOP spike following laser peripheral iridotomy (LPI) and yttrium aluminum garnet (YAG) capsulotomy?

Ans. Usually IOP spike is seen, 4–6 hours after the procedure.

12. What is the importance of sleep time IOP recording?

Ans. IOP is subject to cyclic fluctuations through the day. Diurnal variation in glaucoma was first reported in 1898. Duke-Elder and others reported high IOP on awakening. There is therefore a chance of missing a pressure elevation with single readings. Across sleep stages, IOP is highest during REM sleep and progressively decreases as NREM sleep deepens.

REFERENCES

1. Whitacre MM, Stein R. Sources of error with use of Goldmann-type tonometers. Surv Ophthalmol. 1993;38(1):1-30.
2. Doughty MJ, Zaman ML. Human corneal thickness and its impact on intraocular pressure measures: a review and meta-analysis approach. Surv ophthalmol. 2000;44(5): 367-408.
3. Glaucoma Today. (2004) Robert L. Dynamic contour tonometry. [online] Available from http://glaucomatoday.com/pdfs/0304_10.pdf [Last accessed October, 2024].
4. Kaufmann C, Bachmann LM, Thiel MA. Comparison of dynamic contour tonometry with Goldmann applanation tonometry. Invest Ophthalmol Vis Sci. 2004;45(9): 3118-21.
5. Congdon NG, Broman AT, Bandeen-Roche K, Grover D, Quigley HA. Central corneal thickness and corneal hysteresis associated with glaucoma damage. Am J Ophthalmol. 2006;141(5):868-75.
6. Kontiola A, Puska P. Measuring intraocular pressure with the Pulsair 3000 and Rebound tonometers in elderly patients without an anesthetic. Graefes Arch Clin Exp Ophthalmol. 2004;242(1):3-7.

5.3 OPTIC NERVE HEAD EVALUATION

Talvir Sidhu, Mohit Goyal, Tanuj Dada

INTRODUCTION

Glaucoma is progressive optic neuropathy characterized by degeneration of retinal ganglion cells (RGC) which results in changes in the optic nerve head (ONH). So, ONH evaluation is a key feature for diagnosis of Glaucoma. The characteristic morphologic features of ONH include the following **(Fig. 5.3.1)**:
- Optic disc size and shape
- Neuroretinal rim (NRR)
- Optic cup and cup-disc ratio (CDR)
- Optic disc hemorrhages
- Retinal nerve fiber layer (RNFL) defects

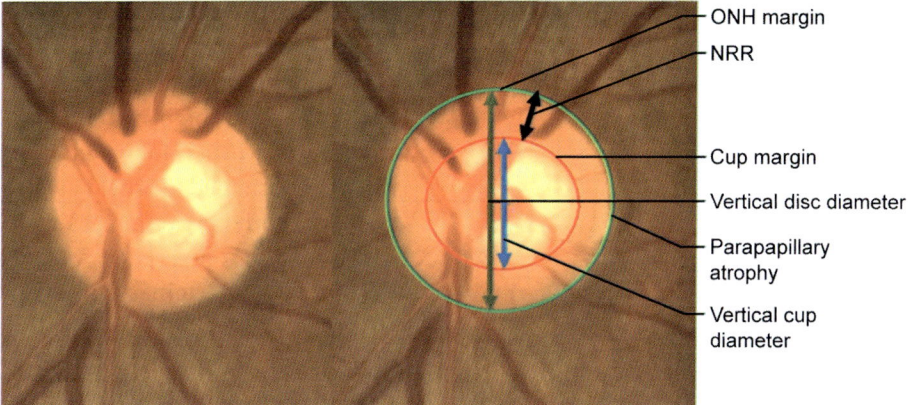

Fig. 5.3.1: Parts of a normal optic nerve head (ONH). (NRR: neuroretinal rim)

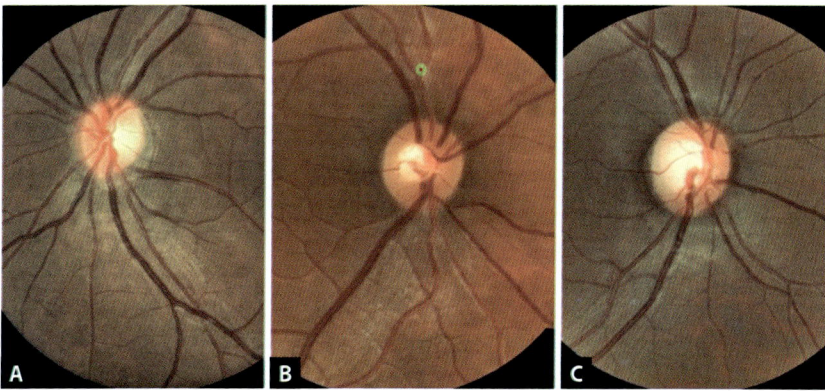

Figs. 5.3.2A to C: (A) A small optic disc with a small cup; (B) Average-sized optic disc; (C) A large optic disc with normal physiological cup.

- Peripapillary chorioretinal atrophy
- Vascular signs

Ophthalmologists need to identify and clinically interpret these ONH features correctly to identify glaucoma patients as well as glaucoma suspects early.

OPTIC DISC SIZE

The outer margin of the optic nerve is formed by the scleral opening from where the axons of the optic nerve pass. ONH evaluation for glaucoma begins with accurately determining the size of the scleral opening/optic disc.

How to Measure Disc Size

- *Direct ophthalmoscope:* The optic disc size can be objectively measured using Welch–Allen direct ophthalmoscope 5-degree aperture, which is similar in size to an average-sized disc. A small disc is smaller than the aperture and large disc falls outside the aperture **(Figs. 5.3.2A to C)**.
- *Slit-lamp biomicroscopy:* Adjust the slit-lamp beam length to match the vertical diameter of the optic disc, then read on the graticule with respective fundus lens correction factor.

- *Volk:* 60 D (0.88×), 66 D (1.0×), 78 D (1.2×), 90 D (1.33×).
- *Nikon:* 60 D (1.03×), 90 D (1.63×).
- Disc size is interpreted as:
  - Small (<1.5 mm)
  - Medium (1.5–2.0 mm)
  - Large (>2.0 mm)

Clinical Implications

- The larger the optic disc size, the larger the cup size and vice versa. A large disc having a large cup may be normal, whereas a small to average size cup in a small disc may suggest glaucoma. So, a large disc may be misdiagnosed as glaucoma due to high CDR and a small disc with glaucoma may be underdiagnosed due to low CDR **(Figs. 5.3.2A to C)**.
- Smaller discs have a greater risk of drusen, pseudo-papilledema and nonarteritic anterior ischemic optic neuropathy (NAION). Large discs may be associated with optic disc coloboma, pits, or morning glory syndrome.
- Disc area is independent of gender and age beyond 3–10 years of age and refractive error within –5 to +5 D.
- In higher hyperopia (>+5 D), disc size is smaller than emmetropic eyes.
- In higher myopia (>–8), disc is larger and more elongated than emmetropic eyes.
- *Race:* Disc size increases with ethnically determined skin pigmentation—i.e., African Americans > Asians > Hispanics > Caucasians.

OPTIC DISC SHAPE

- Disc shape describes the shape of the anterior scleral opening, the internal end of the posterior scleral canal that allows optic nerve axons to exit the eye.
- Normally, the optic disc is slightly vertically oval in shape.
- Disc shape is not correlated with age, sex, or race. In high myopia (>–12 D), disc is more oval, elongated, and more obliquely oriented. Corneal astigmatism is significantly higher in eyes with tilted discs.
- Disc shape determines cup shape and therefore determines our ability to interpret the health of the NRR. The *ISNT rule* applies when the disc is round or vertically ovoid, but it has no merit if the scleral canal is asymmetrically shaped, tilted, or horizontally ovoid **(Figs. 5.3.3A to D)**.

NEURORETINAL RIM

- Neuroretinal rim must be observed before looking at the optic cup.
- Neuroretinal rim area is formed by the ganglion cell axons passing through the optic nerve. Axons from ganglion cells close to the optic disc are arranged more centrally in the optic disc, whereas axons from cells in the retinal periphery are located at the ONH margins.
- *Neuroretinal rim shape:* NRR usually follows *"ISNT rule",* i.e., inferior NRR width is usually most broad, followed by superior NRR, followed by nasal NRR, with the temporal NRR usually being the thinnest sector **(Figs. 5.3.4A and B)**.
- *Neuroretinal rim color:* The normal color of NRR is pink-orange.
- *Neuroretinal rim pallor:* More noticeable in eyes with nonglaucomatous optic neuropathy than in eyes with glaucoma. Pallor extends beyond cupping. Pallor is one of the variables that is helpful to differentiate between glaucomatous and nonglaucomatous optic neuropathy **(Fig. 5.3.5)**.

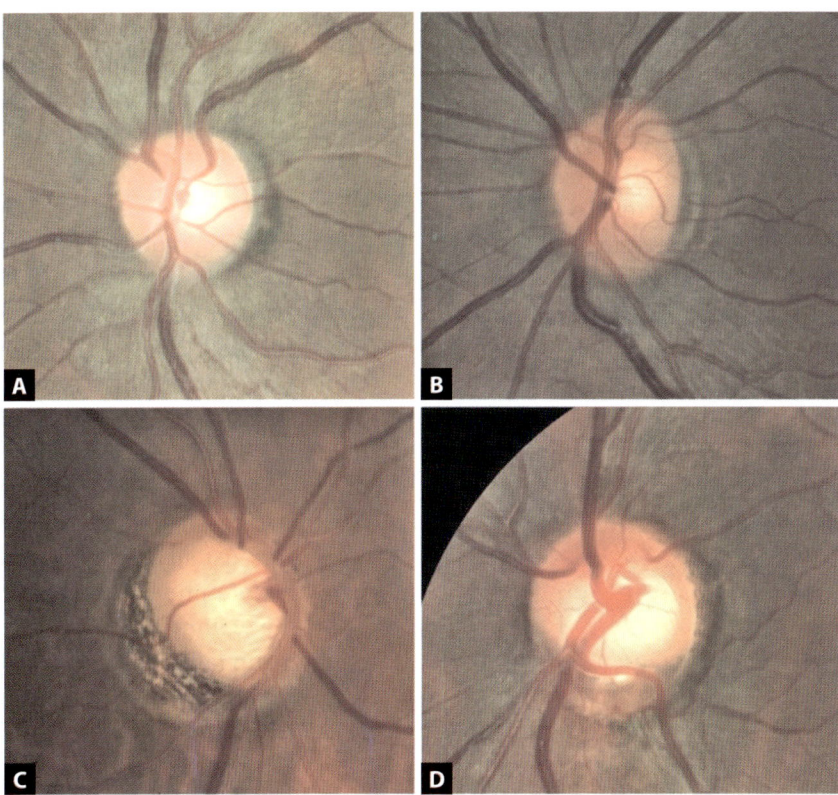

Figs. 5.3.3A to D: (A) Circular disc; (B) Vertically oval, temporally tilted disc; (C) Infero-temporally tilted disc; (D) Inferiorly tilted disc.

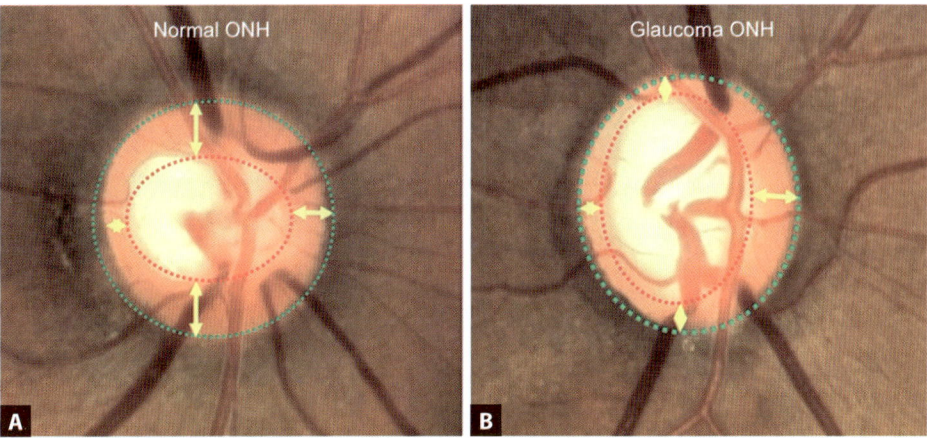

Figs. 5.3.4A and B: (A) A circular optic disc with NRR (yellow arrows) following the ISNT rule—inferior rim > superior rim > nasal rim > temporal rim. The thick NRR makes optic cup (red dotted line) horizontally oval or circular; (B) A vertically oval glaucomatous optic disc showing thinning of NRR in inferior and superior quadrants (ISNT rule not followed—nasal rim is thicker than inferior or superior). The optic cup is vertically oval (red dotted line) due to thin NRR. The color of NRR is pink in both discs. (NRR: neuroretinal rim; ONH: optic nerve head)

Clinical Implications

- *Focal NRR loss* is seen in glaucoma patients where preferential neuroretinal sector rim loss (inferotemporal → superotemporal → temporal horizontal → nasal inferior → nasal superior) correlates with visual field (VF) defect progression.
- *Concentric NRR loss:* A uniform thinning of NRR may be seen in very high IOP conditions such as juvenile open angle glaucoma (JOAG) and congenital glaucoma. Optic atrophy may present with concentric NRR thinning along with NRR pallor **(Figs. 5.3.6A and B)**.

OPTIC CUP

- The inner margin of the NRR is the optic cup.
- *Optic cup size:* The optic cup size depends upon the disc size and the NRR size. Optic cup equals optic disc minus NRR. The margins of the cup are defined by the contour of bending or point of emergence of vessels from inside of disc onto the NRR surface—called the contour cup. Beginners usually confuse the central pale area of optic disc as the optic disc cup—the color cup. Identification of contour cup rather than color cup gives a true estimation of the optic cup and CDR **(Fig. 5.3.7)**.
- *Optic cup shape:* The shape and size of optic cup varies according to the shape and size of the optic disc. In a vertically oval or circular optic disc, the optic cup is horizontally oval because NRR is thick in inferior and superior parts. In a tilted

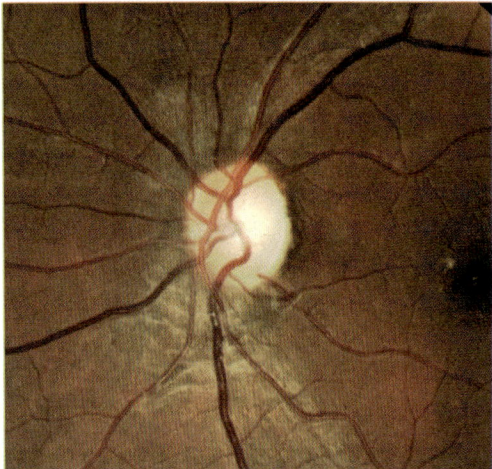

Fig. 5.3.5: Pale NRR + intact NRR = Optic atrophy. (NRR: neuroretinal rim)

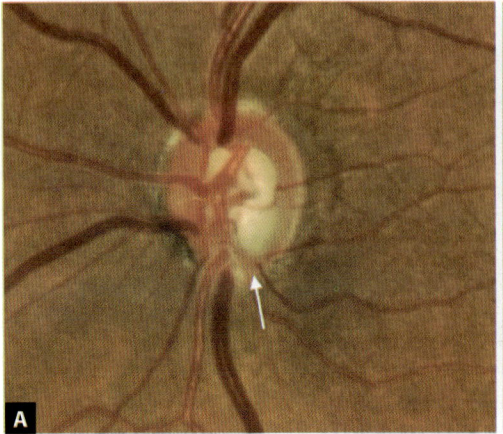

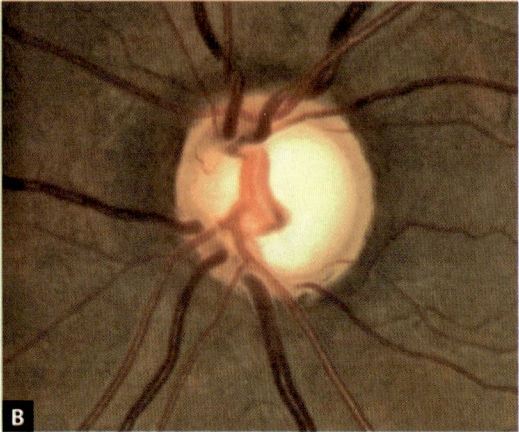

Figs. 5.3.6A and B: (A) Focal NRR loss/focal notch in inferior part of optic disc in glaucoma; (B) Concentric NRR loss in JOAG. (JOAG: juvenile open angle glaucoma; NRR: neuroretinal rim)

disc, the optic cup is also tilted toward the tilt of the optic disc. This may give an impression of NRR thinning in that area.
- *Optic cup depth:* The depth of optic cup is usually proportional to the optic cup size. A large cup is usually deep and a small cup is usually shallow.
- *Vertical cup: Disc ratio*—It is the ratio of size of vertical cup to vertical size of optic disc. Normal CDR in 98% eyes ranges from 0.1 to 0.7. A CDR >0.7 is usually suspected in glaucoma or other pathologic conditions. Optic cup remains constant in size after first years of life. A CDR of 0.6 may be pathologic in a small disc whereas physiological in a large disc. ISNT rule must be checked and mentioned in all optic disc evaluations.
- *Physiological cupping:* Many eyes with large optic disc size or few eyes with normal disc size may have a large cup disc ratio (>0.6) with NRR following ISNT rule. Large CDR or thinner NRR occurs due to spread of ganglion cell axons over a large area in a large, leading to a thinner NRR.

Clinical Implications

- *Color cup versus contour cup* can be confusing especially in older patients having nuclear sclerosis. Glaucomatous changes can be missed if we disregard the contour of vessels **(Fig. 5.3.7)**.
- *Optic cup changes in glaucoma: Focal enlargement* can be due to inferior NRR notch. *Concentric enlargement* of optic cup may be in JOAG/congenital glaucoma/optic atrophy.

OPTIC DISC HEMORRHAGES

- Flame-shaped/splinter-shaped hemorrhages at the margin of disc or within half disc diameter of inferotemporal or superotemporal disc margin. They are usually thin and elongated in the direction of reduced RNFL axons **(Fig. 5.3.8)**.
- Seen in 2-33% of glaucoma cases, usually associated with normal tension glaucoma.
- They disappear after 8-10 weeks.
- Disc hemorrhages result from ischemic damage to the NRR and precede

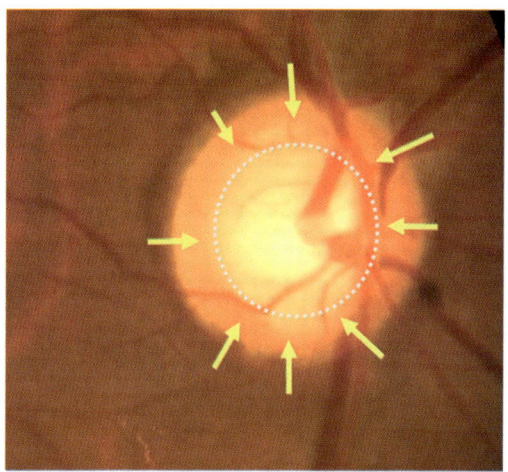

Fig. 5.3.7: Contour cup (yellow arrows)—the bending of vessels is seen. Color cup (white dotted line) is much smaller than contour cup.

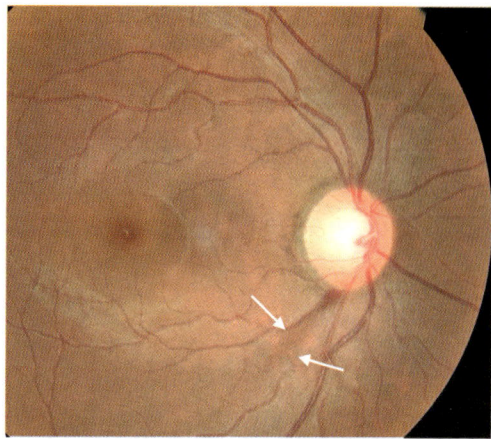

Fig. 5.3.8: Inferotemporal disc hemorrhage with RNFL defect (white arrows) in a case of 45-year-old female with normal tension glaucoma. (RNFL: retinal nerve fiber layer)

formation of new RNFL defects and NRR thinning. They are highly specific for glaucoma and are significant predictors of VF progression.
- A recent posterior vitreous detachment (PVD) may result in similar hemorrhages in diabetics. A careful examination for recent PVD must be done.

RETINAL NERVE FIBER LAYER DEFECTS

- Retinal nerve fiber layer appears as bright striations on the inner surface of the retina, most visible along the superotemporal and inferotemporal arcades. The visibility of RNFL is best in young patients with clear media, using a red-free filter on fundus camera **(Fig. 5.3.9)**.
- Reduced retinal nerve fiber layer defects in glaucoma are associated with NRR thinning in same quadrant of the optic nerve.
- Localized RNFL loss:
  - Localized RNFL defects are seen as wedge-shaped defects in RNFL starting at the optic disc.
  - The wedge defect has a narrow base at the disc and expanding toward temporal side and ending at the horizontal raphe.
  - It is associated with localized NRR loss in the same area adjoining optic disc.
  - Most commonly seen in inferotemporal or superotemporal regions in glaucomatous patients.
  - Nonglaucomatous, localized RNFL loss may also be seen in optic nerve hypoplasia, optic disc drusen, ischemic retinopathy, chronic papilledema, and optic neuritis.
- Diffuse RNFL loss:
  - More difficult to detect than localized but careful intraocular and interocular comparison can detect subtle relative RNFL pattern loss.
  - Increased retinal vessel clarity.
- Retinal nerve fiber layer defects are measured within one disc diameter of the disc margin. Defects or apparent defects further out than this are not classic RNFL defects.

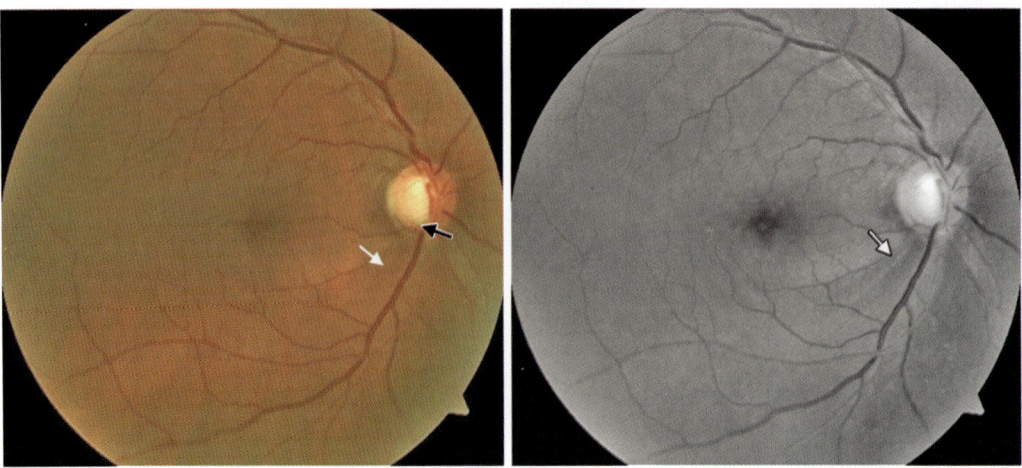

Fig. 5.3.9: Inferotemporal NRR thinning (black arrow) with RNFL defect (white arrow) in color and red free photograph. (NRR: neuroretinal rim; RNFL: retinal nerve fiber layer)

PERIPAPILLARY CHORIORETINAL ATROPHY

- Peripapillary atrophy (PPA) is the area of pigment change due to chorioretinal ischemic degeneration around the optic disc margin formed by changes in retinal pigment epithelium.
- The PPA zone is divided into two—zone β and zone α (**Fig. 5.3.10**).
- *Zone β PPA:*
  - The area of complete absence of retinal pigment epithelium and photoreceptors, near to optic disc, leading to visibility of underlying large choroidal vessels, and sclera-whitish color.
  - Risk factor for glaucoma progression. More commonly seen in myopic open angle glaucoma (OAG).
  - Complete absence of photoreceptors results in absolute scotoma or enlargement of blind spot on perimetry.
- *Zone α PPA:*
  - Area of retinal pigment epithelium (RPE) hypertrophy or change seen as hyperpigmentation or mottled pigmentation outside of β zone.
  - Seen as relative scotoma on perimetry.
  - More common than β zone—can be seen in up to 20% of normal eyes.
- Peripapillary atrophy is observed more frequently in glaucoma patients compared to others.

VASCULAR AND OTHER SIGNS (FIG. 5.3.11)

- *Baring of circumlinear vessels:* The vessels running along the NRR inner margin are left bare as NRR thinning progresses.
- *Overpass phenomenon:* The vessels may seem to float in the cup due to loss of support of thinned NRR.
- *Nasalization of large vessels:* The retinal vessel trunks shift nasally as the NRR thins. The distance of central vascular trunk to NRR is associated with papillomacular bundle and focal NRR loss.
- *Bayoneting of vessels:* Deep cupping is associated with the disappearance of vessels into the cup before emerging out, giving a broken appearance to vessel.
- *Laminar dot sign:* Loss of NRR and supportive tissue inside optic disc leads to visibility of laminar pores.

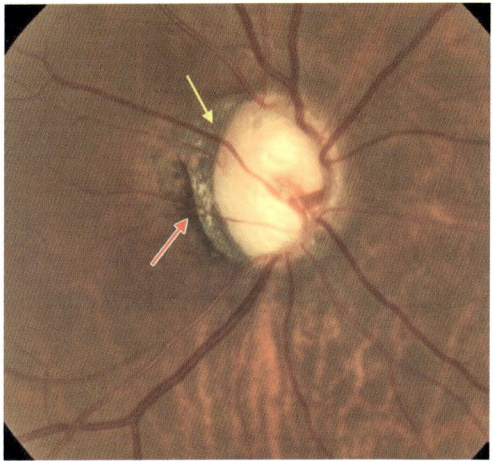

Fig. 5.3.10: Peripapillary atrophy (PPA)— Zone β (yellow arrow), zone α (red arrow).

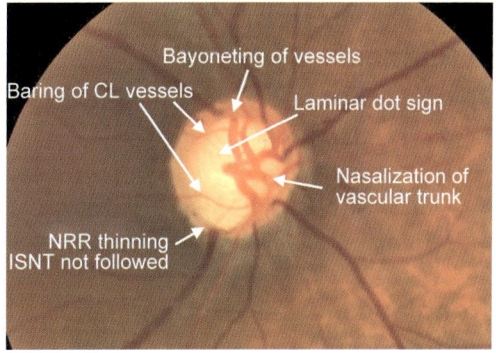

Fig. 5.3.11: Vascular and other signs of glaucoma. (CL: circumlinear; ISNT: inferior > superior > nasal > temporal; NRR: neuroretinal rim)

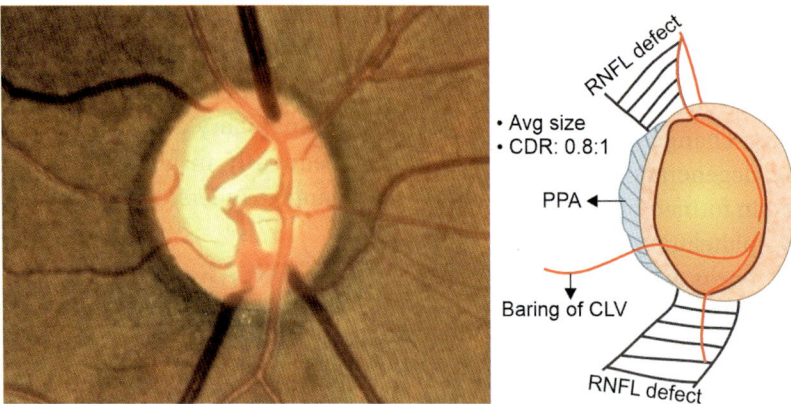

Fig. 5.3.12: Documentation of optic disc in a hand-drawn diagram. (CDR: cup-disc ratio; CLV: circumlinear vessels; PPA: peripapillary atrophy; RNFL: retinal nerve fiber layer)

DOCUMENTATION OF OPTIC NERVE HEAD MORPHOLOGY (FIG. 5.3.12)

- Serial disc photographs
- Disc drawings
- Optical coherence tomography (OCT)

GLAUCOMATOUS VERSUS NONGLAUCOMATOUS OPTIC NEUROPATHY

Table 5.3.1 shows the difference between glaucomatous and nonglaucomatous optic neuropathy.

Optic Nerve Head Findings in Glaucoma

- Greater CDR with vertical elongation with focal or diffuse NRR loss
- Greater frequency of PPA
- Optic disc hemorrhage
- Minimal NRR pallor

Nonglaucomatous Optic Neuropathy

- Pallor that exceeds or extends beyond the cupping.
- In most cases, the optic disc rim thickness tends to follow the classical ISNT rule. However, this rule might not hold true in cases of large optic discs.
- Diffuse rim thinning, although complete loss of the disc rim is rare.
- Usually does *not* have PPA, and if it does, it does not usually progress.

Optic Nerve Head Findings Common in Glaucomatous and Nonglaucomatous Optic Neuropathy

- Decreased retinal arteriole diameter with focal arteriole narrowing
- Reduced RNFL visibility
- Localized RNFL defects
- Enlargement and deepening of optic cup

VIVA QUESTIONS

1. How do you describe the optic disc findings in Figure 5.3.13?

Ans: This is the optic disc photograph of the right eye. The optic disc margins are well defined, vertically oval shape, large size, and parapapillary alpha atrophy is seen near temporal border. The neuroretinal

TABLE 5.3.1: Difference between glaucomatous and nonglaucomatous optic neuropathy.

	Glaucomatous	*Nonglaucomatous*
Age	Mostly elderly	Any age group
Presenting complaints	Mostly asymptomatic; except in advanced stage	Sudden onset decrease in visual function
Visual acuity (VA)	Well-preserved central vision until advanced stage	Early and severe vision loss
Color vision	Not affected until advanced	Affected early
Pupils	No RAPD until advanced stage as relatively symmetrical disease	Often unilateral and asymmetrical involvement; RAPD present
Optic disc	Vertical cupping, splinter disc, and hemorrhages	NRR pallor > cupping
Visual field defects	• Nasal step, arcuate defect, and spares fixation until advanced stage • Good correlation between visual field defects and disc changes	• Central, centrocecal, altitudinal, bitemporal, and hemianopic that respect vertical meridian • Poor correlation between visual field defects and disc changes

(NRR: neuroretinal rim; RAPD: relative afferent pupillary defect)

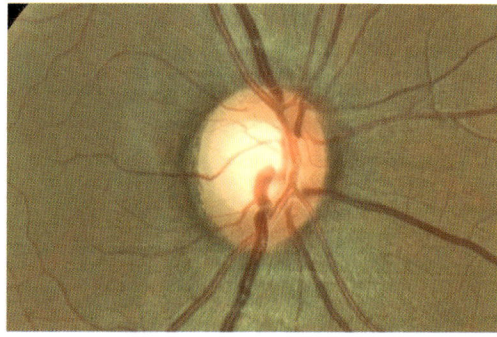

Fig. 5.3.13: Question 1.

rim is intact in all quadrants and follows the ISNT rule. The vertical cup-disc ratio is approximately 0.6:1. The retinal nerve fiber layer is visualized and is normal. *Diagnosis: Physiological cupping.*

2. **What are the signs of glaucoma in optic disc?**
Ans: Refer to text.

3. **How do you differentiate between glaucomatous versus nonglaucomatous optic atrophy?**
Ans: Refer to text.

5.4 PERIMETRY PART 1: KINETIC PERIMETRY— GOLDMANN VISUAL FIELD

Jyoti Shakrawal, Talvir Sidhu, Nikita Gupta

■ INTRODUCTION

Normal Visual Field

An island of vision (the hill) with a central peak in the sea of darkness[1] extends normally as:
- Superiorly—60°
- Nasally—60°
- Inferiorly—75°
- Temporally—90–100°

Visual sensitivity of a given point is related well with the altitude of island. The physiological blind spot represents as a pit/well in the island.

Types of Perimetry (Fig. 5.4.1)

Following types of perimeter are available currently:
- *Static perimetry:*
  - More sensitive
  - *Target:* Static, size usually constant for a test, stimulus intensity varies
  - *Axis:* Tests in *z*-axis also
  - *Printout:* Computerized
  - Three-dimensional, threshold-based test
  - *Examples:* Humphrey visual field (HVF), octopus, white noise campimetry
- *Kinetic perimetry:*
  - Faster
  - *Target:* Mobile, size, and intensity of stimulus can be altered
  - *Axis:* Tests in *x*- and *y*-axis
  - *Printout:* Manual (isopter maps)
  - Two-dimensional
  - *Examples:* Goldmann, confrontation, tangent screen, Lister, octopus kinetic perimetry
- *Combined perimetry:*
  - Both, sensitive and fast
  - For central VF-static
  - For peripheral VF and scotoma-kinetic
  - Usually manual perimetry

■ PRINCIPLE OF KINETIC PERIMETRY

The principle of Goldmann visual field (GVF) involves following points:
- An isopter is plotted, by moving the test target from the nonseeing area (at the rate of 2° per second approximately) to seeing area.
- At the end, an isopter is formed by joining the series of points obtained respective to the stimulus used.
- Size or brightness of the stimulus can be increased or decreased to plot different isopter.
- By using sequential stimuli, reproducibility of the test can be increased.[2]

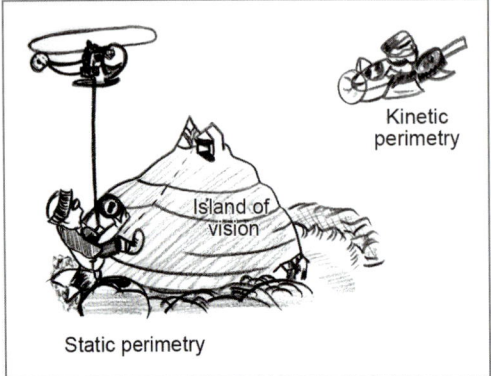

Fig. 5.4.1: The normal hill of vision with comparison of kinetic versus static perimetry.

- For defining a scotoma, the stimulus is placed in the scotoma and move outward until the observer perceives it. It is repeated in all directions to get all edges of the scotoma.

The edges of scotoma might be:
- *Sloping edge:* Brighter stimulus describes a smaller scotoma. Dimmer stimulus describes a large scotoma.
- *Steep edge:* Size of scotoma varies slightly with stimulus.

Target

Three alphanumeric digits represent the target **(Table 5.4.1)**.
- *Size:* By the first *Roman numeral* (0, I, II, III, IV, and V). 0 is the smallest; V is the largest.
- *Brightness:* By *Arabic number* (1, 2, 3, and 4). 1 is the dimmest, 4 is the brightest in 5 decibels (dB) steps **(Table 5.4.2)**.

TABLE 5.4.1: Different sizes of targets used in Goldmann visual field represented by various Roman numeral.

Target	Size
0	1/16 mm^2
I	1/4 mm^2
II	1 mm^2
III	4 mm^2
IV	16 mm^2
V	64 mm^2

TABLE 5.4.2: Different luminance values in apostilbs of targets used in Goldmann visual field represented by various Roman numeral.

Target	1	2	3	4
a	12.5	40	125	400
b	16	50	160	500
c	20	63	200	630
d	25	80	250	800
e	31.5	100	315	1,000

- *Luminance finer calibration:* By *alphabetical letter* (a, b, c, d, and e). a is the dimmest, e is the brightest in 1 dB steps.
- Background illumination, V1e; 31.5 apostilbs.
- Isopter is the line that connects points in a VF that have the same sensitivity to light. It is usually represented as (Roman numeral; Arabic number; letter)/(0–V; 1–4; a–e) and indicated using colors, i.e., red or green or black in the VF.
- The maximum stimulus is V4e (1,000 apostilbs) and it represents maximum outline of the field or absolute scotomas.
- The I4e stimulus indicates far periphery in VF and I2e represents central VF in a normal person.

EXAMINATION METHOD

Indications of Goldmann Visual Field

- Poor vision is <6/18
- Poor performance on automated testing
- Defects outside central 30° of VF
- Residual islands of vision
- Functional visual loss

Technique

Goldmann visual field is performed in the following way **(Fig. 5.4.2)**.

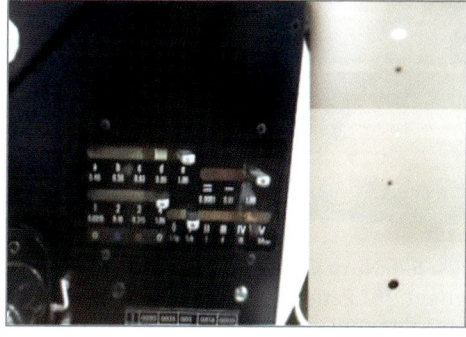

Fig. 5.4.2: Controls for target size and intensity in Goldmann perimetry.

Patient Preparation

- Appropriate refractive correction should be inserted in the lens holder.
- Pupil should not be dilated or pilocarpinized.
- In comfortable position with chin and forehead firmly against the support.
- Should be instructed properly regarding the procedure.

Examination (Figs. 5.4.3A to C)

- Done uniocularly
- Working distance is 30 cm, with examiner sitting opposite viewing via the eyepiece. Examiner should ensure good fixation of the patient during the test by seeing the patient's eye through the telescope **(Fig. 5.4.4)**.
- *Mapping the VF:* Illuminated white target is projected from nonseeing (periphery) to seeing area (center)—centripetally. The patient is instructed to press the buzzer, as they see the target. Start with V4e (largest) target to map the outermost isopter of the VF. Same maneuver is done at every 15–30° interval around 360° VF to examine at least 12 meridians. Three isopters are normally examined—V4e, III4e, and I4e.
- *Mapping the blind spot:* Plot blind spot from nonseeing to seeing area—centrifugally or outward, using at least 8 points (oval, around 10° in diameter, 12–15° temporal to fixation point; 5° below horizontal) using I4e target. Patient will press the buzzer, as they first see the target moving from blind area to seeing area.
- *Mapping a scotoma:* Any area of decreased sensitivity within the VF is mapped from nonseeing to seeing area—centrifugally or outward in at least 8 different clock hours.
- Static testing of central field using GVF:
  - Static target, shown for 1 second
  - *Starts at 2.5° centrally:* 5°, 10°, 15°
  - Circle all points missed.
  - Second reading still missed, mark an X in the circle.
  - Check all 76 points.
  - Kinetically plot out scotoma moving from center to outside in 8 directions or more.
  - Ask to fixate on center, move target within scotoma isopter to look for additional nonseeing points.
  - Recheck X points with increasing intensities (relative/absolute scotoma).

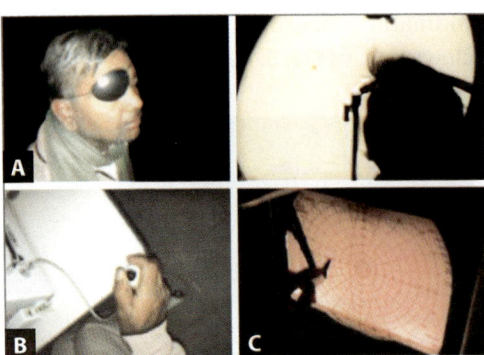

Figs. 5.4.3A to C: (A) Cover the other eye of the patient; (B) Patient pressing the buzzer as the target first comes in seeing area; (C) After patient's response, examiner marks the location of that point on a printout.

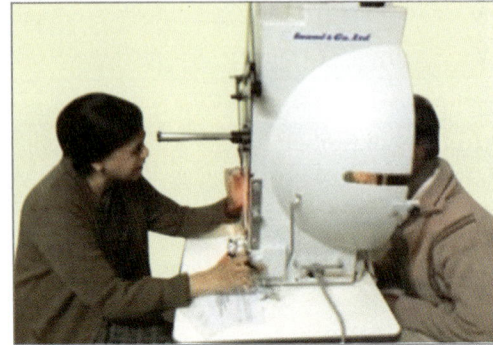

Fig. 5.4.4: During the test, examiner should ensure good fixation of the patient by viewing through the telescope.

INTERPRETATION

Following points are important while interpreting GVF:
- Patient name and age, the date of test, and the eye tested should be noted. Any additional notes such as pupil diameter trial frame addition and fixation quality should be noted.
- Look for the largest peripheral field, topographic map; with target V4e and subsequently at the other isopters and compare with age-matched ranges. In patients older than 50, there may be constriction of largest isopter by 10°.[3]
- Any distortion in the "contours:"
  - The smaller isopters, respective to smaller or dimmer stimulus are known as contours.
  - Check the following:
    - *Margins of contours*: Smooth or irregular?
    - *Restriction*: For example, nasal step in papilledema.
    - *Spacing between the isopters*: Two isopters should not cross each other. Functional overlay is denoted by a very small central field with stacked (close) isopters. Seen in patients with striate cortex lesions.[4]
    - Scotomas present or not?
- *Blind spot:* Enlarged?
- *Central field:* Static testing done or not?
- *Compare both eye fields:* Monocular or binocular defect? If binocular, homonymous or heteronymous?
- *Comments regarding fixation.*

Quantification of a Goldmann Visual Field

Software like Field Digitize 4.20 software (Johns Hopkins Technology Ventures, Baltimore, USA) may be used.

Interpretation of Normal Goldmann Visual Field (Fig. 5.4.5)

- Patient details, date of test
- The largest peripheral isopter (violet color)
- Other isopters are with smooth margins (green and red color). No scotoma present.
- Blind spot
- Central vision

CLINICAL EXAMPLES

Figures 5.4.6 to 5.4.13 give examples of GVF.

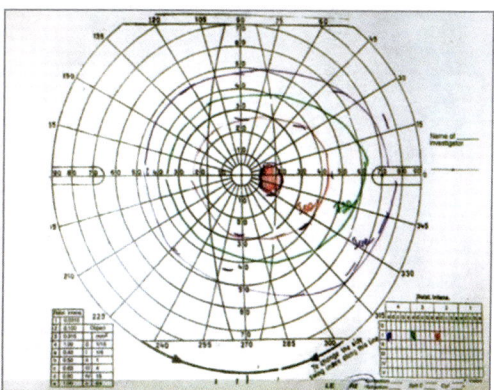

Fig. 5.4.5: Interpreting the normal Goldmann visual field.

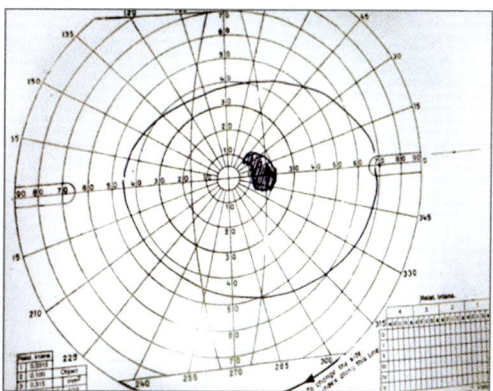

Fig. 5.4.6: Goldmann visual field of a glaucoma patient showing "Seidel's scotoma."

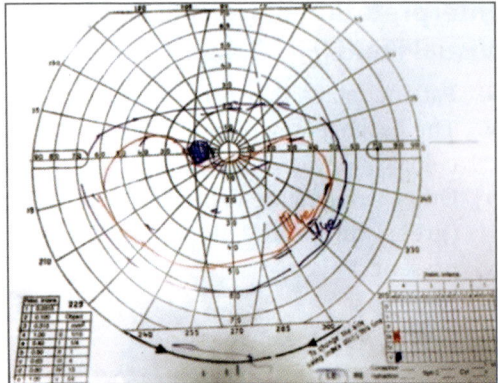

Fig. 5.4.7: Goldmann visual field of glaucoma patient showing baring of blind spot in glaucoma patient with superior visual field loss along with inferior nasal step.

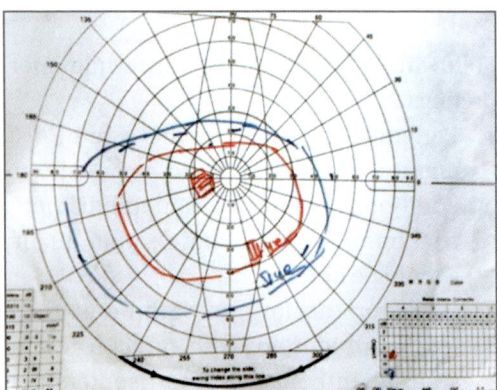

Fig. 5.4.10: Goldmann visual field of a patient with ptosis showing superior field defect.

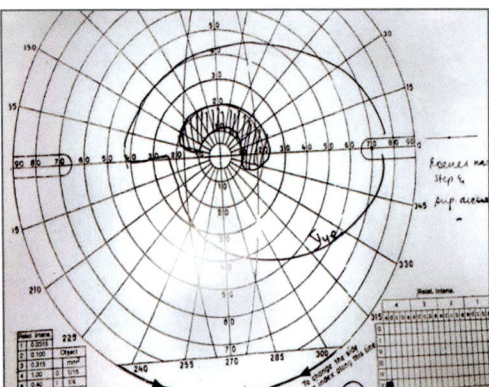

Fig. 5.4.8: Goldmann visual field of glaucoma patient showing Roenne's nasal step and Bjerrum's scotoma.

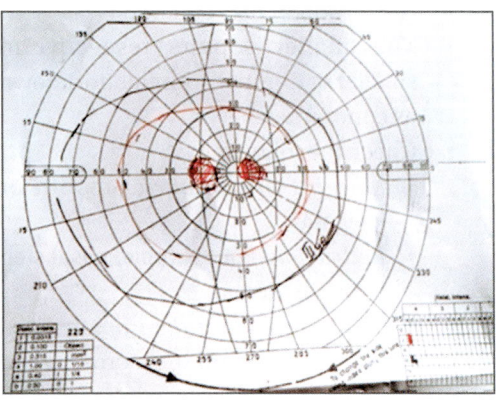

Fig. 5.4.11: Goldmann visual field of a patient with macular scar showing a central scotoma.

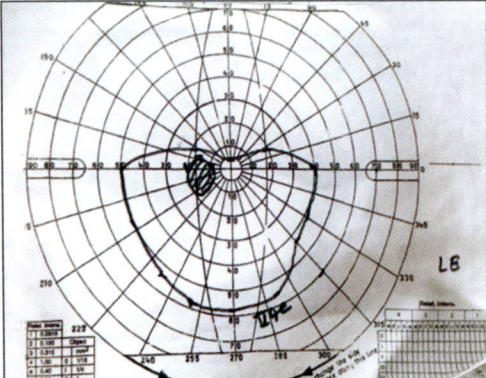

Fig. 5.4.9: Goldmann visual field in advanced glaucoma done with a large-sized (Goldmann size V4e) spot showing superior field defect with inferior nasal step.

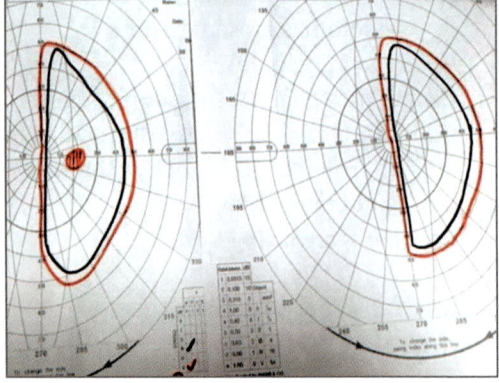

Fig. 5.4.12: Goldmann visual field showing left-sided hemianopia.

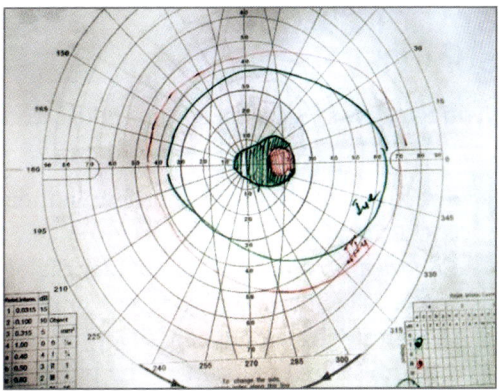

Fig. 5.4.13: Goldmann visual field from optic neuritis, showing centrocecal scotoma.

CONCLUSION

- Goldmann visual field gives an alphanumeric digits coded printout of patients "hill of vision." Always consider the normal hill in thoughts while interpreting these results.
- Always correlate the results of VF with clinical examination.
- Goldmann visual field is also helpful in representing neurological conditions, in addition to glaucomatous field defects.
- Therefore, perimetry not only helps in diagnosis of disease, but also to look for progression of disease and monitoring the therapy.

VIVA QUESTIONS

1. **State the difference between kinetic and static perimetry.**
   Ans: Refer to text.

2. **State the indications of Goldmann visual field.**
   Ans: Refer to text.

3. **How to read a printout of Goldmann visual field?**
   Ans: Refer to text.

4. **How to elaborate the alphanumerical representation of target size?**
   Ans: Refer to text.

REFERENCES

1. Harrington DO, Drake MV. The visual fields: a textbook and atlas of clinical perimetry, 6th edition. St Louis: Mosby; 1990.
2. Gandolfo E, Capris P, Corallo G, Zingirian M. Effects of random presentation on kinetic threshold. Doc Ophthalmol Proc Series. 1985;42:539-43.
3. Grobbel J, Dietzsch J, Johnson CA, Vonthein R, Stingl K, Weleber RG, et al. Normal values for the full visual field, corrected for age- and reaction time, using semiautomated kinetic testing on the octopus 900 perimeter. Transl Vis Sci Technol. 2016;5(2):5.
4. Hickman SJ. Neurological visual field defects. Neuro-ophthalmology. 2011;35:242-50.

5.5 PERIMETRY PART 2: STATIC PERIMETRY— HUMPHREY VISUAL FIELD

Talvir Sidhu, Jyoti Shakrawal, Harika Regani, Tanuj Dada

INTRODUCTION

The HVF is a standard method of automated static perimetry. Therefore, it is also known as standard automated perimetry (SAP), with the protocol of "white-on-white" stimuli.

It has several advantages over GVF such as:
- Less perimetrist subjectivity
- Maintain the uniformity and reproducibility of VFs
- Random presentation of targets is possible
- Calculate the patient's reliability statistical calculation of data at various levels
- Faster

PRINCIPLE

It detects differential light sensitivity (DLS), which is the ability to detect a difference in contrast, between two areas of different contrast (background vs. stimulus). Each point is examined by projecting a stationary stimulus of increasing intensity until the threshold is reached. Threshold is defined as the light intensity at which the retina can visualize a defined intensity of light at least 50% of the time, when projected to the retina.

INDICATIONS OF VISUAL FIELD TESTING

Glaucoma diagnosis and progression.

EXAMINATION METHODS

Components of Humphrey Visual Field (Figs. 5.5.1 and 5.5.2)
- *Perimetric unit:* Consist of a bowl-shaped screen with a matte finish Lambertian surface at 30 cm. The targets projected onto it are seen equally bright in all directions. The background illumination is 31.6 apostilbs.
- *Control unit:* Consist of a computer, dialog screen, keyboard, and printer. Controls the interaction between the operator and the system to evaluate the patient's response. Lastly, give us a printout after data processing. The hard copy consists of symbols and numerical values. The

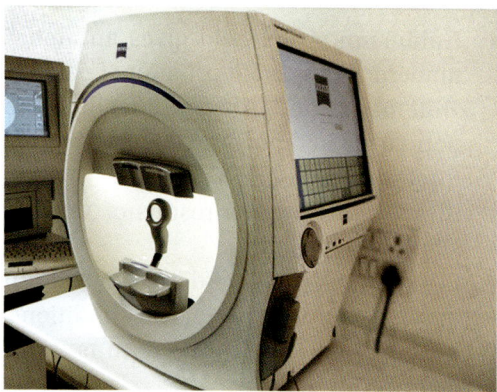

Fig. 5.5.1: Exclusive gaze tracker of Humphrey field analyzer 3 (HFA3).

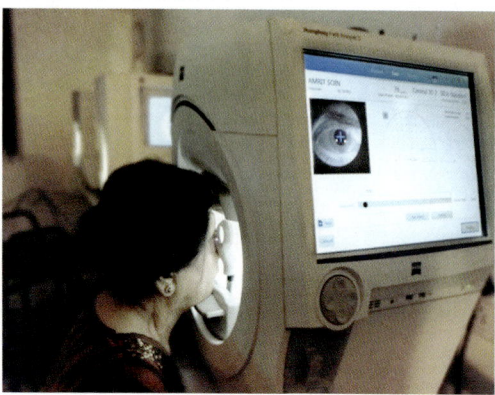

Fig. 5.5.2: Humphrey field analyzer 3 (Carl–Zeiss HFA3).

information is also stored in the computer for future need.

Stimuli

Spots of white light are projected on white background (white-on-white perimetry). The size and intensity combination of the stimuli is fixed for a test.
- Measured light intensity (logarithmic unit) is dB = 0.1 log apostilbs
- Brightest target = 0 dB
- Dimmest target = 50 dB
- *Threshold stimulus*: Target which is bright enough to be seen 50% of the time at a given set of test parameters at a given retinal location.

Parameters of the Test

- *Background luminance:* 31.6 apostilb
- *Background color:* White
- *Stimulus size:* Goldmann size III (4 mm^2)
- *Stimulus color:* White
- *Fixation targets: Central yellow dot*—used in all patients; *Large diamond*—used in patients with macular lesions like age-related macular degeneration (ARMD); *Small diamond* for checking foveal threshold **(Fig. 5.5.3)**.
- *Exposure time:* 0.2 seconds

Testing Strategy

- *Suprathreshold strategy:* A similar intensity bright stimulus (brighter than normal threshold) is used across the entire VF, and the patient's responses are recorded as seen or not seen. Absolute scotomas can be picked. Therefore, used for a rapid screening like the motor vehicle driving tests.[1]
- *Threshold strategy:* First, the threshold is determined at four primary locations

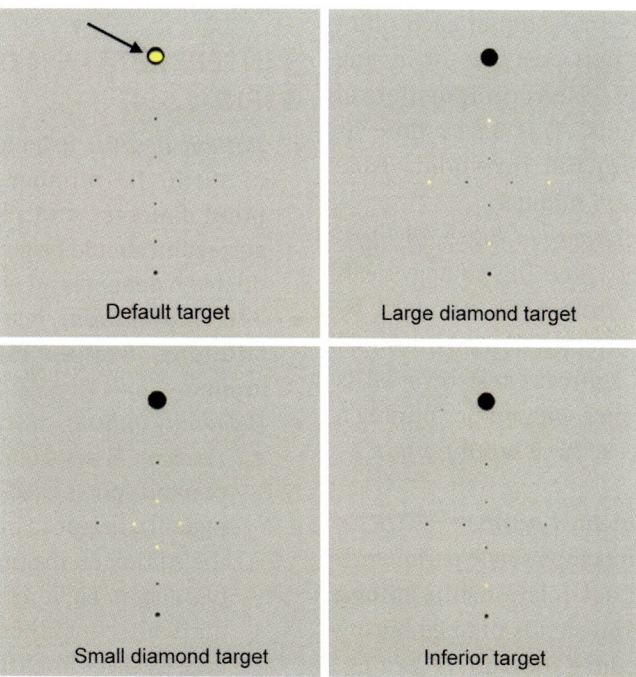

Default target | Large diamond target
Small diamond target | Inferior target

Fig. 5.5.3: Humphrey field analyzer examination targets.

which are symmetrically placed 9° from both, horizontal and vertical meridian. The threshold for each point is then determined in 4 dB up step and 2 dB down steps. Visual sensitivity is estimated at each point by a staircase or bracketing strategy. Used for monitoring glaucoma progression and worsening.

- Strategies for Humphrey visual field are:
  - *Full threshold*: 4-2 dB staircasing is used at four primary points in VF at 9°. Short-term fluctuation in visual sensitivity is also tested at primary points. *Time taken for test:* 15–20 minutes.[2]
  - *Swedish interactive threshold algorithm (SITA) standard*: Time efficient estimation of threshold 12.7° from fovea with 4-2 dB staircasing. It uses Bayesian statistics and calculates the reaction time of the patients, along with VF modeling to determine when testing can stop at each point location. It uses post-test processing for more precise recomputation of all thresholds. This saves time as compared to full threshold. *Time taken for test:* 7 minutes.
  - *Swedish interactive threshold algorithm fast or faster*: This strategy saves more time than SITA standard by using age corrected normal threshold levels and staircase test reversal is done only once without performing a second check. *Time taken for test:* 4–5 minutes.
  - *Tendency oriented perimetry (TOP)* is available on octopus style perimeters. It uses spatial relationship among sensitivity thresholds of neighboring zones to reduce time on VF testing. *Time taken for test:* 2–4 minutes.

TABLE 5.5.1: Commonly used programs for Humphrey visual field (HVF).

30-2	Central 30° tested, 76 points, 6° apart
24-2	Central 24° tested, 54 points, 6° apart; the nasal edge is extended to 30° to detect early nasal steps
24-2 C	Central 24° tested, 54 points 6° apart, along with 10 extramacular points in central 10° for early paracentral scotomas
10-2	Central 10° tested, 68 points, 2° apart (Optic disc/blind spot not mapped as it falls outside central 10°)
5-2	Central 5° tested, 16 points, 2° apart
Macula pattern	16 points, 2° apart (to look for macular split)
Pattern	• Along vertical and horizontal meridian • Grid of points 6° apart, which are 3° on either side of meridian

Programs Used

Table 5.5.1 shows the commonly used programs for Humphrey visual field.

INTERPRETATION OF RESULTS (FIG. 5.5.4)

- *Patient details:* It includes name, date of birth, ID number, eye examined, pupil diameter, and visual acuity. Near correction should be given. Pupil must be dilated if patient is on pilocarpine.
- *Test information:* Test name, strategy, stimulus, fixation target, and background.
- *Reliability indices:*
  - *Fixation losses*: Heijl–Krakau method of blind spot is used—by checking the patient's response by projecting 5% of the stimuli on the previously detected blind spot. Light reflex monitoring by corneal reflex. Gaze monitoring by gaze tracker. Unreliable field if fixation losses of >20%.

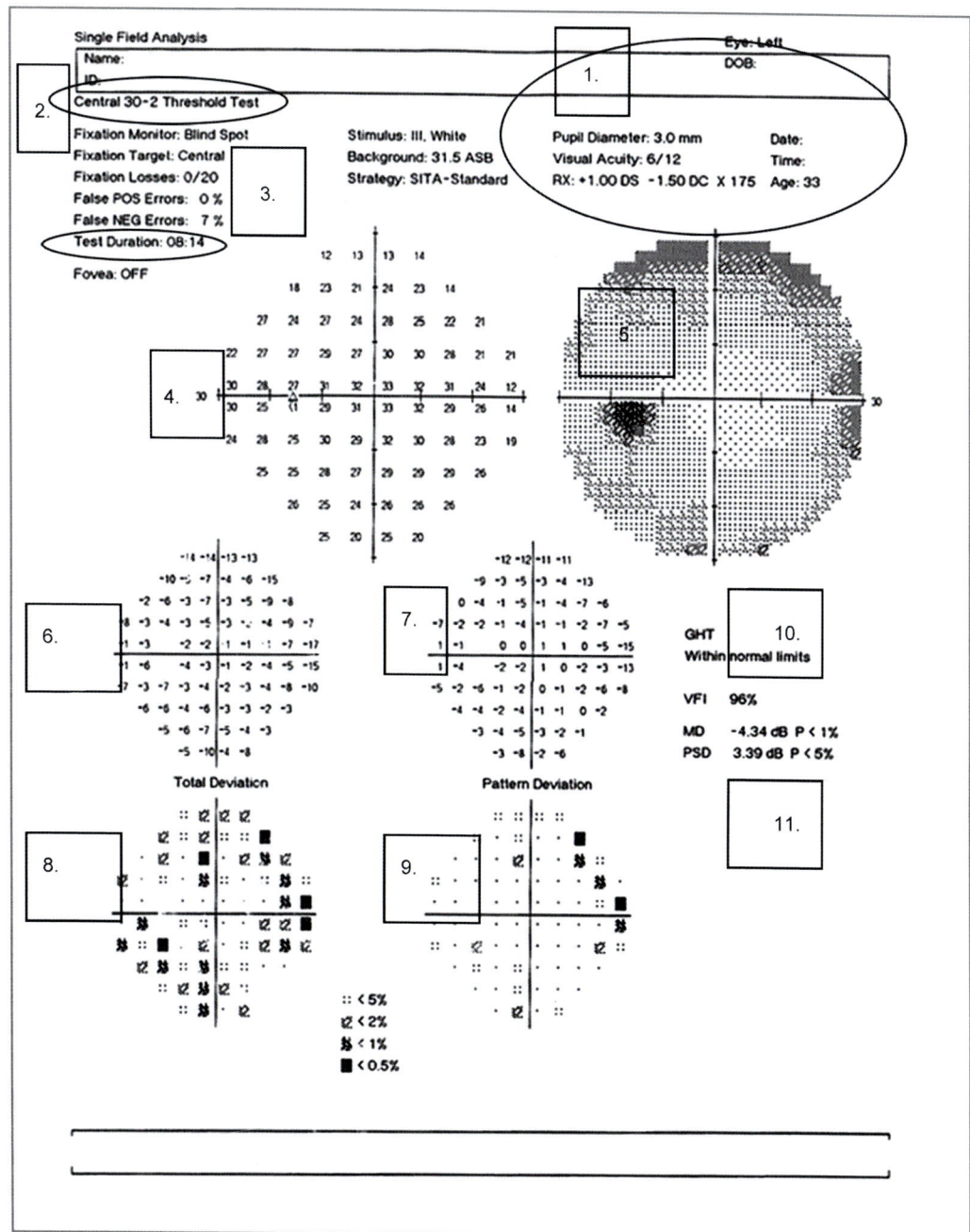

Fig. 5.5.4: Humphrey visual field (HVF) 30-2 showing: 1. Patient's details, 2. Test details, 3. Reliability index, 4. Raw data numerically, 5. Gray scale, 6. Total deviation, 7. Pattern deviation, 8. Total deviation probability plot, 9. Pattern deviation probability plot, 10. Glaucoma hemifield test (GHT), 11. Global indices. (ASB: apostilbs; MD: mean deviation; NEG: negative; POS: positive; PSD: pattern standard deviation; SITA: Swedish interactive threshold algorithm; VFI: visual field index)

- *False positive errors*: Patient responds even when the target is not presented. They are "trigger happy" patients. Unreliable field if >15%. This results in Swiss cheese pattern or white-out of the field.
- *False negative errors*: Patient does not respond to the maximum intensity stimulus on which he had responded previously. It indicates an inattentive patient. Unreliable field if >33%. This results in Cloverleaf pattern of the field.

- *Numerical data:* It shows the measured light sensitivity in dB at a particular test location in that particular patient.
- *Gray scale:* It is calculated from the numeric data itself. Represents the general impression of the VF. Threshold sensitivities are combined into a group of 5 dB each (range 1–40 dB/eight levels of gray).
- *Total deviation and pattern deviation:* Total deviation is the difference between the measured light threshold of the patient (numerical data) and the age-matched normative data for every point tested. Pattern deviation is derived from total deviation by subtracting all threshold values by the 7th highest value. It removes generalized depression of VF due to cataract and adjusts the whole VF to reveal localized scotomas which are more depressed than other points.
- *Total and pattern deviation probability plot:* Probability (p value) of each point being normal is represented by symbols by comparing it to age-matched normal population. Single dot is used for normal points, 4 dots (::) for points with probability of <5% being normal, multiple dot (▨/▧) points have probability of <1–2% being normal and solid black squares (■) have probability of <0.5% being normal. Pattern deviation probability plot depicts the pattern deviation plot in symbols and more accurately represents the deeply depressed scotomas. In cases where the entire total deviation plot is extremely depressed (advanced glaucoma), the machine is unable to derive the pattern deviation.
- *Glaucoma hemifield test (GHT):*[3,4] The machine divides the VF into five zones in superior and inferior quadrants/mirror images of each other and compares corresponding points in superior and inferior areas as glaucoma affects RGC on either side of horizontal meridian. GHT is depicted as:
  - Within normal limits
  - Borderline
  - Outside normal limits
  - General reduction of sensitivity
  - Abnormally high sensitivity
- *Global indices:* Used for staging and follow-up.
  - *Mean deviation (MD)*: It is the average of total deviation values. Ideally, it should be zero. Negative value shows worsening of the field.
  - *Pattern standard deviation (PSD)*: It shows the deviation in the shape of hill of vision. Irregular hill of vision due to focal defects will have higher value. PSD may be low in people where hill of vision is generally depressed rather than being irregular, e.g., advanced glaucoma.
  - *Visual field index (VFI)*: Percentage of the normal VF after adjusting for age-matched.[5] VFI of 100% means normal VF and zero percent means perimetrically blind VF. Whereas, MD is a derivative of total deviation, VFI is based both on total deviation

and pattern deviation probability plots. The VFI algorithm gives more weightage to central macular points than peripheral points, because central macular points have more impact on patients' quality of vision.
- Short-term fluctuation and corrected PSD (CPSD) are seen in full threshold tests.
■ *Abnormality of the report? Anderson's criteria*—Any two out of the three features:
  1. Scotoma is defined as localized defects with cluster of at least three or more points which have sensitivities occurring in <5% of the population and one of which has a sensitivity occurring in <1% of the population. Test locations surrounding the blind spot are to be ignored in this analysis.
  2. The PSD has a value that occurs in <5% of the population.
  3. The GHT is abnormal.
■ Always correlate the VF loss with optic disc NRR loss or fundus exam. Medullated nerve fibers, Branch retinal vein occlusion, Diabetic retinopathy (lasered), chorioretinal scars or retinitis pigmentosa can lead to glaucoma like VF defects.
■ *Grading of VF loss: Hodapp–Parrish–Anderson classification*—Refer to **Table 5.5.2**.

PATTERNS OF VISUAL FIELD LOSS IN GLAUCOMA

- Nasal step
- Arcuate or Bjerrum scotoma
- Paracentral scotoma
- Altitudinal defect
- Generalized loss
- Temporal crescent (rare)

CLINICAL EXAMPLES

Figures 5.5.5 to 5.5.12 give examples of HVF.

VISUAL FIELD PROGRESSION

- Visual field progression is defined by:
  - Development of a new defect.
  - Enlargement/deepening of a pre-existing defect.
  - Diffuse loss of sensitivity.
- *Guided progression analysis software (Humphrey perimeter)* **(Fig. 5.5.13)**
  - The software compares baseline VF to subsequent VFs.
  - Progression analysis is shown as event-based analysis and trend-based analysis.
  - *Event-based analysis* compares the pattern deviation probability plot of the baseline VF tests with current test of the same eye. It identifies points that show progression. Points that

TABLE 5.5.2: Hodapp-Parrish-Anderson classification for visual field loss.

Parameters	Mild	Moderate	Severe
Mean deviation	<–6 dB	<–12 dB	>–12 dB
Points depressed below the 5% probability level	<18	<37	>37
Points depressed below the 10% probability level	<10	<20	>20
Central 5°	No point with sensitivity <15 dB	• No absolute deficit • Only one hemifield with sensitivity <15 dB	• Absolute deficit (0 dB) • Both hemifields with sensitivity <15 dB

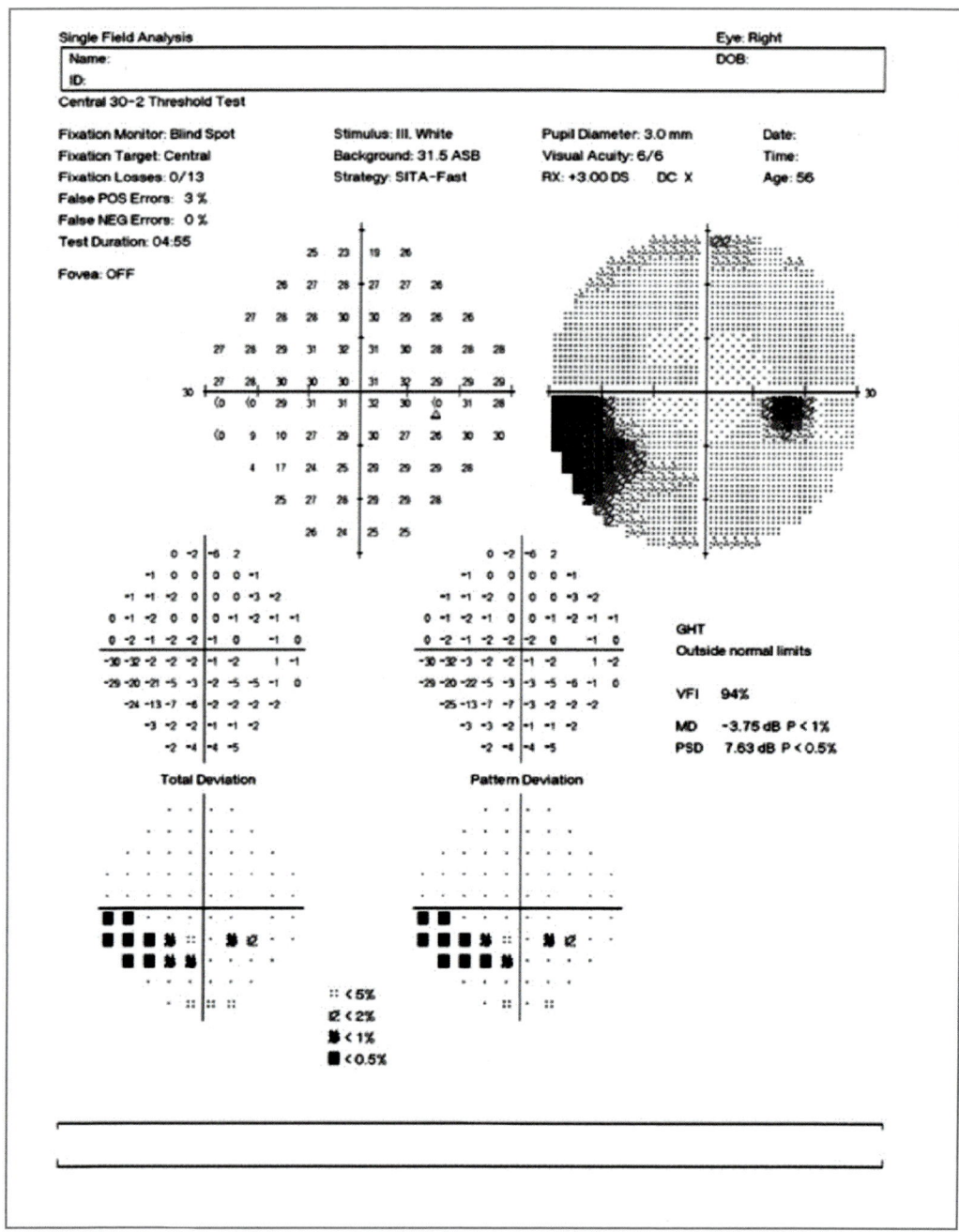

Fig. 5.5.5: Humphrey visual field (HVF) 30-2 of right eye of a patient showing inferior nasal step. (ASB: apostilbs; GHT: glaucoma hemifield test; MD: mean deviation; NEG: negative; POS: positive; PSD: pattern standard deviation; SITA: Swedish interactive threshold algorithm; VFI: visual field index)

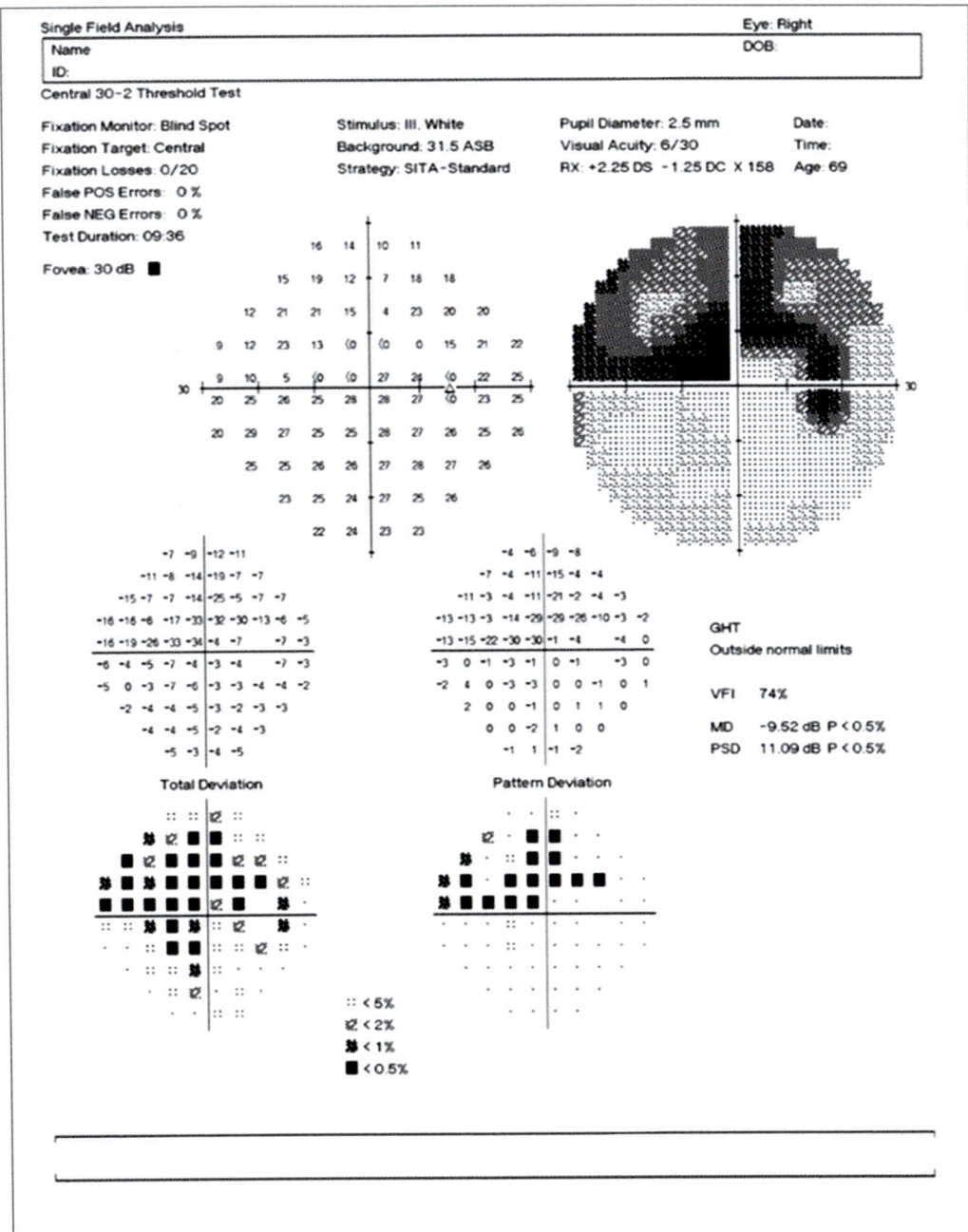

Fig. 5.5.6: Humphrey visual field (HVF) 30-2 of right eye of a patient showing superior nasal step extending further to the blind spot. (ASB: apostilbs; GHT: glaucoma hemifield test; MD: mean deviation; NEG: negative; POS: positive; PSD: pattern standard deviation; SITA: Swedish interactive threshold algorithm; VFI: visual field index)

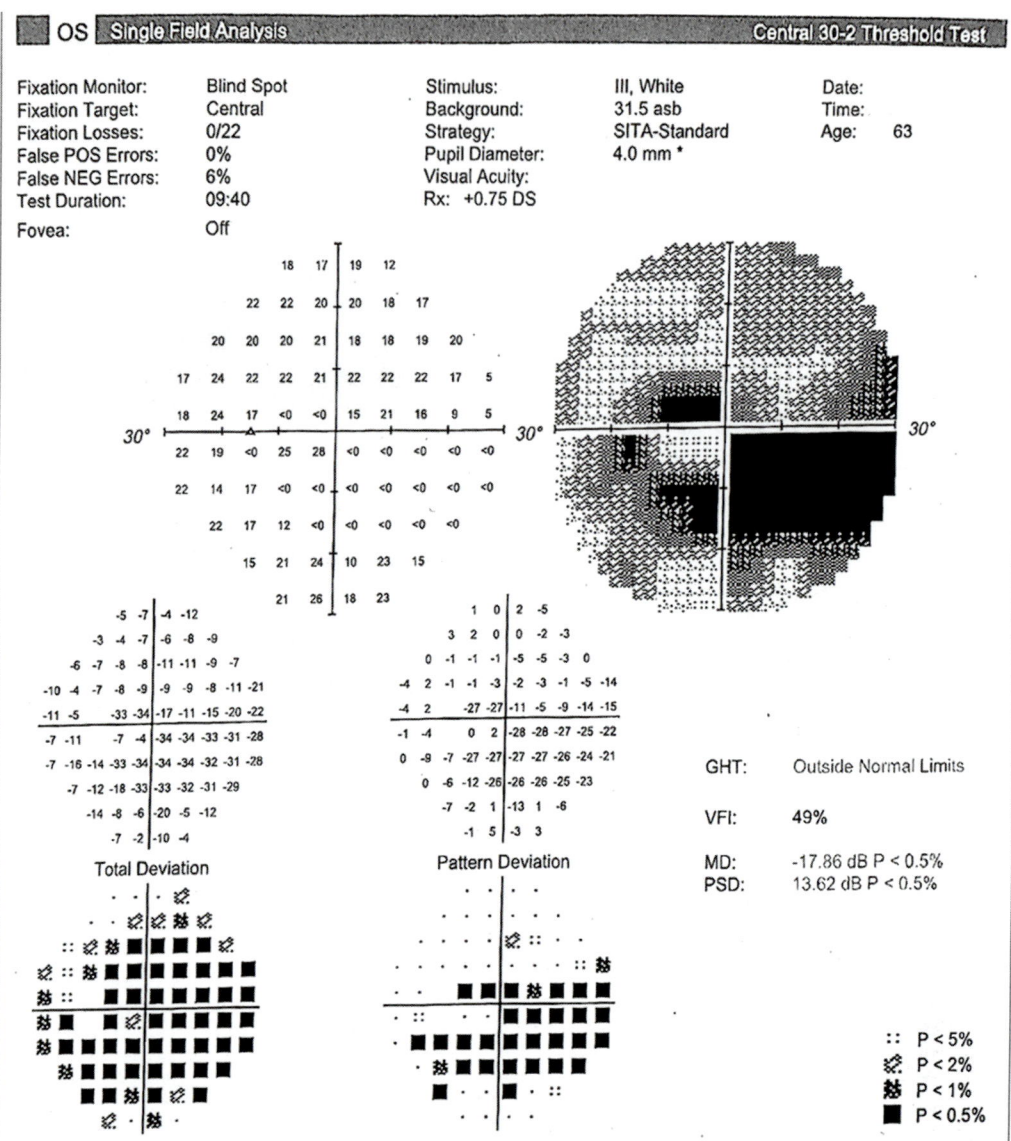

Fig. 5.5.7: Humphrey visual field (HVF) 30-2 of a patient showing inferior arcuate and superior nasal step extending further into the blind spot. (ASB: apostilbs; GHT: glaucoma hemifield test; MD: mean deviation; NEG: negative; POS: positive; PSD: pattern standard deviation; SITA: Swedish interactive threshold algorithm; VFI: visual field index)

show progression in three consecutive tests are marked as black triangle (▲). Points that show progression in two consecutive tests are marked as half-shaded black triangle (◮).

Points that show progression expected <5% of the time at that location in stable glaucoma patients marked as open triangle (△). The VF is marked "Likely Progression" if there is significant

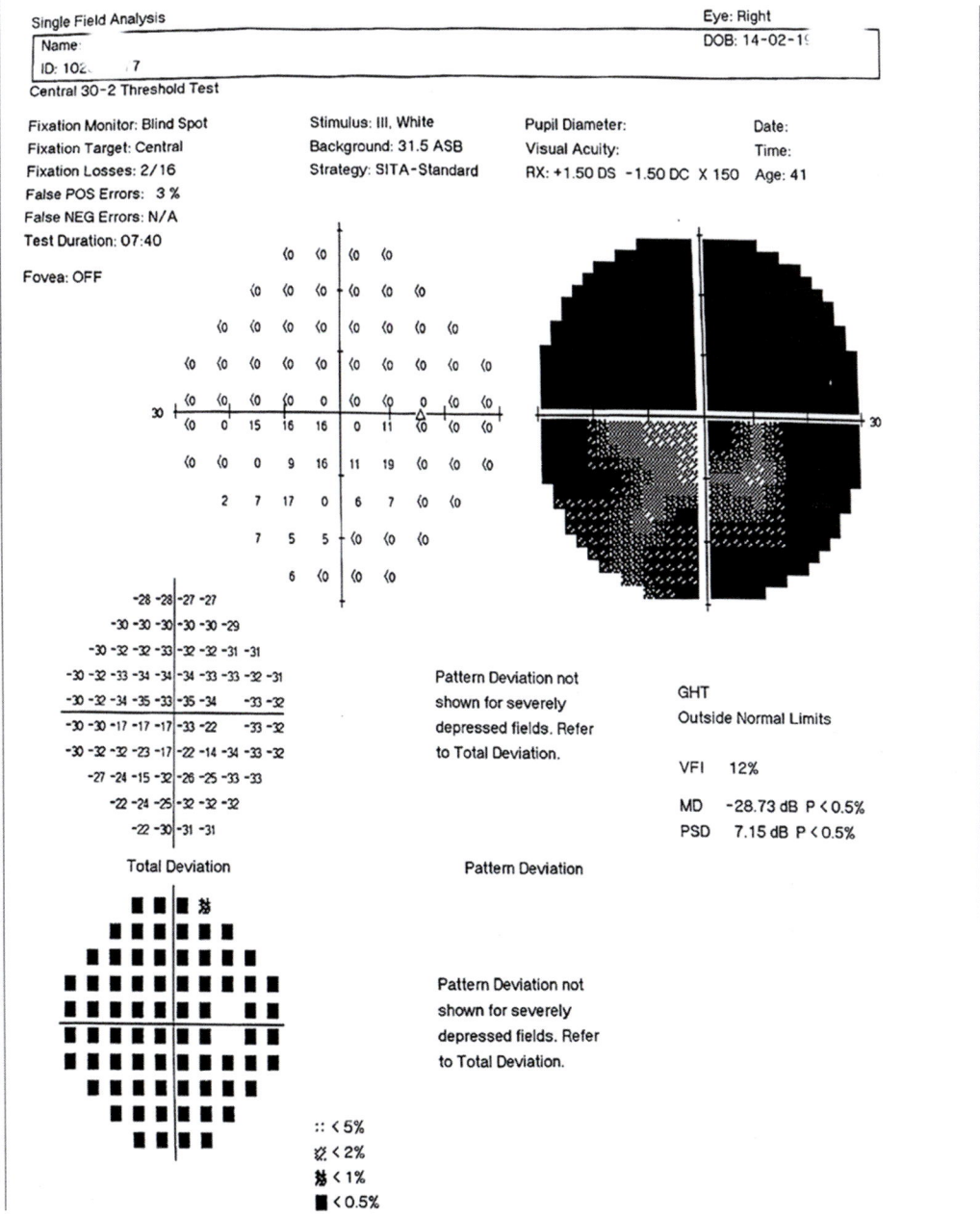

Fig. 5.5.8: Humphrey visual field (HVF) 30-2 of right eye of a patient showing severely depressed fields. Pattern deviation cannot be determined due to severe depression of visual field. (ASB: apostilbs; GHT: glaucoma hemifield test; MD: mean deviation; NEG: negative; POS: positive; PSD: pattern standard deviation; SITA: Swedish interactive threshold algorithm; VFI: visual field index)

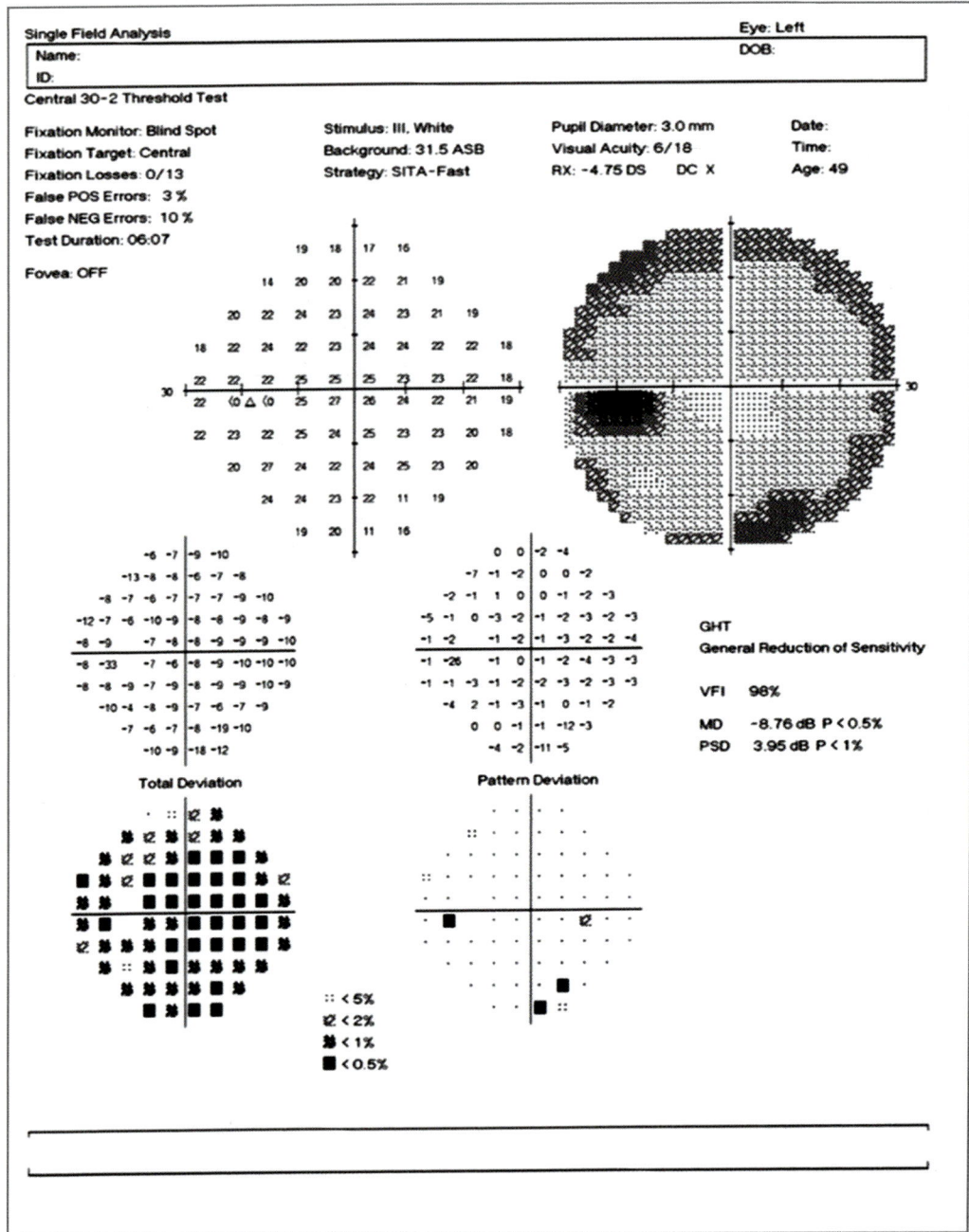

Fig. 5.5.9: Humphrey visual field (HVF) 30-2 of left eye of a patient showing generalized depression in total deviation probability plot, which is not present in pattern deviation probability plot, suggestive of nonglaucomatous defect like cataract. (ASB: apostilbs; GHT: glaucoma hemifield test; MD: mean deviation; NEG: negative; POS: positive; PSD: pattern standard deviation; SITA: Swedish interactive threshold algorithm; VFI: visual field index)

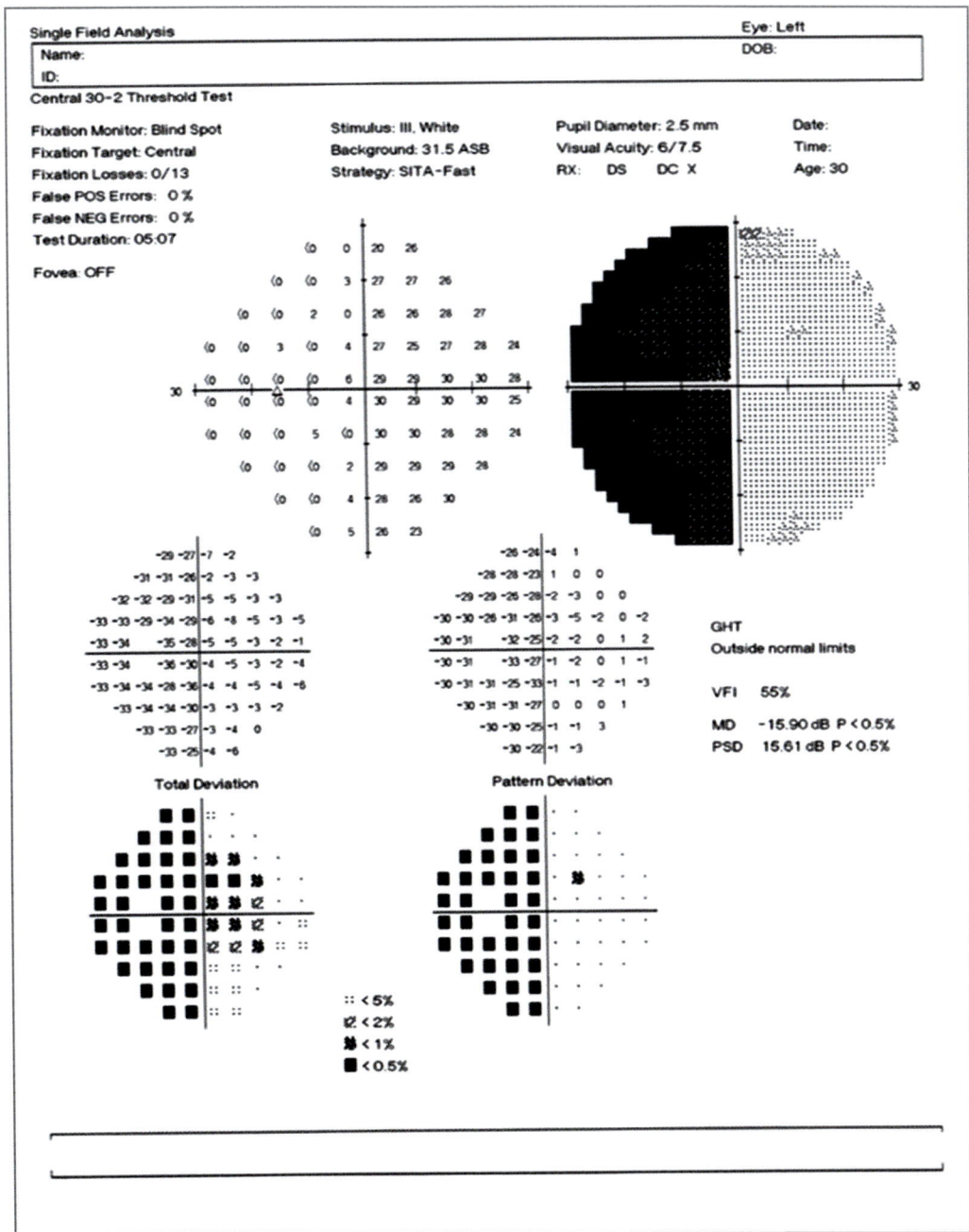

Fig. 5.5.10: Humphrey visual field (HVF) 30-2 of right eye of a patient showing complete temporal hemianopia secondary to pituitary adenoma. (ASB: apostilbs; GHT: glaucoma hemifield test; MD: mean deviation; NEG: negative; POS: positive; PSD: pattern standard deviation; SITA: Swedish interactive threshold algorithm; VFI: visual field index)

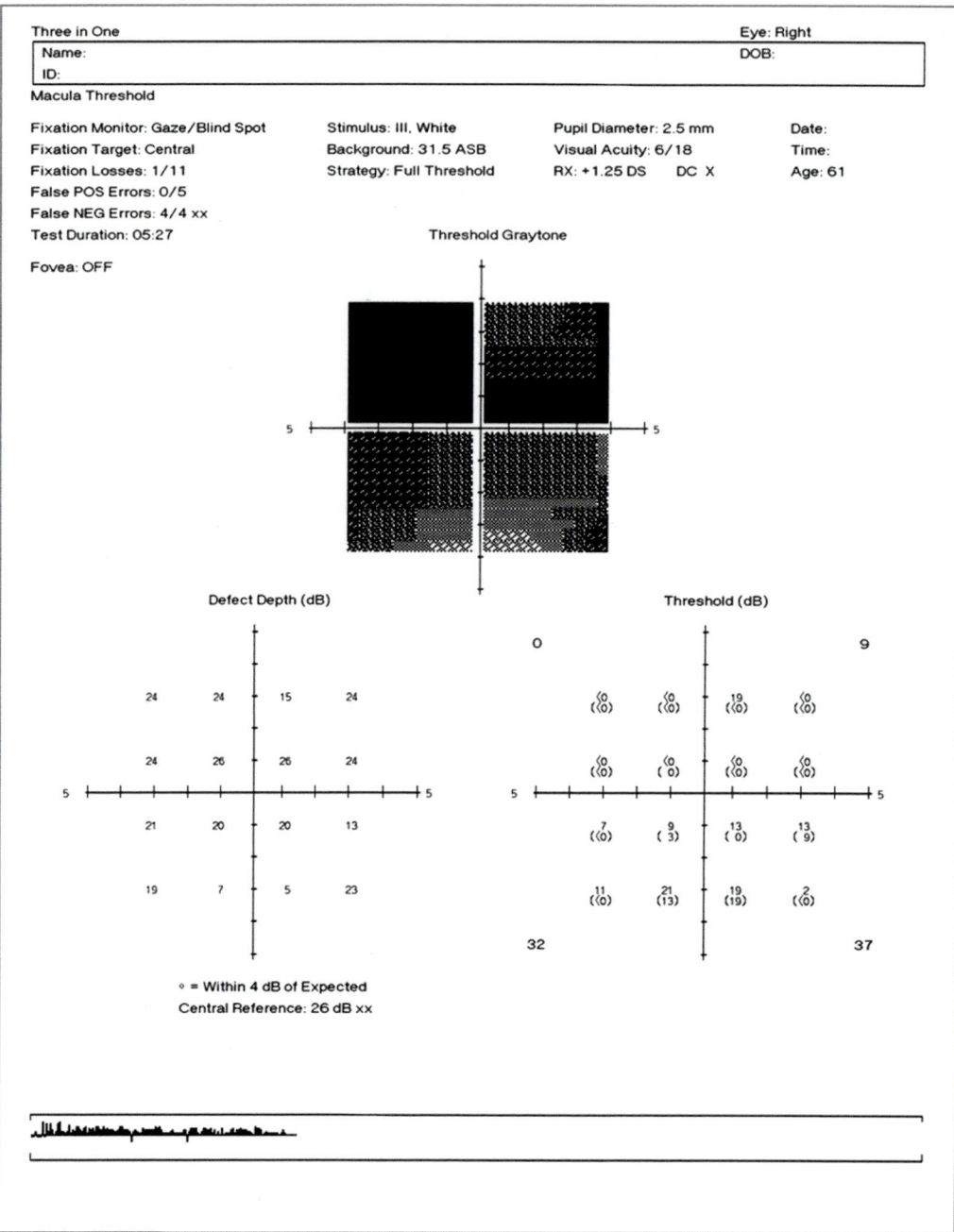

Fig. 5.5.11: Macular threshold test. (ASB: apostilbs; NEG: negative; POS: positive; PSD: pattern standard deviation)

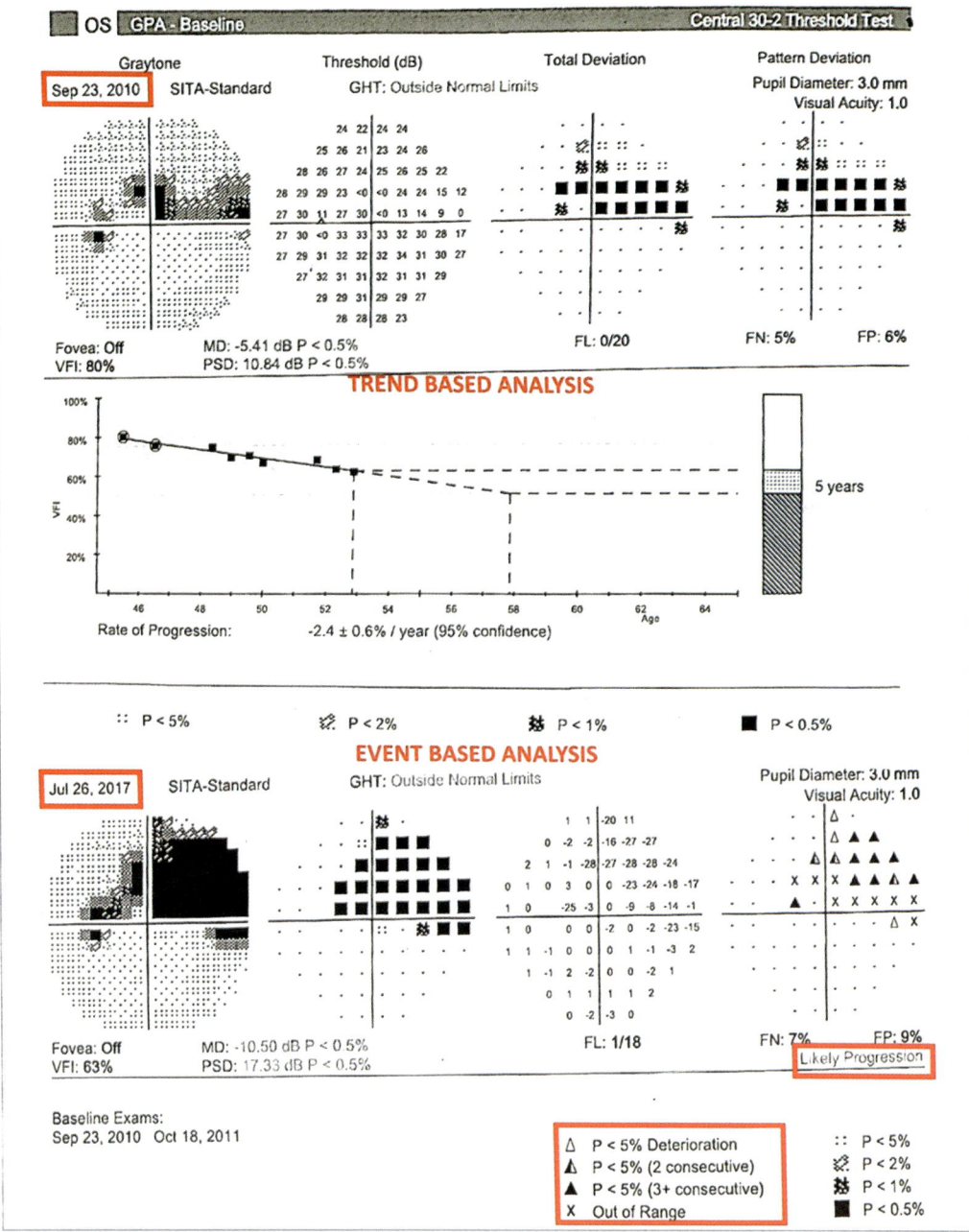

Fig. 5.5.12: Guided progression analysis printout showing event-based analysis and trend-based analysis. (GHT: glaucoma hemifield test; MD: mean deviation; NEG: negative; POS: positive; PSD: pattern standard deviation; SITA: Swedish interactive threshold algorithm; VFI: visual field index)

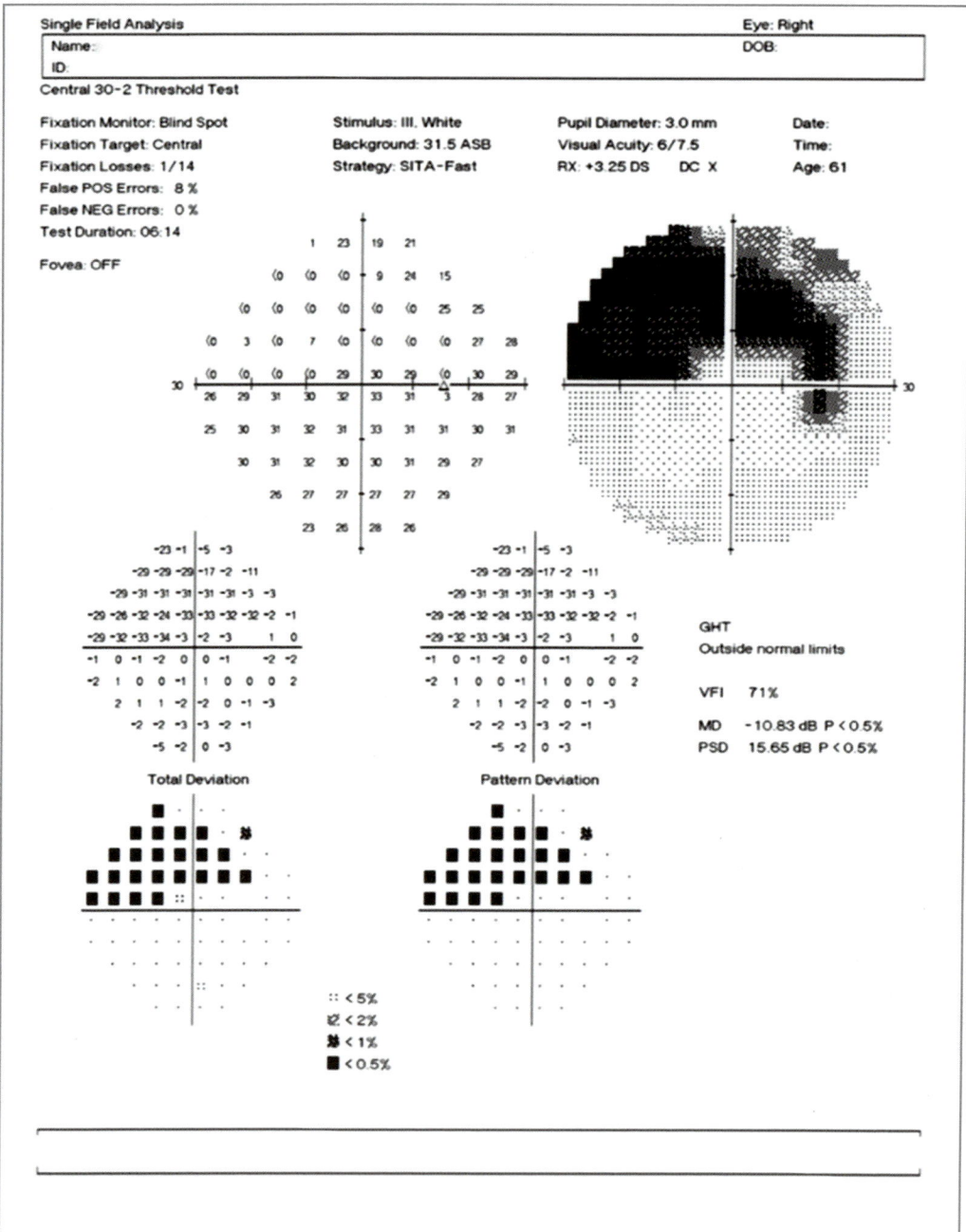

Fig. 5.5.13: Humphrey visual field (HVF) 30-2 of right eye of a patient showing superior arcuate breaking into periphery. (ASB: apostilbs; GHT: glaucoma hemifield test; MD: mean deviation; NEG: negative; POS: positive; PSD: pattern standard deviation; SITA: Swedish interactive threshold algorithm; VFI: visual field index)

change in the same three or more points in three consecutive follow-up tests; and *"Possible Progression"* if there is significant change in the same three or more points in two consecutive follow-up tests.
- *Trend-based analysis* plots the VFI of patient's VFs against time and extrapolates it to show progression in next 5 years. A VF is classified as progressing if a negative slope is significant with a $p < 5\%$.
- *Eyesuite Software (octopus perimeter):* Plots MD with time instead of VFI.
  - A red triangle (▼) that points down identifies significant worsening.
  - A yellow diamond (◆) signals increased fluctuation—a sign for upcoming changes.
  - A green triangle (▲) signals recovery.

■ FREQUENCY OF VISUAL FIELD

- Baseline
- At least six VF examination in the first 2 years.
- After that, once or twice yearly if stable.
- In case, a progression is noted proceed with another confirmatory test.

■ CASE

Reading the printout and interpretation— **Figure 5.5.13** is showing:
- Single field analysis of a patient named. ***, 61-year-old.
- This is a central 30-2 field done using SITA—fast strategy for the right eye with near correction is given and pupil diameter is adequate.
- The VF is reliable.
- Total deviation probability plot shows >3 consecutive points depressed below p value 0.05% suggesting a scotoma in the superior arcuate area.
- Pattern deviation plot also shows a similar defect suggesting localized damage.
- Glaucoma hemifield test is outside normal limits and global indices are abnormal.
- Therefore, given VF shows a superior arcuate scotoma breaking into the periphery, suggestive of glaucomatous damage. Clinical correlation is needed.

■ CONCLUSION

- Standard automated perimetry, being the more sensitive, is the most commonly used method for assessing VF defects in glaucoma.
- Always establish a baseline after first few tests, as there is a learning curve in a patient undergoing VF testing.
- Unexplained visual field defects always raise suspicion of other causes like neurological causes.

■ VIVA QUESTIONS

1. What is a scotoma?
Ans. Refer to text.

2. What is threshold value and how to estimate it?
Ans. Refer to text.

3. What is Swedish interactive threshold algorithm (SITA)?
Ans. Refer to text.

4. How to read Humphrey's visual field printout?
Ans. Refer to text.

5. How is reliability estimated?
Ans. Refer to text.

6. What is Anderson's criteria?
Ans. Refer to text.

REFERENCES

1. Henson DB, Artes PH. New developments in supra-threshold perimetry. Ophthalmic Physiol Opt. 2002;22(5):463-8.
2. Stewart WC, Shields MB, Ollie AR. Full threshold versus quantification of defects for visual field testing in glaucoma. Graefes Arch Clin Exp Ophthalmol. 1989;227(1):51-4.
3. Asman P, Heijl A. Glaucoma Hemifield Test. Automated visual field evaluation. Arch Ophthalmol. 1992;110(6):812-9.
4. Duggan C, Sommer A, Auer C, Burkhard K. Automated differential threshold perimetry for detecting glaucomatous visual field loss. Am J Ophthalmol. 1985;100(3):420-3.
5. Bengtsson B, Heijl A. A visual field index for calculation of glaucoma rate of progression. Am J Ophthalmol. 2008;145(2):343-53.

5.6 ULTRASOUND BIOMICROSCOPY AND ANTERIOR SEGMENT OPTICAL COHERENCE TOMOGRAPHY IN GLAUCOMA

Talvir Sidhu, Saurabh Verma, Tanuj Dada

INTRODUCTION

Ultrasound biomicroscopy (UBM) was first developed by Pavlin and associates as a method to obtain high resolution images of anterior segment in situ.[1] They used 50–100 MHz frequency probe to demonstrate its ability to determine relationship between cornea, angle, iris, zonules, and lens. With time, it has emerged as a useful imaging modality to study other conditions such as adnexal pathology, assessment of trauma, lens position, iris cysts, corneal changes with refractive surgeries, etc.

PRINCIPLE

Ultrasound biomicroscopy **(Fig. 5.6.1)** makes use of a transducer capable of producing very high frequency ultrasound. Conventional ophthalmic ultrasound uses around 10 MHz frequencies. UBM uses frequency between 35–100 MHz. This increases resolution of images but at the expense of depth of penetration and smaller angular field. The higher the frequency of ultrasound used, more the resolution, and lesser the depth and angular field. An axial and lateral resolution up to 25 and 50 microns, respectively, can be achieved. An image up to ciliary zonules and anterior part of lens can be obtained.

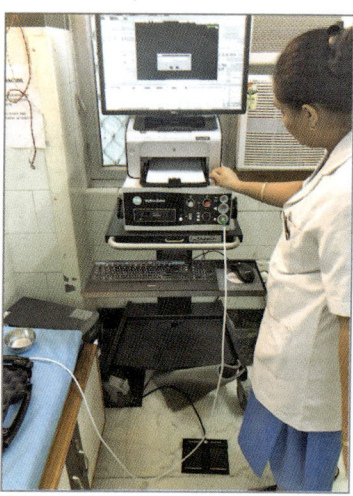

Fig. 5.6.1: Ultrasound biomicroscopy.

TECHNIQUE

After explaining the procedure to the patient in detail, topical anesthesia is given with 0.5% proparacaine or 4% xylocaine. Patient is made to lie in supine position and an eye cup made up of silicon or plastic **(Fig. 5.6.2)**, of sufficient size (must be more than limbal diameter by 1–2 mm) is applied to avoid indentation of the limbal angle structures. Then it is filled with water to create a small water bath. Scanning is performed with ultrasound transducer dipped in water bath.

The transducer is held in such a way that the scanning beam strikes the target tissue as perpendicularly as possible.[2] In a small palpebral aperture, a smaller cup may be used or additionally eye speculum can be applied for opening the eye after instillation of topical anesthetic eyedrops.

USES

- *Glaucoma:* UBM has varied uses in glaucoma.[3] It can be used for visualization of the iris abnormalities, ciliary body, and quantification of angle parameters.
    - *Anterior chamber biometry*: Corneal thickness, anterior chamber depth, posterior chamber depth, intraocular lens (IOL)/lens thickness, etc. **(Figs. 5.6.3A and B)**.

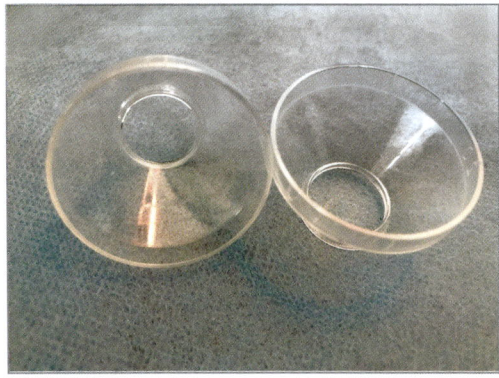

Fig. 5.6.2: Eye cup made up silicon or plastic.

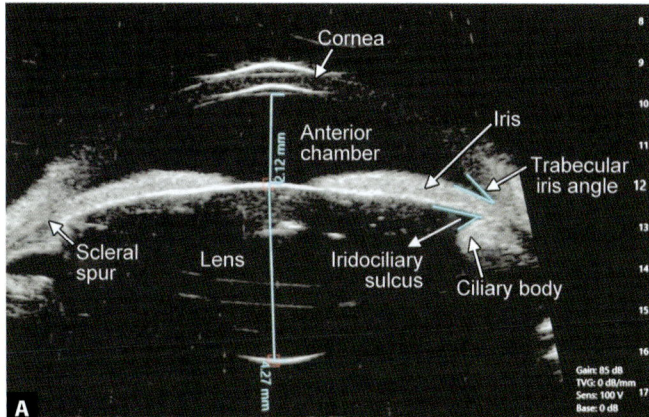

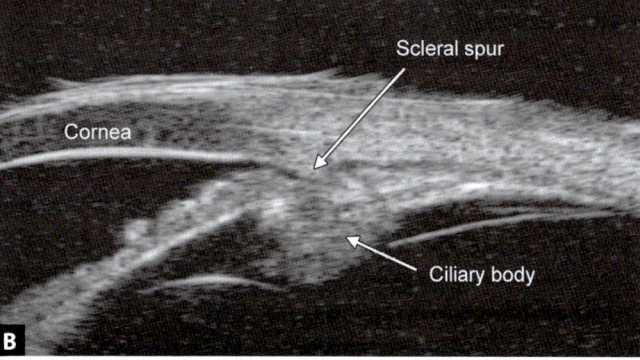

Figs. 5.6.3A and B: (A) Ultrasound biomicroscopy (UBM) scan using 35 MHz showing anterior chamber, lens thickness, and various landmarks as seen on UBM; (B) Angle structures as seen on 50 MHz UBM scan. Biometry can be done using measurements.

- *Angle parameters:* Scleral spur is identified as the inward invagination point where sclera meets the cornea. Identification of scleral spur is key to quantification of angle parameters. Lens vault is the part of lens anterior to the line joining the scleral spur on each side. Trabeculo-iris angle (TIA) is the angle between the TM and iris, starting at the scleral spur. Angle opening distance (AOD) is the distance measured by drawing a perpendicular line between cornea and iris at 500 μm or 750 μm anterior to scleral spur. The trabecular-ciliary process distance (TCPD) is the distance between the corneal endothelium to the ciliary processes **(Figs. 5.6.4A and B)**.
- To determine iris configuration and cause of glaucoma. Open angles usually have a flat iris configuration. *Pigment dispersion syndrome* is characterized by posterior bowing of midperipheral iris called "S-shaped" configuration causing pigment release from posterior surface or iris due to rubbing of iris with lens zonules.
- Primary angle closure is characterized by *occludability of angle* with iridotrabecular contact and may have high lens vault and thick lens **(Figs. 5.6.5A to C)**. *Plateau iris syndrome*: It is characterized by anteriorly directed ciliary processes with obliteration of the iridociliary sulcus and steeply rising root of iris followed by flat iris profile. This is seen "sine wave configuration" of iris on indentation gonioscopy **(Fig. 5.6.6)**.
- To determine patency of iridotomy.
- *To determine functional status of filtering surgery*: UBM can be used to show patency of sclerotomy and peripheral iridotomy. It has been used

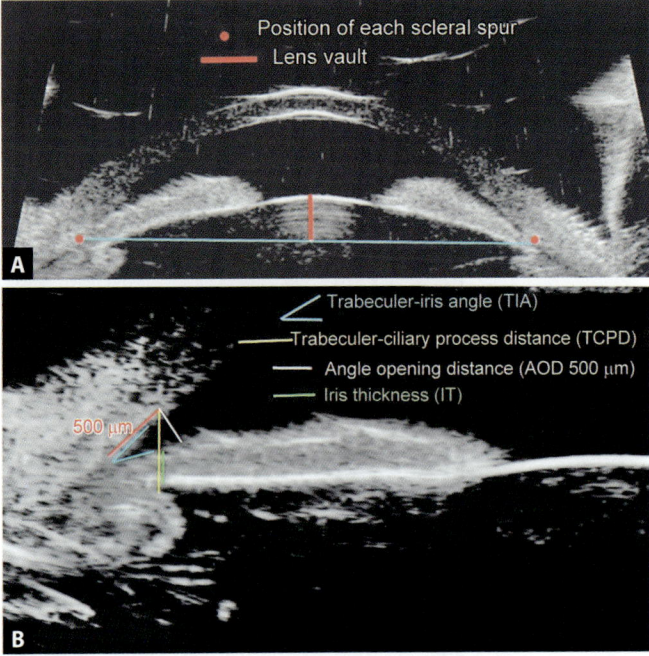

Figs. 5.6.4A and B: Angle parameters measured on ultrasound biomicroscopy.

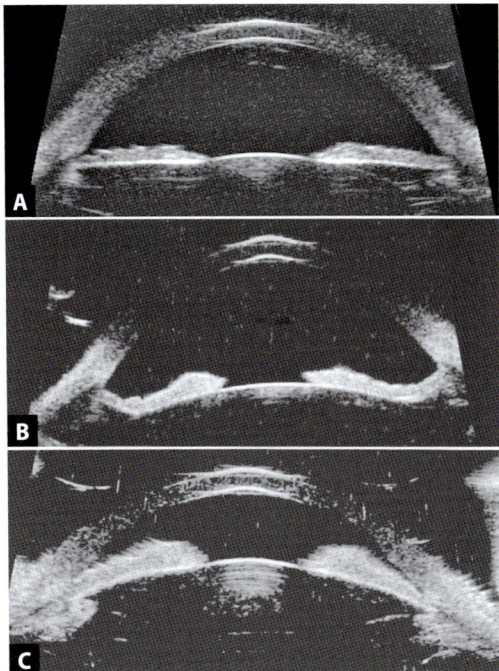

Figs. 5.6.5A to C: (A) Flat iris configuration in a wide open angle; (B) Posterior bowing of midperipheral iris in pigment dispersion syndrome causing a S-shaped iris; (C) Anteriorly bowing iris with iridociliary contact with shallow anterior chamber and increased lens vault in angle closure.

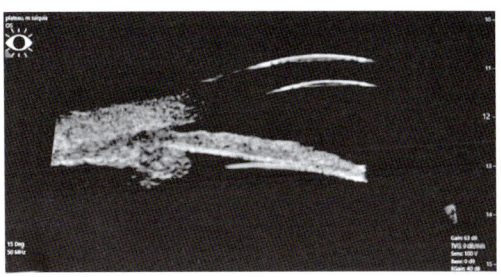

Fig. 5.6.6: Obliteration of iridociliary sulcus in plateau iris.

to study characteristics of blebs based on their height and reflectivity.
- It is a very good procedure for determining presence and extent of shallow choroidal detachments and cyclodialysis clefts **(Fig. 5.6.7)**.

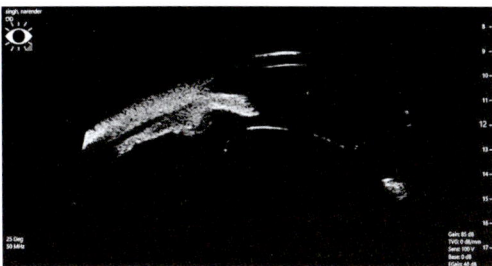

Fig. 5.6.7: Ultrasound biomicroscopy showing shallow choroidal detachment (CD).

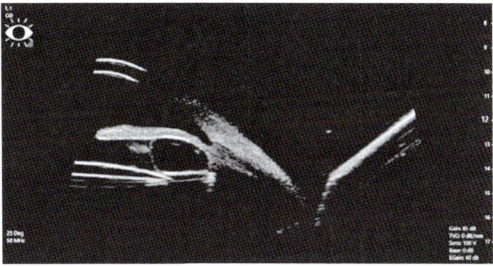

Fig. 5.6.8: Iris cyst causing localized shallowing of anterior chamber.

- To evaluate cysts and tumors of iris, ciliary body, and angle. It can be used to determine exact location, dimension, thickness of wall, and internal characteristics of cysts and tumors[4] **(Fig. 5.6.8)**.
- *To evaluate tumors of ocular surface*: It is a very useful tool for evaluating dimensions and intraocular extension of ocular surface tumors.
- *To evaluate eyelid lesions*: It is a useful tool to determine tissue characteristics depth of eyelid lesions.[5,6]
- *To evaluate aponeurotic ptosis*: It can be used for measuring thickness of levator palpebrae aponeurosis which is thinned out in aponeurotic ptosis.[7]
- *To evaluate corneal conditions*: It has been used to examine sclerocornea, corneal dystrophy, limbal dermoids, etc.[8,9]
- *To evaluate eyes with retinoblastoma*: UBM is a sensitive method for studying ciliary region, anterior retina, and anterior

segment in eyes with retinoblastoma. It is useful for better staging of advanced disease.[10]
- To evaluate extent of anterior proliferative vitreoretinopathy (PVR) in cases with retinal detachment.
- To determine capsular support in patients with dropped IOL or lens.
- To examine any foreign body impacted in the region of ciliary body.
- To study anterior segment details in patients with corneal opacity.
- To rule out cases with lens subluxation in nondilating pupil.
- To study stability of sulcus fixated IOL.
- To study capsular defects in patients with posterior polar cataract.

LIMITATIONS

- It is a contact procedure.
- Cannot be done in eyes with perforations and open globe injuries.
- Application of cup may distort angle structures during examination.

VIVA QUESTIONS

1. What is the role of UBM in limbal dermoid?
Ans. Limbal dermoid is choristoma more commonly seen in the temporal quadrant. It involves variable thickness of corneal stroma and may even extend into anterior chamber. It is difficult to ascertain depth of involvement with slit lamp because of opaque nature of lesion. Surgical management varies according to size and depth of lesion. A superficial lesion can be managed with shave excision or lamellar keratoplasty where as a deep lesion might require penetrating keratoplasty. Sometimes, it can be associated with disorganization of internal structures, which is a relative contraindication for any surgery. UBM can help in accurate measurement of depth and dimensions of dermoid thus helping in proper management of dermoid.[11]

2. What is the role of UBM in corneal hydrops?
Ans. Ultrasound biomicrosopy has been used in qualitative and quantitative evaluation of morphology of corneal hydrops.[12] Descemet membrane (DM) tear can be visualized and its edges and length can be quantified. After intracameral air or gas injection, UBM can also be used to visualize DM apposition, apposition of gas bubble to tear edges, and resolution of corneal edema and cysts. UBM-based studies have shown significant correlation between length of DM tear and corneal thickness in corneal hydrops.

3. State differences between UBM and ASOCT.
Ans. Table 5.6.1 shows differences between UBM and ASOCT.

4. Role of UBM in evaluation of filtering Bleb.
Ans. Ultrasound biomicroscopy has been used for evaluating function and morphology of subconjunctival filtering bleb. It has shown to predict a functioning or a nonfunctioning bleb in 66 and 75% cases, respectively.[13] However, ASOCT has proven to be superior in evaluating bleb function. MacWhae et al. classified bleb functioning as good, fair, and poor, based on presence of a patent pathway and presence or absence of cavities in bleb. UBM has also been used to study bleb status after laser suture lysis.

5. Role of UBM in PVR.
Ans. Ultrasound biomicroscopy can be used to evaluate anterior PVR. Different patterns which can be identified are dots and cords, echo augmentation, and central displacement of retina along with circumferential contraction.[14]

TABLE 5.6.1: Differences between ultrasound biomicroscopy (UBM) and anterior segment optical coherence tomography.

UBM	Anterior segment optical coherence tomography (ASOCT)
Makes use of 35–100 MHz ultrasound to visualize eye structures	Based on optical principle and makes use 1,310 nm wavelength
Can visualize beyond iris. Ciliary body and processes can be seen	Cannot visualize beyond anterior limiting membrane of iris
Image quality is worse than ASOCT	Better quality image
Contact procedure	Noncontact procedure
• Axial resolution: 25 microns • Lateral resolution: 50 microns	• Axial resolution: 5 microns • Lateral resolution: 15 microns

6. What is pseudoplateau iris (PPI)?

Ans. Pseudoplateau iris is a rare cause of glaucoma and is difficult to be differentiated from plateau iris clinically. In PPI, presence of a single large or multiple small iridociliary sulcus cysts result in narrowing of angle. Clinically, S-shaped configuration of iris can be seen in both. Bumpy appearance of peripheral iris on slit lamp or gonioscopic examination points toward PPI but is not always evident. UBM is very useful in diagnosing PPI as cysts can be easily visualized with it. Rupturing the cysts with neodymium-doped yttrium aluminum garnet (Nd:YAG) laser or needle is an effective treatment.[15]

7. State features of malignant glaucoma in UBM.

Ans. Ultrasound biomicroscopy of eyes during malignant glaucoma shows anterior rotation of ciliary processes. They press against periphery of lens in phakic patients or anterior hyaloid phase in aphakic patients thus preventing anterior flow of aqueous.

UBM-based studies have also shown that lens size in such patients is often smaller than normal which allows for easy anterior movement.[16]

REFERENCES

1. Pavlin CJ, Harasiewicz K, Sherar MD, Foster FS. Clinical use of ultrasound biomicroscopy. Ophthalmology. 1991;98(3):287-95.
2. Ishikawa H, Schuman J. Anterior segment imaging: ultrasound biomicroscopy. Ophthalmol. Clin N Am. 2004;17(1):7-20.
3. Dada T, Gadia R, Sharma A, Ichhpujani P, Bali SJ, Bhartiya S, et al. Ultrasound biomicroscopy in glaucoma. Surv Ophthalmol. 2011;56(5):433-50.
4. Conway RM. Ultrasound biomicroscopy: role in diagnosis and management in 130 consecutive patients evaluated for anterior segment tumours. Br J Ophthalmol. 2005; 89(8):950-5.
5. Kikkawa DO, Ochabski R, Weinreb RN. Ultrasound biomicroscopy of eyelid lesions. Ophthalmologica. 2003;217(1):20-3.
6. Smyth CJ, Möllby R, Wadström T. Phenomenon of hot-cold hemolysis: chelator-induced lysis of sphingomyelinase-treated erythrocytes. Infect Immun. 1975;12(5):1104-11.
7. Hoşal BM, Ayer NG, Zilelioğlu G, Elhan AH. Ultrasound biomicroscopy of the levator aponeurosis in congenital and aponeurotic blepharoptosis. Ophthal Plast Reconstr Surg. 2004;20(4):308-11.
8. Kim T, Cohen EJ, Schnall BM, Affel EL, Eagle RC Jr. Ultrasound biomicroscopy and histopathology of sclerocornea. Cornea. 1998;17(4):443-5.
9. Castelo Branco B, Chalita MRC, Casanova FH, Castelo Branco AB, Allemann N, de Freitas D. Posterior amorphous corneal dystrophy: ultrasound biomicroscopy findings in two cases. Cornea. 2002;21(2):220-2.
10. Vasquez LM, Giuliari GP, Halliday W, Pavlin CJ, Gallie BL, Heon E. Ultrasound biomicroscopy in the management of retinoblastoma. Eye. 2011;25(2):141-7.
11. Lanzl IM, Augsburger JJ, Hertle RW, Rapuano C, Correa-Melling Z, Santa Cruz C. The role

of ultrasound biomicroscopy in surgical planning for limbal dermoids. Cornea. 1998;17(6):604-6.
12. Sharma N, Mannan R, Jhanji V, Agarwal T, Pruthi A, Titiyal JS, et al. Ultrasound biomicroscopy-guided assessment of acute corneal hydrops. Ophthalmology. 2011; 118(11):2166-71.
13. Wu Q, Zhang Y, Song B, Lu B, Guan JH. [Evaluation of the bleb morphology and the function of post filtration surgery using slit-lamp adapted optical coherence tomography and ultrasound biomicroscopy in glaucoma patients]. Zhonghua Yan Ke Za Zhi Chin J Ophthalmol. 2008;44(5):402-7.
14. Liu W, Wu Q, Huang S. [Examination of anterior proliferative vitreoretinopathy with ultrasound biomicroscopy]. Zhonghua Yan Ke Za Zhi Chin J Ophthalmol. 1998;34(4):264-6, 17.
15. Shukla S, Damji KF, Harasymowycz P, Chialant D, Kent JS, Chevrier R, et al. Clinical features distinguishing angle closure from pseudoplateau versus plateau iris. Br J Ophthalmol. 2008;92(3):340-4.
16. Shahid H, Salmon JF. Malignant Glaucoma: A Review of the Modern Literature. J Ophthalmol. 2012;2012:1-6.

5.7 OPTICAL COHERENCE TOMOGRAPHY IN GLAUCOMA—INTERPRETATION

Talvir Sidhu, Jyoti Shakrawal, Ritu Nagpal, Tanuj Dada

INTRODUCTION

Optical coherence tomography is a noninvasive tool for preperimetric glaucoma detection, quantification of RNFL loss, and detecting early progression. Besides, quantitative parameters provided by it are useful for monitoring disease progression. The details of OCT, its principle, and uses have been discussed elsewhere (chapter on ASOCT). This chapter will discuss a few examples of OCT analysis in glaucoma **(Fig. 5.7.1)**.

OPTICAL COHERENCE TOMOGRAPHY PARAMETERS IN GLAUCOMA

Following parameters are extremely useful for glaucoma diagnosis and progression.
- *Retinal nerve fiber layer parameters*
- *Macular thickness with ganglion cell thickness*
- *Optic nerve parameters*

Commonly used machines in glaucoma for OCT are:

- *Zeiss Cirrus OCT*
- *Heidelberg Spectralis OCT*
- *Optovue RTVue OCT*

RETINAL NERVE FIBER LAYER ANALYSIS

Basis: The RNFL is formed by the retinal ganglion cell axons seen as bright and fine striations in the inner retinal layer. The RNFL axons are distributed characteristically along the horizontal/temporal raphe. The RNFL layer superior to the horizontal raphe ends in the superotemporal optic disc and inferior RNFL ends in inferotemporal optic disc. The RNFL arising in macula goes directly to the temporal optic disc forming the papillomacular bundle. The RNFL defects in glaucoma are therefore associated with corresponding optic NRR thinning/notch in superotemporal or inferotemporal quadrants. The RNFL defects start at the optic disc and fan like a wedge-like defect along the superior or inferior arcade.

The RNFL is measured in OCT in three ways:
1. *Retinal nerve fiber layer thickness and deviation maps:* The patient's actual thickness of RNFL around the optic disc is shown in color coding in the *RNFL thickness map.* The thicker areas seen as

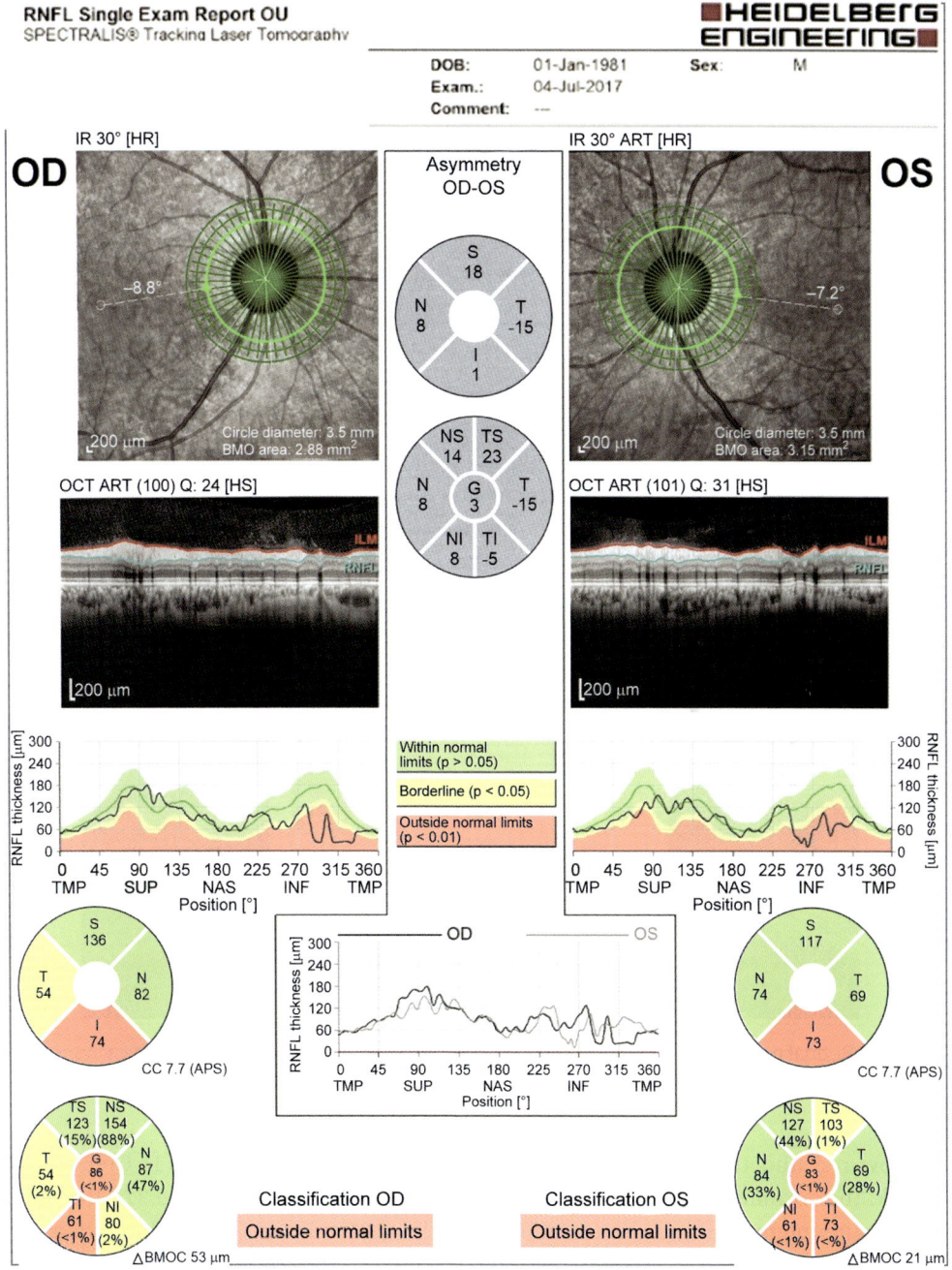

Fig. 5.7.1

Contd...

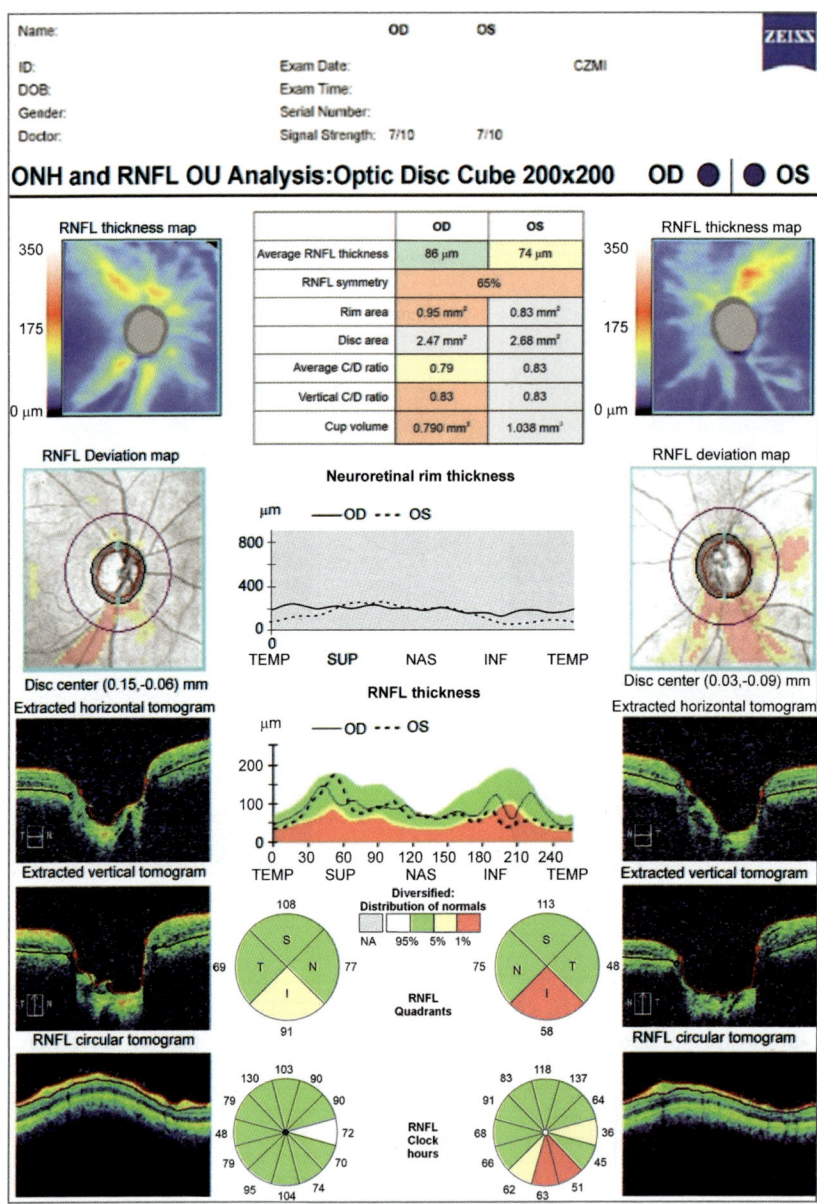

Fig. 5.7.1: Retinal nerve fiber layer (RNFL) analysis printouts of Heidelberg Spectralis optical coherence tomography (OCT) and Zeiss Cirrus OCT.

yellow-red and thinner areas as blue-black. The normal RNFL is seen as yellow-red in superotemporal and inferotemporal quadrants, while any RNFL defects are seen as dark areas of RNFL thinning. The

RNFL deviation map: (1) Centration of optic disc in RNFL circle, (2) The outline of the NRR, and (3) The thin retinal areas (compared to normative data) are marked red-yellow.

Caution: The RNFL thickness map must be checked for areas of missing scan (seen as black areas), which may happen due to blinking or tear film abnormalities or media opacities. This might lead to an abnormally interpreted scan (see **Figures 5.7.2A to C***).*

2. *Temporal-superior-nasal-inferior-temporal (TSNIT) graph of RNFL thickness:* The RNFL thickness in each eye is measured at a fixed 3.46 mm circle in Cirrus OCT, 3.45 mm in RTVue, and 3.5/4.1/4.7 circles in Spectralis OCT. The thickness of the RNFL along this circle is divided into four quadrants (temporal-superior-nasal-inferior) to get a TSNIT graph and compared with age matched controls. The normal TSNIT graph shows a double hump pattern due to superotemporal and inferotemporal RNFL being thicker/peaking than other quadrants. The double hump pattern is lost in glaucoma (see **Figure 5.7.5**).

   Caution: The RNFL thickness never approaches zero in any quadrants, even in advanced glaucoma. If it so happens, it may be due to missing scan data in that area or poor segmentation.

3. *Retinal nerve fiber layer clock hour and quadrant graphs:* In addition to the above graphs, RNFL is also shown in circular four-quadrant and clock hour maps (see **Figure 5.7.6**).

The color coding of the entire scan is done based upon normative database (see **Figure 5.7.7**).

- Green—90% of normative values (normal value)
- Yellow—1–5% of lower normative values (borderline value)
- Red—Lowest 1% of the normative data (abnormal value)
- Gray—normative data not available
- White—Thickest 5% of normative values (thicker than normal)

MACULAR THICKNESS ANALYSIS

Basis: The ganglion cell loss in glaucoma is seen in arcuate shape corresponding to the RNFL loss/optic disc NRR loss. Macula map thickness is used to study changes in the retinal ganglion cell layer (GCL). The GCL contains amacrine cells along with retinal ganglions. The inner plexiform layer (IPL) consists of the synaptic layer between bipolar cell and ganglion cells. About 30–50% ganglion cells are present within ±8 degrees of macula. The RNFL layer contains the RGC axons. Due to similar reflectivity of the IPL and ganglion cell complex (GCC) in OCT scans, the machines combine the GCL and IPL to give ganglion cell-inner plexiform layer (GCIPL) thickness map. Cirrus OCT gives GCIPL thickness scans and Spectralis OCT gives total retinal thickness as well as each layer separately.

- *GCIPL thickness (Cirrus OCT):* Temporal Raphe sign on GCIPL test in Cirrus OCT is seen in patients having GCC thinning in one hemifield resulting in thinning of GCC thickness along the horizontal raphe. This is highly sensitive and specific for glaucoma (see **Figure 5.7.10**).
- *Total macular thickness and hemispheric asymmetry (Spectralis OCT):* The total macular thickness is shown in a color-coded map with hot colors like yellow-red as thick areas and blue as thinner areas. RNFL defects are usually seen as thinner areas starting from optic disc. The GCL thinning due to glaucoma also leads to thinning of total macular thickness. Macular thickness hemispheric asymmetry between superior and inferior hemisphere is analyzed for glaucoma diagnosis on macular thickness scans by Spectralis OCT.

OPTIC NERVE HEAD ANALYSIS

Optic disc cube scans of 200 × 200 cube is done centered on the optic disc. OCT identifies the optic disc margin as the Bruch's membrane opening (BMO). The machine measures the distance from the BMO to the internal limiting membrane and measures the NRR thickness in various quadrants. The data is shown in TSNIT graph and plotted against the age-matched normative data to show normal and abnormal.

HOW TO READ RETINAL NERVE FIBER LAYER PRINTOUT

Table 5.7.1 shows the method of how to read retinal nerve fiber layer printout.

TABLE 5.7.1: How to read retinal nerve fiber layer (RNFL) printout.

S. no.	Parameter	Figure
1.	*Patient information:* The name of the patient and age must be matched to the report for appropriate age matching by the machine	
2.	*Quality scores:* Acceptable signal strength is different in different machines: • ≥6 in Cirrus (0–10) • Q score >15 in Spectralis (0–40) • Signal strength index (SSI) >45 in RTVue (0–100) Poor quality scores give unreliable OCT readings leading to false impression of progression	
3.A	• *RNFL thickness map* is the actual thickness of patient's retina around optic disc. Check for broken scan or any black areas due to tear film abnormality or dry eye. Also, check for any RNFL defects • *RNFL deviation map:* It shows: (A) Centration of optic disc in RNFL circle, (B) The outline of the neuroretinal rim, and (C) the thin retinal areas (compared to normative data) are marked red-yellow **(Figs. 5.7.2A to C)**	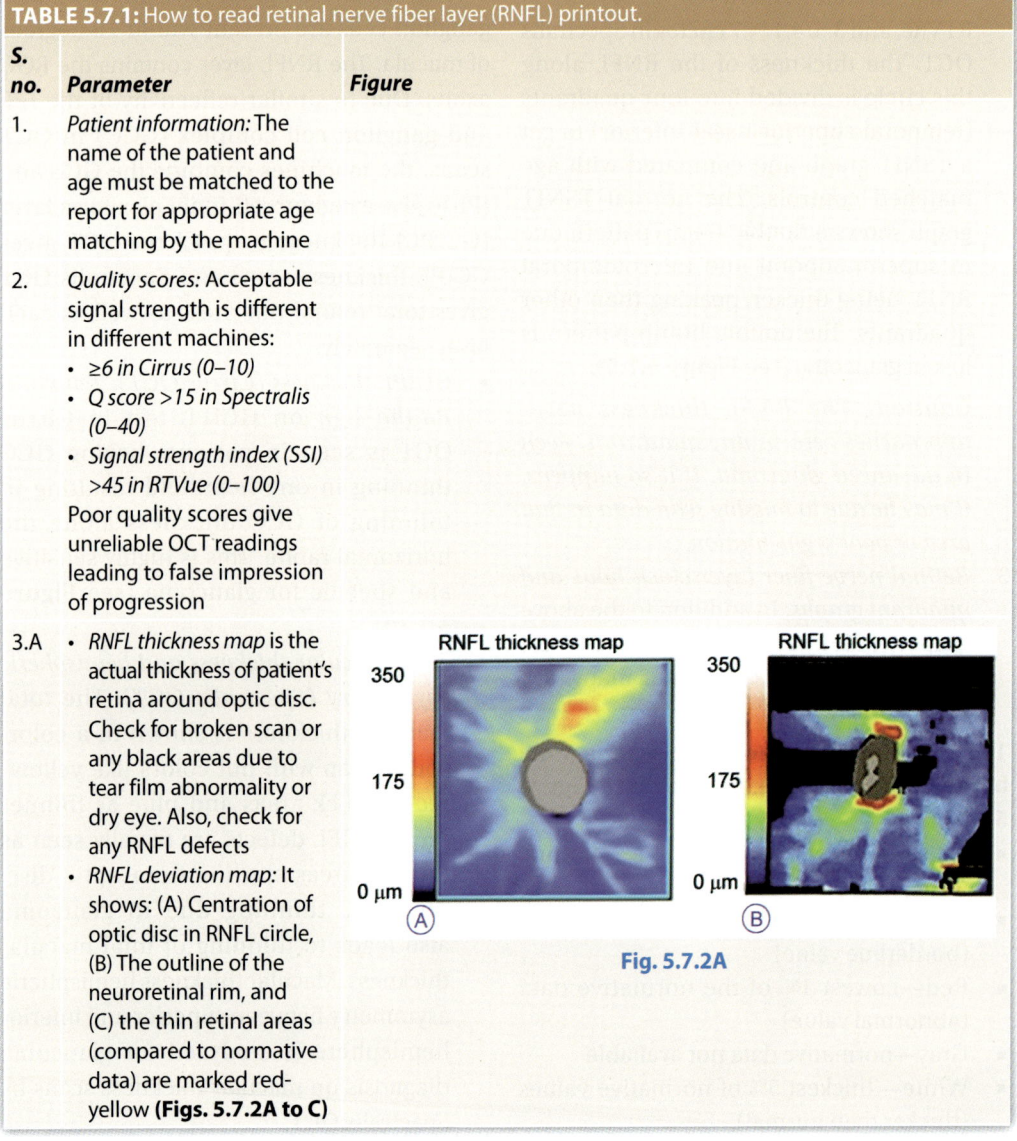 Fig. 5.7.2A

Contd...

Contd...

S. no.	Parameter	Figure
		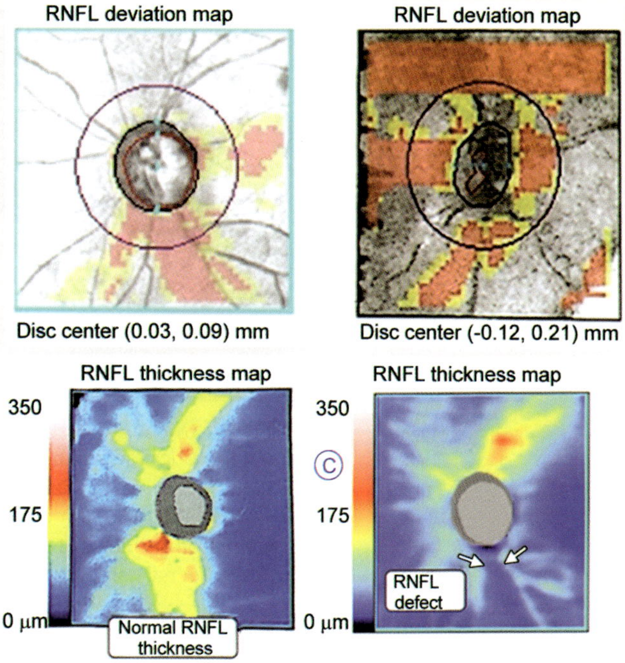 *Figs. 5.7.2B and C* **Figs. 5.7.2A to C:** (A) Normal retinal nerve fiber layer (RNFL) thickness map; (B) Abnormal/broken thickness and deviation map; (C) Normal versus RNFL defect.
3.B	*Quality of scan: Extracted tomograms:* Show the placement of reference lines used by optical coherence tomography (OCT) machine to segment the scan and calculate RNFL thickness. If the reference lines are not properly placed, the values given by machine are false **(Fig. 5.7.3)**	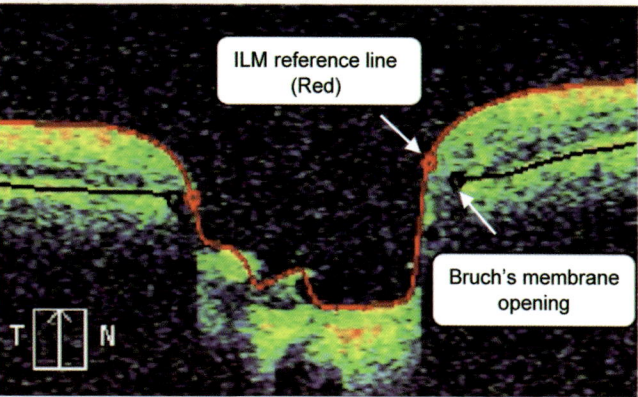

Contd...

Contd...

S. no.	Parameter	Figure

4.	• Key parameters are shown in a table with each parameter being color coded as green (normal), yellow (borderline), red (abnormal), white (above normal range), and gray (normative data not available)
	• Normative data is not available for very small or very large optic nerve heads, hence marked gray. (Average disc area: 1.58–1.88 mm²) **(Fig. 5.7.4)**
	• Interocular asymmetry:
	  – *Cirrus*: Interocular asymmetry of >9 µm difference may be indicative of early glaucoma
	  – *Spectralis*: Difference of >6 µm for RNFL global average has high sensitivity and specificity to detect glaucoma
		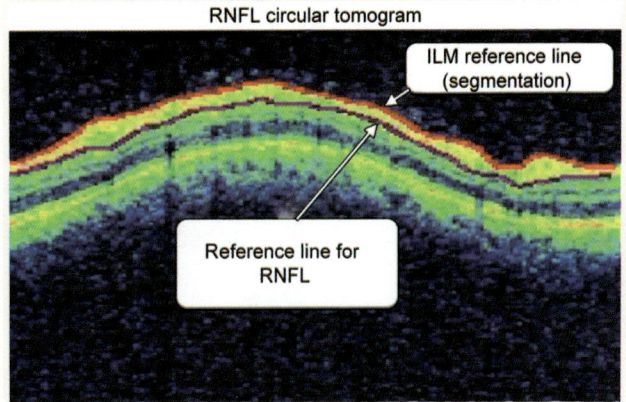
		Fig. 5.7.3: The reference lines for internal limiting membrane (ILM) and optic disc Bruch's membrane opening are shown for calculation of NRR thickness in extracted vertical and horizontal tomogram. The RNFL tomogram shows the reference lines for segmentation and calculating RNFL thickness. (NRR: neuroretinal rim; RNFL: retinal nerve fiber layer)
		
		|
			OD	OS

Average RNFL thickness	86 µm	74 µm
RNFL symmetry	65%	
Rim area	0.95 mm²	0.83 mm²
Disc area	2.47 mm²	2.68 mm²
Average C/D ratio	0.79	0.83
Vertical C/D ratio	0.83	0.83
Cup volume	0.790 mm³	1.038 mm³ | **Fig. 5.7.4:** Key parameters studied in a RNFL and ONH scan of Cirrus OCT. (C/D: cup-disc ratio; RNFL: retinal nerve fiber layer; OCT: optical coherence tomography; ONH: optic nerve head)

Contd...

Contd...

S. no.	Parameter	Figure
5.A, B	Neuroretinal rim thickness and RNFL thickness temporal-superior-nasal-inferior-temporal (TSNIT) graphs: The NRR and RNFL TSNIT plots of the patients' eyes are shown as straight and dotted lines overlapped upon a green yellow and red color coded double hump pattern. Green area represents the 5–95th percentile of normative data and yellow shows the <5th percentile of normative data (borderline) and red area shows <1st percentile of normative data (abnormally low values) **(Fig. 5.7.5)**	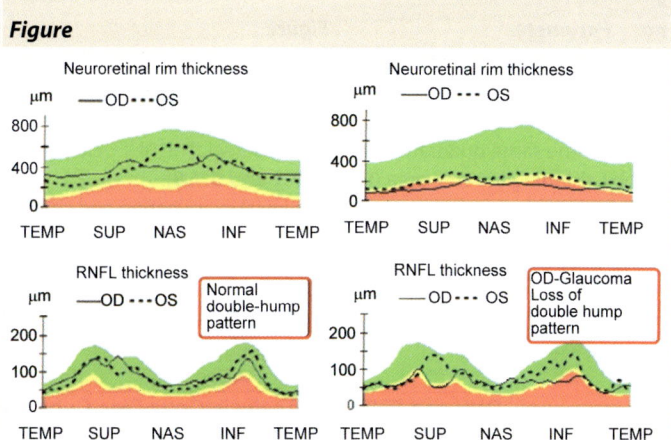 **Fig. 5.7.5:** Normal and glaucoma NRR and RNFL TSNIT maps. (RNFL: retinal nerve fiber layer; NRR: neuroretinal rim; TSNIT: temporal-superior-nasal-inferior-temporal)
5.C	RNFL quadrant and clock hour maps also show the color-coded thickness of the RNFL with standard green yellow-red color coding **(Fig. 5.7.6)**	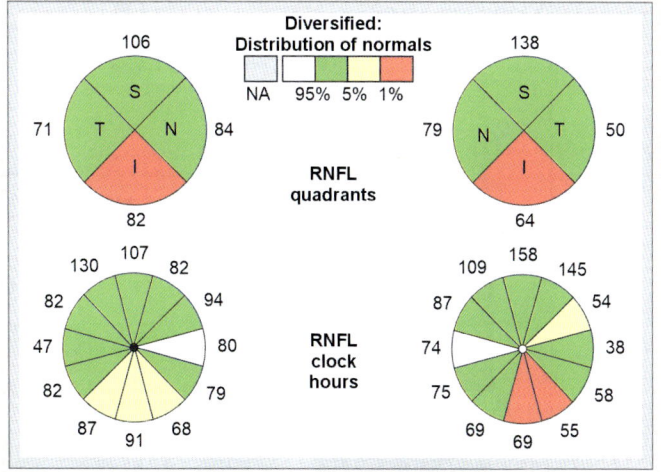 **Fig. 5.7.6:** RNFL quadrant and clock hour maps. (RNFL: retinal nerve fiber layer)

How to confirm glaucoma:
- Good quality scan:
  - Acceptable quality scores
  - The RNFL thickness map is complete without black areas or broken scan. Reference lines of extracted tomogram are not deviated.
- Look at the RNFL thickness in the RNFL thickness map to look for wedge defect. Same area is marked red or yellow in RNFL deviation map.

Contd...

Contd...

S. no.	Parameter	Figure
	• **Check key parameters:** The RNFL average thickness may be marked red or yellow in the same eye, with lower RNFL symmetry, enlarged vertical cup-disc (CD) ratio. • The TSNIT neuroretinal rim (NRR) and RNFL graphs lose the double hump pattern and dip into the red area in the same quadrants as the RNFL defect. The RNFL clock hour and quadrant maps also highlight RNFL thinning in same area **(Figs. 5.7.7 and 5.7.8)**. • **Clinical correlation:** Always do repeat clinical examination and check visual field of the patient to confirm the same.	

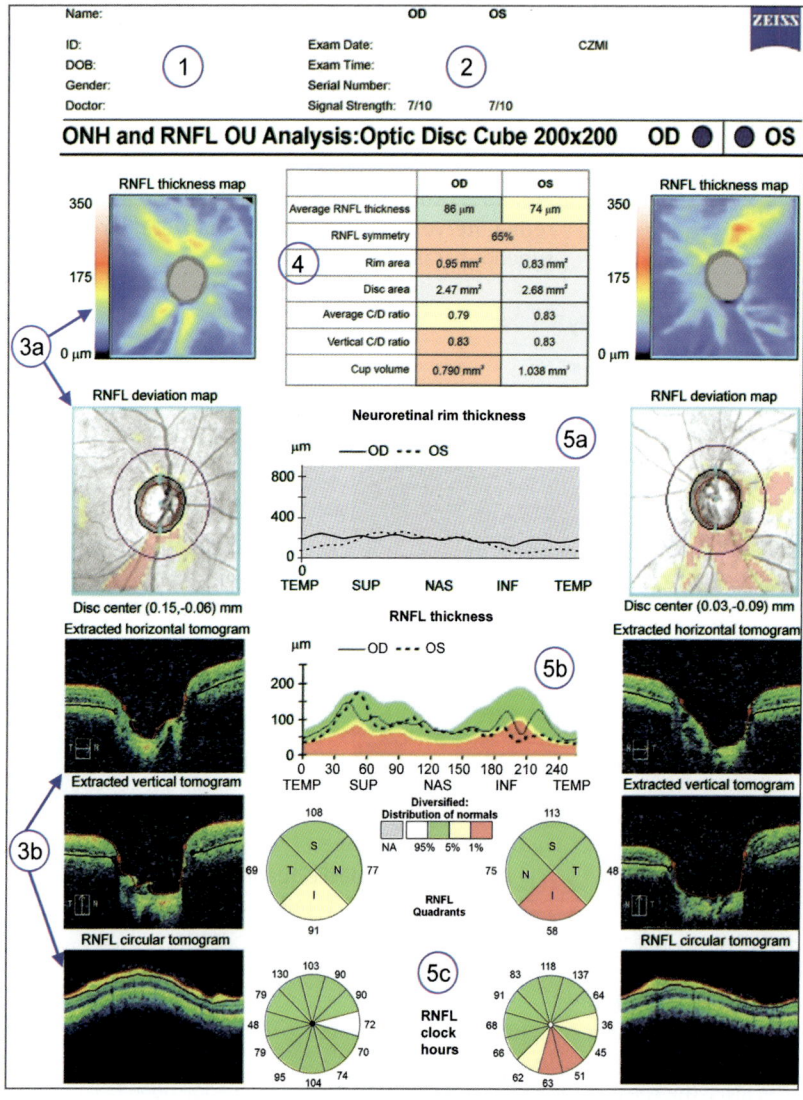

Fig. 5.7.7: ONH and RNFL analysis report on a Cirrus OCT. (C/D: cup-disc ratio; OCT: optical coherence tomography; ONH: optic nerve head; RNFL: retinal nerve fiber layer)

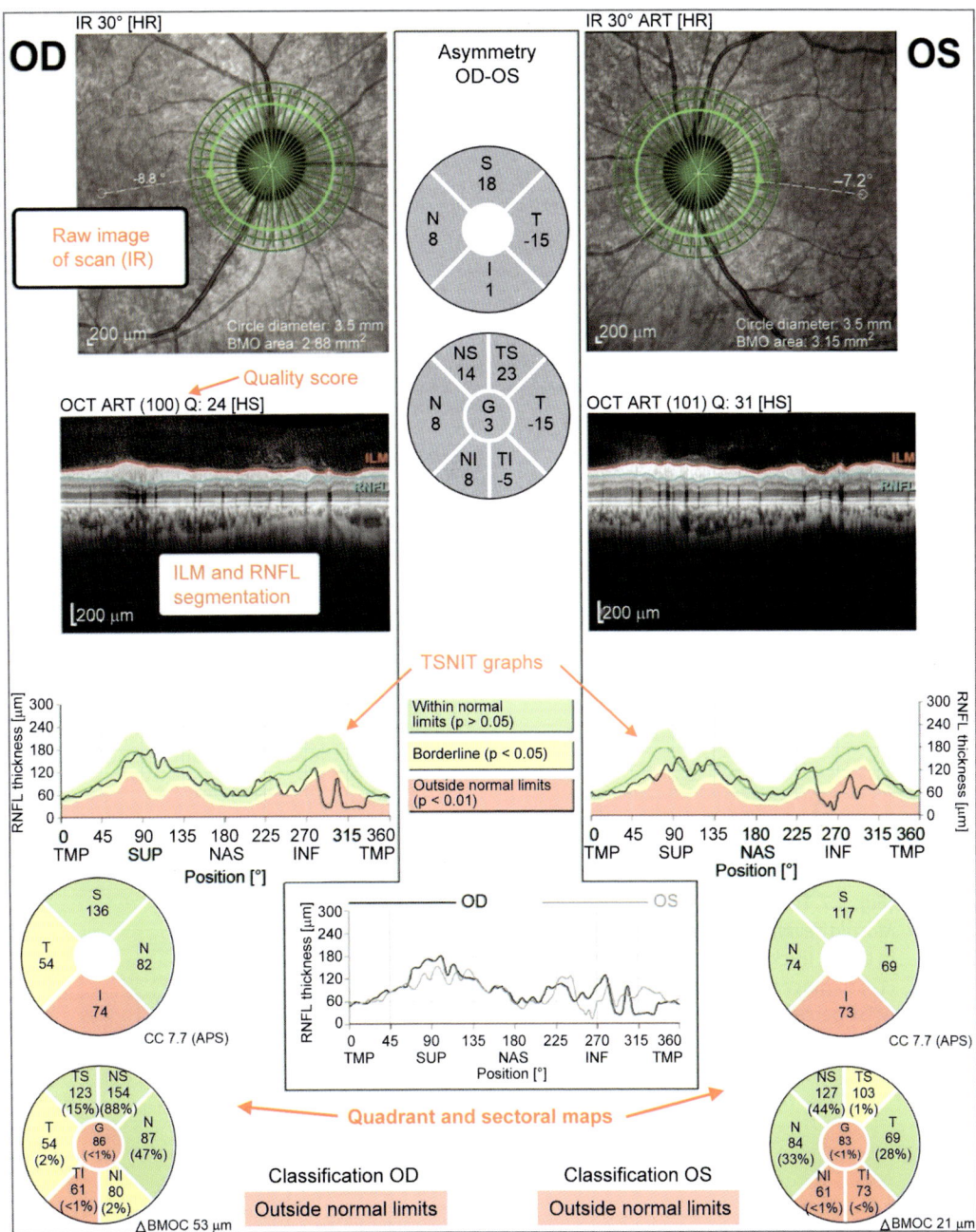

Fig. 5.7.8: RNFL analysis using spectralis OCT. (ILM: internal limiting membrane; TSNIT: temporal-superior-nasal-inferior-temporal; OCT: optical coherence tomography; RNFL: retinal nerve fiber layer)

HOW TO READ A MACULA/GANGLION CELL ANALYSIS PRINTOUT

Table 5.7.2 shows how to read a macula/ganglion cell analysis printout.

TABLE 5.7.2: How to read a macula/ganglion cell analysis printout.

S. no.	Parameter	Figure
1.	• Patient information and quality scores • The name of the patient and age must be matched to the report for appropriate age matching by the machine • Acceptable quality scores should be seen	
2.	*Horizontal macular tomogram* **(Fig. 5.7.9):** The tomogram should be centered over the fovea. It also shows any other abnormalities in macula	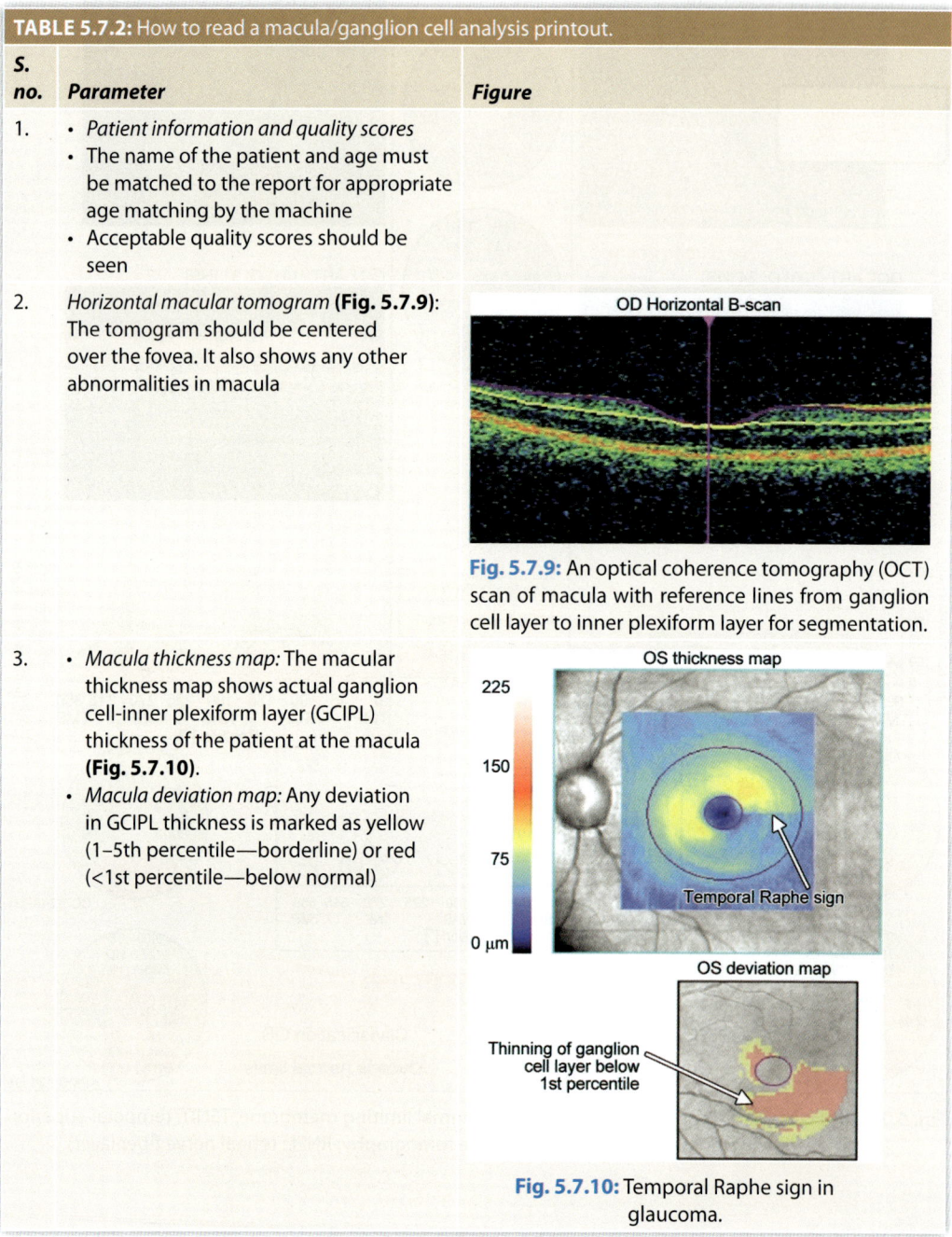 **Fig. 5.7.9:** An optical coherence tomography (OCT) scan of macula with reference lines from ganglion cell layer to inner plexiform layer for segmentation.
3.	• *Macula thickness map:* The macular thickness map shows actual ganglion cell-inner plexiform layer (GCIPL) thickness of the patient at the macula **(Fig. 5.7.10).** • *Macula deviation map:* Any deviation in GCIPL thickness is marked as yellow (1–5th percentile—borderline) or red (<1st percentile—below normal)	**Fig. 5.7.10:** Temporal Raphe sign in glaucoma.

Contd...

Contd...

S. no.	Parameter	Figure
4.	• Sector maps **(Fig. 5.7.11)** • Average and minimum GCIPL thickness **(Figs. 5.7.12 to 5.7.14)**	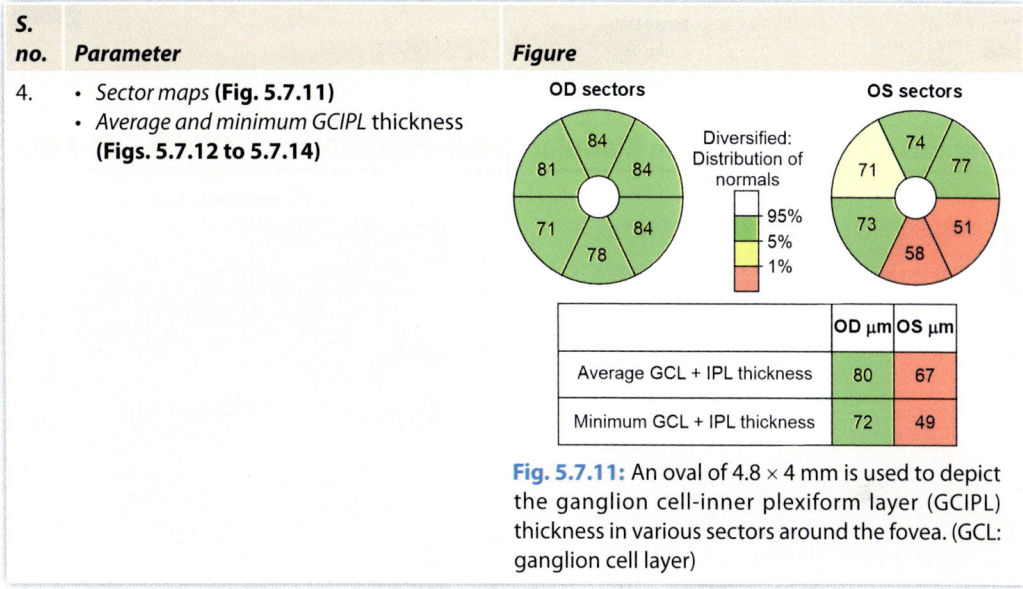 **Fig. 5.7.11:** An oval of 4.8 × 4 mm is used to depict the ganglion cell-inner plexiform layer (GCIPL) thickness in various sectors around the fovea. (GCL: ganglion cell layer)

OPTIC NERVE HEAD ANALYSIS (FIG. 5.7.15)

The optic disc minimum rim width analysis is provided by Spectralis OCT. Cirrus OCT gives optic disc analysis along with RNFL scan.
- Check the quality scores and patient information.
- Check the centration of scan and reference lines of Bruch's membrane opening and internal limiting membrane (ILM) in each sector.
- TSNIT graph of the NRR thickness shows the deviation of NRR compared to color-coded normative data. The sectoral NRR thickness is also provided.
- Always correlate clinically.

PITFALLS OF OPTICAL COHERENCE TOMOGRAPHY

- *Floor effect:* In advanced glaucoma, the structural damage becomes so profound that further progression is difficult to assess by structural test like OCT. This is called floor effect. This happens due to already thin RNFL with predominant residual glial tissues being picked up on segmentation by OCT. Here, VF tests (functional imaging) gives better results.
- *Red disease:* A *false positive diagnosis* of a normal person as glaucoma due to poor scan quality or segmentation errors.
- *Green disease:* A *false negative diagnosis*, i.e., a glaucomatous disc is marked green on OCT. It is the inability of OCT machine to pick up glaucoma.
- *Segmentation errors:* Segmentation done by the machine may be faulty due to poor OCT scan or abnormalities like vitreous traction. This may lead to abnormal values in OCT.
- *Artifacts:* Patient-related artifacts such as tilted optic disc with shifted RNFL peaks, media opacities like cataract/posterior capsule opacification/vitreous opacities, etc., may lead to faulty OCT scans.

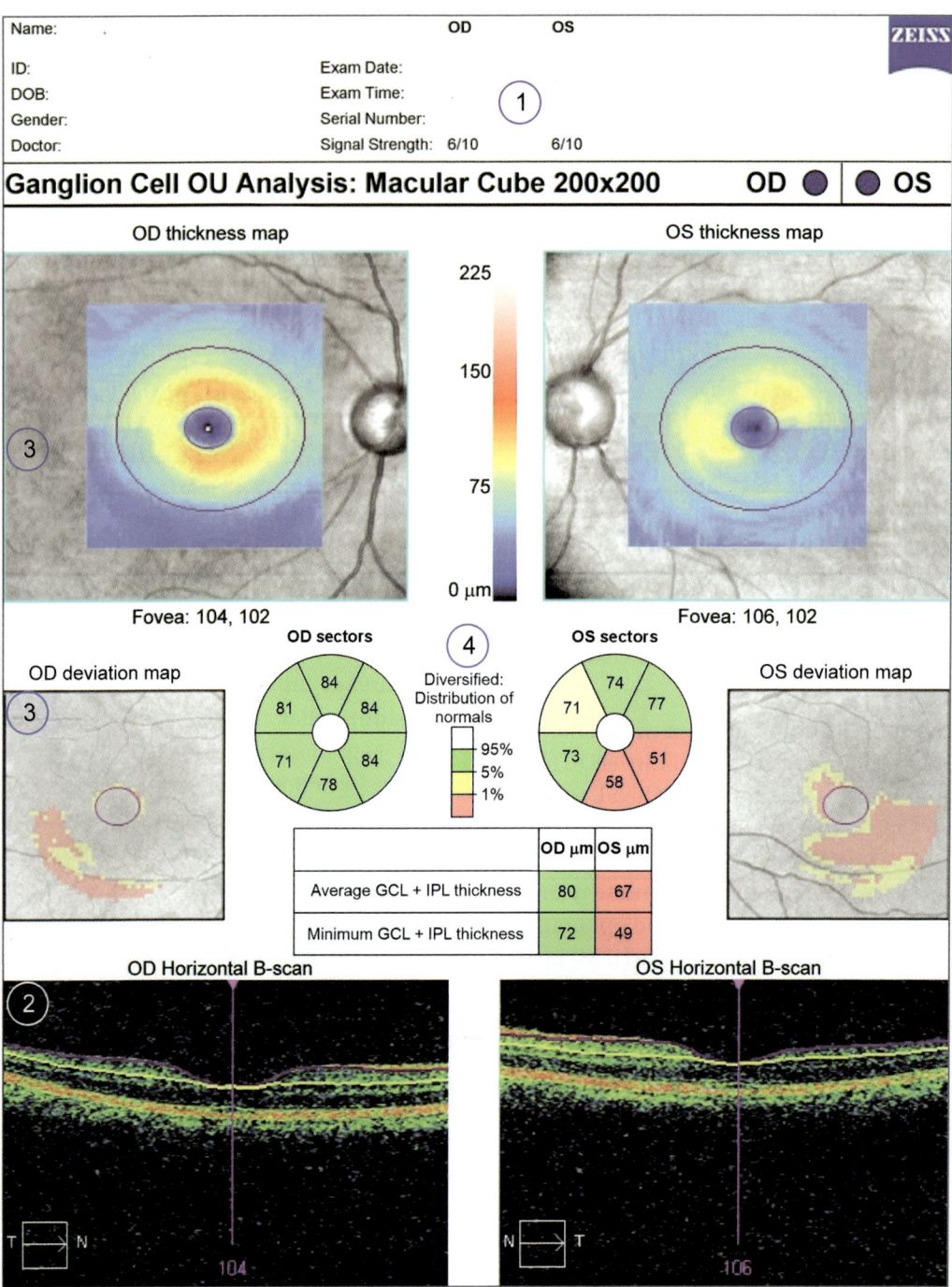

Fig. 5.7.12: Ganglion cell-inner plexiform layer (GCIPL) analysis report printout using Cirrus OCT. (GCL: ganglion cell layer; OCT: optical coherence tomography)

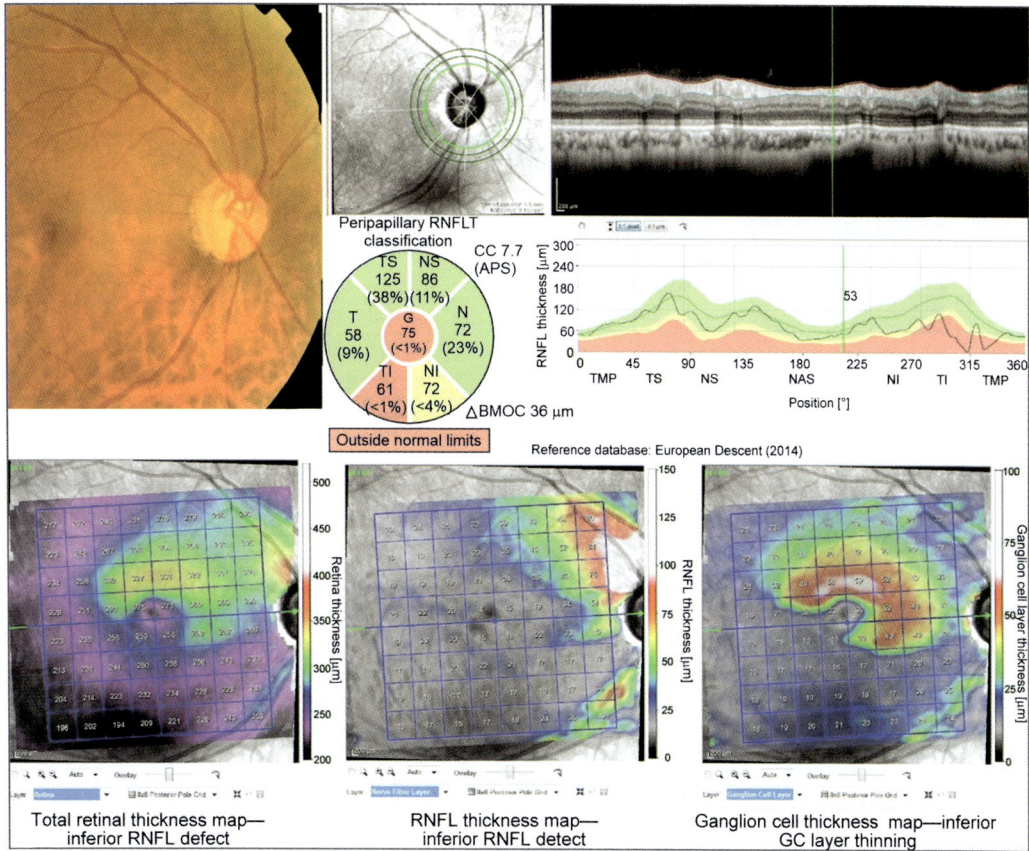

Fig. 5.7.13: Spectralis OCT imaging of the given optic disc with inferior notch. RNFL scanning shows inferotemporal RNFL thinning. Spectralis OCT machine can assess each layer of retina separately and give an overlay thickness map in each cubic area along with pseudo-color-coded thickness map. (OCT: optical coherence tomography; RNFL: retinal nerve fiber layer)

GLAUCOMA PROGRESSION IN OPTICAL COHERENCE TOMOGRAPHY

Guided progression analysis: Two types of analysis are done **(Fig. 5.7.16)**:
1. *Event-based analysis:* Compares two recent scans to two baseline scans. A change seen only once is highlighted in yellow as "possible loss." Any change seen in subsequent scan is highlighted in red as "likely loss."
2. *Trend-based analysis:* Average RNFL thickness values are plotted with time to look for rate of change or progression of RNFL thinning. If there is thinning more than expected test-retest variability, the circle is marked as "possible loss." If the similar change is found in subsequent scan, the circle is colored in red as "likely loss."

VIVA QUESTIONS

1. **How would you interpret the given RNFL OCT scan?**
Ans: Refer to text.

SECTION 1: Appliances and Instruments

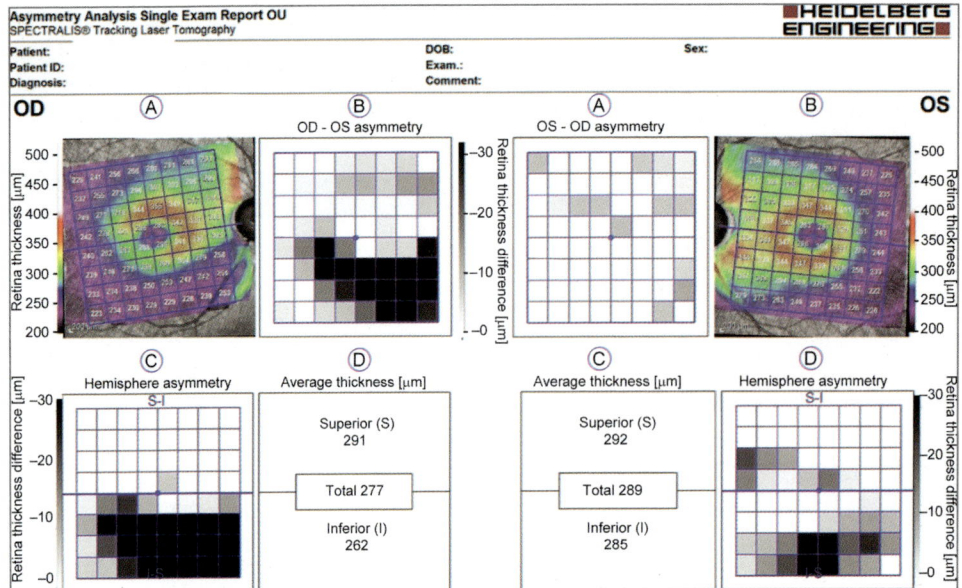

Figs. 5.7.14A to D: Ganglion cell analysis showing inferotemporal thinning. (A) Thickness map showing posterior pole retinal thickness in an 8 × 8 mm grid; (B) OD-OS asymmetry map showing asymmetry in the thickness, between the two eyes (Color scale—the large difference is indicated by darker gray color); (C) Hemisphere asymmetry analysis map showing asymmetry between the two hemispheres; (D) Average thickness, along with superior and inferior hemisphere mean thickness.

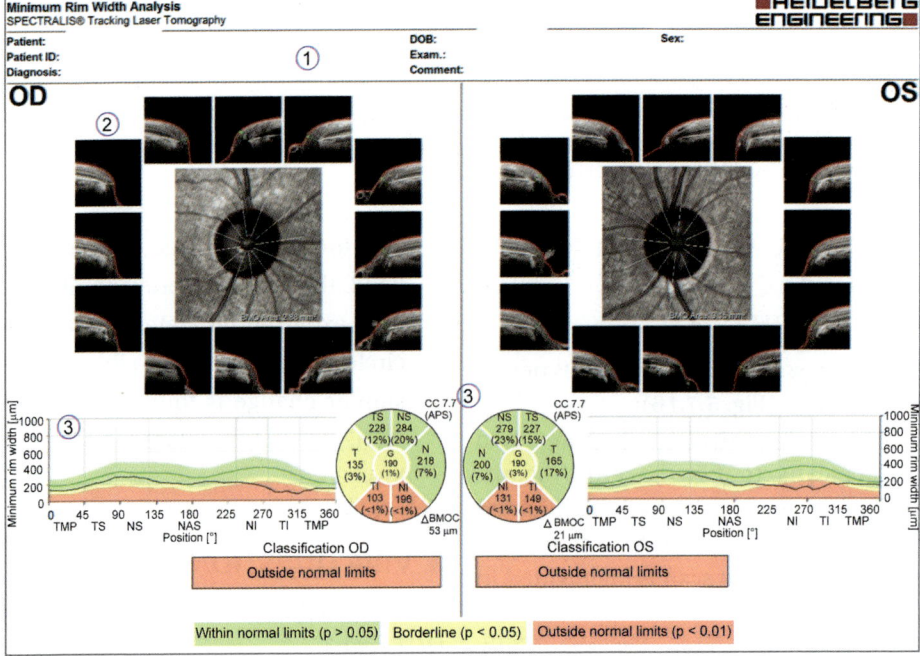

Fig. 5.7.15: Minimum rim width analysis for neuroretinal rim by Spectralis optical coherence tomography.

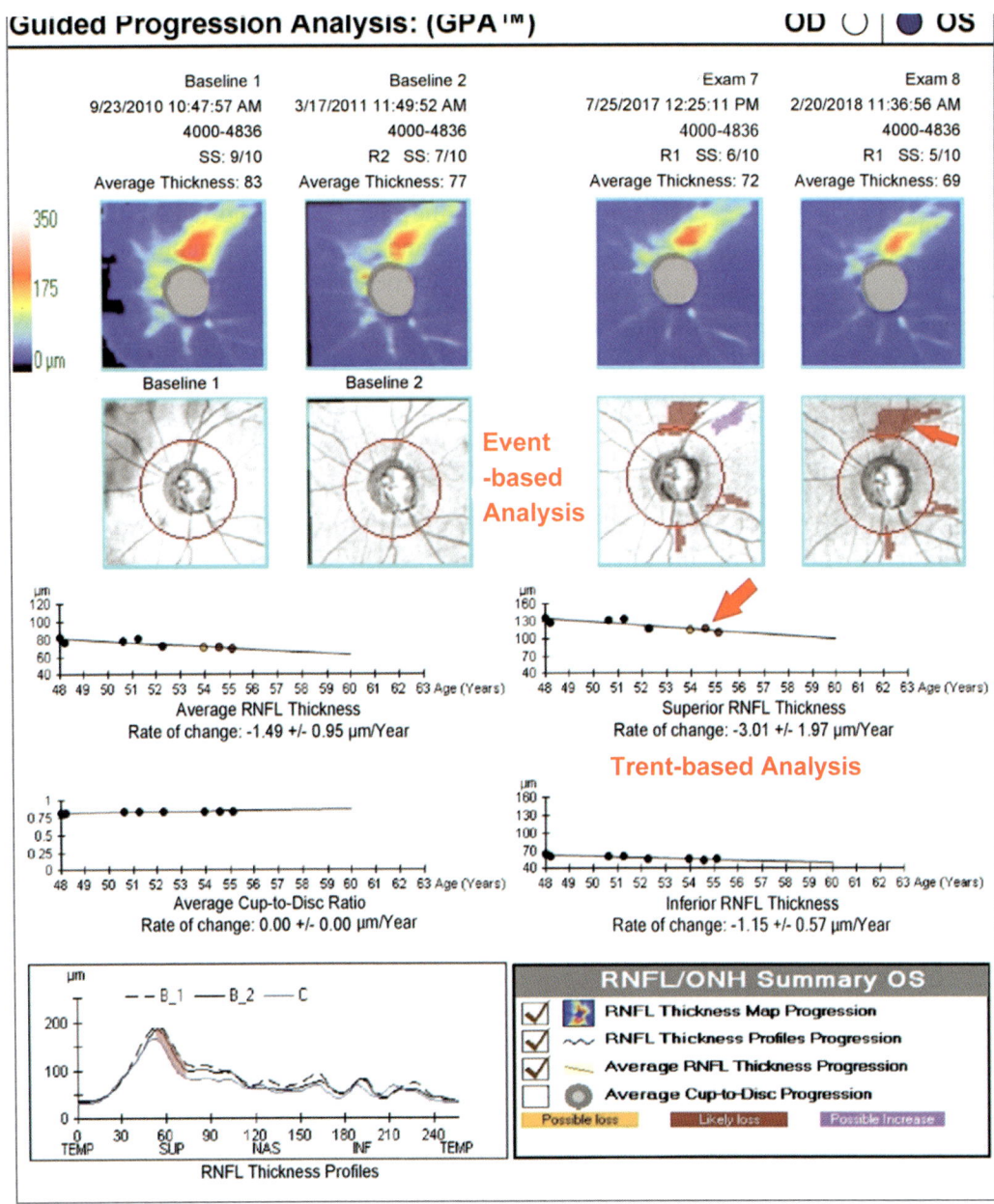

Fig. 5.7.16: Guided progression analysis of serial RNFL scans showing progressive superior RNFL thinning (red arrows) in event-based and trend-based analysis. (RNFL: retinal nerve fiber layer)

2. What is the principle of OCT?
Ans: Refer to text.

3. How is glaucoma progression seen in OCT?
Ans: Refer to text.

5.8 HEIDELBERG RETINA TOMOGRAPH

Gaurav Garg, Jyoti Shakrawal

INTRODUCTION

With the recent advances, diagnosis of glaucoma which was previously just based on clinical assessment is shifting to newer modalities such as VF testing for progression, various imaging methods for RNFL, and optic disc characteristics. Optic disc evaluation is always a subjective finding. Heidelberg retina tomograph (HRT, Heidelberg Engineering, Heidelberg Germany) is an imaging technique for topographical assessment of optic disc **(Fig. 5.8.1)**. HRT gives us an objective and reproducible method of documentation. It is based on confocal scanning laser ophthalmoscopy (CSLO) principle for 3D acquisition of optic disc.[1]

PRINCIPLE

In CSLO-HRT, uses a 670 nm diode-laser light beam for the quantitative imaging of the following:
- Optic disc

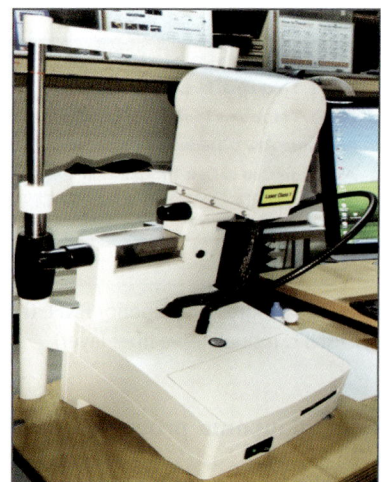

Fig. 5.8.1: Heidelberg retina tomograph 3 (HRT3).

- The retinal nerve fiber layer
- Posterior pole

The procedure does not require dilatation of pupil and take less than a minute to image an eye. The periodic laser beam is deflected by the oscillating mirrors and reflected light is detected by the light-sensitive detector **(Fig. 5.8.2)**. Based on the intensity of reflected light, sequentially scan of optic disc are obtained.

SCANS

- Successive 2D scans of optic disc are acquired.
- The depth of 4.0 mm, with approximately 16–64 reflectance images.
- Each consecutive scan is about 0.0625 deeper.
- These scans are combined to give a 3D contour map of the optic disc.
- 15 × 15° is imaged in a scan.
- Lateral resolution is 10 µm.
- After image acquisition, the contour line is drawn at the scleral ring inner border, either manually as in HRT II, which gives a subjective variation[2] or automated as in HRT III **(Table 5.8.1)**.
- A reference plane is automatically generated as the contour line is drawn, which is parallel and 50 µm below the retinal surface **(Fig. 5.8.3)**. The reference plane helps in dividing the optic disc into rim and cup area. The color-coded images are used as:
  - Green—Rim
  - Blur—Rim slope
  - Red—Cup

EXAMINATION

- The patient is allowed to sit in front of the machine.

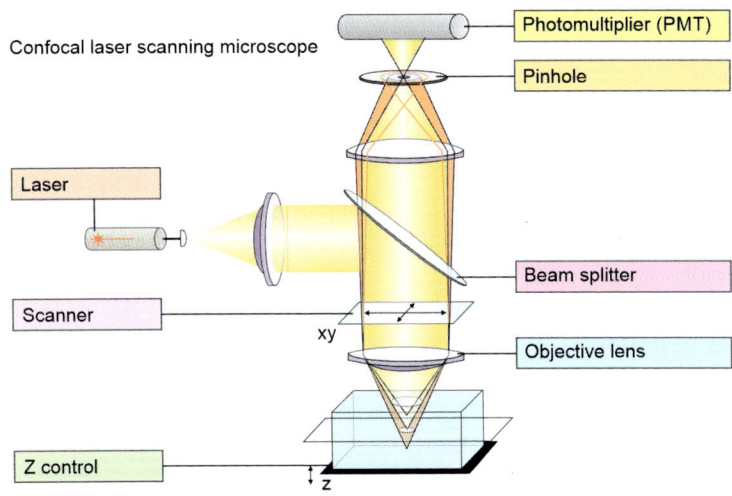

Fig. 5.8.2: Optics of confocal scanning laser ophthalmoscopy (CSLO).

TABLE 5.8.1: Comparison between Heidelberg retina tomograph (HRT) II versus HRT III.

Parameters	HRT II	HRT III
Normative data for more field regression analysis (MRA)	110 subjects	733 Caucasian, 215 African American, and 100 Asian Indians
Contour line	Manual	Automated
Subjective variation	Present	Absent
Glaucoma probability score (GPS)	Absent	Present
Confocal images acquired	32	64

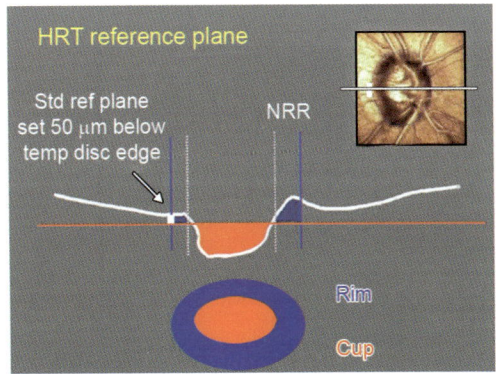

Fig. 5.8.3: Reference plane is located 50 µm below the mean height of the surface along the contour line. (HRT: Heidelberg retina tomograph; NRR: neuroretinal rim)

- No mydriasis is required.
- Internal fixation target is given.
- Refractive error of >1 diopter cylinder is corrected.
- The diode laser is aimed via the pinhole onto the retina.
- Smaller the aperture size, higher will be the resolution.

INTERPRETATION OF PRINTOUT

A standard deviation (SD) value is obtained in each scan, which gives the idea of image quality of the scan. SD value:
- ≤20 µm: Excellent

- *20–30 μm:* Good
- *30–40 μm:* Acceptable

Patient Data (Fig. 5.8.4)

- Provides information on exam type as baseline or follow-up.
- Demographic information (patient name, age, gender, date of birth, etc.).
- Information including image quality score and focus position.

Topography Image

- Pseudocolor image
- Gives disc size, shape, and location of the cup
- Neuroretinal rim appears green, sloping NRR appears blue, and cup appears red.

Reflectance Image

- Pseudocolor image.

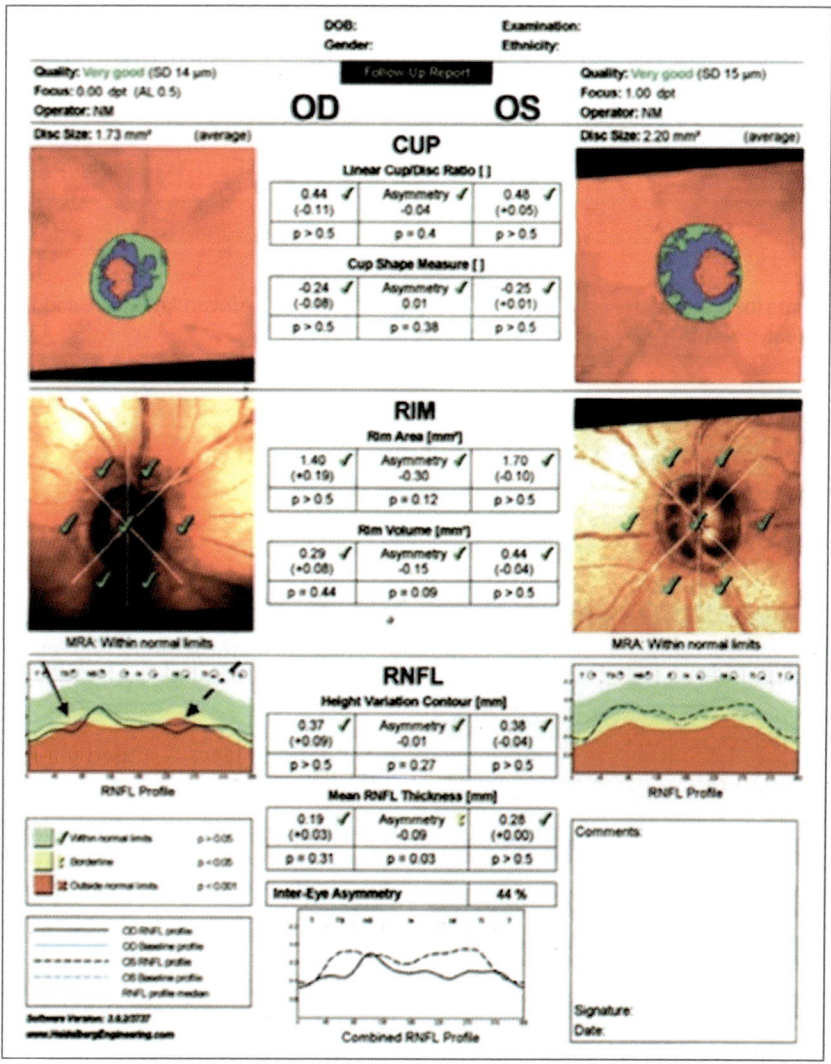

Fig. 5.8.4: Normal Heidelberg retina tomograph printout.

- The optic disc is divided into six sectors and is compared to a standard database.
- All sectors are then classified with Moorefield's regression analysis (MRA), as within:
  - Normal limits (✓)
  - Borderline (!)
  - Outside normal limits (✗)

Retinal Nerve Fiber Layer Graph

- The color-coded graph in which reference plane is indicated by the red line and retinal surface height by the green line.
- The profile starts 0 as temporal and moves superior, nasal, and inferior to temporal again.
- It provides a calculation of the thickness of the nerve fiber layer (NFL).
- Normally, the appearance is "double hump appearance."

Stereometric Analysis of Optic Disc (Table 5.8.2)

- About 75–90% sensitivity
- About 80–97% specificity
  - Optic disc:
    - Area (mm^2): It is the area bounded by the contour line.
  - Optic cup:
    - Area (mm^2): It is the area bounded by the contour line, which is located below the reference plane.
    - Volume (mm^3): It is the volume bounded by the contour line, which is located below the reference plane.
  - Neuroretinal rim:
    - Area (mm^2): It is the area bounded by the contour line and located above the reference plane.
    - Volume (mm^2): It is the volume bounded by the contour line and located above the reference plane.
  - Cup/disc area ratio: The ratio between the cup area to disc area.
  - Linear cup/disc ratio: The square root of the ratio between cup area to disc area.
  - Cup-shaped measure: It is the measure of the overall 3D shape of optic disc cup. Independent of the reference plane and optic disc size.
  - Height variation contour: It is the height difference between the maximum elevated and maximum depressed point of the contour line.

TABLE 5.8.2: Normative stereometric parameter.[3]

Parameters	Normal	Early defect	Moderate defect	Advanced defect
Disc area (mm^2)	2.257 ± 0.563	2.345 ± 0.569	2.310 ± 0.554	2.261 ± 0.461
Cup area (mm^2)	0.768 ± 0.505	0.953 ± 0.594	1.051 ± 0.647	1.445 ± 0.562
Rim area (mm^2)	1.489 ± 0.291	1.393 ± 0.340	1.260 ± 0.415	0.817 ± 0.334
Cup volume (mm^3)	0.240 ± 0.245	0.294 ± 0.270	0.334 ± 0.318	0.543 ± 0.425
Rim volume (mm^3)	0.362 ± 0.124	0.323 ± 0.156	0.262 ± 0.139	0.128 ± 0.096
Cup/disc ratio	0.314 ± 0.152	0.380 ± 0.179	0.430 ± 0.203	0.621 ± 0.189
Mean cup depth (mm)	0.262 ± 0.118	0.279 ± 0.115	0.289 ± 0.130	0.366 ± 0.182
Maximum cup depth (mm)	0.679 ± 0.223	0.680 ± 0.210	0.674 ± 0.249	0.720 ± 0.276
Cup shape measure	−0.181 ± 0.092	−0.147 ± 0.098	−0.122 ± 0.095	−0.036 ± 0.096
Height variation contour (mm)	0.384 ± 0.087	0.364 ± 0.100	0.330 ± 0.108	0.256 ± 0.090
Mean RNFL thickness (mm)	0.384 ± 0.063	0.217 ± 0.076	0.182 ± 0.086	0.013 ± 0.061
RNFL cross sectional area (mm^2)	1.282 ± 0.328	1.155 ± 0.396	0.957 ± 0.440	0.679 ± 0.302

- **Mean RNFL thickness:** Mean thickness of RNFL along the contour line.

Moorfield's Regression Analysis

- Histogram representation **(Fig. 5.8.5)**
- Depends on the reference plane, disc area.
- Compares the patient's data (global and local rim area) with an age-matched normative data.
- Rim area is coded as green and cup area as red.
- Four white lines represent 50%, 95%, 99%, and 99.9% prediction interval.

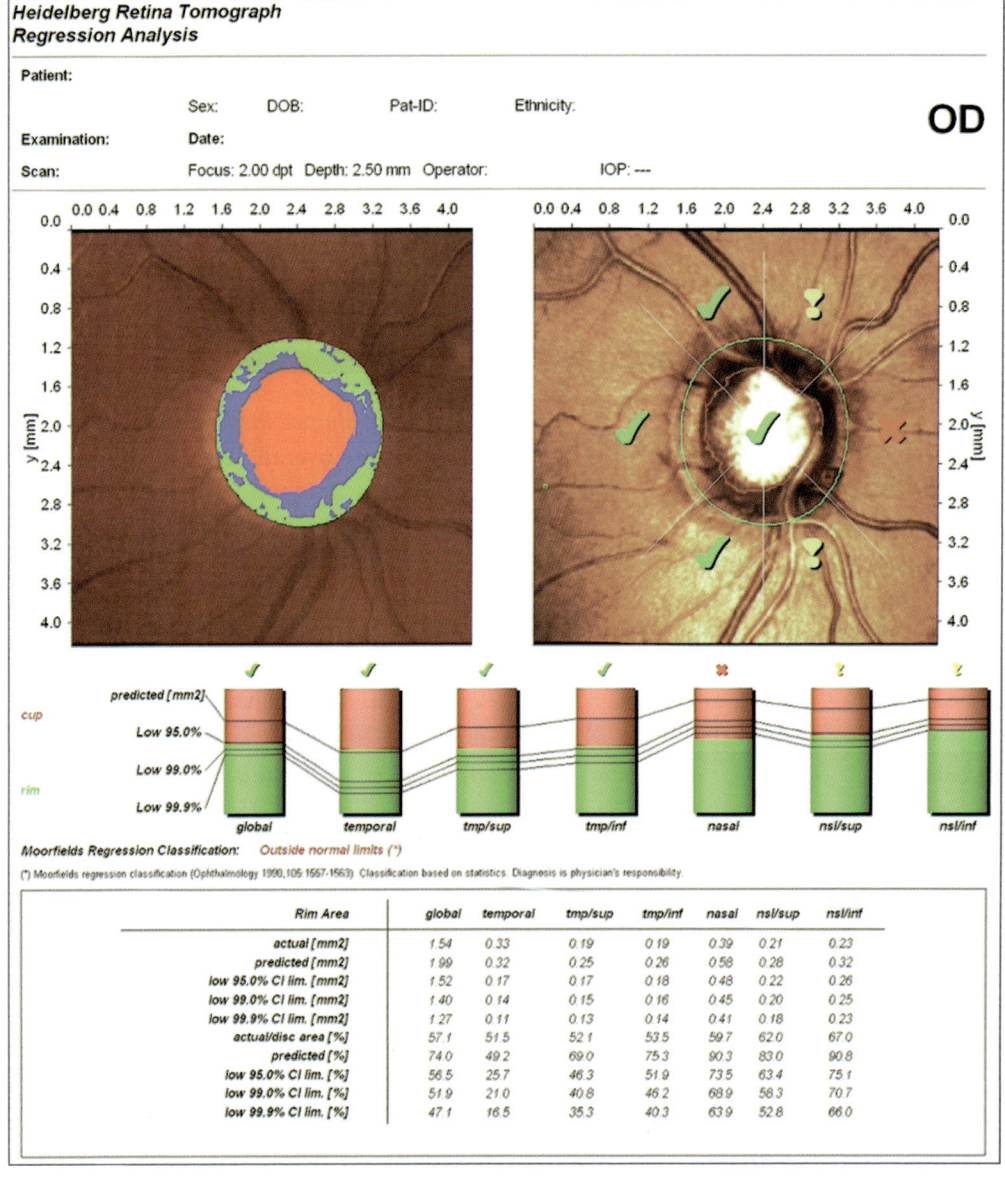

Fig. 5.8.5: Moorefield's regression analysis.

Glaucoma Probability Score

- *Based on five parameters:* Cup size, cup depth, optic nerve rim steepness, horizontal RNFL, and vertical RNFL curvature.
- Does not depend on the reference plane.
- All sectors are then classified same as in MRA as, within normal limits, borderline, and outside normal limits **(Fig. 5.8.6)**.

MONITORING THE PROGRESSION

Progression can be measured by comparing ONH stereometric parameters of different scans done on follow-ups.

Progression Analysis with Change Probability Map

- *Top row:* Sequential topographic images

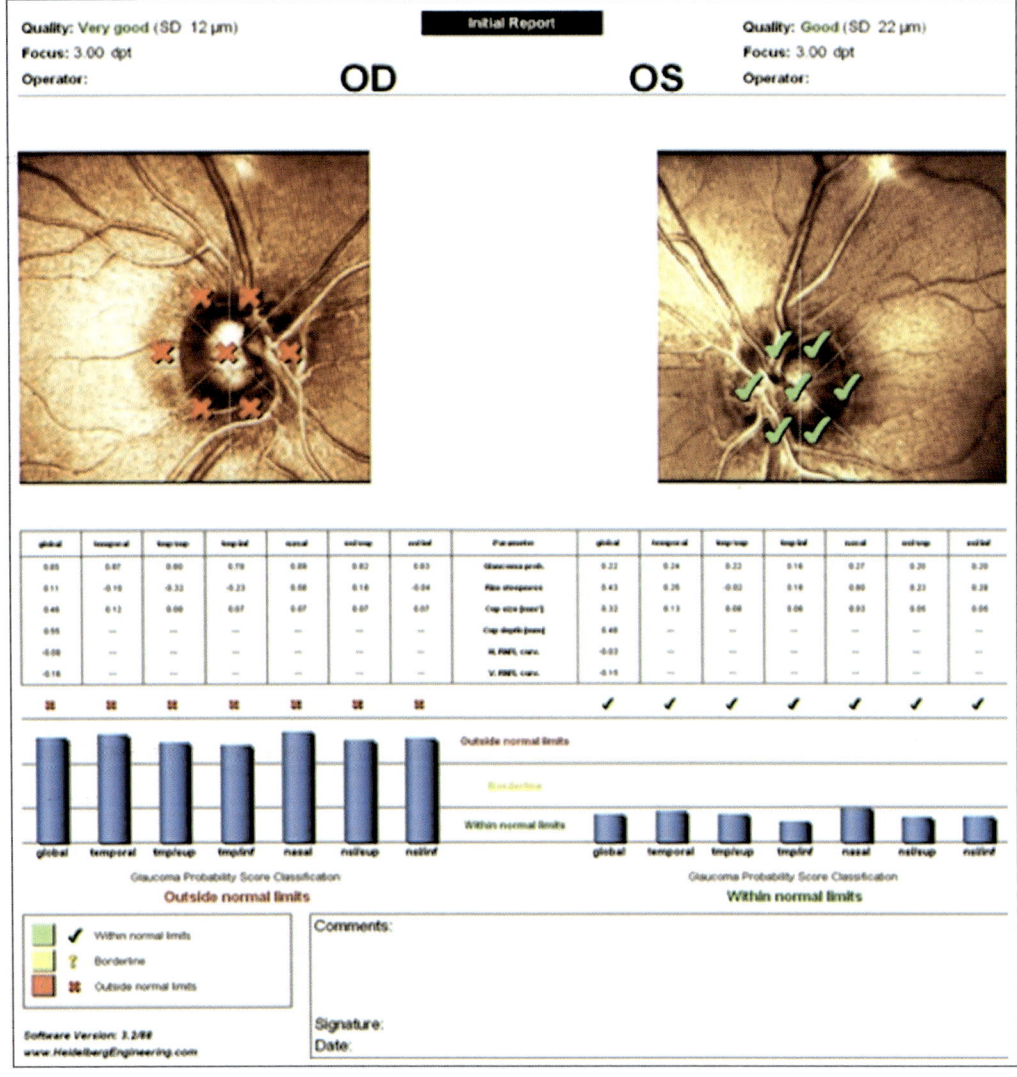

Fig. 5.8.6: Glaucoma probability score (GPS).

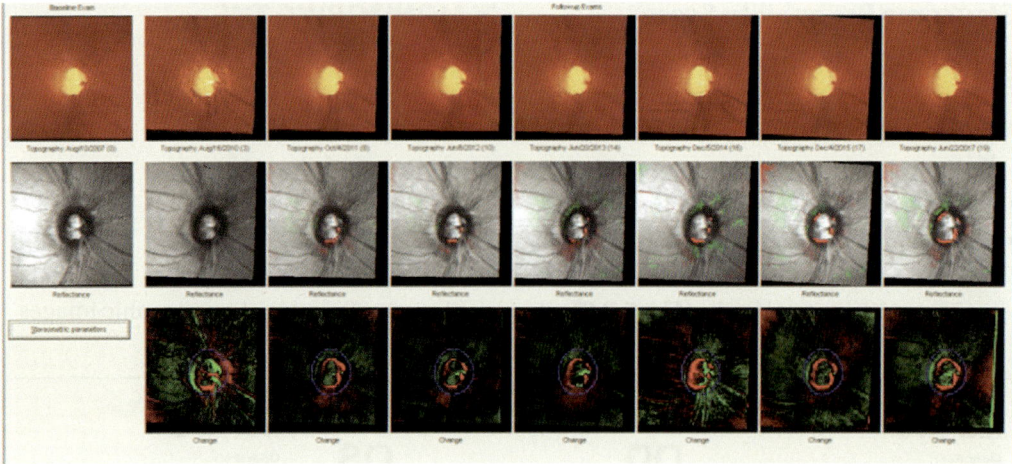

Fig. 5.8.7: Progression analysis with change probability map.

- *Second row:* Sequential reflectance images
- *Third row:* Appears after capturing fourth follow-up scan which starts flagging significance level if the same area is showing a similar change in at least two consecutive examinations progression is suspected, and if in three consecutive examinations progression is confirmed **(Fig. 5.8.7)**.

CASE (FIG. 5.8.8)

This is a HRT, "OU report" printout of patient named........., age.......
- The quality of the scan is very good with 0.00 dpt focus. This gives us information on both eyes of a glaucoma patient on a single paper.
- The OD disc is larger, whereas the OS disc is average size.
- The linear cup/disc ratio is 0.87 and 0.82 in both eyes, with a cup shape measure of −0.01 and −0.05. The NRR area is 0.81 mm^2 each with the volume of 0.09 mm^3. The RNFL height variation contour shows 0.23 mm variation for both eyes with mean RNFL thickness of 0.04 mm and 0.09 mm in OD and OS.
- For all these parameters, classification as within normal limits (green mark), borderline (yellow mark), outside normal limits (red mark), and the degree of asymmetry is also written. For both the eyes, NRR area and volume are below normal limits. In most of the sectors, MRA results are outside normal limits.
- This HRT concludes inferotemporal RNFL defect of retina (right eye), as seen in stereophotograph of RE similarly.

CONCLUSION

Heidelberg retina tomography provides quick and noninvasive reproducible, objective measurements of the optic disc and RNFL. It helps both in detecting early glaucomatous changes and its progression.

VIVA QUESTIONS

1. **What is the principle of HRT?**
   Ans: Refer to text.
2. **How to read an HRT printout?**
   Ans: Refer to text.
3. **What is the significance of green, yellow, and red color coding?**
   Ans: Refer to text.

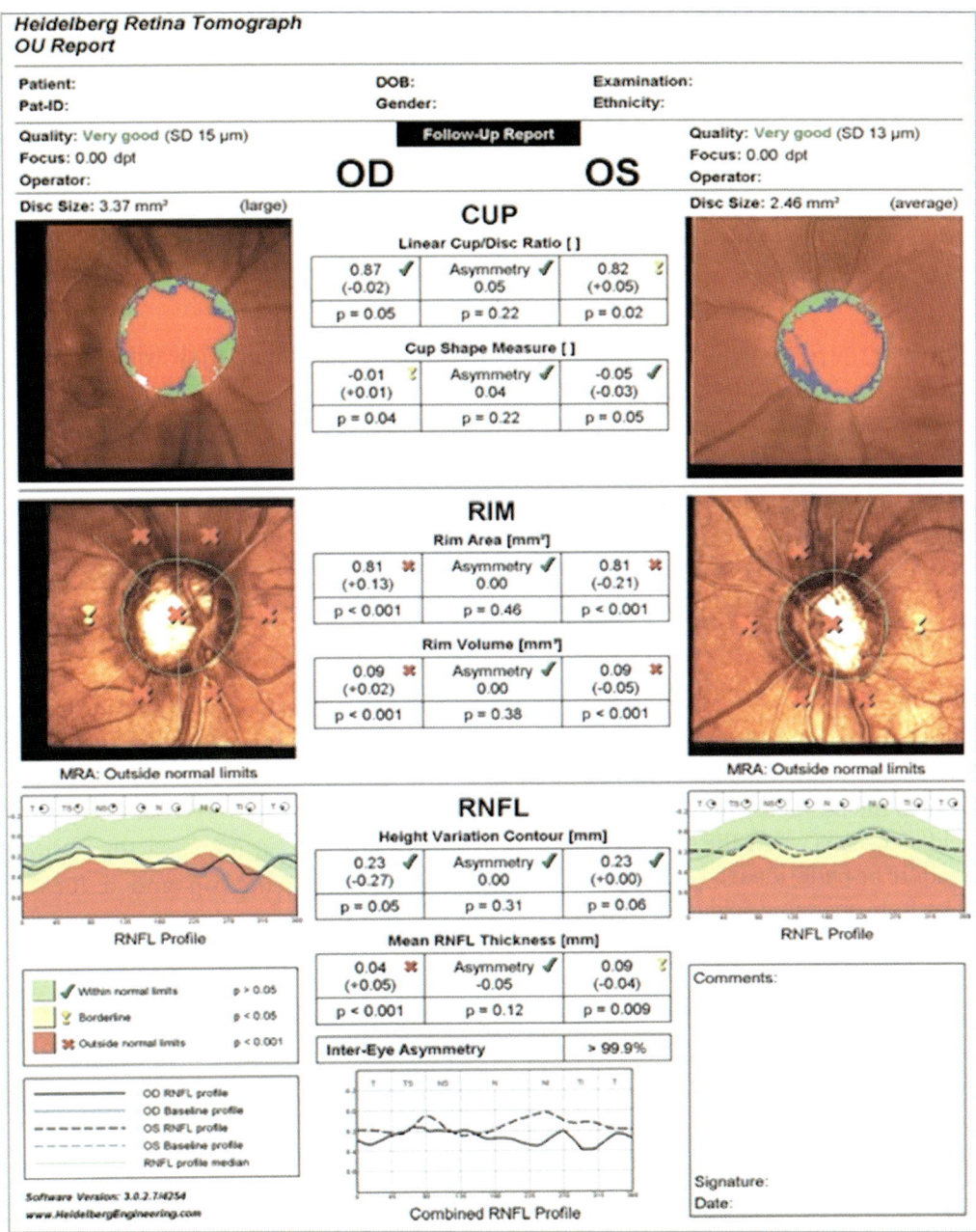

Fig. 5.8.8: Glaucoma probability score (GPS) report.

REFERENCES

1. Quigley HA, Katz J, Derick RJ, Gilbert D, Sommer A. An evaluation of optic disc and nerve fiber layer examinations in monitoring progression of early glaucoma damage. Ophthalmology. 1992;99(1):19-28.
2. Miglior S, Albé E, Guareschi M, Rossetti L, Orzalesi N. Intraobserver and interobserver

reproducibility in the evaluation of optic disc stereometric parameters by Heidelberg Retina Tomograph. Ophthalmology. 2002; 109(6):1072-7.

3. Burk R. Laser Scanning Tomographie: Interpretation der Ausdrucke des Heidelberg Retina Tomographen HRT II. Z Prakt Augenheilkd. 2001;22:183-90.

5.9 INSTRUMENTS USED IN GLAUCOMA SURGERIES

Vatsalya Venkatraman, Pranita Sahay, Jyoti Shakrawal

■ INTRODUCTION

Surgical intervention for glaucoma includes chiefly trabeculectomy and trabeculotomy.

Most instruments required for this procedure are routine except for a few additional ones. The following details will give you a comprehensive idea regarding the appearance and use of each instrument required during the procedure.

■ WIRE SPECULUM

This instrument is an essential need for almost all ophthalmologic surgeries. It aids to keep the lids apart so one can get a clear field of the area where the surgical procedure needs to be performed. It keeps the eyelashes away from operating field **(Fig. 5.9.1)**.

■ PLAIN FORCEPS

It is a blunt forceps without any tooth. Its tip has serrations **(Fig. 5.9.2)**.

Uses

- For holding conjunctiva, scleral flap, or skin
- For holding sutures while tying

■ SUPERIOR RECTUS HOLDING FORCEPS

It is a toothed S-shaped forceps especially designed to fit into the orbit while trying to grasp the muscle belly while passing the bridle suture **(Fig. 5.9.3)**.

■ LIMS FORCEPS

It is also a toothed forceps to hold the limbus or scleral flap or sutures **(Fig. 5.9.4)**.

■ ARTERY (HEMOSTATIC) FORCEPS

It is a blunt tipped forceps with multiple serrations near the tip and a locking

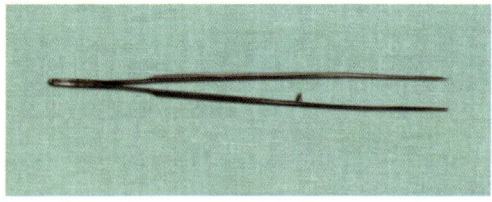

Fig. 5.9.2: Plain forceps.

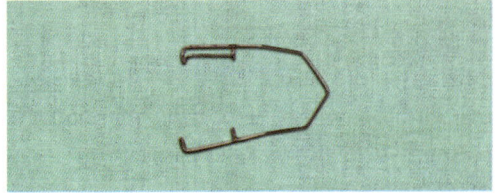

Fig. 5.9.1: Wire speculum.

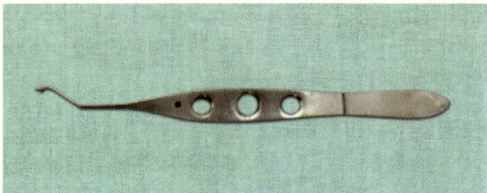

Fig. 5.9.3: Superior rectus holding forceps.

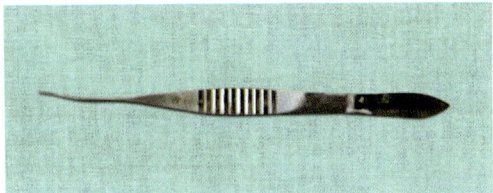

Fig. 5.9.4: Lim forceps.

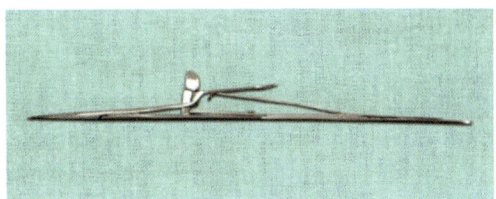

Fig. 5.9.7: Arruga needle holder.

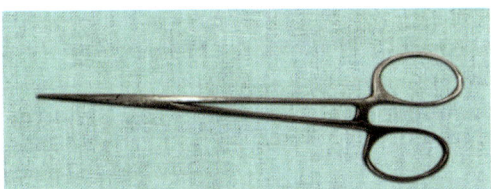

Fig. 5.9.5: Artery (hemostatic) forceps.

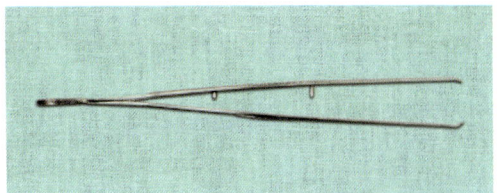

Fig. 5.9.8: Globe holding forceps.

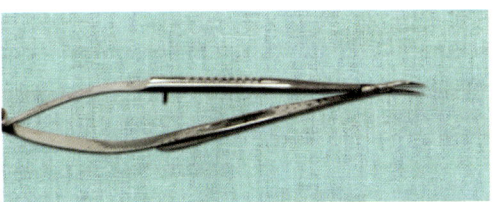

Fig. 5.9.6: Barraquer needle holder.

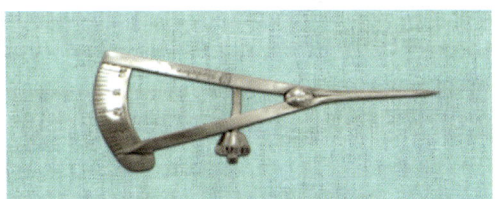

Fig. 5.9.9: Castroviejo caliper.

mechanism on the other end. It is available in various sizes **(Fig. 5.9.5)**.

Uses
- To hold the bleeders during the surgery
- To tie the fixation suture.

BARRAQUER NEEDLE HOLDER

It is a needle holder with fine serrations at the jaw for better grip while passing sutures through the conjunctiva, cornea, and sclera **(Fig. 5.9.6)**.

ARRUGA NEEDLE HOLDER

It is a large needle holder with one end being flat for placement of the surgeon's thumb and the other end having serrations for better grip of the suture. In glaucoma surgery, it is used to pass the superior rectus bridle suture **(Fig. 5.9.7)**.

GLOBE HOLDING FORCEPS

The tip of this forceps is toothed for better grip while holding conjunctiva and episcleral tissue near the limbus. It can also be used while mitomycin application **(Fig. 5.9.8)**.

CASTROVIEJO MARKING CALIPERS

It measures from 0 to 15 mm in 0.25 increments. It consists of a standard caliper handle and an adjustable screw in the center. The center of the tips measures the size of the objects that needs to be measured. In trabeculectomy, this instrument is used to measure the size of scleral flap **(Fig. 5.9.9)**.

CRESCENT BLADE

It is a blunt tipped instrument with beveled edges and having cut-splitting action on both the sides. It is used for faster dissection of the scleral flap in trabeculectomy (**Fig. 5.9.10**).

MICROVITREORETINAL BLADE

It is a fine straight instrument with triangular knife at its distal end having cutting edge on both the sides. It is used to make side port entry at the limbus. Also, used while making ostium (**Fig. 5.9.11**).

VANAS SCISSORS

It is a fine scissor working on spring action used for cutting fine sutures. Also, for cutting tissue while making ostium (**Fig. 5.9.12**).

CASTROVIEJO CORNEOSCLERAL SCISSORS

It is a fine curved scissor working on spring action used to cut the scleral tissue flap or for conjunctival dissection (**Fig. 5.9.13**).

KELLY'S PUNCH

This instrument is used to perform the sclerotomy to drain the excess fluid from the anterior chamber. It has a serrated squeeze handle for precise control. The advantage here is one does not have to hold the scleral flap during the procedure (**Fig. 5.9.14**).

WESTCOTT CONJUNCTIVAL SCISSORS

It is a stout scissor with straight/curved blades for conjunctival dissection (**Fig. 5.9.15**).

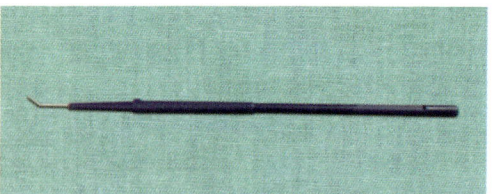

Fig. 5.9.10: Crescent blade.

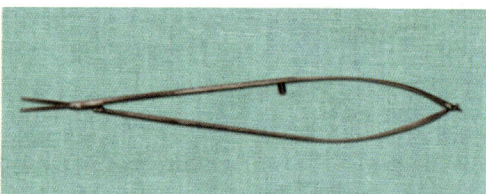

Fig. 5.9.13: Castroviejo corneoscleral scissors.

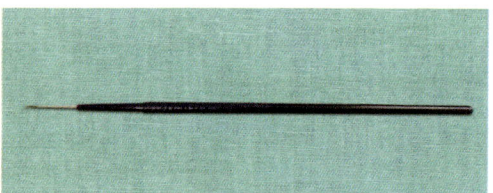

Fig. 5.9.11: Microvitreoretinal (MVR) blade.

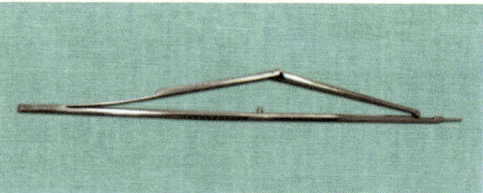

Fig. 5.9.14: Kelly's punch.

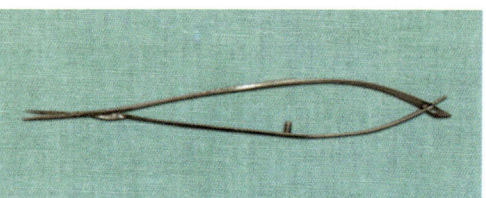

Fig. 5.9.12: Vanas scissors.

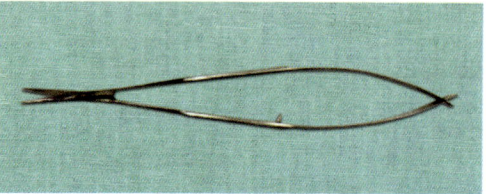

Fig. 5.9.15: Westcott conjunctival scissors.

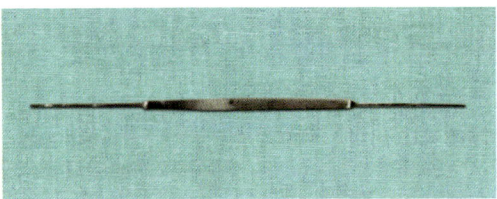

Fig. 5.9.16: Dastoor iris repositor.

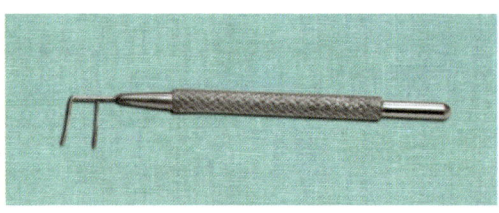

Fig. 5.9.18: Harms trabeculotome.

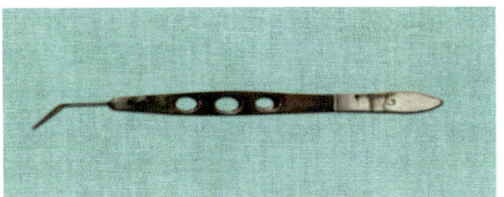

Fig. 5.9.17: McPherson's forceps.

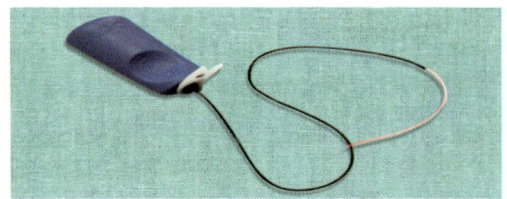

Fig. 5.9.19: Illuminated microcatheter.

DASTOOR IRIS REPOSITOR

It is a flat and straight/curved blade with blunt edges used for repositioning the iris back in the anterior chamber. In trabeculectomy, it can be used to send the iris back after iridotomy to prevent ostium from block **(Fig. 5.9.16)**.

KELMAN-MCPHERSON FORCEPS

It is a fine sharp tipped nontoothed forceps with angulation to hold sutures while tying. Also, can be used for mitomycin application or holding conjunctiva **(Fig. 5.9.17)**.

HARMS TRABECULOTOME

It is of both sides, right sided and left sided. This instrument is used to manually catheterize the Schlemm's canal for about 120° approximately (trabeculotomy) along with trabeculectomy **(Fig. 5.9.18)**.

ILLUMINATED MICROCATHETER

It is used for 360° catheterization of the Schlemm's canal. It has an atraumatic tip for smooth passage along with an illumination source at the tip, which acts as a guide through the canal **(Fig. 5.9.19)**.

CHAPTER 6

Squint and Neuro-Ophthalmology

6.1 HESS CHART/LEES SCREEN

Ritu Nagpal, Mousumi Bannerjee, Anin Sethi, Pallavi Singh

■ INTRODUCTION

A Hess chart is plotted to aid in the diagnosis and monitoring of a patient with incomitant strabismus, such as an extraocular muscle palsy (e.g., third, fourth, or sixth nerve paresis) or a mechanical or myopathic limitation (e.g., thyroid ophthalmopathy, blowout fracture, or myasthenia gravis).[1]

The chart is commonly prepared using either the Lees or Hess screen, which facilitates plotting of the dissociated ocular position as a measure of extraocular muscle action.

Information provided by the Hess chart should be regarded in the context of other investigations such as the field of binocular single vision (BSV).

Following points must be remembered:
- *Principle:* It is based on the haploscopic principle. Here two targets are projected, examiner points one target and the subject is asked to superimpose it with the point **(Fig. 6.1.1)**.
- Both Hering's law of equal innervation and Sherrington's law of reciprocal innervation are utilized in this test:[2]
  • *Hering's law of equal innervation*: An equal and simultaneous innervation flows from the brain to the pair of

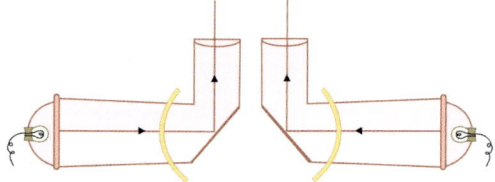

Fig. 6.1.1: Haploscopic principle.

muscles of both eyes (yoke muscle), which contract simultaneously in different binocular movements.
  • Sherrington's law of reciprocal innervation states that "When a muscle contracts, its direct antagonist relaxes to an equal extent allowing smooth movement".
- *Dissociation of two eyes is through colors.*
- *Prerequisites for testing*: Patient should have the following:
  • A proper understanding of the procedure
  • Patient's visual acuity must be good.
  • Patient must have a central fixation.
  • Normal retinal correspondence (NRC)

■ HESS SCREEN

- The Hess screen **(Fig. 6.1.2)** contains a tangent pattern displayed on a dark-gray background.

- Next, the goggles are changed.
- Red points of lights are illuminated at selected positions on the screen.
- The patient is instructed to match these points using a green pointer.
- If the patient is orthophoric, the red and green lights superimpose in all the positions of gaze.
- The goggles are then reversed and the procedure repeated.

LEES SCREEN

- It consists of two opalescent glass screens positioned at 90° to each other. Dissociation of the eyes is achieved by a two-sided plane mirror that bisects these two screens **(Figs. 6.1.3A to C)**.
- Each of the eyes can see only one of the two screens.
- Each screen has a tangent pattern, which is revealed only when the screen is illuminated.
- The patient faces the nonilluminated screen.
- The chin positioned over the chin rest.
- Using a pointer, the examiner indicates a target point on the illuminated tangent pattern and the patient places the pointer on the nonilluminated screen, at a position supposed to be superimposed on the spot pointed by the examiner.
- The nonilluminated screen is briefly illuminated by the examiner using a footswitch to facilitate recording of the dot indicated by the patient.
- When the procedure has been completed for one eye, the patient is rotated through 90° to face the previously illuminated screen and the procedure repeated.

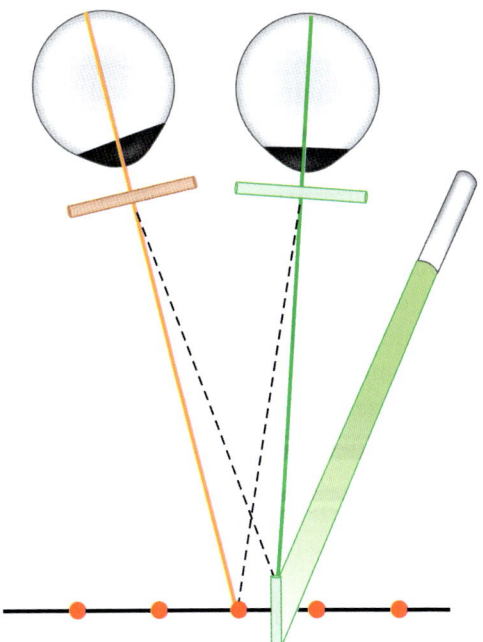

Fig. 6.1.2: Hess charting.

- The cardinal positions are indicated by use of red lights that can be illuminated through a control panel.
- The cardinal positions are illuminated both in the central (which is 15° from the primary position) as well as the peripheral field (30°).
- Within the screen, each square represents 5° of ocular rotation.
- The testing procedure includes:
  - The test is performed with each eye fixating in turn.
  - It is done at 50 cm.
  - The patient wears red and green glasses. The eyes are dissociated by the use of reversible goggles incorporating a red and a green lens, the red lens in front of the fixating eye and the green lens on the nonfixating eye.
  - Green glass is placed over the eye to be tested.
  - The chart has electronically operated board with small red lights.

INTERPRETATION

- The eye with paretic muscle is represented by the smaller chart **(Figs. 6.1.4 to 6.1.8)**,

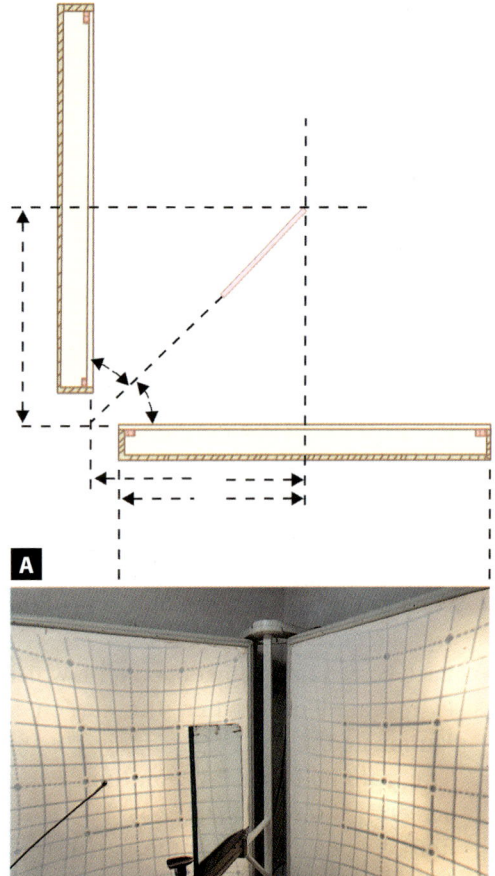

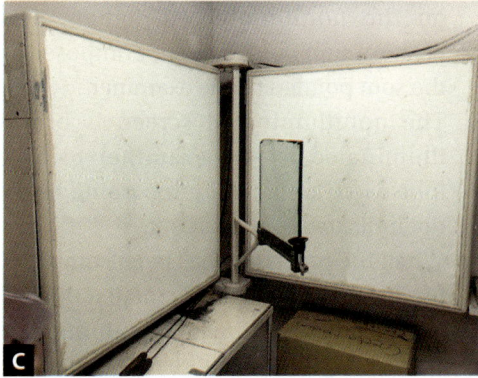

Figs. 6.1.3A to C: Lees screen.

while the eye with overacting yoke muscle is represented by the larger chart.
- The maximum restriction will be seen in the smaller chart along the direction of action of the paretic muscle while maximum expansion will be seen in the larger chart along action of the yoke muscle.
- In comitant deviation, the fields are of similar size and shape while in case of incomitant deviation it varies in shape and size.
- *If compressed, consider mechanical causes.*
- The angle of deviation is measured by the difference between the plotted point and the template in any position of gaze.

■ VIVA QUESTIONS

1. Can the Hess/Lees chart be used in all types of strabismus?
Ans. It is useful in incomitant strabismus only.

2. What is the difference between Hess screen and Lees screen?
Ans. See text, the fundamental difference is in the method of dissociation. While in Hess chart the dissociation is achieved by using color glasses; in case of Lees screen it is achieved by the use of a bisecting two-sided plane mirror bisecting the two opalescent glass screens placed at right angles to each other, bisected by a two-sided plane mirror.

3. What are the uses of Hess chart?
Ans. The uses of Hess chart are:
- To monitor progress
- Treatment plan
- Evaluating the results of incomitant strabismus

4. Is Hess chart alone useful for assessing incomitant strabismus?
Ans. No, it has to be interpreted along with other tests.

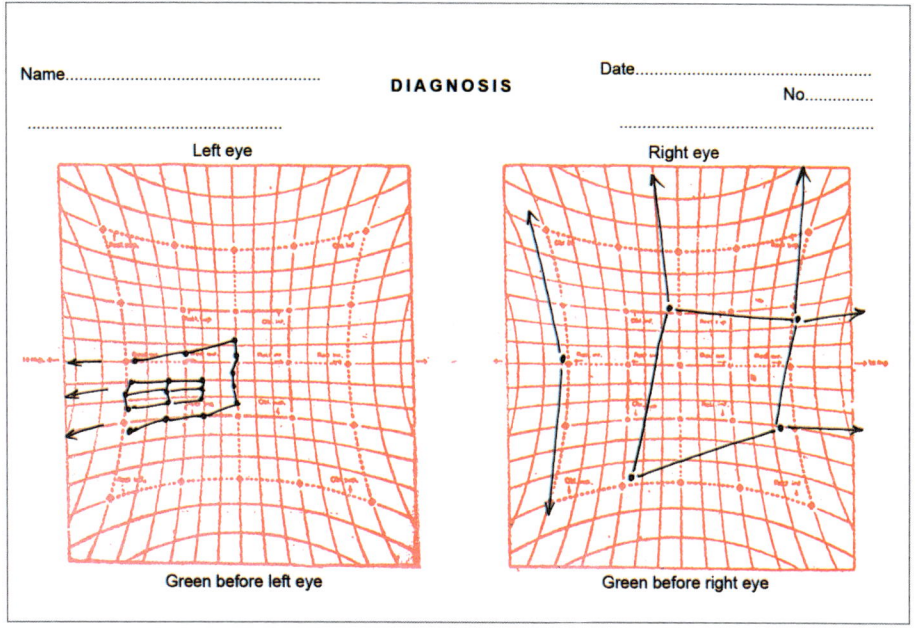

Fig. 6.1.4: Hess chart of left third nerve palsy. Note the underaction of superior rectus, medial rectus, inferior rectus and inferior oblique, and overaction of ipsilateral antagonist lateral rectus and superior oblique.

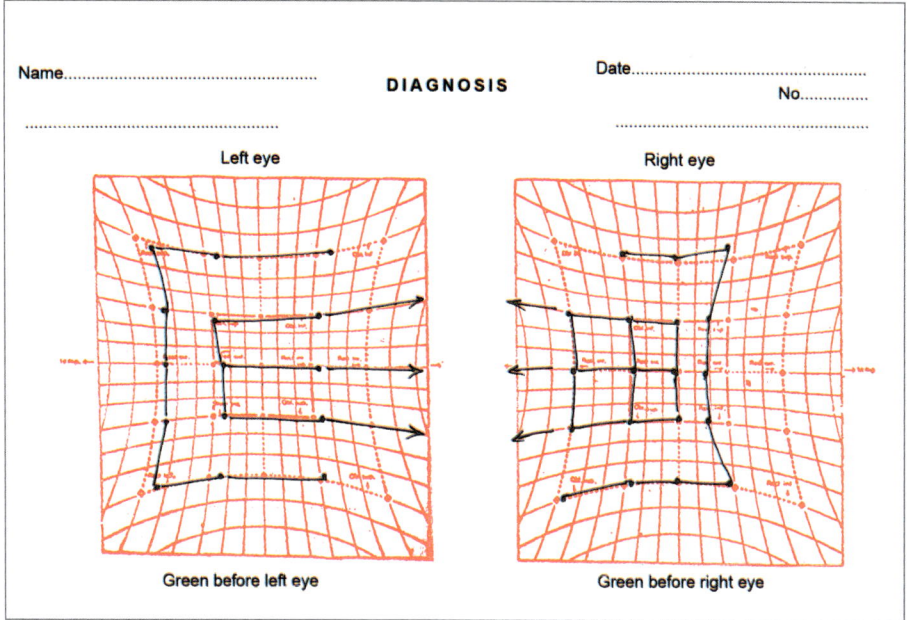

Fig. 6.1.5: Hess chart of right sixth nerve palsy. Note the underaction of lateral rectus, overaction of medial rectus and overaction of the contralateral yoke, medial rectus.

SECTION 1: Appliances and Instruments

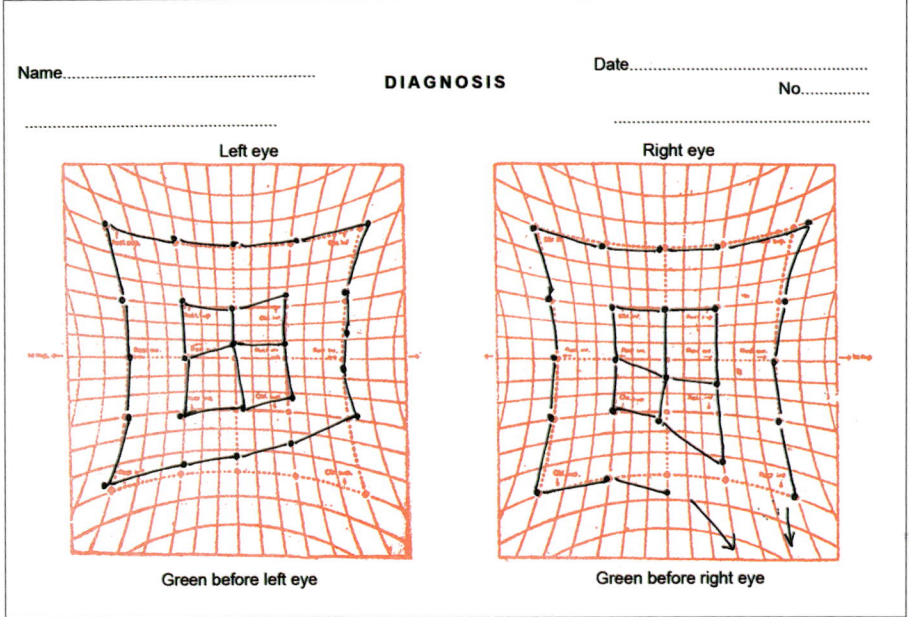

Fig. 6.1.6: Hess chart of left superior oblique palsy. Note underaction in the direction of action of superior oblique (depression in adduction) and overaction of ipsilateral antagonist inferior oblique, causing overelevation in adduction. Also note the overaction of contralateral yoke muscles.

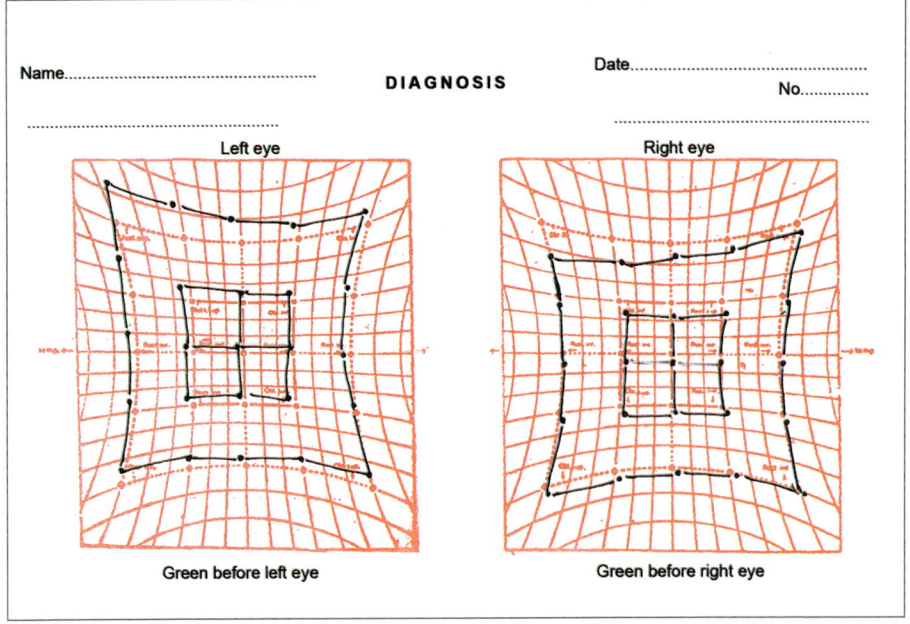

Fig. 6.1.7: Hess chart of right Brown's syndrome, which is characterized by limitation of elevation in adduction, with normal elevation in abduction and divergence in upgaze.

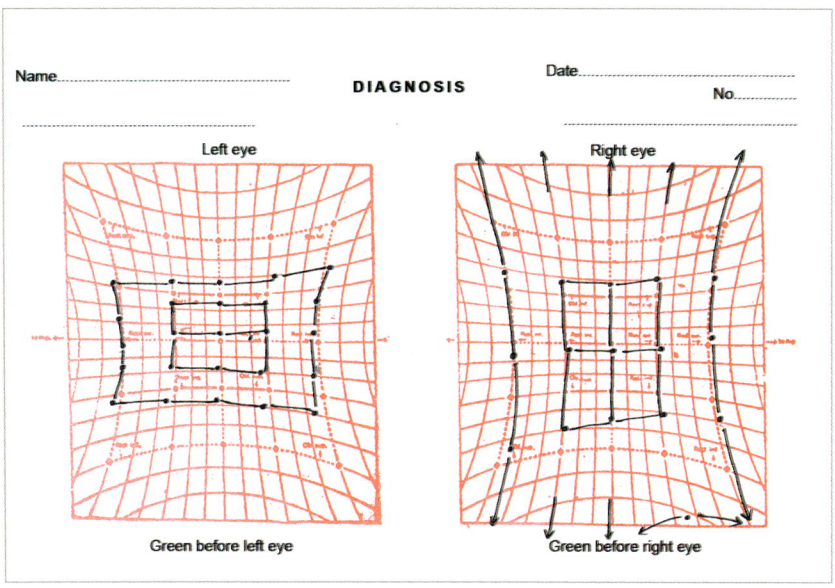

Fig. 6.1.8: Hess chart of orbital flow fracture.

5. What are the prerequisites for using the Hess charts?
Ans. Refer to text.

6. What does the shape of the Hess chart indicate?
Ans. A charts with sloping edges points to A or V pattern.

7. What happens to Hess chart over time?
Ans. It becomes uniform.

8. What does a compressed chart suggest?
Ans. Mechanical cause.

9. How can the amount of deviation be measured with Hess chart?
Ans. The amount of deviation can be calculated by measuring the gap between the pointer and the dot, taking into consideration that each small square subtends an angle of 5°. The torsional measurements can be calculated by using a specially adapted linear pointer.

10. What is the clinical significance of the outer field?
Ans. The outer field is useful in the detection of a small amount of incomitant strabismus where the central field can be normal.

11. Original Hess chart.
Ans. The original Hess chart consisted of a black cloth of 80 × 80 cm with the tangent coordinates stitched as red embroidered dots. The pointer was 50 cm long with a green arrow at its end.[1]

12. Interpret Figure 6.1.4.
Ans. Steps to interpretation:
1. Smaller chart indicates the eye with the paretic muscle—left eye.
2. Larger chart indicates the eye with overacting yoke muscle—right eye.
3. Smaller chart shows a greater limitation in the main direction of muscle: In this case the medial rectus, superior rectus, inferior rectus, and inferior oblique (IO) of the left eye show underaction (can be noted by inward displacement of dots, therefore the whole curve).

4. An overaction of the left lateral rectus is seen (outward displacement of the dots).
5. In the larger field of right eye, maximum displacement can be seen in the primary direction of action of the contralateral synergist. Hence overaction of the all muscles can be seen except the right medial rectus and inferior rectus ("yokes" of spared muscles).
6. This is a case of left third nerve palsy.

13. Interpret Figure 6.1.5.

Ans. Steps to interpretation:
1. Both fields are similar in size this denotes that either it is a comitant squint or both eyes may be involved. The chart as mentioned above shows incomitance; hence probably both eyes are involved.
2. In both eyes, overaction of the medial rectus is seen, and underaction of lateral rectus is seen (more apparent in the outer field).
3. Also the right eye shows more underaction of the lateral rectus than the left eye.
4. This is a case of bilateral asymmetric sixth nerve palsy.

14. Interpret Figure 6.1.6.

Ans. Steps to interpretation:
1. The smaller field of the left eye denotes that the affected eye is left eye.
2. Underaction of the left eye superior oblique (SO) is noted.
3. Overaction of the ipsilateral antagonist the left IO is noted.
4. The right field shows the larger secondary deviation—right hypotropia (Hering's law) and the greatest enlargement is in the field of action of the right inferior rectus (contralateral synergist—Sherrington's law).
5. This is a case of left SO palsy.

15. Interpret Figure 6.1.7.

Ans. Steps to interpretation:
1. Hypotropia of the right eye can be seen.
2. The right eye shows impairment of elevation in adduction whereas elevation is normal in the abduction.
3. An increase in exotropia is seen in upgaze with the same amount of deviation in primary position and downgaze denoting a Y pattern.
4. This is a case of right eye Brown's syndrome.

16. Interpret Figure 6.1.8.

Ans. Steps to interpretation:
1. The smaller field of the left eye denotes that the affected eye is the left eye.
2. Left eye denotes a hypotropia with a limitation of elevation.
3. The amount of deviation increases in the upgaze or downgaze.
4. This denotes an entrapment of the left inferior rectus at the equator postorbital floor fracture of the left eye.

■ REFERENCES

1. Roper-Hall G. The Hess screen test. Am Orthopt J. 2006;56:166-74.
2. The Principles of Hess Chart. [online] Available from http://www.mrcophth.com/commonhesschart/principlesofhesschart.html [Last accessed October, 2024].

6.2 SYNOPTOPHORE

Pallavi Singh, Vatika Jain, Pranita Sahay

■ INTRODUCTION

Synoptophore, derived from the Greek language (syn = with, ops = eye, phoros = bearing), is an orthoptic instrument used for both motor and sensory evaluation of strabismus. It is also used for the nonsurgical treatment of strabismus in the form of orthoptic exercises.

■ PRINCIPLE

Synoptophore is based on the haploscopic principle, which states that *there is a division of physical space into two separate areas of visual space, each of which is visible to one eye only.*

■ HISTORY

In 1838, the first stereoscope was constructed by Sir Charles Wheatstone. Subsequently, Claud Worth made the amblyoscope, to evaluate and stimulate binocular vision. The slides used in these earlier devices for determining the extent of simultaneous perception and measuring the area of suppression were developed by MC Maddox. Nowadays, Clement Clarke's major synoptophore is the most commonly used version.

Older versions include Moorfields synoptophore, Lyle-Major amblyoscope, and Curpax-Major amblyoscope.

■ DESIGN

The instrument has a base that contains the electrical components and controls **(Fig. 6.2.1)**. Attached to the base are scales for measuring vergence movements. Supported at the base are two optical tubes that contain a light source; high-intensity light for after

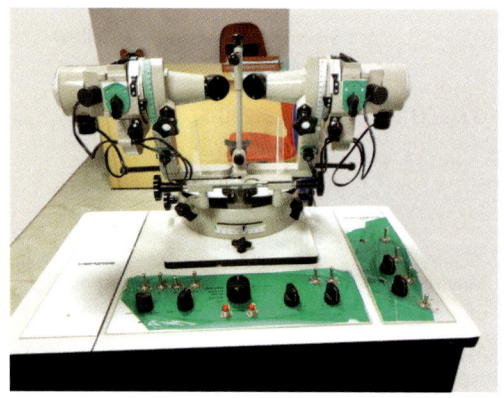

Fig. 6.2.1: Synoptophore.

image test and Haidinger's brushes and a low-intensity light; a slide carrier; various scales, and control knobs for measuring horizontal, vertical, and torsional deviations; a reflecting mirror and an eyepiece with a +6.5 D convex lens. Plus lenses in the eyepiece ensure relaxation of patient's accommodation and the image appears to come from the distance. Accommodation can be induced by placing —3 D lenses in the lens holder placed in front of the eyepiece. Degrees and prism diopters (Δ) are used as scales on the synoptophore to measure displacement.

■ USES

Diagnostic Uses

- To measure interpupillary distance (IPD)
- To measure the angle of deviation, primary and secondary deviations
- To assess anomalous retinal correspondence (ARC).
- To measure angle kappa (K), accommodative convergence/accommodation (AC/A) ratio
- To assess various grades and anomalies of binocular vision

TABLE 6.2.1: Different types of slides in synoptophore.

Series	Use	Binding
A	Maddox test	White
D	Stereoscopic vision	Yellow
F	Fusion	Green
G and H	Simultaneous perception	Red
S	Automatic flashing, after images, haidinger brushes	Blue
Mayou series of 8	Simultaneous perception	Orange

Note: The strict following of color codes for different types of slides are rarely followed nowadays.

TABLE 6.2.2: Angle subtended by different slides in synoptophore.

Slide size	Angle subtended
Foveal	1°
Macular	1°–3°
Paramacular	3°–5°
Peripheral	>5°

- To measure fusional reserve
- To assess special functions such as adaptability to function in aniseikonia with the help of special slides, appreciation of entopic phenomenon (visual effects whose source is within the eye itself) with Haidinger's brushes
- After image testing

Therapeutic Uses

- For various orthoptic exercises
- To treat convergence insufficiency
- To improve fusional reserve
- To combat suppression and ARC

TYPES OF SLIDES

A wide variety of slides are used as summarized in **Table 6.2.1**. The size of each slide has been calculated to subtend a different angle at the nodal point of the eye **(Table 6.2.2)**.

MEASUREMENTS

Interpupillary Distance Measurement

Interpupillary distance measurement is the first step before starting any measurement of strabismus. Set all the scales to zero, put the slides of foveal fixation, and ask the patient to look into the right picture with his right eye and then align the corneal reflection with the white line on the top of the tube by closing your right eye. Repeat similarly for the left eye of the subject, note down the IPD, and lock it for further measurements.

Angle of Deviation

Objective Angle of Deviation

Objective angle of deviation can be measured based on the principles of either the Hirschberg's test or the alternate cover test. The patient should be sitting comfortably and in the correct position in front of the instrument. The IPD is then adjusted, and the first-grade targets are inserted. In the Hirschberg's test, the patient looks at the center of the target slides, and the angle of slide carrier is adjusted to make corneal reflection symmetrical (in the center of the pupillary area in both eyes), and the deviation is measured. For measuring the angle of deviation by the alternate cover test, the lion or car is placed in front of the fixing eye and the cage or gate in front of the nonfixing eye. The arms are set to zero, and the patient is fixing at the center of the slide; when the fixing light in front of the fixing eye is turned off, the nonfixing eye will immediately take fixation. It will move either inwards (in exotropia), outwards (in esotropia), and upwards or downwards to take fixation. If the nonfixing eye moves out to take fixation, the arm is moved into a more convergent or less divergent position and so on for other deviations as well. The alternate flashing is continued and the tube adjusted until there is no movement in either eye on fixation. The reading on the horizontal scale and vertical scale in front of the nonfixing arm represents the objective angle of deviation.

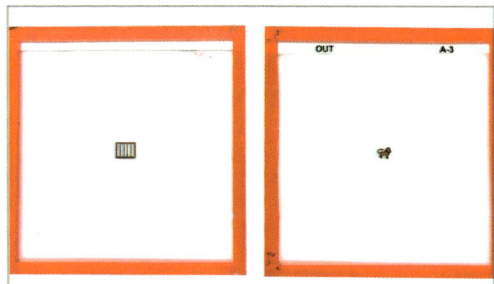

Fig. 6.2.2: Simultaneous perception slides.

Subjective Angle of Deviation

First measure the objective angle of deviation, if the patient sees superimposition (the lion in the cage) at the objective angle, it is the same as the subjective angle. If this is not the case, the patient is asked to superimpose the two slides by adjusting the angle between two slides by the handle. Reading on the scale will give the subjective angle of deviation.

Angle of Anomaly

- If subjective and objective angles of deviation are same, it is called normal retinal correspondence, and if they are different, it is called ARC.
- The difference between the subjective and objective angle of deviation is the angle of anomaly. For instance, if a patient has an objective angle of deviation of 25Δ base out (BO) and a subjective angle of 10ΔBO, his angle of anomaly is 15Δ.
- If the objective angle is equal to the angle of anomaly, i.e., subjective angle is zero, it is called a harmonious ARC.
- If objective angle exceeds the angle of anomaly, it is known as unharmonious ARC.

Measurement of Cyclodeviation

It can only be measured subjectively. Simultaneous perception slides (**Fig. 6.2.2**) are used, the patient is asked to look at each slide in turn and is asked whether the cage appears level or tilted. A cyclodeviation is present if the image appears to be tilted. If with the right eye focusing, the cage's right-hand side is lower than the left-hand side, incyclophoria or tropia is present. It is important to note that the tilt of the image is in the direction opposite to the tilt of the eye. The deviation is corrected with the torsional deviation screw and the amount of deviation is measured from the scale.

Grades of Binocular Single Vision

There are three grades (**Fig. 6.2.3**) of BSV:
1. *The first grade of BSV:* Simultaneous perception (usually red slides)
2. *The second grade of BSV:* Binocular fusion (usually green slides)
3. *The third grade of BSV:* Stereopsis (usually yellow slides)

Simultaneous Perception

Simultaneous perception is the ability to perceive two images, one formed on each retina simultaneously. The smaller picture, i.e., the lion, is kept in the slide holder in front of the fixing eye, while the bigger picture is kept in front of the fellow eye. The slides (**Fig. 6.2.4**) are designed so that the patient puts something into something, e.g., a lion in a cage. Either parafoveal, foveal, or

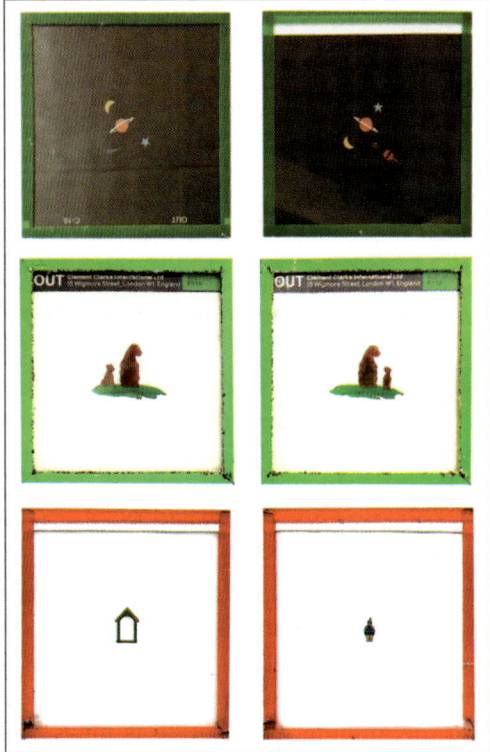

Fig. 6.2.3: Slides used for testing different grades of binocular single vision.

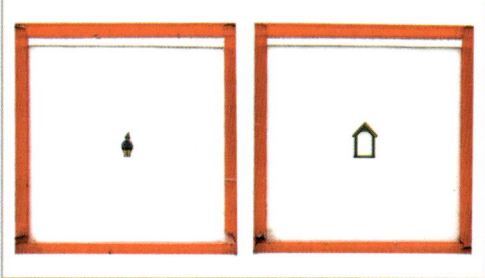

Fig. 6.2.4: Slides used for testing simultaneous perception.

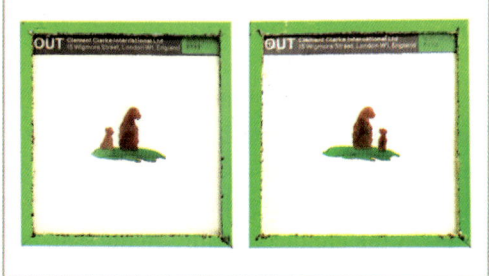

Fig. 6.2.5: Slides for testing binocular fusion.

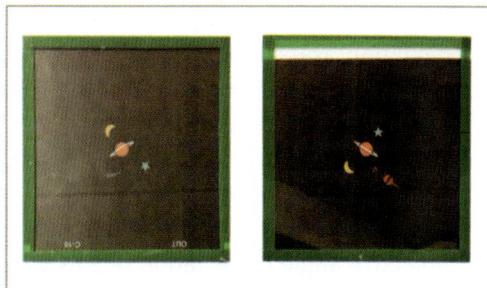

Fig. 6.2.6: Slides used to test stereopsis.

macular slides may be used. If the patient sees the lion in the cage, he is using each eye simultaneously and has a grade 1 binocular vision.

Binocular Fusion

Sensory fusion is the ability to fuse two slightly dissimilar images and perceive them as one. These consist of targets, which are mainly the same, but each has a different control on it **(Fig. 6.2.5)**. A grade 2 target will show a picture of a rabbit with no tail and clutching flowers to one eye, and the other eye will see a picture of the same rabbit, but it would have a tail, and held in its hand would be a stem without flowers. The patient has a grade 2 binocular vision if he fuses these images and confirms seeing a tailed rabbit clutching a bunch of flowers by a stem.

Stereopsis

Stereopsis is the perception of depth based on binocular image disparity. Images of the same object are hypothetically taken from slightly different angles, to denote depth perception. These slides **(Fig. 6.2.6)** have slightly disparate targets; the fusion of these minutely dissimilar images by the brain creates the perception of depth or stereopsis. If fused correctly, a three-dimensional image is perceived.

Torsion

Maddox slides (white binding) help in the assessment of nine positions of gaze. Horizontal and vertical deviations are assessed by the usual method. However, the torsional control is rotated until the patient is satisfied that it superimposes in the center of the green surroundings and all lines should run parallel.

Afterimage Test

Afterimage test is a fovea-to-fovea sensory test used to measure ARC. Special slides **(Fig. 6.2.7)** that present the retina with a linear strobe of light (one vertical and one horizontal) are used. The center of the linear strobe light is masked to spare the fovea; thus, the afterimage line has a break in the middle. Stronger 12 V lamps are used to stimulate the fovea for fixation in dense amblyopia.

Determination of Fusional Amplitudes

After determining the objective angle and presence of first and second grades of binocular vision, the examiner blocks the arms at the objective angle (divided equally between both arms). Utilizing the horizontal vergence controls, both arms are first diverged/converged (depending on whether divergence or convergence fusional amplitude is being measured) and the point of fusion breakage is noted. The arms are then reversed to a less divergent/converged position, and the point of fusion recovery is noted. The recovery point is usually 2–4 ΔD below breakpoint. Fusional amplitude should be tested slowly as vergence movements are slow and tonic.

Orthoptic Exercises

Orthoptics is the training process of an individual to obtain the best possible binocular interaction in the form of BSV. For the treatment of convergence/divergence insufficiency, fusional reserve and all grades of BSV are first assessed. Stereoscopic slides are used as they are the strongest stimulation for fusion. The patient first fuses the slides; tubes are then converged until the patient can sustain fusion; when diplopia occurs, the patient is asked to try to fuse the images. This exercise is continued for 5 minutes at each weekly visit, and the patient is given a home exercise in the form of pencil convergence exercise and physiological diplopia exercise (stereogram card) before he comes for the next visit.

Haidinger Brushes

The concept of Haidinger brushes was first described in 1844 by Austrian physicist Wilhelm Karl von Haidinger. It is an entoptic phenomenon appreciated by macula (entoptic phenomenon are visual responses generating from within the eye). It appears as an hourglass pattern subtending the angle of 3° on macula.

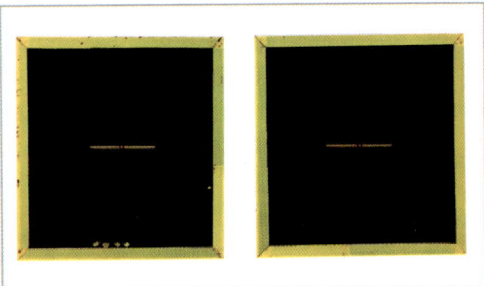

Fig. 6.2.7: Slides used for afterimage testing.

It is used for the treatment and diagnosis of eccentric fixation. It was also used for amblyopia management in adjunct to occlusion.

The normal eye of patient is occluded. A rotating polarized plate backlit with a bright light is projected in front of the eccentric eye. The pattern is shown in clockwise and anticlockwise direction. The speed of the brushes is eventually increased.

The patient appreciates the Haidinger brush with his macula and then looks at the test object in such a way that the Haidinger brush overlaps the test object.

■ VIVA QUESTIONS

1. **Grades of binocularity and their age of development.**
Ans. Refer to text.

2. **Principle of synoptophore.**
Ans. Refer to text.

3. **Amblyopia therapy on synoptophore.**
Ans. Amblyopia therapy is performed on synoptophore using Haidinger brushes.

4. **What is "instrument convergence"?**
Ans. Even though targets are placed at optical infinity in the synoptophore by using +6.0 D or +6.5 D lenses in the eyepiece, proximal convergence comes into play while measuring deviations (especially horizontal) and fusional vergences. This might distort the values obtained for the said measurements.

5. **Different angles.**
Ans.
- *Angle alpha:* The angle between the optical axis and the visual axis; a positive angle (corneal reflection placed nasally) leads to pseudodivergent squint; negative angle (corneal reflections placed temporally) leads to pseudoconvergent squint.
- *Angle gamma:* The angle between the axis and the fixation axis
- *Angle kappa:* The angle between the midpupillary line and visual axis

6.3 TESTS FOR BINOCULAR VISION AND STEREOPSIS

Pallavi Singh, Shreya Nayak, Pranita Sahay

■ TEST FOR BINOCULAR VISION

Bagolini Glasses

- Most physiological test for binocularity
- The striated glasses have striations at 45° and 135° (**Fig. 6.3.1A**).
- A point source of light is shown to the patient.
- The glasses convert a point source of light into a straight light. The following responses can be obtained (**Figs. 6.3.1B to E**).
- *Symmetrical cross response:* Seen normally in the absence of manifest squint; in patients with manifest squint a symmetrical cross response suggests harmonious ARC.
- *Diplopia response* is seen in case of manifest squint without suppression.
- *Suppression* absence of any one slant line is seen in case of suppression.
- *Central scotoma:* A central scotoma can be seen in case of fixation point scotoma in manifest squint with ARC.

■ MADDOX ROD TEST

Double Maddox rod test is similar to the Bagolini's test, here Maddox rod is used.

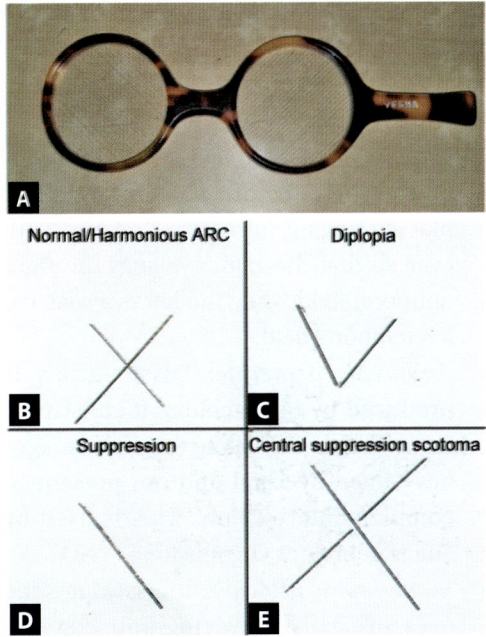

Figs. 6.3.1A to E: (A) Bagolini glasses; (B to E) responses obtained. (ARC: anomalous retinal correspondence)

A Maddox rod has multiple cylinders to convert a point source of light to a straight line.

Maddox rods are placed in horizontal and vertical orientations and a point source of light is shown to the patient. The patient perceives the point source of light as a straight line.

WORTH FOUR-DOT TEST— RED–GREEN GLASSES

The test uses red–green glasses for dissociation of the two eyes. It is done at a distance of 6 m.

The chart consists of four colored dots. Two green on either side, one red on top, and white below **(Figs. 6.3.2A to E)**. The patient is made to wear the red glass before right eye and green glass before the left eye. The following responses can be seen.

Four dots: In normal binocular response without squint, all four dots are seen.

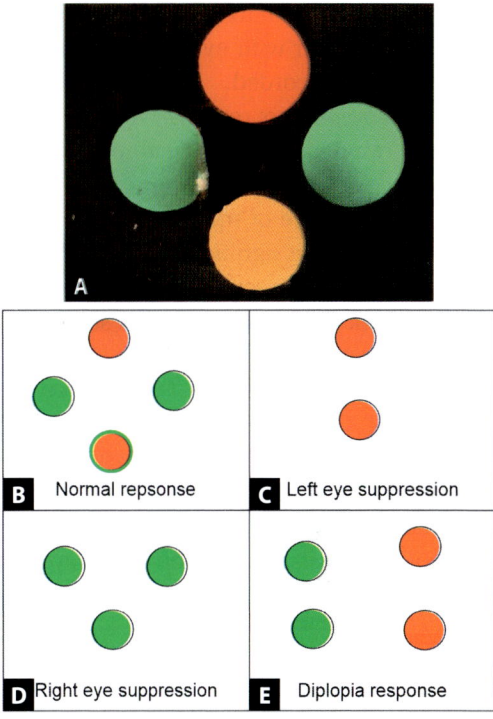

Figs. 6.3.2A to E: (A) Worth four-dot test; (B to E) responses obtained.

In the presence of manifest deviation, this response suggests harmonious ARC.

Five dots: This response is obtained in patients with manifest deviation with NRC without suppression. Patient sees three green dots and two red dots.

Presence of either two red dots or three green dots: In patients with right eye suppression only three green dots are seen and patient with left eye suppression sees two red dots.

AFTERIMAGE TEST

- The foveae of both eyes are stimulated with straight line, horizontal for right eye and vertical for left eye.
- Central portion is black to provide fixation and to protect the fovea.

- Patient then visualizes the afterimage in a darkroom or with eyes closed and the response is recorded.
- *Symmetrical cross response:* Symmetrical cross response is the normal response in absence of squint.
- In the presence of squint a symmetrical cross response signifies normal bifoveal fixation. Irrespective of the type of deviation, symmetrical cross is seen with normal retinal correspondence (NRC).
- *Asymmetrical crossing:* This is seen in cases of ARC. The amount of separation between the two lines gives the subjective angle of deviation.
- *Single line response:* If any one line is absent, then it suggests suppression of that eye.

SYNAPTOPHORE

Discussed in detail in the **Part 6.2**.

STEREOPSIS DEFINITION

Stereopsis is defined as the relative positioning of visual objects in depth, i.e., in the third dimension.

PHYSIOLOGIC BASIS OF STEREOPSIS

Wheatstone in 1838 was the first to understand that stereopsis occurs when horizontally disparate retinal elements are stimulated simultaneously and the fused image lies within the Panum's area of single binocular vision. Vertical displacement produces no stereopsis.

Stereopsis is lacking in infants <3 months of age, and develops to adult levels by about the 6th month of life.

PRINCIPLE OF TESTS FOR STEREOPSIS

As a principle, all tests for stereopsis provide disparate images to each eye. They fundamentally differ in their methodology of dissociating the two images. The commonly used dissociation methodologies are described below:

- *Haploscopic principle:* Used in synoptophore where the dissociation occurs by placing angled mirrors in front of both eyes so that the right eye sees the right temporal field while the left eye sees the left temporal field.
- *Anaglyph principle:* Dissociation is produced by using colors. It consists of stereograms in which the half images have been overlaid and are present in complementary colors. This is used by The Netherlands Organization (TNO).
- *Vectographic principle:* It dissociates the eyes optically. A vectograph consists of Polaroid material on which two stereopaired images are etched in such a way that each target is polarized 90° with reference to the other. This is used in titmus fly test and Randot stereopsis test. It avoids the color tint annoyance as seen in anaglyph.
- *Panographic principle:* At times, children do not comply with wearing polaroid or red–green glasses, and it is needed to observe the position of the eyes while the patient is being tested. To overcome this, Lang reported a real-time stereogram where a different image is provided to each eye through cylindrical lamination/gratings on the surface of stereoscopic random dot plates used in Lang test.

TESTS FOR NEAR STEREOACUITY

The Netherlands Organization Test

- Based on anaglyph principle[1]
- *Equipment:* Seven plates booklet **(Fig. 6.3.3)** and red-green spectacles **(Fig. 6.3.4)**

CHAPTER 6: Squint and Neuro-Ophthalmology

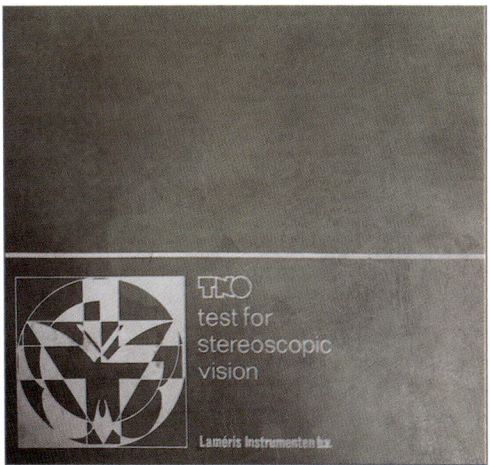

Fig. 6.3.3: The Netherlands Organization (TNO) test, seven plates booklet.

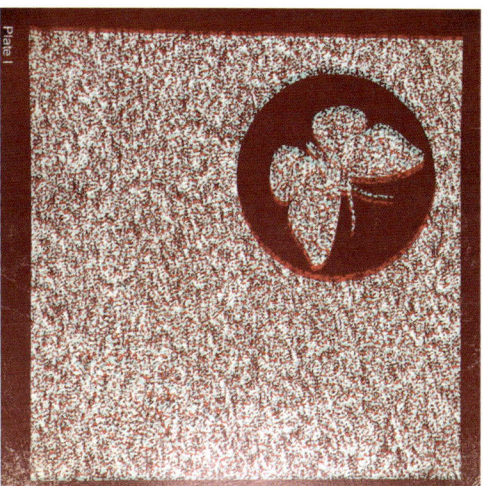

Fig. 6.3.5: The Netherlands Organization (TNO) plate I—two butterflies are present, one can be seen monocularly and the other is only seen in stereopsis.

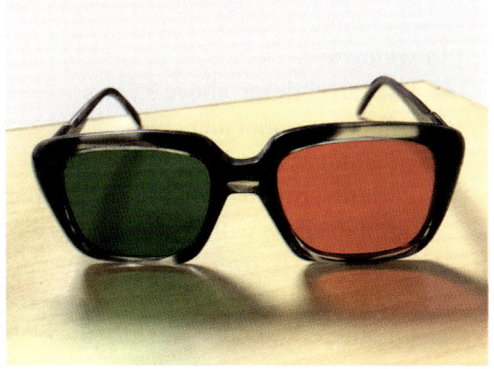

Fig. 6.3.4: Red–green spectacles.

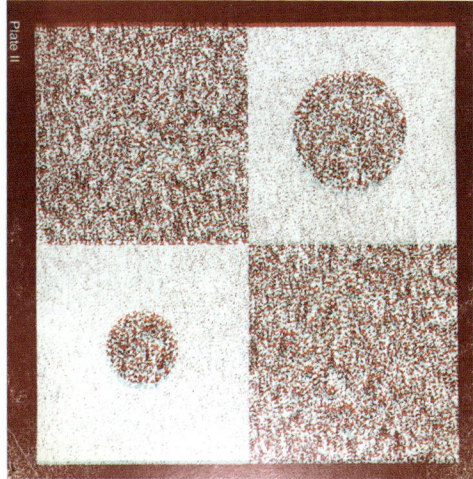

Fig. 6.3.6: The Netherlands Organization (TNO) plate II—four discs, two are seen monocularly and two require stereopsis.

- *Seven plates with test figures:*[2]
  - *Plates I-III*, screening plates, to establish gross stereopsis, tells if stereopsis is present or not **(Figs. 6.3.5 to 6.3.7)**
  - *Plate IV* is a suppression test **(Fig. 6.3.8)**
  - *Plates V-VII* are for quantitative examination for exact determination of stereoacuity **(Figs. 6.3.9A to C)**
- *Method:* Plates are presented at 40 cm from the subject, well-lit room
- *Advantage:*
  - Can be used in children (2.5–5 years)
- *Disadvantages:*
  - Tests only near stereoacuity.
  - Color tint annoyance

Titmus Stereotest

- Based on vectographic principle that uses crossed polarized filters located at the axis of 45° and 135° in front of either eye

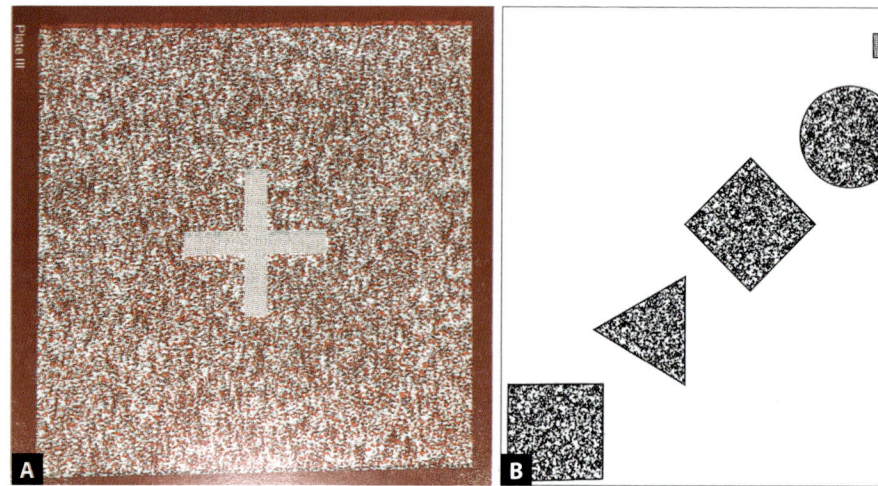

Figs. 6.3.7A and B: The Netherlands Organization (TNO) plate III—four hidden shapes (O, □, Δ, ∨) are arranged around a centrally placed cross. The child is first asked to look at one of the example in the opposite page (B) and find the corresponding one in the test plate (A).

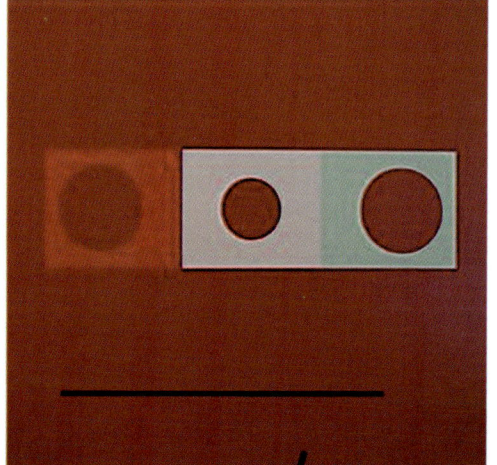

Fig. 6.3.8: The Netherlands Organization (TNO) plate IV—this is a suppression test. There are three discs, one seen by the right eye, one by the left, and one is seen binocularly.

- *Equipment:* Stereo housefly card or circles or animal test plates, and polarized glasses
- Children can be asked to touch the wings of the fly.
- *Uses:* For screening and fine depth perception in strabismus

- *Advantages:*
  - Used in children above 3 years
  - Offers no monocular clues
- *Disadvantages:*
  - Patients might choose the correct animal/circle without seeing stereoscopically. To overcome this, they are asked to see it monocularly and asked for difference or one can turn the plate vertically by 90°, which would block the stereoscopic effect.
  - Only tests for near stereoacuity.

Stereo Butterfly Test

Equipment: Like titmus fly test but it has a hidden configuration of a butterfly.

Randot Stereotest

- Randot stereotest **(Fig. 6.3.10)** is based on vectographic principle. The arrangement of dots eliminates monocular cues for stereopsis. However, the introduction of shapes and form in the random dots facilitates global stereopsis. This allows for elimination of false results, which

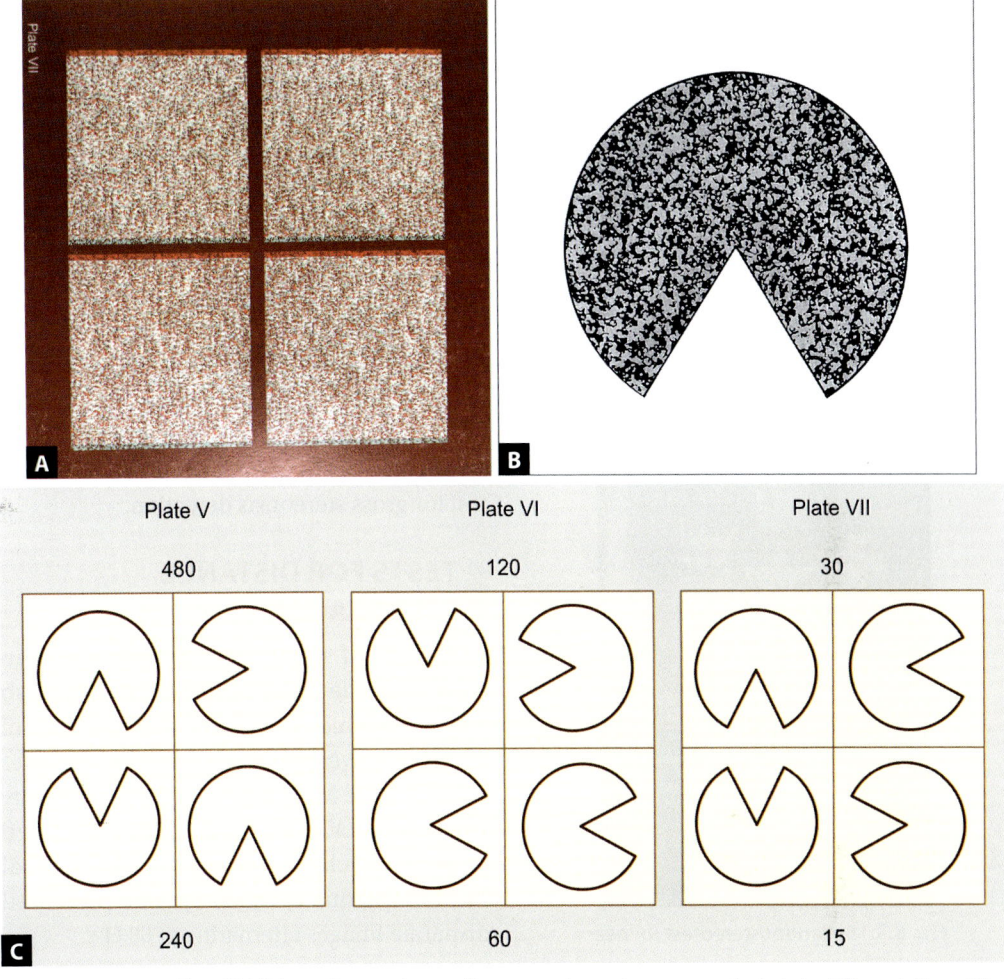

Figs. 6.3.9A to C: Plate V–VII here the test items (Pac-man shapes) are presented at six different disparities ranging from 15 to 480 seconds of arc.

can be produced by correspondence of ambiguous localized areas within the Panum's area.
- It evaluates the depth perception by requiring patients to identify six geometric forms from random dot backgrounds (500–20 seconds of arc) **(Figs. 6.3.11A and B)**.[3]
- Random dot patterns necessitate the person to recognize images from a background. The distance between the image and background in question does not affect the judgment of the individual, as both are in immediate juxtaposition.
- The test images can be recognized only with polarized three-dimensional (3D) viewing glasses **(Fig. 6.3.12)**.
- It consists of the graded circle test (400–20 seconds of arc) and animal test for children (400–100 seconds of arc) **(Fig. 6.3.13; Tables 6.3.1 and 6.3.2)**.
- *Equipment:* Plates with random dot stereograms

- *Uses*: Screening and fine depth perception in strabismus.
- *Advantages*:
  - Used in children above 3 years of age
  - Offers no monocular clues
- *Disadvantage:* Only tests near stereoacuity.

Lang Test

- Based on panographic presentation of a plate on random dot pattern
- Two types have been described:

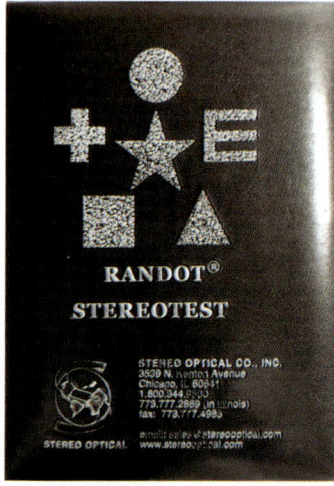

Fig. 6.3.10: Randot stereotest for near.

1. Lang stereotest I with a star, a cat, and a car **(Fig. 6.3.14)**; children as young as 6 months of age can be tested, as the child looks at a particular form helping us to draw the inference.
2. Lang stereotest II is performed with a moon, a truck, and an elephant.

Lang Two-Pencil Test

No equipment is needed in this test. The patient is asked to hold a pencil in his hand and asked to touch the pencil tip-to-tip in the examiner's hand rapidly. This test has 100% sensitivity. It is frequently used as a screening test for gross stereopsis detection.

TESTS FOR DISTANCE STEREOACUITY

Two types of stereo tests were available in older days, the first one being AO vectograph stereotest, which was dissociating because of the need to wear polarized glasses. The latter one being the Mentor Binocular Visual Acuity Testing (BVAT) system, a computerized system, which contained a liquid crystal shutter aperture for each eye and presented disparate images alternating at 60 Hz.

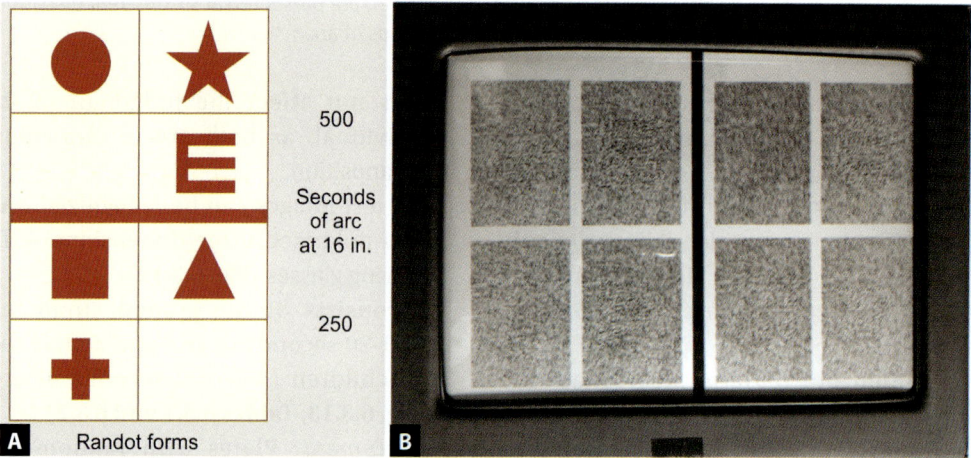

Figs. 6.3.11A and B: Identify six geometric forms (A) from background dots and (B) in Randot stereotest.

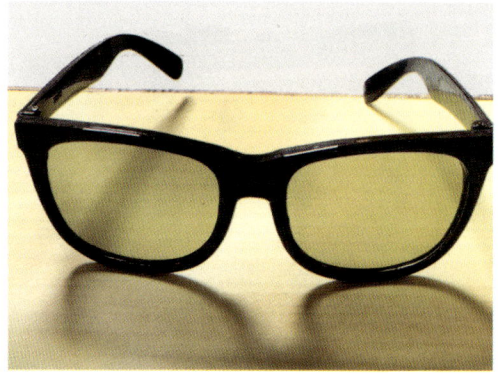

Fig. 6.3.12: Polarized three-dimensional viewing glasses for Randot stereotest.

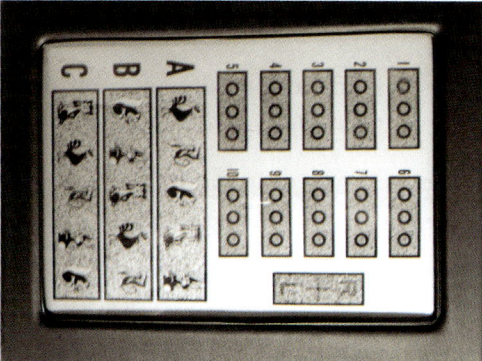

Fig. 6.3.13: Graded circle and animals of Randot stereotest.

TABLE 6.3.1: Graded circle interpretation of Randot stereotest.

	Scoring key	Seconds of arc at 16 in.
1	L	400
2	R	200
3	L	140
4	M	100
5	R	70
6	M	50
7	L	40
8	R	30
9	M	25
10	R	20

Both these tests have become obsolete now. Currently used tests include **(Tables 6.3.3 and 6.3.4)**:

TABLE 6.3.2: Animal test interpretation of Randot stereotest.

Scoring key	Seconds of arc at 16 in.	Shepard percentage	Verhoff distance
A Cat	400	15%	0.1
B Rabbit	200	30%	0.2
C Monkey	100	50%	0.3

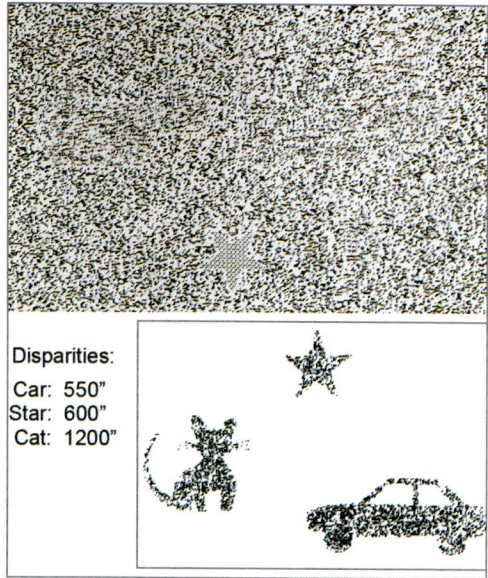

Fig. 6.3.14: Lang's stereotest I consisting of a card with pictures of a cat, a star, and a car.

- *Frisby–Davis distance test*:
  - This is a test to evaluate real depth in a free space and was designed by JP Frisby and H Davis **(Fig. 6.3.15)**.
- *Equipment*: Box containing four back illuminated various plastic objects mounted on rods pointing towards the observer. They are all translucent but also opaque enough to cover the rods giving the shapes a free-floating appearance **(Fig. 6.3.13)**.
- *Advantages*:
  - Can be used in children 3 years and above

TABLE 6.3.3: Grade of stereopsis in different tests.

Test	Grade of stereopsis (unit-second of arc)
Titmus fly test	• Fly: 3,500 • Graded circle test: 800-40 • Animal test: 400, 200, 100
The Netherlands Organization (TNO) test	15–480
Stereo Butterfly test	• Upper wings: 2,000 • Lower wings: 1,150 • Abdomen: 700
Random dot test	400–20
Lang stereo I	• Car: 550 • Star: 600 • Cat: 1,200
Lang stereo II	• Moon: 200 • Truck: 400 • Elephant: 600
Lang two-pencil	3,000–5,000
Synoptophore	720–90

TABLE 6.3.4: Grade of stereopsis for distance.

Test	Grade of stereopsis (unit-second of arc)
Frisby–Davis distance stereotest	5–50s at 6 m
Distance Randot test	400–60

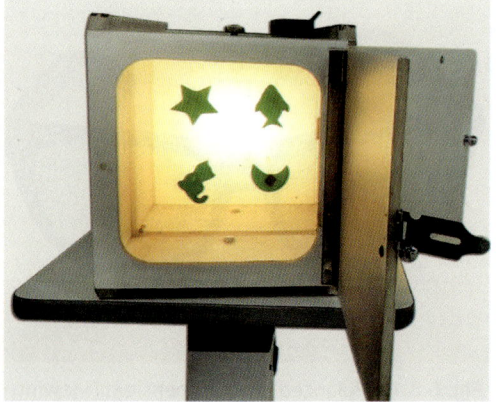

Fig. 6.3.15: Frisby–Davis stereoacuity test for distance.

- Repeated testing possible without the patient guessing
- Possible to teach the patients before the test
- Not using stereograms or any polarized/tinted glasses, which may break fusion
- *Distance Randot test:*
  - Similar to near vectographic Randot test
  - *Advantages*:
    - Gives no monocular clues
    - Worsening of distance stereoacuity in patients with intermittent exotropia is an indicator of poor control and necessitates early surgery.

NEWER ADVANCES IN STEREOACUITY TESTS

Three-dimensional Testing

Computer-based 3D images are shown both at near and at a distance, in front (conventional) and behind (proposed) the background image on a 3D monitor. It was also combined with liquid-crystal display (LCD) type shutter glasses to separate the stereoscopic images.

REFERENCES

1. Om Tao (2018). TNO Anaglyph Stereo Test. [online] Available from http://www.omtao.in/product/tno-anaglyph-stereo-test/ [Last accessed October, 2024].
2. Good-Lite. TNO Anaglyph Stereo Test. [online] Available from https://www.good-lite.com/cw3/Assets/documents/884TNO%20Instructions-web.pdf [Last accessed February 2019].
3. Stereo Optical (2018). Randot® Stereotest. [online] Available from https://www.stereooptical.com/products/stereotests-color-tests/randot/ [Last accessed October, 2024].

6.4 INSTRUMENTS FOR SQUINT SURGERY

Pranita Sahay, Devesh Kumawat, Divya Agarwal, Karthika Bhaskaran

SELF-RETAINING BARRAQUER EYE SPECULUM (FIG. 6.4.1)

This lid speculum has a screw that helps in giving desired exposure of the surgical site, which can be changed as per the surgery or surgeon's choice.

The disadvantage is that the screw increases pressure over the eyeball and thereby increases the intraocular pressure. Hence it is not advisable in perforated cases.

Uses

- All intraocular surgeries such as cataract surgery, glaucoma surgery, keratoplasty, buckling, and other vitreoretinal surgery.
- Extraocular surgeries such as squint surgery and pterygium removal.
- Removal of conjunctival and corneal foreign body.
- Examination of children and patients with severe blepharospasm.

Artery (Hemostatic) Forceps (Fig. 6.4.2)

It is a blunt-tipped forceps with multiple serrations near the tip and a locking mechanism near the other end. It is available in various sizes small, medium, and large. The small-sized forceps are called mosquito forceps and are the most commonly used variety in ophthalmic surgeries.

Uses

- Holding the bleeders during surgery
- To crush the muscle before cutting in squint surgery

GREEN'S HOOK (FIG. 6.4.3)

Green's hook has a straight shaft with flat-ended, hooked tip. It is used for hooking the muscle during squint or enucleation surgery.

JAMESON'S HOOK (FIG. 6.4.4)

Jameson's hook has a straight shaft with flat hooked end and paddle-shaped tip. It is used for retrieving the rectus muscles at their insertion site during squint or enucleation surgery.

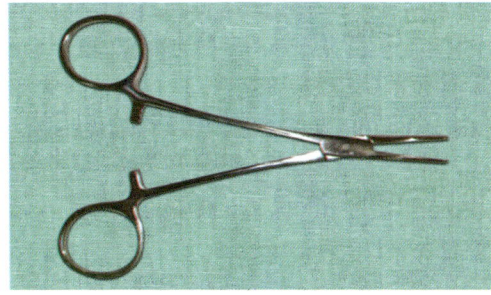

Fig. 6.4.2: Artery (hemostatic) forceps.

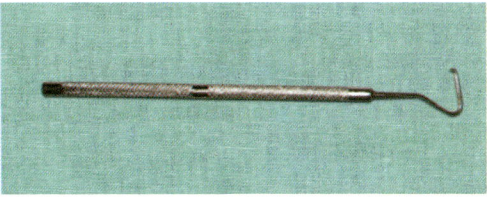

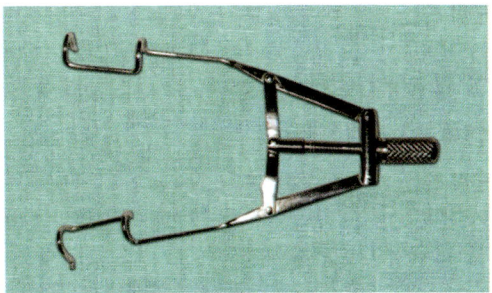

Fig. 6.4.1: Self-retaining Barraquer eye speculum.

Fig. 6.4.3: Green's hook.

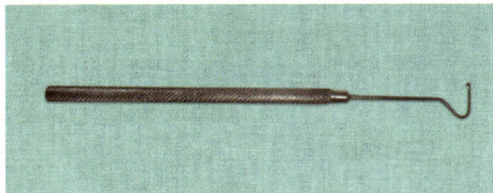

Fig. 6.4.4: Jameson's hook.

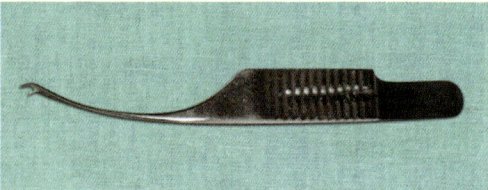

Fig. 6.4.7: Colibri forceps.

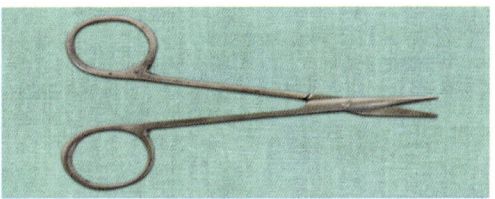

Fig. 6.4.5: Stevens tenotomy scissors.

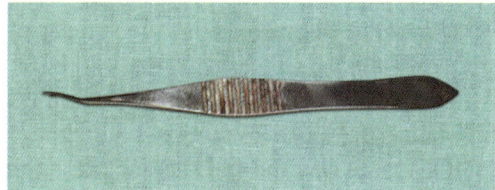

Fig. 6.4.8: Lim's forceps

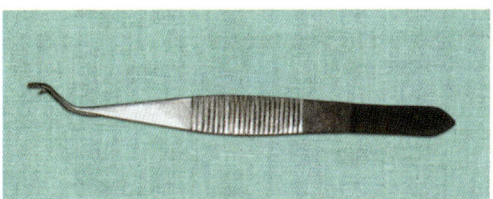

Fig. 6.4.6: Superior rectus holding forceps.

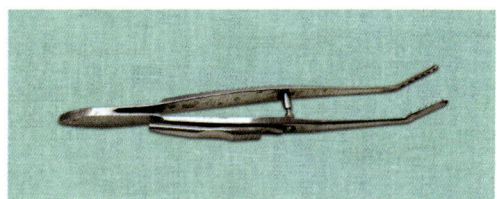

Fig. 6.4.9: Jameson muscle forceps.

PLAIN STRAIGHT SCISSORS/ PLAIN CURVED SCISSORS/ STEVENS TENOTOMY SCISSORS (FIGS. 6.4.5)

Stevens tenotomy scissors is a plain scissors with blunt end and comes in two designs: Straight and curved.

Uses

- For cutting the muscle
- For blunt dissection of the soft tissue in squint and oculoplasty procedures

SUPERIOR RECTUS HOLDING FORCEPS (FIG. 6.4.6)

This is a toothed forceps with "S"-shaped curve specially designed to fit into the orbit while trying to grasp the muscle belly.

COLIBRI FORCEPS (FIG. 6.4.7)

Colibri forceps is a fine-toothed forceps for holding flaps of cornea or sclera and rarely the iris.

LIM'S FORCEPS (FIG. 6.4.8)

Lim's forceps is also a toothed forceps for holding the cornea or sclera and rarely the iris.

JAMESON MUSCLE FORCEPS (FIG. 6.4.9)

Jameson muscle forceps has a flat, serrated handle with a side lock, and four teeth in one jaw that fit into holes in the opposing jaw. It is used to clamp the muscle before resection.

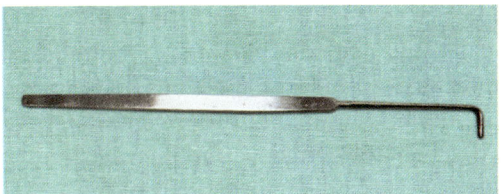

Fig. 6.4.10: Von Graefe hook.

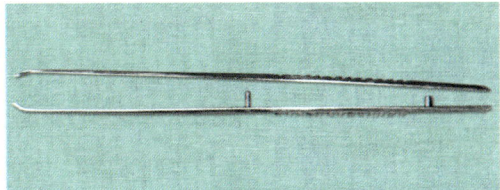

Fig. 6.4.11: Pierse Hoskin forceps/Globe fixation forceps.

VON GRAEFE HOOK/LENS HOOK (FIG. 6.4.10)

This is used as an alternative to muscle hook or to retract the conjunctiva during squint surgery.

PIERSE HOSKIN FORCEPS/GLOBE FIXATION FORCEPS (FIG. 6.4.11)

Toothed tip of the forceps helps to provide better grip for holding the tissues.

Uses

- Holds muscle stump, episcleral tissue and conjunctiva near limbus.
- For holding the globe during forced duction test (FDT)

VIVA QUESTIONS

1. What are the complications of squint surgery?

Ans. Intraoperative:
- Intraoperative bleed
- Scleral perforation
- Splitting of muscle fibers
- Lost muscle/slipped muscle
- Oculocardiac reflex

Postoperative:
- Diplopia
- Anterior segment ischemia
- Postoperative endophthalmitis/subconjunctival abscess
- Foreign body granuloma at the suture site
- Conjunctival inclusion cyst
- Conjunctival scarring
- Fat adherence can be caused by a violation of Tenon's capsule with prolapse of orbital fat. This causes a fibro-fatty scar leading to a restrictive strabismus.
- Corneal/scleral dellen
- Eyelid retraction or ptosis after surgery on vertical recti
- A lost muscle occurs when the muscle slips free of the sutures
- Residual/consecutive strabismus

2. What are the normal insertions of recti muscles from the limbus?

Ans.
- *Medial rectus:* 5.3 mm (3.6–7.0)
- *Inferior rectus:* 6.8 mm (4.8–8.5)
- *Lateral rectus:* 6.9 mm (5.4–8.5)
- *Superior rectus:* 7.9 mm (6.2–9.2)

3. What are the types of IO weakening procedures?

Ans.
- Fink's recession
- Parks recession
- Elliot and Nankin procedure
- Modified Elliot and Nankin procedure
- Pure anteropositioning
- Total anterior positioning
- Anterior nasal transposition (Stager's)
- Myectomy
- Extirpation
- Disinsertion
- Denervation

4. What are the types of IO strengthening procedures?

Ans.
- IO resection
- IO advancement

5. What are the types of SO weakening procedures?

Ans.
- Tenotomy
- Tenectomy
- Silicon expander lengthening
- Loop tenotomy
- Chicken suture
- Recession
- Translational recession
- Split-tendon lengthening.

6. What are the types of SO strengthening procedures?

Ans.
- SO tuck
- Harada-Ito procedure

7. What are the various weakening procedures on recti?

Ans.
- Conventional recession
- Hang-back recession
- Slanting recession
- Adjustable recession
- Marginal myotomy
- Faden procedure
- Myectomy
- Disinsertion

8. What are the various strengthening procedures on recti?

Ans.
- Resection
- Advancement
- Plication
- Transposition of adjacent muscles

9. What is oculocardiac reflex?

Ans. Bradycardia associated with stretching of extraocular muscles during strabismus surgery, or compression of the eye ball is called the oculocardiac reflex. The reflex is mediated by nerve connections between the ophthalmic branch of the trigeminal nerve via the ciliary ganglion, and the vagus nerve of the parasympathetic nervous system.

10. What are the common causes of residual/recurrent strabismus?

Ans. *Preoperative:*
- Very large deviation
- Difficulty in measuring deviation of very young children and uncooperative patients.

Intraoperative:
- Faulty marking during surgery
- Splitting of muscle fibers during surgery

Postoperative: Scar stretch

11. What are the common causes of consecutive strabismus?

Ans. *Preoperative:* Difficulty in measuring deviation of very young children and uncooperative patients

Intraoperative:
- Faulty marking during surgery
- Lost muscle

Postoperative:
- Slipped/lost muscle
- Scar stretch

12. What is Knapp procedure?

Ans.
- Full tendon width transposition of the horizontal recti to the superior rectus; it is done in cases of monocular elevation deficit.
- Inverse Knapp is the full tendon width transposition of the horizontal recti to the inferior rectus. It is done in double depressor palsy or inferior rectus palsy.

13. What is FDT?

Ans. Forced duction test assesses passive movement of the globe. This test helps in differentiating between neurogenic and mechanical limitation of ocular movements. After topical/general anesthesia, the eye is held at the limbus with Pierse Hoskin/Globe Fixation forceps. Patient is asked to look in the direction of the movement limitation (to relax the muscle and prevent false-positive results). The globe is then passively moved away from the direction of the muscle to be tested. If resistance is encountered, FDT is positive and the cause is mechanical. If no restriction is felt, a neurogenic cause is considered.

14. What is active force generation test (AFGT)?

Ans. Active force generation test assesses active movement of the globe. In a case of known mechanical limitation of eye movement, it helps assess whether the muscle acting in the field of limitation is paretic or normal. After topical/general anesthesia, the eye is held at the limbus with forceps. Patient is asked to look in the direction of the movement limitation. A normal muscle produces a tug on the globe, which can be felt by the examiner.

SECTION 2: Basic Sciences

7. Pathology Basics
8. Ocular Microbiology
9. Community Ophthalmology

CHAPTER 7

Pathology Basics

Seema Kashyap, Siddhi Goel, Suman Lata, Prafulla Kumar Maharana

■ INTRODUCTION

Histopathological examination of the tissue specimen is vital to know the disease process affecting the different ocular structures. It is essential to be aware of the basic histopathology of the essential structures of the eye. It is often an essential component of postgraduate and fellowship examinations.

This chapter deals with a few fundamental aspects of ocular histopathology and examples of common clinical conditions where histopathology plays a vital role in diagnosis, management, and prognostication of cases.

■ COMMON FINDINGS IN PATHOLOGY

The following components are typically seen in the presence of any disease process:[1]

Polymorphonuclear Leukocytes

Polymorphonuclear leukocytes are characterized by:
- A typical multilobulated nucleus
- Abundant eosinophilic cytoplasm
- Occasionally, intracytoplasmic granules which are nothing but proteolytic enzymes

Mast Cells

Mast cells are characterized by:
- Single nucleus
- Bigger than the polymorphonuclear leukocytes
- Intracytoplasmic pink and red granules (characteristic)
- These granules contain heparin, histamine, and prostaglandins.
- Important mediators of allergic conjunctivitis reactions

Lymphocytes

Lymphocytes are characterized by:
- A very large dark staining nucleus with scanty cytoplasm
- Condensed coarse chromatin
- Play an important role in chronic inflammation and autoimmune disorders

Plasma Cells

Plasma cells are characterized by:
- These are modified altered B lymphocytes
- These are oval in shape
- The nucleus is eccentric with a cartwheel or "clockface arrangement" (nucleus is at one pole of the cell)
- Abundant amphophilic cytoplasm
- A paranuclear pale area is characteristic
- Produce antibodies

■ GRANULOMATOUS REACTION

A granulomatous reaction usually occurs in response to some chronic low-grade infections (such as tuberculosis or aspergillosis) or a foreign body or chronic uveitis (sarcoidosis).

The inflammatory cells primarily consist of macrophages, lymphocytes, and plasma cells. One of the characteristic features is the formation of epithelioid cell granulomas along with multinucleated giant cells.[1]

PYOGENIC GRANULOMA

- Clinically a pyogenic granuloma is characterized by a fleshy, granular, red mass primarily in the conjunctiva. Unlike the name suggests, it does not contain any pus, hence a misnomer.
- Histopathologically, it is a lobulated lesion with a rich, vascular network within a loose fibrous connective tissue along with inflammatory cells. Surface is often ulcerated.[1]

NEOPLASIA

The different types of changes seen are:[1]
- *Hypertrophy:* Increase in size of cells
- *Hyperplasia:* Increase in the number of cells
- *Hyperkeratosis:* Hyperkeratosis, generally, refers to a thickening of the keratin-containing outer layer of the skin. In the eye, there is thickening of the conjunctiva.
- *Parakeratosis:* Retention of the nucleus in superficial layers of skin or conjunctiva.
- *Metaplasia:* It is the transformation of one cell type to another cell type.
- *Examples:*
  - *Keratinization of ocular surface:* In Stevens–Johnson syndrome (SJS), ocular cicatricial pemphigoid (OCP), and severe dry eye, the columnar epithelium of conjunctiva is transformed into the stratified squamous keratinized epithelium.
  - Metaplasia of retinal pigment epithelium (RPE) in proliferative vitreoretinopathy (PVR)

- Metaplasia of lens epithelium after cataract or posterior capsular opacification (PCO)
- *Dysplasia:* It is an abnormal proliferation of atypical squamous epithelial cells of the conjunctiva. They are classified as mild, moderate, or severe dysplasia depending on the thickness involved. When it involves the entire thickness of the epithelium without any breach in the underlying basement membrane, it is called as carcinoma in situ.
- *Mitotic figures:* Instead of a nucleus, the chromosomes are visible as tangled, dark-staining threads called mitotic figures, which are generally present in malignant tumors.
- *Atrophy:* It means a decrease in the size of a body part, tissue or an individual cell. It can occur following any disease or loss of trophic support due to another disease. It can be physiological (e.g., atrophy of lacrimal gland with increasing age) or it can be pathological [RPE atrophy in age-related macular degeneration (ARMD)].
- *Apoptosis:* Apoptosis is programed cell death that occurs in healthy tissue. Examples include loss of tissue/organs during embryogenesis.
- *Necrosis:* It is the death of cells in an organ or tissue due to disease, injury, or failure of blood supply. Inflammation is always there. Examples include aseptic necrosis in retinoblastoma (RB) when tumor growth exceeds the blood supply.

SPECIMENS RECEIVED IN OCULAR PATHOLOGY

- *Eyeball:* Evisceration, enucleation, exenteration
- *Eyelid:* Biopsy
- *Lacrimal gland:* Biopsy
- *Conjunctiva:* Biopsy, excised lesion, impression cytology

- *Cornea:* Lamellar keratoplasty (LK), full thickness (penetrating keratoplasty), impression cytology, and corneal biopsy in keratitis
  - *Optic nerve:* Enucleation
  - *Temporal artery biopsy:* Giant cell arteritis
  - *Aqueous tap:* In non-Hodgkins lymphoma (NHL), retinoblastoma (RB), and malignant melanoma (MM) cases
  - *Vitreous tap:* Vitrectomy in endophthalmitis
  - *Retinal:* Rare as in retinal tumors, or retinitis

TISSUE PREPARATION

Fixatives Used

- *Formalin:* 10% buffered formalin is the most commonly used fixative. The advantage of formalin is that it has prolonged chemical stability.[1]

  Time for fixation:
  - Minimum period for a 4-mm thick specimen—8 hours, 6 mm thick specimen—24 hours
  - Large specimen to be cut into thin slices for fixation
  - Eyeball to be cut after 24–48 hours
- *Glutaraldehyde:* It is used for scanning electron microscopy (SEM) and transmission electron microscopy (TEM).

Preparation of Tissue

- *Paraffin embedding:* It is the most commonly used method. The tissue is embedded in paraffin wax. The wax serves two purposes; firstly, it allows the sample to adhere to the slide and secondly, it stabilizes the tissue during sectioning. Paraffin-prepared blocks can be stored indefinitely.[1]
- *Fresh/frozen sections:* In frozen section, fresh tissue is immediately transported in saline to the laboratory, frozen and embedded in a special medium, and multiple sections are taken using a cryostat. Sections are stained and report is given within 20–30 minutes while the patient is still under anesthesia. It is extremely useful in cases when immediate histopathology report is required as in Mohs' micrographic surgery, to know whether the margins are involved in eyelid tumor surgery in the evaluation of intracellular fat as seen in sebaceous carcinoma, and for immunohistochemical studies.[1]
- *Plastic embedding:* The tissue is embedded in an epoxy resin such as araldite. It is used in TEM.[1]

GROSS EXAMINATION (MACROSCOPIC EXAMINATION)

Dimensions: It is the first step. The specimen is measured and its description regarding its shape, size, texture, external and cut surface characteristics are noted.

Usually, the following things are recorded (e.g., in case of an enucleated globe) **(Fig. 7.1)**:[1]
- The maximum dimensions are measured:
  - Anteroposterior (normal 22–24 mm)

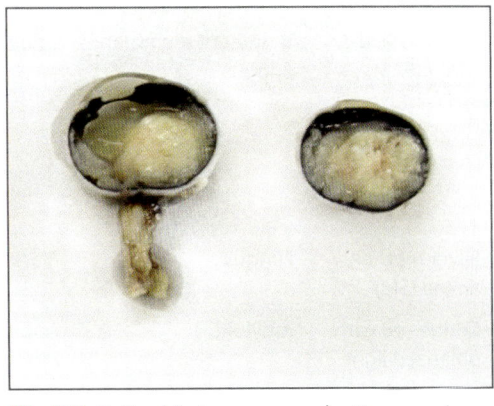

Fig. 7.1: Retinoblastoma—enucleation specimen showing an intraocular retinoblastoma with optic nerve infiltration.

- Horizontal (normal 23.5 mm)
- Vertical (normal 23 mm)

Transillumination: For this, light is projected from behind the globe to look for the location of mass lesions within the globe.

The eye is then cut in a way revealing the most prominent tumor areas that include the pupil as well as the optic nerve. This half of the globe along with optic nerve is submitted for the routine examination and is termed as the pupillary-optic disc portion (PO). The remaining cut portions of the globe are called calottes, as they resemble the shape of caps. Each calotte is cut serially to maximize the tissue examined.

Special Stains

Commonly used special stains and their uses are depicted in **Table 7.1**.

TABLE 7.1: Special stains in ocular histopathology.

Stain	Target	Color	Diagnostic use
Alcian blue	Mucopolysaccharides	Blue	Macular corneal dystrophy (**Fig. 7.2**)
Colloidal iron	Mucopolysaccharides	Blue	Macular corneal dystrophy (**Fig. 7.3**)
Alizarin red	Chelates calcium	Red	Detects calcification like in band-shaped keratopathy
Von Kossa	Calcium	Black or brown black	Calcific band keratopathy
Bodian	Axons	Black	Optic atrophy
Loyez	Myelin	Black	Demyelinating diseases (multiple sclerosis), optic atrophy
Masson trichrome	Connective tissue hyaline material	• Red—muscle • Green—connective tissue • Nuclei—blue	• Granular corneal dystrophy (**Fig. 7.4**) • Thyroid eye disease (muscle)
Periodic acid–Schiff (PAS)	Basement membranes Fungus	Bright pink	• *Cornea:* Epithelial basement membrane, Descemet's membrane • *Lens:* Capsule • *Retina:* Internal limiting membrane (ILM) • Fungal elements
Silver methen-amine (SM)	Fungus	Black	Fungal hyphae in a light-green background
Congo red with polarized light	Amyloid	Apple-green birefringence	Lattice corneal dystrophy (**Fig. 7.5**)
Perl's Prussian blue	Iron	Dark blue	• Intraocular foreign body • Fleischer ring

Contd...

Contd...

Stain	Target	Color	Diagnostic use
Van Gieson	Elastic fibers	Gray	Elastic tissue like in giant cell arteritis
Ziehl–Neelsen	Acid-fast bacilli	Pink-beaded rods	Detects *Mycobacterium*, *Nocardia* species in inflammatory tissue and in granulomatous lesions
Oil Red O	Lipid	Red	Fat within cells, sebaceous carcinoma
Fontana–Masson	Melanin and argentaffin cells	Black	Melanin pigments in malignant melanoma and carcinoid tumor

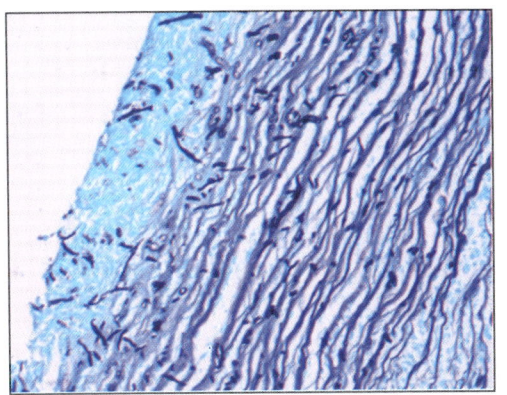

Fig. 7.2: Silver methenamine stain reveals black-colored septate fungal hyphae with acute angle branching in mycotic keratitis.

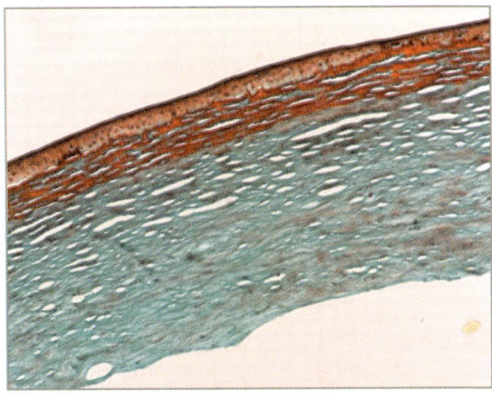

Fig. 7.4: Granular dystrophy—stromal deposits take up a brilliant red color on Masson's trichrome stain.

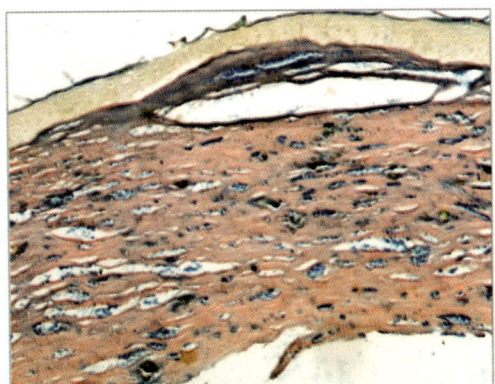

Fig. 7.3: Macular dystrophy—acid mucopolysaccharides are seen in the keratocytes, which take up a Prussian blue color by colloidal iron stain.

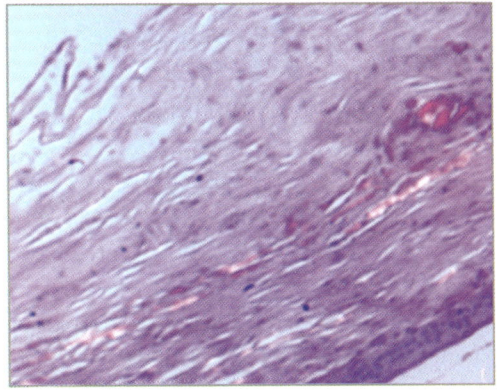

Fig. 7.5: Lattice dystrophy—apple-green birefringence is demonstrated on Congo red stain in polarized light in the corneal stroma.

Example: Macular corneal dystrophy (MCD) is characterized by deposit of mucopolysaccharides in the stroma, in the keratocytes, beneath the epithelium and endothelium in advanced cases. The stains commonly used are colloidal iron or Alcian blue, both of which stain the mucopolysaccharides blue.[1]

Silver methenamine stains fungal hyphae black in color against a green background **(Fig. 7.1)**.

IMMUNOHISTOCHEMISTRY

Immunohistochemistry involves accurate identification of cells by using an antigen-specific antibody against the antigens present within/on the cells. Specific stains are used to label the antibody and visualize under a light microscope or a fluorescence microscope. The commonly used antibodies are summarized in **Table 7.2**.[1]

TABLE 7.2: Summary of immunohistochemistry antibodies.

Antibody	Antigen	Diagnostic use	Ocular example
Muscle-specific actin, desmin	Contractile filaments in smooth and striated muscle	Smooth muscle-derived tumors	Leiomyosarcoma
Desmin, myogenin, MYOD1	Intermediate filaments in smooth and striated muscle	Muscle-derived tumors	Rhabdomyosarcoma
Cytokeratin (CK 7)	High-molecular-weight glycoprotein epithelial cells	Metastatic adenocarcinomas, adnexal skin tumors	Metastatic carcinoma to orbit
LCA, B cell (CD20), CD3 (T cell), MPO, macrophage (CD68)	Components of T and B cells, macrophages	Hematological malignancies	Lymphomas, leukemias
Cytokeratin/CAM 5.2/AE1/AE3	Intermediate filaments in epithelial cells	Epithelial-derived carcinomas	Squamous cell carcinoma, sebaceous cell carcinoma
Epithelial membrane antigen (EMA)	Epithelial cells and carcinomas	Epithelial derived carcinomas	Sebaceous cell carcinoma, meningioma
Factor VIII-related antigen	Endothelial cell	Vascular tumors	Ocular angiosarcoma
Glial fibrillar acidic protein (GFAP)	Glial cell constituents	Glial cells and astrocytes origin tumors	Glioma of optic nerve
HMB45/Melan-A	Intracytoplasmic antigen in melanocytes	Tumors of melanocytic origin	Malignant melanomas
S-100	Neural crest cells	Peripheral nerve tumors	Schwannomas, melanoma
Vimentin, smooth muscle antigen (SMA)	• Intermediate filaments • Cells of mesenchymal origin	Spindle cell tumors	Fibrous histiocytoma
Glucose transporter 1 (GLUT 1)	Microvascular endothelium	Tumors of vascular origin	Infantile hemangioma

Electron Microscopy

Transmission electron microscopy is useful in identifying cell organelles and viral particles at a very high magnification of up to 100,000×. SEM is useful for the evaluation of structures like corneal endothelium.[1]

Molecular Methods

Polymerase Chain Reaction

Polymerase chain reaction (PCR) identifies DNA or RNA sequences specific to particular pathogenic organisms or cellular components. The most significant advantage of PCR is that it requires a tiny amount of sample. The nuclear chromatin is lyzed into individual sequences, and the desired sequence is amplified followed by its rapid detection using various electrophoresis methods.[1]

In Situ Hybridization

Similar to PCR the nuclear chromatin is segregated into fragments, which are detected by immunohistochemical techniques in routine light microscopy. Using this, the exact location of the protein fragments can be visualized within the tissue.[1]

Flow Cytometry[1]

Flow cytometry is useful in identification of various cell types such as B and T cells. Fluorescent antibodies specific to the antigens of different cell types are used for identification.[1]

COMMON PATHOLOGICAL LESIONS IN OPHTHALMOLOGY

Dermoid Cyst (Fig. 7.6)

- These are benign teratomas present since birth.
- Clinically they are most commonly seen

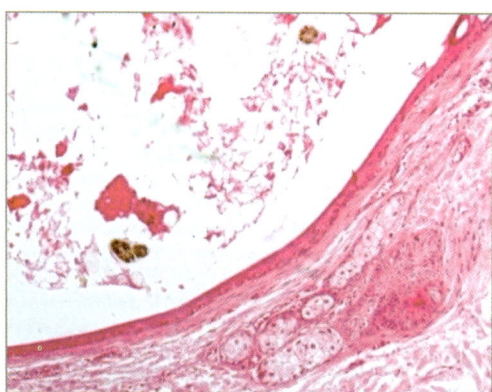

Fig. 7.6: Dermoid cyst—the cyst wall is lined by stratified squamous epithelium with hair follicle and epidermal appendages in its wall with desquamated keratin in its lumen.

  in superotemporal quadrant of the eye, followed by superonasal quadrant.
- *Histologically:* It is lined by the stratified squamous epithelium and contains adnexal structures such as sebaceous glands and hair follicles in its wall. The lumen may contain pultaceous material, hair shafts and thyroid, bone, tooth, and other epidermal-derived structures in case of benign teratoma.
- Appendages are a rule for a fully matured cyst and differentiate it from the epidermoid cyst and sebaceous cyst.
- Rupture of cyst during removal provokes a foreign body giant cell reaction and thus removal of cyst should be done.

Pigmented Tumors

Benign tumors of nevus cells are called melanocytic nevi. These can be of the following types:
- *Intradermal nevus:*
  - It is the most common type of nevus.
  - Presents as an elevated mass, brown to black (**Fig. 7.7**)
  - Histologically, nevus cells are arranged in the form of nests and cords and

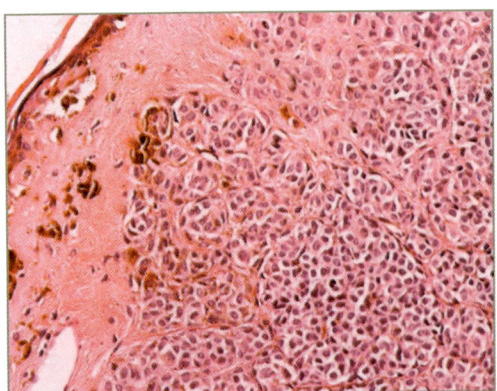

Fig. 7.7: Intradermal nevus showing benign nests of nevus cells with melanin in its superficial cells.

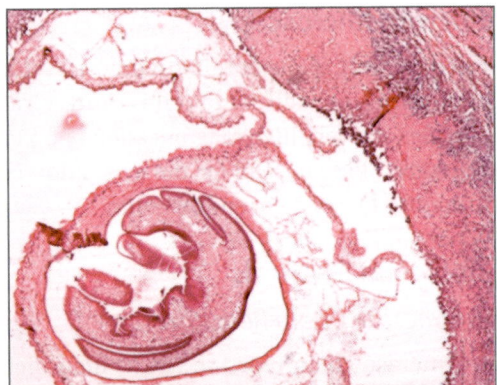

Fig. 7.8: Cysticercosis—body of a cysticercus larva with multiple papillary infoldings.

are located entirely in the dermis. Cells contain a moderate amount of cytoplasm and melanin. The nuclei mature as they go deeper in the dermis and cells become smaller, with less cytoplasm and less melanin and lie in a well-defined mass. Still lower down the nevus cells appear spindle-shaped. Maturation is regarded as an evidence of benignity. There is no malignant potential.

- *Congenital nevus:*
  - Larger in size than acquired nevus
  - Differentiated from acquired nevus on the basis of histology
  - Presence of nevus cells in lower reticular dermis/subcutaneous fat
- *Compound nevus:*
  - Both intradermal and junctional component
  - Malignant potential is related to the junctional component.
- *Nevus of Ota:*
  - Bluish-gray discoloration of periorbital skin with the sclera
  - Heterochromia or choroidal nevi may be present.
  - Fusiform, bipolar, heavily pigmented melanocyte in the dermis.
- *Junctional nevus:*
  - Nevus cells are at the junction of epithelium and dermis.
  - Low malignant potential

Cysticercosis (Fig. 7.8)

Cysticercosis is caused by the larvae of the pork tapeworm, *Taenia solium, Cysticercus cellulosae*. The preferred tissues by the larvae are subcutaneous tissue, skeletal muscles, brain, and eye. Microscopically the scolex consists of a sucker and multiple papillary infoldings of tegument. The larvae contain a perioral double row of hooklets.[1]

The wall of the cyst shows characteristic histologic appearance, with three distinct layers:
1. *Outer layer/cuticular layer*: Corrugated containing multiple microtrichia, which are nothing but hair-like protrusions. This layer remains in contact with the host surface.
2. Middle layer, which is very thin and cellular.
3. Inner layer, which is thick and contains a network of multiple small canaliculi.

Chalazion (Fig. 7.9)

A chalazion is a chronic lipogranulomatous inflammation of the sebaceous glands (Zeis

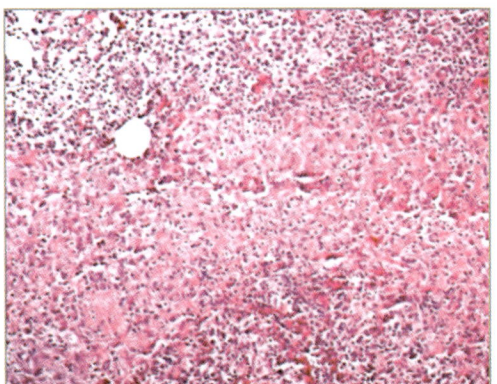

Fig. 7.9: Chalazion—microscopic examination reveals lipogranulomatous inflammation comprising plasma cells, lymphocytes, histiocytes, giant cells, and ill-defined epithelioid cell granuloma. Lipid dissolved during processing is seen as a large vacuolated area.

and Meibomian glands), resulting in a hard painless eyelid nodule. Microscopically, the essential lesion is the formation of focal granuloma centered around clear spaces (lipid vacuoles) discharged from sebaceous glands.

The lipid deposits can be stained using Oil Red O stain on frozen section. The granuloma contains giant cells, epithelioid cells, plasma cells, and lymphocytes.[1]

Differential diagnosis:
- Tuberculosis
- Sarcoidosis
- Fungal infections
- Parasitic infections

Intraocular Tumors

Retinoblastoma

Retinoblastoma is the most common intraocular tumor seen in the pediatric age-group. It arises from the nucleated retinal layers. The average age of presentation is 13 months. Six percent may be familial and 50% of these may be bilateral. Around 94% of the RBs are sporadic.

- *Endophytic RB:* This form grows from the inner surface of the retina, and can be easily seen with ophthalmoscopy.
- *Exophytic RB:* This form grows from the outer surface of retina toward the choroid.
- *Mixed, endo-exophytic:* Most common type
- *Diffuse infiltrating RB:* It is a rare (1–2%) histologic form of RB characterized by diffuse infiltration of the retina without a tumor mass.

Histology reveals cells with a large basophilic nucleus of variable size and shape and scanty cytoplasm. Mitotic figures are numerous **(Figs. 7.10A to D)**. Rosettes are highly characteristic of RBs seen in well-differentiated RBs. Flexner–Wintersteiner rosette is formed by cuboidal cells, which are lined up around an empty central lumen. Special stains reveal acid mucopolysaccharides in the lumen. Homer-Wright rosettes are less common, and cells are not arranged around a lumen. The cells send out cytoplasmic processes and are lined up around cobweb-like eosinophilic material. Well-differentiated RB has a better prognosis.[1]

Endophytic RBs tend to spread anteriorly by seeding into vitreous and aqueous. Aqueous seeding may stimulate a hypopyon. Deposits may appear on iris and in anterior chamber angle and produce secondary angle-closure glaucoma. Anterior uveal invasion leads to hematogenous disease or regional lymphatic spread.

Poorly differentiated RB is composed of cells with a large basophilic nucleus of variable size and shape and scanty cytoplasm. No rosettes are identified. Mitotic figures are numerous. Necrotic RBs result in liberation of DNA from tumor nuclei. This DNA is preferentially absorbed by blood vessels.

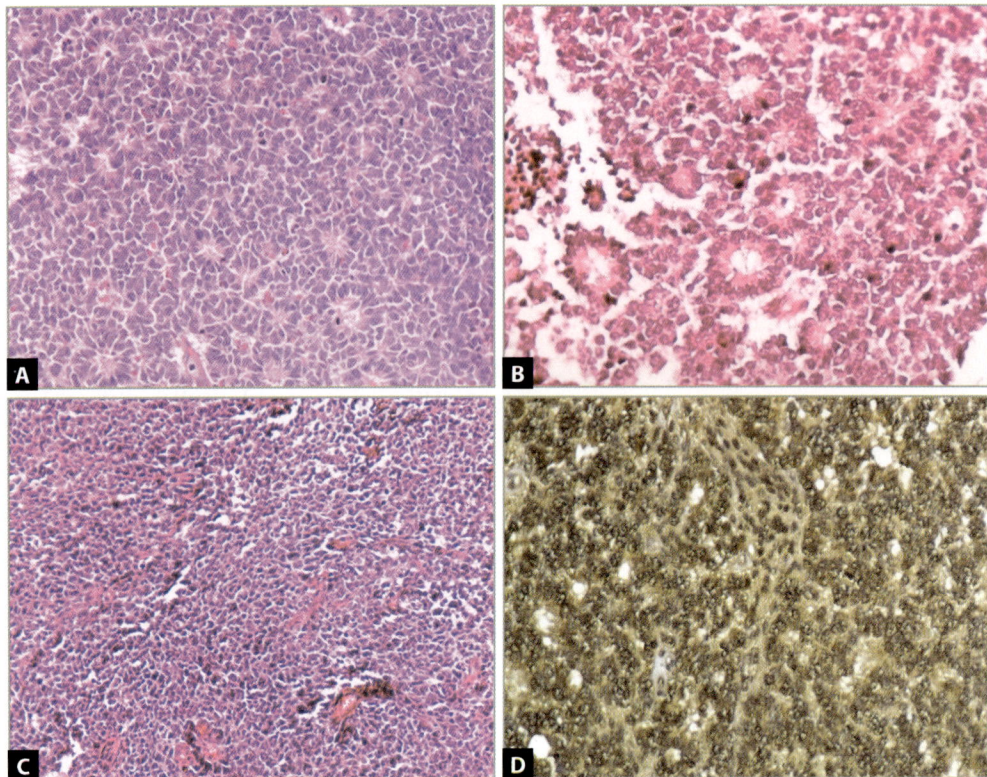

Figs. 7.10A to D: (A) Retinoblastoma—hematoxylin and eosin section from a well-differentiated retinoblastoma showing numerous Homer-Wright rosettes. In these rosettes, the pink material in the center represents tangle of processes of tumor cells; (B) Retinoblastoma—section shows Flexner–Wintersteiner rosettes with a central lumen; (C) Poorly differentiated retinoblastoma; (D) Immunohistochemical stain synaptophysin shows cytoplasmic positivity in the tumor cells.

Retinoblastoma, extraocular spread: Extraocular spread may occur to orbit and brain. All RBs show a striking tendency to invade the optic disc. Optic nerve involvement increases the mortality to 15% when the invasion is up to lamina cribrosa. This increases up to 65% when the resected margin is involved. Once in the nerve, the tumor can reach chiasma through nerve bundles or subarachnoid space through the pia. The access to subarachnoid space can occur via central retinal vessels. Histopathological high-risk factors like massive choroidal invasion, optic nerve retrolaminar region and cut end involvement, iris and ciliary body involvement, and scleral and extrascleral invasion should be looked for in the histopathology sections for adjuvant chemotherapy **(Figs. 7.11A and B)**.[1]

Uveal Malignant Melanoma

Malignant melanoma of the uveal tract is rare. It originates most commonly from choroid, followed by ciliary body and iris. The prognosis is poor with hematogenous spread mainly to the liver, lung, and bone. Microscopically based on the cell type they

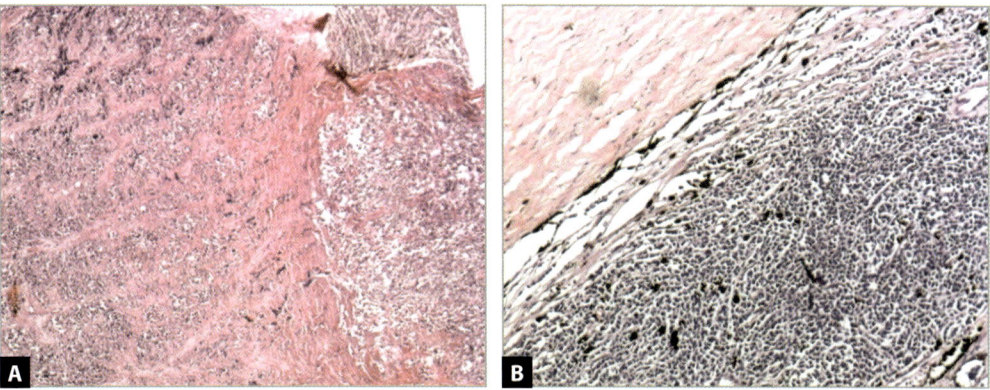

Figs. 7.11A and B: (A) Optic nerve head and retrolaminar invasion; (B) Massive choroidal invasion.

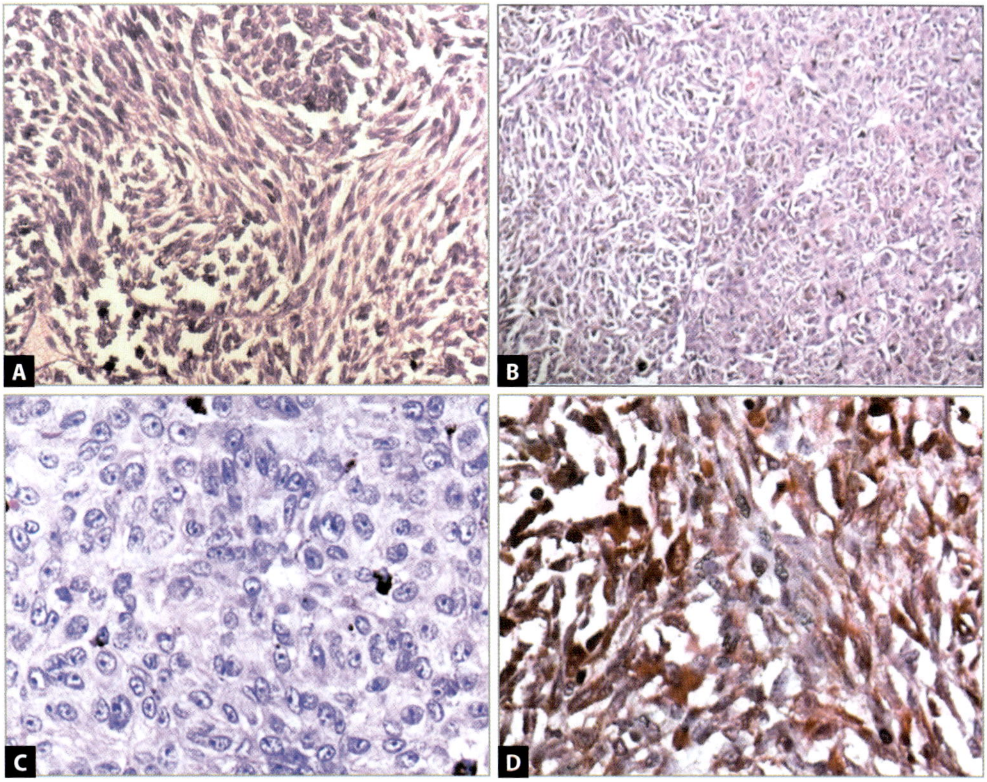

Figs. 7.12A to D: (A) Spindle-cell melanoma; (B) Mixed-cell melanoma; (C) Epithelioid cell melanoma; (D) Cytoplasmic HMB45 positivity in melanoma cells.

are classified into spindle cell type, mixed cell type, and epithelioid cell type **(Figs. 7.12A to D)**. Immunohistochemical stain HMB45, Melan A, and S-100 are positive in the tumor cells. Spindle cell type has the best prognosis while epithelioid has the worst prognosis.[1]

Basal Cell Carcinoma (Fig. 7.13)

Basal cell carcinoma (BCC) is the most common malignant eyelid tumor worldwide. It usually occurs in elderly patients. However, it occurs in equal frequency to squamous cell carcinoma (SCC) and sebaceous cell carcinoma in India (33% of each). Most frequently involves the lower lid followed by upper lid, inner canthus, and lateral canthus. Clinically nodulo-ulcerative, pigmented, sclerosing, or morphea types are described. The tumor tends to be locally invasive and almost never metastasizes. Prognosis is good with complete excision.

Microscopically BCC shows small, moderate- or large-sized groups of basaloid cells in papillary dermis with peripheral palisading **(Fig. 7.13)**. Pleomorphism and mitotic figures are often found in these cells. The surrounding and intervening dermis undergoes desmoplasia, fibroblasts become large, bizarre, and the mesenchymal tissue becomes loose.

Microscopic variants of BCC: Depending on the differentiation pattern, the tumor may be keratotic with parakeratotic cells and horn cysts; cystic BCC with cystic spaces within tumors lobules; and adenoid BCC, which shows the formation of tubular, gland-like structures. The cells are arranged in a lace-like pattern. The morphea or sclerosing pattern shows elongated strands of basaloid cells embedded in a fibrous stroma.

Squamous Cell Carcinoma

Keratoacanthoma

Keratoacanthoma is a benign tumor characterized by rapid growth (months) and hyperkeratosis. It is ovoid-shaped with a central keratin core. Spontaneous resolution can occur, but surgical excision is effective. Gross appearance includes a well-defined nodule with central umbilication containing keratinized core and a smooth, rounded peripheral surface.[1]

Premalignant Lesions

Actinic/solar/senile keratosis: Precancerous changes in the epidermis follow overexposure to sunlight. The characteristic clinical appearance consists of a nonelevated, variable-sized plaque with irregular margins. The management consists of excision.[1]

Squamous Cell Carcinoma

Squamous cell carcinoma can occur due to chronic sun exposure, exposure to ionizing radiation, chronic irritation, and infection by human papillomavirus (HPV).

Clinically, the most common presentation is as a nodule, which may ulcerate.

Grossly, the tumor appears as a heavily keratinized or ulcerated mass with irregular edges.

Microscopically, the appearance depends upon the grade of differentiation. A well-differentiated tumor has the formation of characteristic keratin pearls along with features

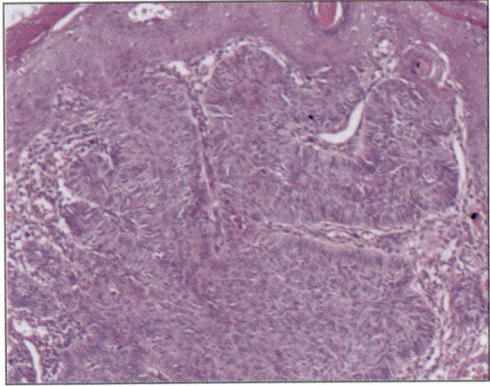

Fig. 7.13: Basal cell carcinoma—irregular islands of basophilic tumor cells arising from basal layer of the epidermis with characteristic peripheral palisading of tumor cells.

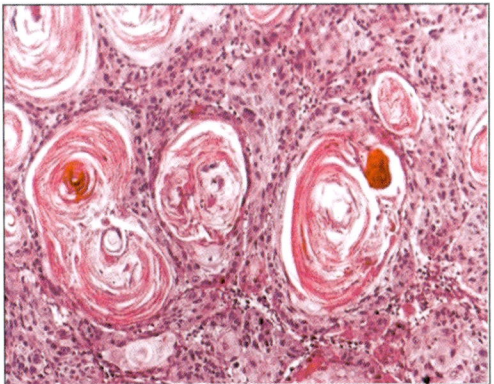

Fig. 7.14: Hematoxylin and eosin stain reveals numerous pearls in a well-differentiated squamous cell carcinoma.

of metaplasia. Keratin pearl is a focus of central keratinization within concentric layers of abnormal squamous cells around it **(Fig. 7.14)**. In doubtful cases, immunohistochemistry is done using cytokeratins such as CAM 5.2, AE1, and AE3, which helps in diagnosis. In poorly differentiated type, nest-like squamous differentiation is lost, but intercellular bridges are still identified. Sometimes individual cell keratinization is seen. Spindle-cell type carries the worst prognosis among all types.[1]

Sebaceous Cell Carcinoma

Sebaceous cell carcinoma usually arises from pilosebaceous follicles and sebaceous glands (Meibomian and Zeiss). Clinically it presents as a yellow nodule, which may be ulcerated, along with the presence of telangiectatic blood vessels. The other mode of the presentation includes plaque-like lesion, chronic blepharoconjunctivitis, and recurrent eyelid inflammation. Lymph node and distant metastasis can occur in advanced cases.

Though BCC is most common worldwide, sebaceous gland carcinoma is seen more frequently in Asian and Asian Indian population. Sebaceous carcinomas are usually nodular in form and are unilateral, but their ability to spread within the epidermis simulates a chronic blepharoconjunctivitis (masquerade syndrome).

Clinically presents as a yellow nodule that may or may not be ulcerated, if the diagnosis is delayed. It is more common in the elderly, females, and the upper lid.[1]

For special stain Oil Red O, frozen section is preferred as normal tissue processing, which removes fat, an important finding for the diagnosis. Grossly, the tumor appears as a pale yellow nodular lesion. Microscopically characterized by the presence of lobule, surrounded by a single cuboidal basal layer. The center of the lobule contains foamy cells. These cells have characteristic lipid-laden foamy cytoplasm and a small nucleus. In the neck of the follicle, the cells fragment to release lipid into the ducts (holocrine secretion) **(Figs. 7.15A and B)**.

In a well-differentiated sebaceous gland carcinoma, the morphology is lobular, and the center of the lobule contains foamy cells. The basal cells may fail to differentiate into foamy cells and the lobules are filled with small basophilic cells.

In moderately differentiated tumors, the basal cells predominate and the cytoplasm contains small circular spaces, which represent the lipid globules, which were removed during paraffin processing.

In poorly differentiated tumors, lipid spaces are rare.

In advanced cases, the tumor infiltrates the eyelids extensively.[1]

Rhinosporidiosis

Rhinosporidiosis is a granulomatous disease caused by aquatic protistan parasite *Rhinosporidium seeberi*. It primarily affects the mucous membrane including conjunctiva. The nasal form is the most common clinical type accounting for 70% of the cases.[1]

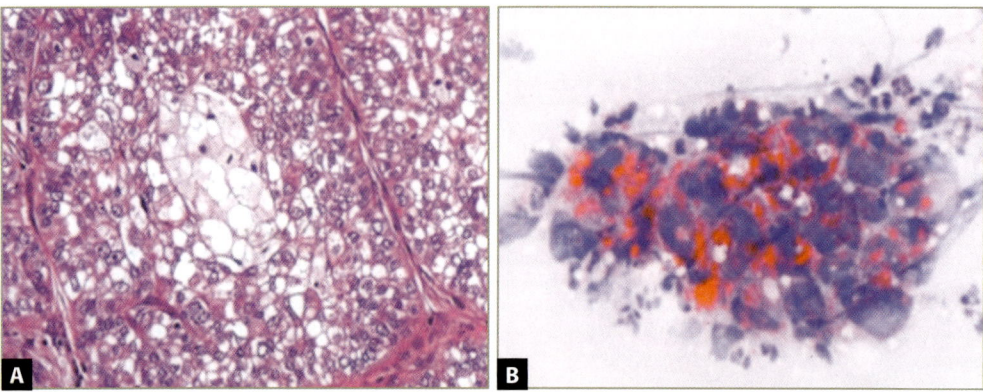

Figs. 7.15A and B: (A) Sebaceous cell carcinoma—well-differentiated sebaceous cell carcinoma showing sebaceous differentiation in the center of a tumor island; (B) Aspirate from a lid mass shows orange-colored intracytoplasmic lipids as seen on Oil Red O stain.

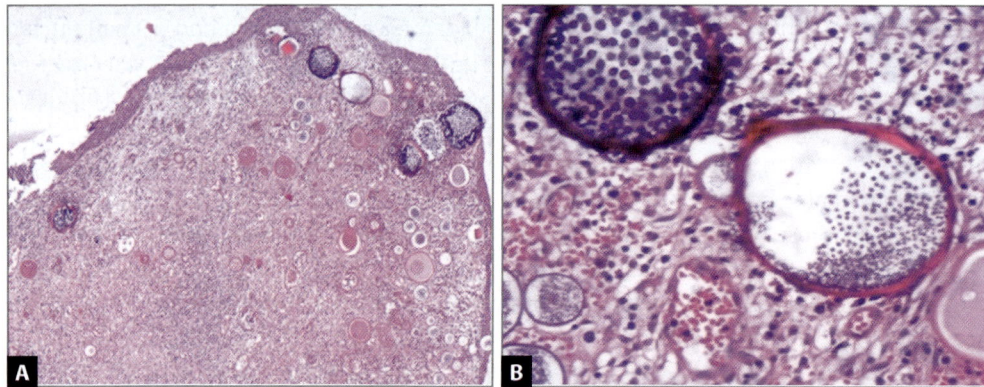

Figs. 7.16A and B: Rhinosporidiosis—low power and high-power images show numerous sporangia of *Rhinosporidiosis seeberi* in the conjunctival stroma.

Infection of the palpebral conjunctiva occurs in around 15% of the cases. In conjunctiva and lid, it leads to the formation of a solitary, friable mass lesion. Histological examination demonstrates thick-walled sacs or sporangia. The sporangium contains numerous spores (size of an erythrocyte). A granulomatous response may be seen. Spores and sporangia can be seen on conventional sections and are highlighted by periodic acid–Schiff (PAS) or methenamine silver stain **(Figs. 16A and B)**. Usually, surgery is required as there is no response to antibiotics.[1]

Lacrimal Gland Tumor

The tumor can arise either from the acinar (adenocarcinoma) or the ductal (pleomorphic adenomas/adenocarcinomas) part of the lacrimal gland.

Pleomorphic Adenoma

Pleomorphic adenoma is the most common lacrimal gland tumor. It accounts for 50% of the epithelial tumors of the lacrimal gland. The term pleomorphic is used as it contains cells arising from epithelium as well as mesenchyme. It is also called as mixed tumor because of this mixed cells of origin.[1]

Macroscopic examination: Grossly, it appears as a single, solid mass, gray-white in color, with a bosselated surface. On cut section, mucoid cystic spaces and hemorrhage can be seen.

Microscopic examination: Microscopically, the tissues show two different components as described below:
1. *Epithelial component:* Characterized by the formation of a glandular pattern with cords and ducts; the ducts may contain eosinophilic proteinaceous material within the lumen.
2. *Stromal component:* Characterized by the formation of connective tissue components such as fibrous with myxoid areas, and rarely fat and cartilage within the tumor **(Fig. 7.17)**; the mass is usually surrounded by a pseudocapsule, formed due to fibrous condensation around the mass as it grows over a while.[1]

Malignant Lacrimal Gland Tumor

Malignant lesions are characterized by rapid onset, rapid progression, and presence of pain in contrast to a benign tumor.

Adenoid cystic carcinoma (ACC): ACC is the most common malignant tumor of the lacrimal gland.

Macroscopic examination: It appears as a pale-gray mass.

Microscopic examination: It may form a cribriform, solid or tubular pattern depending upon the arrangement of ducts and myxoid material. Cribriform is the most common variant. The pathognomonic appearance is called *"Swiss cheese"* appearance **(Figs. 7.18A and B)**. This appearance is caused by the

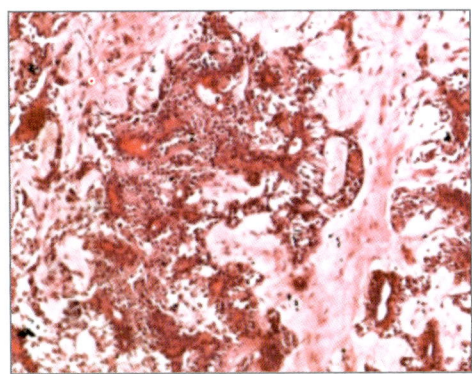

Fig. 7.17: Pleomorphic adenoma—histology shows a characteristic biphasic pattern consisting of a pale myomatous stroma and cellular area containing epithelial element.

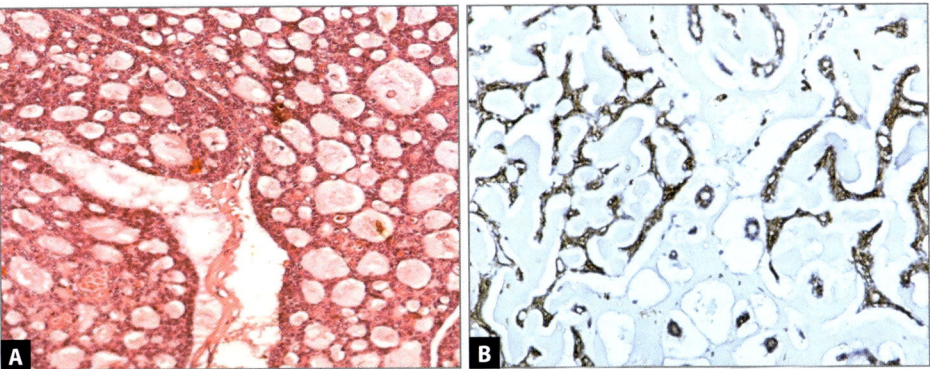

Figs. 7.18A and B: Adenoid cystic carcinoma—characteristic Swiss cheese pattern or cribriform appearance of the tumor on microscopic examination; (B) Immunohistochemical stain c-Kit is positive in the tumor cells.

presence of solid cords of hyperchromatic cuboidal cells with a high mitotic rate surrounding cystic spaces containing myxoid material, which are PAS-positive.[1] The other characteristic findings include peripheral perineurial invasion, squamous differentiation, and cystic changes. It can be graded into three grades depending upon the proportion of the solid component.

1. *Grade 1:* Primarily tubular or cribriform with an occasional solid component
2. *Grade 2:* Primarily cribriform or mixed with solid component <50%
3. *Grade 3:* Solid component >50%[1]

Adenocarcinoma: Similar to ACC, but the pattern is that of solid masses of tumor tissue.

REFERENCE

1. Sehu KW, Lee WR. Ophthalmic Pathology: An Illustrated Guide for Clinicians. New Jersey: Wiley; 2008. p. 290.

CHAPTER 8: Ocular Microbiology

Siddhi Goel, Nishat Hussain Ahmed, Geeta Satpathy

INTRODUCTION

Microbiology has an invaluable role in the management of ocular infection. Several terms are essential to understanding the basic concepts of ocular microbiology. These are described as follows:

- *Primary infection:* When the organism infects the eye for the first time
- *Secondary infection:* When the infection by a microorganism occurs in an already infected eye with a different microorganism; the example includes bacterial infection over and above in a case of mycotic keratitis. The most common pattern seen in the eye is a superadded fungal infection in a patient with bacterial keratitis.
- *Reinfection:* When the same organism causes the infection again
- *Reactivation:* When the organism remains dormant for a variable period in any of the organs and causes infection by reactivation under various conditions of stress. Recurrent herpes simplex keratitis is the best example of such reactivation.
- *Latent period:* The time gap between infection to infectiousness
- *Incubation period:* The period between infection and onset of the disease
- *Nosocomial infection:* When a patient acquires an infection during the hospital stay; the infection may be acquired from slit-lamp, applanation tonometer, hands of hospital staff, prosthesis, tap water, etc.
- *Iatrogenic infection:* It is a physician-induced infection due to therapy; a typical example is hepatitis B infection or human immunodeficiency virus (HIV) following blood transfusion.
- *Carriers:* They are persons who harbor the pathogenic organism without actually manifesting the disease; however, they can transmit the infection to others.

ROLE OF MICROBIOLOGY IN OPHTHALMOLOGY

The normal ocular surface flora consists of a wide range of organisms mainly due to the nutrient-rich nature of it. The microorganisms can either be saprophytes or commensals; both the group of organisms do not produce disease in the immunocompetent host. The eye is exposed to the atmosphere throughout the waking hours and their proximity with skin, nasopharynx, and paranasal sinuses make them vulnerable to contamination.

Ocular infections can be self-limiting requiring only symptomatic treatment while some may be mild, which can be managed with empirical therapy and there may be some which are potentially blinding infections, which need urgent attention and systemic antimicrobial therapy based on antimicrobial sensitivity.

Infections of the lid and adnexa are common and caused by the proliferation of the local flora or infection by a virulent organism.

However, infection of the globe requires a breach of the natural barriers, either by trauma, surgery, or other risk factors. Sometimes, the infection may be endogenous, which comes from other parts of the body through the bloodstream or lymphatic system. The best example of endogenous infection is metastatic endophthalmitis.

There are multiple barriers to ocular infections **(Table 8.1)**.[1] For ocular infections to occur, a breach in these defense mechanisms is essential. Various infectious diseases of the eye include:[2]

- Conjunctivitis
- Infective keratitis
- Endophthalmitis
- Panophthalmitis
- Infectious uveitis
- Orbital cellulitis
- Infections of the lacrimal system like dacryocystitis and dacryoadenitis
- Adnexal infections like blepharitis, meibomitis, etc.
- Iatrogenic infections (postsurgery)

The various organisms implicated in ocular infections can be classified as prokaryotes or eukaryotes **(Table 8.2)**. Prokaryotic cells are primitive cells that lack any nucleus or membrane-bound organelles; in contrast, eukaryotic cells contain nucleus as well as membrane-bound organelles.

TABLE 8.1: Barriers to ocular infections.

Anatomical	• Bony orbit • Eyelids • Eyelashes • Epithelial barrier of cornea and conjunctiva
Mechanical	• Blink reflex • Lacrimal drainage system • Tear film lipid layer
Antimicrobial defense	• Tear film constituents like mucin, immunoglobulin A (IgA), complement proteins, lactoferrin, lysozyme, beta-lysin and ceruloplasmin • Conjunctiva-associated lymphoid tissue (CALT) consisting of both B and T lymphocytes • IgA and glycocalyx crosslinks on anterior surface of cornea

TABLE 8.2: Classification of microorganisms causing ocular infections.

Prokaryotes	Eukaryotes
Bacteria	**Fungi**
Gram-positive cocci	*Fusarium* species
Staphylococcus aureus	*Candida* species
Staphylococcus epidermidis	*Aspergillus* species
Streptococcus pneumoniae	*Acremonium* species
Streptococcus pyogenes	
Streptococcus viridans	*Alternaria* species
Enterococcus species	*Penicillium* species
Peptostreptococcus species	*Bipolaris* species
Gram-positive bacilli	**Parasites**
Corynebacterium diphtheriae	*Acanthamoeba* species
Clostridium species	
Bacillus species	*Microsporidia*
Gram-negative cocci/ Coccobacilli	*Onchocerca volvulus*
Neisseria gonorrhoeae	*Leishmania braziliensis*
Moraxella species	
Acinetobacter species	*Trypanosoma* species
Gram-negative bacilli	
Pseudomonas aeruginosa	*Toxoplasma*
Escherichia coli	
Klebsiella species	
Proteus species	
Serratia marcescens	

Contd...

Contd...

Prokaryotes	Eukaryotes
Filamentous bacteria	
Actinomyces	
Nocardia	
Mycobacterium	
Streptomyces	
Spirochetes	
Treponema pallidum	
Borrelia	
Leptospira	
Mycoplasma	
Rickettsia and *Chlamydia*	

MICROBIOLOGY METHODS

The various methods used to identify the causative organism include various stains to identify the morphology of the organism and culture media to grow these organisms.

Sample Collection and Transport

Appropriate collection and transport of specimen is the first important step in diagnosing ocular infections. Since the specimens available from ocular infection are very small and the load of infectious organisms is less, extra care should be taken while obtaining samples. It is recommended to obtain dual swabs, one for smear examination and one for culture. The commonly used specimens in ocular infections are:
- A swab from the lids
- Conjunctival swab
- Corneal scraping
- Aqueous tap
- Vitreous tap/biopsy
- Explanted intraocular lens (IOL)
- Infected scleral bands, buckle, etc.
- Contact lens solution and case
- Infected corneal button
- Regurgitated material from canaliculi/sac
- Discharge from orbital and lacrimal sinuses/fistula or nasal cavity

In cases where patient-side inoculation is not possible, transport media are used. Example of such transport media include Amies transport medium without charcoal that allows the sample to be stored for about 24 hours. For transport of specimens in suspected viral infection the sample must be transferred in ice, more so when a significant delay is expected.

Microscopy

The various methods of microscopy used to identify organisms included potassium hydroxide (KOH) wet mount preparation, Gram's stain, Giemsa stain, and special stains such as Ziehl–Neelsen (acid-fast stain) and modified Grocott–Gomori methenamine silver nitrate stain.[3] Microscopy done directly from the clinical specimen is called primary microscopy, whereas secondary microscopy is smear examination done on the growth obtained upon culture.

Gram's Staining

Gram staining is a differential staining technique named after Danish bacteriologist Hans Christian Gram,[4] who developed the technique. Depending on the cell wall properties, the bacteria are categorized into two groups, i.e., gram-positive or gram-negative.

Procedure

- Take a clean glass slide.
- Make a thin smear and allow it to air dry.
- Heat fixation is done by passing the slide over the flame several times so that the

heat is unbearable by touching the slide on the dorsum of the hand.
- Pour crystal violet (primary dye) on the smear and wait for 1 minute.
- Wash under running tap water.
- Stain with gram's iodine for 1 minute.
- Wash under running tap water.
- Decolorize with acetone for 2–4 seconds.
- Wash the slide and apply safranin (counter-stain) for 1–2 minutes.
- Blot dry and observe under 100× (oil immersion) objective of the microscope.

Principle and Interpretation

Thicker peptidoglycan layer and acidic protoplasm of the gram-positive bacteria allow them to retain the basic primary dye against decolorization, whereas thinner peptidoglycan layer and labile outer membrane in gram-negative bacteria permit decolorization. Thus, a gram-positive bacteria will appear blue as it will retain the gentian violet–iodine complex. In contrast, a gram-negative will appear blue–purple as it will lose its gentian violet–iodine complex in the decolorization step and appear pink after counterstaining with safranin. The gram-positive bacteria appear purple due to retention of primary dye and gram-negative bacteria appear pink due to counter-stain. Also, the smear should be assessed for inflammatory cells, arrangement, and shape of the bacteria, and their uniformity of staining.

Clinical Application

- Gram-stained smear showing pus cells and gram-positive cocci in clusters suggest staphylococcal infection **(Fig. 8.1)**.
- Gram-stained smear showing pus cells and gram-positive cocci in pairs surrounded by a clear halo suggest *Streptococcus pneumoniae*.

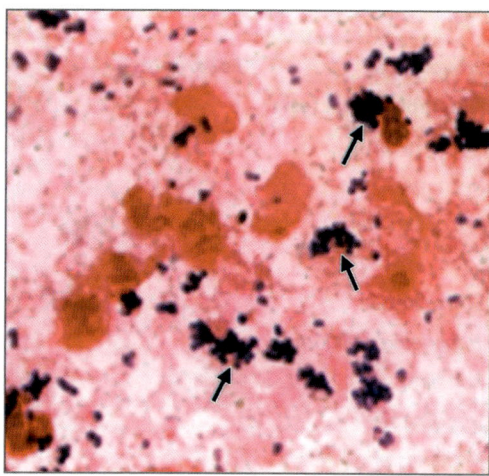

Fig. 8.1: Gram-positive cocci in clusters suggestive of *Staphylococcus* species.

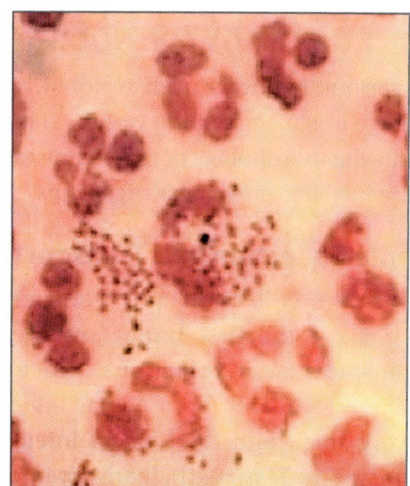

Fig. 8.2: Gram-negative cocci, mostly intracellular.

- Gram-stain smear showing pus cells and gram-negative intracellular and extracellular cocci in pairs (diplococci) suggest *Neisseria* infection **(Fig. 8.2)**.

Potassium Hydroxide Wet Mount

Potassium hydroxide mounts are used for detection of fungal elements in patient's specimens.

Procedure

- Take a clean glass slide.
- Place the specimen in the center of the slide.
- Put one drop of 10% KOH on the specimen.
- Put a coverslip while avoiding any air bubbles.
- Incubate at room temperature for 30–90 minutes to allow clearing of the specimen.
- Screen under 10× objective of the microscope for the presence of fungal elements.
- Confirm the findings by examining under 40× objective.

Principle and Interpretation

Potassium hydroxide digests the animal cells leaving behind the fungal elements intact. KOH helps in loosening the corneal stromal lamellae and exposing more fungal filaments. Fungal elements can be appreciated as refractile, septate or aseptate hyphae **(Fig. 8.3)** yeast cells or conidia with specific morphology. KOH mount also helps to identify *Acanthamoeba*.

Clinical Application

- Septate hyphae with V-shaped acute angle branching is suggestive of infection with *Aspergillus* species.
- Aseptate hyphae with irregular or right-angled branching are suggestive of infection with *Rhizopus/Mucor*.

Figures 8.4A to H depict the characteristics of common fungi implicated in ocular infections.

Ziehl–Neelsen (Acid-Fast) Stain

Ziehl–Neelsen stain is a special stain used for the identification of suspected *Mycobacteria*, *Actinomyces*, or *Nocardia*.

Procedure

- Flame the slide to hit fix (as described above).
- Flood the entire slide with carbol fuchsin.
- The slides are then heated slowly with a Bunsen burner until steaming. The steaming is maintained for 5 minutes using low or intermittent heat.
- Wash the slide with water.
- Using 3% acid alcohol, flood the slide and allow to decolorize for 5 minutes.
- Wash the slide with water.
- Flood the slide with methylene blue (counterstain) for 1 minute.
- Wash the slide with water.

Principle and Interpretation

Mycobacteria with few strains of *Nocardia* resist decolorization by a strong acid (hence the name acid-fast) after staining with basic carbol fuchsin. These organisms have unique lipid-rich cell walls that resist decolorization. Acid-fast organism appears red against a blue background.

Clinical Application

Mycobacteria are acid-fast, *Nocardia* stain variably, whereas *Actinomyces* are nonacid-fast.

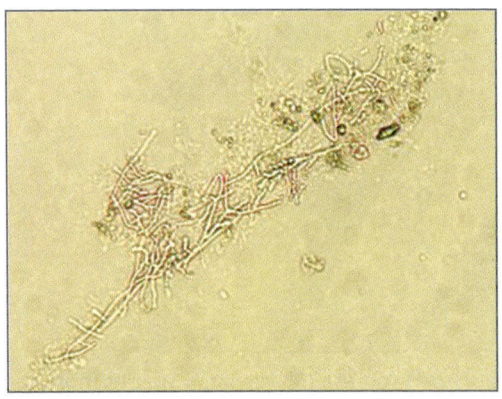

Fig. 8.3: Potassium hydroxide (KOH) mount showing fungal hyphae.

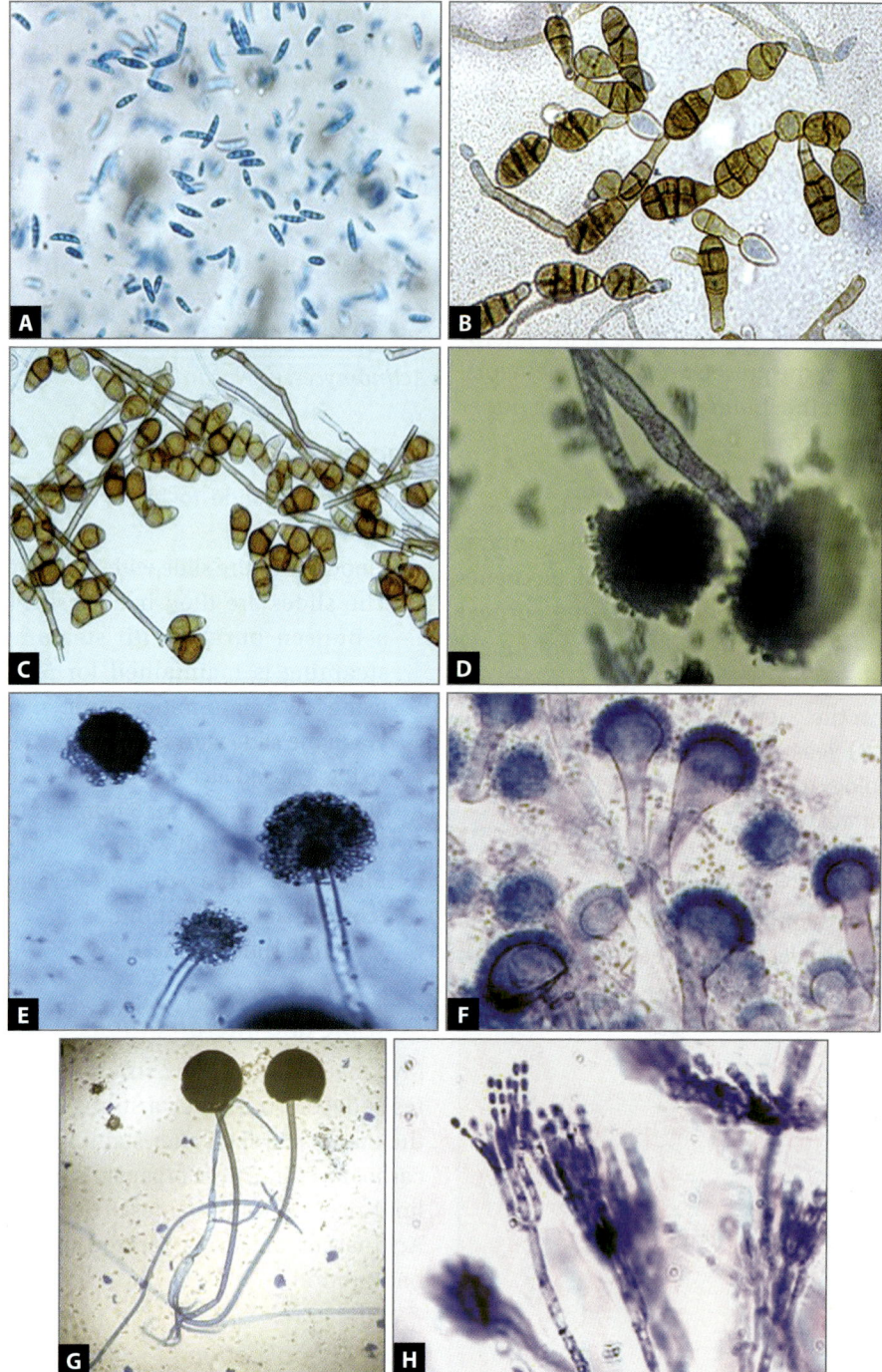

Figs. 8.4A to H: (A) *Fusarium* species (note the sickle-shaped spores); (B) *Alternaria* species (note the vertically and horizontally divided spores); (C) *Curvularia* species; (D) *Aspergillus flavus*; (E) *Aspergillus niger*; (F) *Aspergillus fumigatus*; (G) *Rhizopus* species; (H) *Penicillium* species.

Culture

Culture is the gold standard tool for diagnosing bacterial and fungal infections. Most organisms appear on culture media with distinct characteristics, which helps in easy identification of causative pathogen. The features to be noted while studying the colonies on solid media include shape, size, elevation, margins, surface, edges, color, structure, and consistency.

Culture Media

In ocular microbiology, the commonly used culture media are:
- *Nutrient agar:* It is a type of basic media that support the growth of most nonfastidious bacteria.
- *Blood agar:* It is a type of enriched media, which is used to grow nutritionally exacting (fastidious) bacteria. This contains 5-10% (by volume) blood added to a blood agar base.
- *Chocolate agar:* It is also an enriched media also known as heated blood agar or lysed blood agar.
- *Thioglycollate broth:* It is a liquid medium used for growth of anaerobic organisms.
- *Sabouraud's dextrose agar (SDA):* It is a nonselective medium for growth of fungi **(Fig. 8.5)**.
- *Lowenstein-Jensen (LJ) medium*: It is a selective medium, which is designed to suppress the growth of some microorganisms while allowing the growth of others. LJ medium is used to recover *Mycobacterium tuberculosis* and is made selective by incorporating malachite green.

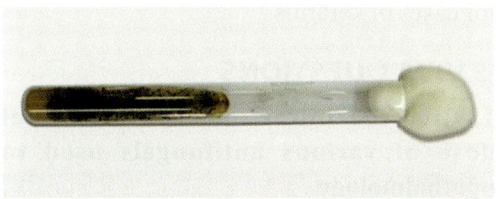

Fig. 8.5: Sabouraud's dextrose agar depicting fungal growth.

Culture Techniques[5]

For aerobic bacterial cultures, all media are incubated at 37°C for 48-72 hours. Chocolate agar is incubated in 3-5% CO_2 in a candle jar or CO_2 incubator. For anaerobic bacterial cultures, anaerobic chamber or anaerobic jar with a gas pack is required. Anaerobic cultures are incubated at least for 5 days before discarding. SDA requires a temperature of 25°-27°C and a biochemical oxygen demand (BOD) incubator. Fungal cultures are incubated for at least 2 weeks before a specimen is considered negative. The *Mycobacteria* may take as long as 4-6 weeks to grow. *Acanthamoeba* species are grown on non-nutrient agar with an overlay of *Escherichia coli* and are incubated at 37°C for 2 weeks. Once the culture shows positive growth, the organisms are subjected to various procedures like microscopy, biochemical tests, subcultures to special media, etc. for identification.

Antimicrobial Susceptibility Testing

The pathogenic microorganisms, especially bacteria, are known to develop resistance to antibiotics or may be insensitive to a particular antibiotic. Thus, susceptibility testing is a must at least for all bacterial pathogens.[6] It helps in determining the most effective drug that can be used for treatment. The two commonly used methods are disc diffusion method and broth dilution.

Disc diffusion method is the most widely used method; it is easy to perform, cost-effective, and reasonably accurate. It consists of using a standard disc of filter paper impregnated with a standard strength of antibiotic under investigation. Dilution method is mostly employed to titrate the therapeutic dose of antibiotic. Susceptibility testing against antifungal drugs can be performed for various fungi by broth or agar dilution methods, where minimum inhibitory concentration (MIC) is determined or by the disc diffusion method.

MOLECULAR METHODS

Molecular methods, especially polymerase chain reaction (PCR), are highly sensitive and specific in diagnosing ocular infections. PCR involves using a pair of priming complementary sequences (oligonucleotide primers), through which multiple copies of a targeted chimeric gene are obtained. The three major steps involved are denaturation, annealing, and elongation. It is particularly useful in diagnosing infections due to organisms, which are difficult to isolate by traditional techniques like culture including viruses, Microsporidia, *Chlamydia*, etc. or those organisms that take a long time to grow, such as *M. tuberculosis*.

IMMUNODIAGNOSTIC METHODS

These tests are useful for detection of *Chlamydia* antigen by immunofluorescence in conjunctival swabs and that of herpes simplex virus (HSV) in corneal scrapings. Antibody detection is also sometimes helpful in ocular manifestations of systemic diseases like syphilis, toxoplasmosis, etc. The direct immunofluorescence (DIF) assay involves fixing the specimens with methanol on a slide and staining with monoclonal immunoglobulin G (IgG) Ab conjugated with fluorescein according to manufacturer instructions. DIF is more sensitive and more reliable than Giemsa staining for detection of *Chlamydia trachomatis* in the conjunctiva samples of patients with follicular conjunctivitis.[7] Indirect immunofluorescent antibody techniques are a useful tool detection of HSV and have a high sensitivity (97%) and specificity (73%) when compared to HSV cultures.[8]

IN VIVO CONFOCAL MICROSCOPY

In vivo confocal microscopy (IVCM) is a noninvasive technique for direct visualization of pathogen throughout the entire depth of the cornea. IVCM allows for rapid identification of fungi and *Acanthamoeba*. The fungal branching angle detected in IVCM imaging of keratitis can be used to differentiate between fungal species, with a 90° angle reported in *Fusarium* species and 45° in *Aspergillus* species.[9] There is increasing evidence that keratitis caused by *Aspergillus* species may have worse clinical outcomes, have higher risk of serious complications such as corneal perforation, and respond less well to natamycin therapy compared with *Fusarium* species. Therefore, IVCM is a useful tool to distinguish between the two species early on in the clinical course. It is particularly useful when corneal infiltrates are deep-seated. It can also be used to monitor the patients' response based on the density of organisms before and after the treatment. However, there are limitations in its widespread use as it requires the expensive machine and expertise in confocal microscopy along with excellent patient cooperation. Moreover, it can only be used for cases of keratitis.

VIVA QUESTIONS

1. Give the intrastromal/intracameral dose of various antifungals used in ophthalmology.

Ans.
- *Amphotericin B:* 5–7.5 µg/0.1 mL

TABLE 8.3: Classification of antifungals.

Class of drug	Examples
Antibiotics	• Polyenes—amphotericin B, nystatin, natamycin • Echinocandins—caspofungin, micafungin • Heterocyclic benzofuran— griseofulvin
Antimetabolites	Flucytosine
Azoles	• Imidazoles—clotrimazole, econazole, miconazole, ketoconazole • Triazoles—fluconazole, itraconazole, voriconazole, posaconazole
Allylamine	Terbinafine

- *Natamycin:* 1 μg/0.1 mL
- *Voriconazole:* 50–100 μg/0.1 mL

2. **Classify various antifungals.**
Ans. Refer to **Table 8.3**.

REFERENCES

1. Klotz SA, Penn CC, Negvesky GJ, Butrus SI. Fungal and Parasitic Infections of the Eye. Clin Microbiol Rev. 2000;13:662-85.
2. Armstrong RA. The microbiology of the eye. Ophthalmic Physiol Opt. 2000;20(6):429-41.
3. Ahmed NH, Satapathy G. Primary microscopy as a point of care test in ophthalmology. Ocular Microbiol DOS Times. 2016;22(3):47-50.
4. Gram HC. "Über die isolierte Färbung der Schizomyceten in Schnitt-und Trocken-präparaten" (in German). Fortschritte der Medizin. 1884;2:185-9.
5. Ahmed NH, Satapathy G. Ocular infections: microbiological perspective. Ocular Microbiol DOS Times. 2017;22(4):35-42.
6. CLSI. Performance Standards for Antimicrobial Susceptibility Testing; Twenty-Third Informational Supplement. CLSI document M100-S26. Wayne: Clinical and Laboratory Standards Institute; 2016.
7. Abedinyfar Z, Doustdar F, Amoli FA, Goudarzi H, Fallah F. Comparison of Direct Immunofluorescence (DIF) Method and Giemsa Staining with PCR Method for Detection of *Chlamydia trachomatis* in Patients with Follicular Conjunctivitis. J Med Microb Diagn. 2016;5(4):216-60.
8. Schwab IR, Raju VK, McClung J. Indirect immunofluorescent antibody diagnosis of herpes simplex with upper tarsal and corneal scrapings. Ophthalmology. 1986;93(6):752-6.
9. Chidambaram JD, Prajna NV, Larke N, Macleod D, Srikanthi P, Lanjewar S, et al. In vivo confocal microscopy appearance of *Fusarium* and *Aspergillus* species in fungal keratitis. Br J Ophthalmol. 2017;101(8):1119-23.

CHAPTER 9

Community Ophthalmology

9.1 BLINDNESS: DEFINITION, BURDEN, PREVENTION, AND REHABILITATION

Vivek Gupta, Pallavi Shukla, Suraj S Senjam, Meenakshi Wadhwani, Praveen Vashist

■ DEFINITION

Standardized measurement and classification of visual impairment and blindness are vital to ensuring the correct comparison of the burden of them across regions and countries. An initial definition recommended by the 1948 World Health Organization (WHO) Expert Committee on Health Statistics was a central visual acuity (VA) of 6/60 (20/200) or worse with the best correcting lens, or widest diameter of visual field no greater than 20°. The definition has changed over the years and before 2006, the definition endorsed by the WHO under ICD-10 (International Statistical Classification of Diseases and Related Health Problems-10) was based on best-corrected visual acuity (BCVA) of less than 3/60 in better eye or a visual field of under 10°. In 2006, the definition was changed to reflect the importance of refractive errors as a cause of blindness. The standardized definition adopted by WHO since 2006 is as shown in **Table 9.1.1**.[1] Thus, the current definition of blindness by WHO is *"presenting visual acuity (PVA) of less than 20/400 (3/60) or a visual field of no greater than 10° in radius around central point of fixation in the better eye".* The term "low vision" was present in ICD-10 before 2006. This term was replaced by category 1 and 2. This was done so since the term "low vision" is commonly used to identify patients who need low-vision care and services (as described later in the chapter) and has a different definition.

In India, the National Programme for Control of Blindness (NPCB) used to define blindness as "presenting distance visual acuity less than 20/200 (6/60) in the better eye" or decrease in field of vision to <20° around the central point of fixation in the better eye. However, with this definition in place, it was difficult to compare the blindness data of India with the worldwide statistics. As a result, there used to be wide disparity in estimation of blindness and visual impairment as per WHO and NPCB. Another implication of this definition was that uncorrected refractive error (URE) emerged as an important cause of blindness as per Indian data. This also decreased the emphasis on other causes of blindness such as glaucoma and posterior segment diseases.[2] After due considerations, the definition of blindness in India was changed in 2017 as *"presenting distance VA less than 3/60 (20/400) in the better eye or limitation of field of vision <10° from center of fixation".*[3]

TABLE 9.1.1: Definition of blindness after the 2006 revision of ICD-10.

Category	Presenting visual acuity (PVA) for distance vision	
	Worse than	Equal to or better than
Category 0, early or mild, or no visual impairment (EVI)	–	6/18
Category 1, moderate visual impairment (MVI)	6/18 3/10 (0.3) 20/70	6/60 1/10 (0.1) 20/200
Category 2, severe visual impairment (SVI)	6/60 1/10 (0.1) 20/200	3/60 1/20 (0.05) 20/400
Category 3, blindness: OR Visual field 10° or less radius around central point of fixation in the better eye	3/60 1/20 (0.05) 20/400	1/60 1/50 (0.02) 20/1200 or counts finger (CF) at 1 m
Category 4, blindness: OR Visual field 10° or less radius around central point of fixation in the better eye	1/60 1/50 (0.02) 20/1,200	Light perception
Category 5, blindness: OR Visual field 10° or less radius around central point of fixation in the better eye	No light perception	
Category 9, unspecified or undetermined		

BURDEN

Globally, around 216.6 million are estimated to be suffering from moderate-to-severe visual impairment and another 36 million are estimated to be suffering from blindness in 2015. The trends in blindness in India are displayed in **Table 9.1.2**.

In India, there were 7.2 million (<3/60 vision) blind people in 1990, which have increased to 8.8 million in 2015. India is home to almost a quarter of the total 36 million blind people globally.

Causes of Blindness and Visual Impairment

The major causes of blindness (<3/60 vision) in India as reported by the National Blindness Survey of 2001 in population aged 50 years and above are given in **Table 9.1.3**.

The National Blindness and Visual Impairment Survey 2015–2019 was conducted in order to provide the evidence about the present status of blindness and visual impairment in India. The survey was planned by the Ministry of Health and Family Welfare, Government of India. Dr Rajendra Prasad Centre for Ophthalmic Sciences, AIIMS, New Delhi was responsible for planning and executing the field work, monitoring, analysis and report writing of the survey. The survey was conducted in partnership with various reputed Eye Health Institutes of the country.

The survey was conducted in aged ≥50 years population using rapid assessment of avoidable blindness (RAAB) strategy in

TABLE 9.1.2: Trends in the prevalence of blindness.

Survey	Definition	50+ years	All ages
ICMR survey 1974	<6/60 in better eye	–	1.38%
WHO-NPCB National Blindness Survey (1986–89) across all ages	<6/60 in better eye	–	1.49%
NPCB National Blindness Survey (1999–2001) in population aged 50 years or more	Presenting vision <6/60 in better eye	8.5%	–
	BCVA <6/60 in better eye	4.3%	1.1%
National Blindness Survey (2006–07) in population aged 50 years or more	Presenting vision <6/60 in better eye	8.0%	–
	BCVA <6/60 in better eye	5.9%	1.0%

(BCVA: best-corrected visual acuity; ICMR: Indian Council of Medical Research; NPCB: National Programme for Control Blindness; WHO: World Health Organization)

TABLE 9.1.3: Major causes of blindness.

Cause	Percent of blindness <6/60
Cataract	62.6
Refractive errors	19.7
Glaucoma	5.8
Post. Seg. disorders	4.7
Corneal blindness	0.9
Surgical complication	1.2
Others	5

31 districts of 24 States/Union Territories of India from September 2015 to June 2018. The key findings are described in **Table 9.1.4**.

Avoidable blindness includes blindness that is either preventable or treatable—refractive errors, cataract, aphakia, cataract surgical complications, trachoma, corneal opacities, and diabetic retinopathy. Approximately 80–90% of blindness in India is considered avoidable. The profile of blindness has changed and infectious causes such as trachoma, which were the most important causes of blindness at the time of independence have decreased in importance. Trachoma is on the verge of elimination with <5% prevalence of active trachoma infection in children.

- *Cataract:* Cataract surgical rate (CSR) measures cataract surgeries per million population per year. India has a CSR of approximately 5,000/million. The cataract surgical coverage (CSC) measures among the persons who are suffering from cataract-related blindness, what proportion has been operated and was 82.3% in 2007 for India among persons having vision less than 3/60. *In the 2007 survey, 64% of all cataract surgeries and 82% of surgeries conducted in last 5 years* were with intraocular lens (IOL) implantation. Currently over 6,500,000 cataract surgeries occur annually in India.
- *Refractive errors:* Nearly 11.0% children in schools and 8% children in community suffer from refractive errors. Burden is higher in urban children as compared to rural and in students of private schools as compared to government schools. School vision screening and distribution of free spectacles are the major strategy for control. Presbyopia is also an important condition affecting all persons aged 50+ years.

TABLE 9.1.4: Key findings of the National Blindness and Visual Impairment Survey 2015–2019.

Indicators	Percentage
Prevalence of blindness in all age groups	0.36
Prevalence of blindness in population aged ≥50 years	1.99
Prevalence of severe visual impairment (SVI) in all age groups	0.35
Prevalence of SVI in population aged ≥50 years	1.96
Prevalence of early visual impairment (EVI) in all age groups	1.84
Prevalence of MVI in population aged ≥50 years	9.81
Prevalence of EVI in all age groups	2.92
Prevalence of EVI in population aged ≥50 years	12.92
Prevalence of moderate severe visual impairment (MSVI) in all age groups	2.19
Prevalence of MSVI in population aged ≥50 years	11.77
Prevalence of visual impairment (VI – Blindness + MSVI) in all age groups	2.55
Prevalence of visual impairment (VI – Blindness + MSVI) in population aged ≥50 years	13.76
Major causes of blindness in population aged ≥50 years	
Cataract	66.2
Corneal opacity (including trachomatous)	8.2
Cataract surgical complications (including PCO)	7.2
Posterior segment disease (excluding DR and ARMD)	5.9
Glaucoma	5.5
Major causes of visual impairment in population aged ≥50 years	
Cataract	71.2
Refractive error	13.4
Cataract surgical complications (including PCO)	5.9

Contd...

Contd...

Indicators	Percentage
Major causes of blindness in population aged 0–49 years	
Corneal opacity	37.5
All globe/CNS abnormality (Amblyopia)	25.0
Phthisis	12.5
Other/undetermined	25.0
Major causes of visual impairment in population aged 0–49 years	
Refractive error	29.6
Cataract	25.4
All globe/CNS abnormality (Amblyopia)	15.5
Corneal opacity	14.1
Cataract surgical coverage (persons) in population aged ≥50 years	
Visual acuity <3/60	93.2
Visual acuity <6/18	74.0
Proportion of intraocular lense (IOL) cataract surgery in population aged ≥50 years	
With intraocular lense	94.2
Visual outcomes (BCVA) after cataract surgery in population aged ≥50 years	
Very good (can see 6/12)	73.4
Good (cannot see 6/12 but can see 6/18)	10.5
Borderline (cannot see 6/18 but can see 6/60)	7.6
Poor (cannot see 6/60)	8.5

(ARMD: age-related macular degeneration; BCVA: best-corrected visual acuity; CNS: central nervous system; DR: diabetic retinopathy; PCO: posterior capsular opacification)

- *Corneal blindness:* In India, approximately 1–1.2 million are affected by bilateral corneal blindness and another 5–6 million have unilateral corneal involvement. The annual rise is estimated to be 50,000 cases. We need 100,000 keratoplasties and collection of 200,000 corneas per year in

India. Setting of eye collection centers, eye banks, training of surgeons in corneal transplantation, promoting eye donation through public awareness, and hospital-based cornea retrieval program (HCRP) are some key strategies.

- *Glaucoma:* Prevalence of glaucoma ranges from 1 to 4% among 40+ years population in India of which approximately one-third is angle closure glaucoma. An important issue is that over 90% of people with glaucoma remain undiagnosed. Compliance among patients diagnosed with glaucoma is poor. Opportunistic screening in eye clinics is advised as is family-based screening among blood relatives of diagnosed patients. Glaucoma screening is also advised in comprehensive eye camps.
- *Diabetic retinopathy:* India is the diabetic capital of the world and the diabetic retinopathy is also rising. The prevalence of *diabetic retinopathy* in India is estimated as 16.37% in 40+ year aged population. Risk factors include uncontrolled blood glucose levels, longer duration of disease, concurrent dyslipidemia, being overweight, use of insulin, and presence of comorbid diabetic complications. Annual retinal screening of patients with diabetes is the recommended strategy for early diagnosis, alongside ensuring blood sugar control for prevention.
- *Childhood blindness and retinopathy of prematurity (ROP):* Childhood blindness is estimated to affect 0.8/1,000 children in India. Of this, one-fifth is attributable to corneal scars, one-fifth to pediatric cataract and glaucoma, and rest to other causes. ROP is increasing in India due to opening of a large number of private as well as government neonatal intensive care units (NICUs), and increasing survival of prematurely born children (<30 weeks, 1,500 g birth weight). Approximately 10% of childhood blindness in India can be attributed to ROP. Under the Rashtriya Bal Swasthya Karyakram (RBSK), weekly ROP screening of infants by ophthalmologist is recommended in case of (1) low birth weight <2,000 g; (2) gestation <35 weeks; and (3) infants having risk factors—sepsis, hypotension, apnea, poor weight gain, anemia, and blood transfusion.

PREVENTION

The objective of "prevention" is to prevent development or progression of disease and its complications. It comprises health promotion, preservation, and restoration.

Primary Prevention

Primary preservation refers to preventing development of risk factors for blindness. This often includes health education and health promotion interventions. Some primary prevention strategies for prevention of blindness and visual impairment include:

- *Corneal blindness:* Preventing ocular injuries.
- *Trachoma:* Facial hygiene and environmental sanitation interventions.
- *UREs:* Evidence is emerging toward increasing outdoor activity for prevention of myopia.
- *Diabetic retinopathy:* Encouraging healthy behaviors that prevent development of diabetes mellitus through lifestyle interventions and environmental modifications will prevent diabetic retinopathy.
- *Glaucoma:* Cessation of smoking in high-risk groups and observance of the glaucoma awareness week.

Secondary Prevention

Secondary prevention includes early diagnosis and treatment of blinding conditions. This includes screening and case finding interventions. This also includes interventions aimed to improving the access eye care services such as development of vision centers, ensuring availability of refractive services, and availability of eye surgeries. Some of secondary prevention strategies for prevention of blindness and visual impairment include:
- *Corneal blindness:* Vitamin A supplementation to prevent keratomalacia, measles vaccination to prevent vitamin A deficiency precipitated by measles infections, improving quality of antenatal care, intranatal practices, and essential newborn care to prevent ophthalmia neonatorum, involving local volunteers to ensure immediate referral of ocular injuries, and setting up of eye collection centers, eye banks, and keratoplasty units.
- *Trachoma:* Mass drug administration with azithromycin and surgical interventions for trichiasis.
- *UREs:* School vision screening programs for early detection and presbyopia spectacle dispensing.
- *Diabetic retinopathy:* Promoting treatment and ensuring blood sugar control among patients with diabetes, screening programs for diabetic retinopathy, improving cross-referral linkages between diabetes treatment clinic and ophthalmology clinics, and provisioning treatment of diabetic retinopathy.
- *Cataract:* Cataract screening camps, ensuring cataract surgeries.
- *Glaucoma:* Implementing opportunistic screening, family member screening, screening for glaucoma after cataract surgeries, provisioning antiglaucoma medications, training physicians in awareness, etc.
- *ROP:* ROP screening in NICUs.

TERTIARY PREVENTION (REHABILITATION)

Tertiary prevention targets minimizing complications of illness and limiting visual disabilities and helping a person to utilize the remaining vision to the fullest through visual rehabilitation. There are multiple components of rehabilitation, which are discussed in the following text.

Low Vision and Rehabilitation

The concept of visual disability has now extended beyond simple anatomical impairments or disease. It is recognized now that multiple other personal, social, and environmental factors are extremely important for an individual's functioning and daily living skills. Under the International Classification of Functioning (ICF), following concepts are used currently:
- *Impairments:* These are problems in physiological body function of the eye (vision, color vision, stereopsis, etc.) or alterations in anatomical structures of the eye (ulceration, lens opacities, etc.).
- *Activity limitations:* Due to the impairment of vision, a person may find difficulty in performing various activities. At the same time, with the same type of visual impairment, another person may be still able to perform the same activities.
- *Participation restrictions:* Due to the impairment, an individual may not be able to participate in various social, vocational, educational, or other types of activities.

Disability includes all these three above-mentioned concepts. *Also* use of the term "handicap" is discouraged.

It has been observed that majority of individuals, who are visually impaired or blind even after best correction person still have useful residual vision. These are the target group for low vision and rehabilitation activities.[4,5]

The term *"functional low vision"* was introduced in 1989 as "a level of vision that with standard correction hinders an individual in the planning and/or execution of a task, but which permits enhancement of the functional vision through the use of optical or nonoptical devices, environmental modifications, and/or techniques". WHO redefined functional low vision in 2005, as *"VA of less than 6/18 to light perception, or a visual field of <10° from the point of fixation, after treatment and refractive correction, in the better eye, which is useful or potentially useful for planning and/or execution of a task"*.

The WHO in 1993 defined *low vision* as "person with low vision is one who has impairment of visual functioning even after treatment and/or standard refractive correction, and has a VA of less than 6/18 to light perception, or a visual field of <10° from the point of fixation, but who uses, or is potentially able to use, vision for the planning and/or execution of a task".

Magnitude of low vision: The data on low vision across the globe is extremely lacking. These include people with visual impairment due to causes other than UREs, cataract, and corneal opacities. Roughly, it may be estimated that nearly 20% of visual impairment can account for low vision. As per the 2010 global estimates on blindness and visual impairment, 285 million individuals had visual impairment.[6] It has been estimated that among children <15 years of age, 1.4 million need vision rehabilitation interventions.[7] Scenario in India is no better. Functional low vision prevalence of 1.05% was reported in the Andhra Pradesh Eye Disease study (APEDS), which translates to approximately 12 million in India.[8,9]

Visual Disability Certification

In January 2018, updated guidelines have been notified by the Ministry of Social Justice and Empowerment, Government of India for assessing quantum of visual disability for certification purposes. These are based on two criteria: (1) VA and (2) field of vision.

As per the act, a medical authority has been defined and it should include one ophthalmologist. Vision assessment should be done using Snellen chart after best possible correction (medical, surgical, or usual or conventional spectacles). Under the provisions of the act, a temporary certificate can be issued, if condition is likely to worsen while clearly mentioning the period after which reassessment should be done **(Table 9.1.5)**.

Low-Vision Rehabilitation

Visual rehabilitation is defined as interventions that help in achieving optimized functioning and reduce disability in individuals with visual disability. The major focus of these interventions is helping person with visual disability to be independent, and help them participate in various activities in their home or community, and to help them live independently.

Community-based rehabilitation (CBR) is an important strategy for implementing rehabilitation. It focuses involving the entire community in the rehabilitation process by engaging families, peers, local community groups, social organizations, local self-governments, and other community-based organizations in addition to various governmental organizations. Rehabilitation also

TABLE 9.1.5: Guidelines for grading the visual disability under the RPWD Act 2016, based on best-corrected visual acuity and fields of vision.

Better eye	Worse eye best corrected	Percent impairment
6/6–6/18	6/6–6/18	0
	6/24–6/60	10
	Less than 6/60–3/60	20
	Less than 3/60, no light perception	30
6/24–6/60 or visual field <40° up to 20° around center of fixation or hemianopia involving macula	6/24–6/60	40
	Less than 6/60–3/60	50
	Less than 3/60 to no light perception	60
Less than 6/60 to 3/60 or visual field <20° up to 10° around center of fixation	Less than 6/60–3/60	70
	Less than 3/60–no light perception	80
Less than 3/60 to 1/60 or visual field <10° around center of fixation	Less than 3/60–no light perception	90
Only HMCF, only light perception, no light perception	Only HMCF, only light perception, no light perception	100

(HMCF: hand movements close to face; RPWD: Rights of Persons with Disabilities)

requires policy level action on the part of the government to ensure adequate opportunities are available and support is provided to persons needing rehabilitation services. In simple words, visual rehabilitation is a cross-sectoral exercise with much wider scope beyond the eye care sector.

Low-vision services include low-vision aids and rehabilitative services. Setting up of low-vision services involves following six main steps:

1. *Needs assessment:* It is done through retrospective analysis of available hospital data, subspecialty outpatient department (OPD), disability certification data, community-based studies, and surveys of blind school. Sometimes the only data, which is available is through nongovernment organizations (NGOs) working for the blind.
2. *Situation analysis:* Assessment of human resource availability, infrastructure, and equipment availability need to be done beforehand. Space needs to be identified where these services shall be provided.
3. *Capacity building and training-human resource:* Short-term training on optical, nonoptical, adaptive, orientation, and mobility and activity of daily living (ADLs), home-based care, vocational counseling, and assistance for certification.
4. *Networking with other organizations:* Networking is essential in bringing about a significant change. It requires support of various sectors, community, and many departments. The activities should no longer be restricted to clinic-based rehabilitation, but also CBR.
5. *Equipment and assistive devices:* WHO has a standard list for low-vision assistive devices. These equipment can be made available locally or with the external support. Government also makes provision of such equipment through

scheme of Assistance to Disabled Persons for Purchase or Fitting of Aids or Appliances (ADIP). Under this scheme, a separate list for the visually disability is included.[10,11] Multiple types of optical devices are available, which work through principles of enlargement or object, enhancement of contrast, selective fixation, or magnification that can be achieved electronically or optically. Apart from optical devices, there are certain nonoptical aids as well, which can be of considerable help for the visually disabled:

a. *Relative size devices:* These include devices such as large print books, large typewriters, etc., which increase the size of object to be viewed.
b. *Positioning and posture devices:* These devices provide more comfort to the disabled in doing vision related work at length.
c. *Light and illumination modification:* These devices increase illumination, control glare, and restrict certain wavelength to increase clarity.
d. *Writing and communication devices* in the form of typoscopes, writing guide, and signature guide.
e. *Mobility assistive devices:* Canes, smart cane, broad-beam lights, and dog guide assist the visually disabled in walking from place to place without seeking assistance from others.
f. *Visual substitution devices:* These devices are helpful in making their day-to-day activities easier, e.g., talking clocks, Braille, and Notex.

6. *Monitoring:* Last but not the least is the program monitoring. It must be integral part of the low-vision services. It includes efficiency indicators and effectiveness indicators. Efficiency indicators include number of patients registered, number of examined and number prescribed aids, number of patients rehabilitated, etc. Effectiveness indicator includes—quality of life, occupational or educational performance, improvement in ADLs, etc. The Indian Visual Function Questionnaire (Ind-VFQ) is also used to study and track changes in visual function over time.

Visual rehabilitation is multidisciplinary in activities. It involves a wide range of professionals. Various professional along with their engagements is listed in **Table 9.1.6**.[12,13]

Community-based Low-Vision Rehabilitation Matrix

The CBR matrix developed by the WHO consists of five components—each with five elements. These help in identifying the nature of services that are needed by a specific person and also help in identifying the nature of services that can be offered to a specific person within a CBR program. The matrix also helps clarify the roles of CBR organizations that are not directly related to patients suffering from low vision such as advocacy and community mobilization **(Flowchart 9.1.1)**.

VISION 2020: THE RIGHT TO SIGHT

Vision 2020: The Right to Sight is a joint global initiative of WHO and IAPB (International Agency for Prevention of Blindness) for elimination of avoidable blindness by 2020. Five priority diseases under Vision 2020 (Global) are—(1) cataract, (2) refractive errors, (3) onchocerciasis, (4) childhood blindness, and (5) trachoma.

A "Vision 2020: The Right to Sight India" initiative has also been launched at the

TABLE 9.1.6: Low-vision professionals and their roles.

Professional	Roles
Ophthalmologists	• Examination and diagnosis of eye disease • Treatment of eye disease • Medication • Surgery
Optometrist	• Low-vision examination • Treatment of refractive error • Eye glasses • Contact lenses • Treatment of low vision • Modification of lighting and contrast
Occupational therapist	• Low-vision rehabilitation examination • Low-vision rehabilitation • Management of multiple disabilities
Vision rehabilitation therapists or rehabilitation teachers	• Low-vision rehabilitation examination • Low-vision rehabilitation, Braille reading instruction
Orientation and mobility specialist	• Orientation and mobility examination • Orientation and mobility
Teachers of the visually impaired	Special education of children with low vision and blindness
Low-vision therapist	• Low-vision therapist examination • Low-vision therapist
Social worker	Individual and group counseling, facilitate access to resources, and support services

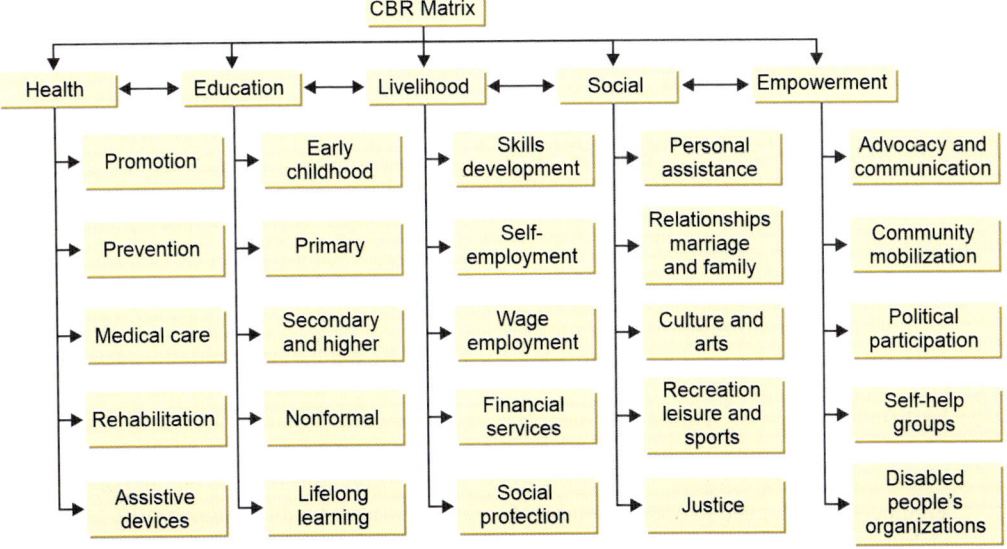

Flowchart 9.1.1: The community-based rehabilitation (CBR) matrix.

country level. Diseases included under Vision 2020: The Right to Sight India are:
- Cataract
- Refractive errors and low vision
- Childhood blindness
- Trachoma
- Corneal blindness
- Diabetic retinopathy
- Glaucoma

NATIONAL PROGRAMME FOR CONTROL OF BLINDNESS AND VISUAL IMPAIRMENT

The NPCB was launched in 1976. The program had set a target of reducing the blindness prevalence from 1.4 to 0.3% by the year 2000. This target was subsequently shifted to 2020. The name of the program has been revised to National Programme for Control of Blindness and Visual Impairment (NPCB & VI) along with the change in definition of blindness in 2016. Under the National Health Policy of 2017, a target of reducing the prevalence of blindness to 0.25/1,000 by 2025 and disease burden by one-third from current levels has been announced. The government of India has also endorsed the Global Action Plan for Universal Eye Health developed by the WHO. The Global Action Plan has set a target of reduction in prevalence of avoidable visual impairment by 25% by the year 2019 (target 2.4%) from the baseline of 2010 (baseline 3.2%).

REFERENCES

1. World Health Organization. List of official ICD-10 updates ratified October 2006. Geneva: WHO; 2006.
2. Vashist P, Senjam SS, Gupta V, Gupta N, Kumar A. Definition of blindness under National Programme for Control of Blindness: Do we need to revise it? Indian J Ophthalmol. 2017;65(2):92-6.
3. Leat SJ, Fryer A, Rumney NJ. Outcome of low vision aid provision: the effectiveness of low vision clinic. Optom Vis Sci. 1994;71(3):199-206.
4. Goodrich G, Bailey I. A history of the field of vision rehabilitation from the perspective of low vision. In: Silverstone B, Lang M, Rosenthal B, Faye E (Eds). The Lighthouse Handbook on Vision Impairment and Vision Rehabilitation. New York: Oxford University Press; 2000. pp. 675-708.
5. Pascolini D, Mariotti SP. Global estimates of visual impairment: 2010. Br J Ophthalmol. 2012;96:614-8.
6. WHO. Vision Impairment and Blindness. [online] Available from www.who.iny/mediacentre/factsheets/fs282/en/ [Last accessed January, 2019].
7. Dandona R, Dandona L. Review of findings of the Andhra Pradesh Eye Disease Study: policy implications for eye care services. Indian J Ophthalmol. 2001;49(4):215-34.
8. World Health Organization. Rehabilitation. [online] Available from www.who.int/rehabilitation/en/ [Last accessed October, 2024].
9. World Health Organization. WHO framework on rehabilitation services: expert meeting. [online] Available from www.who.int/rehabilitation/expert-meeting-june17/en/ [Last accessed October, 2024].
10. ADIP Scheme. National Board of Examination in Rehabilitation. [online] Available from www.niepmdexaminationsnber.com/documents/niepmd_scheme.pdf [Last accessed October, 2024].
11. Whittaker SG, Scheiman M. Low Vision Rehabilitation: A Practical Guide for Occupational Therapists, Second edition. Thorofare: Slack Incorporated Publishers; 2015.
12. WHO. About the community-based rehabilitation (CBR) matrix. [online] Available from: www.who.int/disabilities/ cbr/matrix/en/ [Last accessed January, 2019].
13. Johnson GJ (Ed). The Epidemiology of Eye Diseases. London: Imperial College Press; 2012.

9.2 SURVEY METHODS IN OPHTHALMOLOGY

Vivek Gupta, Meenakshi Wadhwani, Praveen Vashist, Suraj S Senjam

INTRODUCTION

Eye health surveys are instrumental tools in ophthalmic epidemiology and community eye health. Survey data have proven indispensable in situation analysis, development planning, program management, and decision-making at all levels. Very often the health systems in developing countries are not adequately developed and the data generated routine reporting mechanisms is not adequate for programmatic planning or evaluations. Ophthalmic surveys fill this gap. The basic premise in any survey is that systematic data collection from an adequate number of participants, who are representative of a larger reference population, can yield valid information about the entire reference population. However, a rigorous methodology and execution with population-based data collection and a sufficiently large sample size are key aspects of a survey. The most common design of ophthalmological surveys is cross-sectional studies. Results of surveys have shaped India's NPCB and have provided extremely useful data the world over. Some of the landmark ophthalmic surveys in India include the National Trachoma Pilot Project Survey, ICMR National Survey of Blindness, Andhra Pradesh Eye Disease Study (APEDs), Aravind Comprehensive Eye Study (ACES), and the National Blindness Surveys of 1989, 2001, and 2007.

USES OF OPHTHALMOLOGICAL SURVEYS

The most common uses of surveys include:
- Assessment of the magnitude of blindness and visual impairment
- Assessment of the major causes of blindness and visual impairment
- Assess trends in magnitude and causes over time and across regions.
- Identify the magnitude of treated and untreated visual impairment.
- Estimate indicators of healthcare utilization such as CSC.
- Assessing barriers to utilization of eye health services
- Generate hypothesis about possible relationships between eye health status and risk factors.
- Evaluating the effectiveness of health programs and interventions in reducing blindness and visual impairment.

Survey Approaches

Conventional ophthalmological surveys usually included very detailed data collection about ocular symptoms, vision, and included detailed ophthalmic examination. Conducting extensive eye examination in population-based surveys also decreases participation rates. This makes comprehensive surveys very resource-intensive, time-intensive, and expensive. Since 1990s, there has been a trend toward developing rapid assessment survey methodologies. Rapid ophthalmological survey methodologies have been developed for cataract, onchocerciasis, and trachoma and now for blindness and visual impairment. The surveys become rapid by leveraging local resources, simplifying sampling methodology, omitting detailed history-taking, simplifying ocular examination, and automating data management and analysis. These rapid surveys aim to generate data that satisfies the needs of a program manager for planning and evaluation of ongoing eye care programs. Some of these standard approaches include Rapid Assessment of Cataract Surgical Services (RACSS), Rapid Assessment of Avoidable Blindness (RAAB), Rapid Assessment method for Refractive Errors (RARE), Trachoma Rapid Assessment (TRA), Rapid Assessment of Visual Impairment (RAVI), etc. The RAAB surveys have become especially popular due to their low cost and rapidity and have been extensively conducted all over the world. The 2007 and the 2015 National Blindness Surveys of India are also based on the RAAB methodology.

CONDUCT OF AN EYE HEALTH SURVEY

Objectives

This first step is to clarify the focus and the priority conditions that are the target of the survey. Objectives should be unambiguous and precise, and having clarity in objectives makes the entire survey methodology much more focused.

Objectives of the National Blindness Survey of India 2015–2018 include:
- To determine the prevalence of blindness (including avoidable blindness) among the 50+ population
- To identify the major causes of blindness (including avoidable blindness)
- To ascertain the visual outcomes after cataract surgery among operated cases
- To estimate the CSC
- To ascertain barriers for uptake of cataract surgery
- To assess the prevalence of diabetes and diabetic retinopathy in the study population
- The proportion of people with known diabetes who have had a previous fundus examination

Survey Instruments

The survey instruments include not only the eye examination equipment, but also the survey questionnaire or the examination record (proforma). Comprehensive surveys require more extensive equipment depending on the objectives framed. The survey questionnaire and examination records are carefully designed to ensure simplicity in language, avoiding leading and double-barreled questions, and having a proper flow. Responses are restricted to only a certain set of possible values (closed-ended) wherever possible. Questionnaires are broken down in logical sections by grouping questions of similar type together. Having a well-designed questionnaire goes a long way toward avoiding information biases in the survey. The equipment needed for trachoma prevalence surveys are torchlight and corneal loupe. The National Blindness Survey India involves the following survey instruments:

- *Equipment:*
  - Snellen 6 m single optotypes of 6/12, 6/18, and 6/60
  - One tape or rope of 6 m (20 ft) with a knot or ring in the middle at 3 m (10 ft)
  - Torch with focused light and spare batteries
  - Direct ophthalmoscope with spare batteries
  - Occluder with pinhole, preferably with multiple holes (of size 0.5–1 mm)
  - *Indirect ophthalmoscope*: For evaluation of diabetic retinopathy
- Timetable listing all population units and the dates they will be visited by which team
- Maps of the entire survey area with all selected population units marked
- Forms
- The RAAB survey records; staple exactly as many forms as the total number of

persons 50+ to be examined per cluster together to form one bundle for each cluster
- Referral slips for hospital
- Tally sheet of participants enumerated, dilated, examined, referred, and gender
- *Cluster summary form:* Include survey area, the number and the name of the population area, the date of examination, and the name and signature of the team leader
- One set of coding instructions and a set of instructions for examiners
- Map of population unit to be divided in segments
- Basic medicines to treat common minor ailments
- Necessary stationary and bags.

Study Area

The study area refers to the geographical area in which the survey will be conducted and to which the results of the survey can be generalized. This may be the entire country, a state, a district or a village, or a city. This has an important bearing on the sampling methodology since potentially any person living in the survey area is a potential participant of the survey. The selected survey areas should be safe and accessible. Survey should not be done in an area where the safety of field staff cannot be guaranteed. India's National Blindness Surveys are done to represent entire India as the Study Area.

In the trachoma prevalence surveys, the districts were chosen to be representative of former hyperendemic areas of the country.

Study Population

The entire population of the study area often constitutes the study population. Many population groups exist in the study area who would be extremely difficult to include in the survey. These would include for example the incarcerated populations, migratory labor, army personnel, etc. It is required clearly to enunciate the target study population for the survey and list out their selection criteria. In the RAAB survey, the study population consists of all individuals aged 50 years or more who are usual residents of the selected study area. Residency has been defined as usual resident of the area over the last 6 months. Any visitors are excluded from the study population. In the trachoma surveys, the entire usual resident population comprises the study population—individuals aged 1-9 years are the study population for active trachoma infection prevalence assessment while older residents are the study population for assessment of trachoma sequelae.

Sample Size

Sample size is vital that a proper sample size estimation is done before survey is initiated. The standard formula used to calculate the sampling method for ophthalmic surveys is:

Sample size for prevalence survey

$$= \frac{Z_a^2 \times p \times (100 - p)}{d^2} \times \text{Deff} \times \left[\frac{(100 + NR)}{100}\right]$$

The formula includes:
- *Prevalence (p%):* The estimated or assumed or anticipated prevalence of the disease (p) expressed as a% of population affected by the disease. In case, there are multiple ocular disorders under consideration, the prevalence of an important disease with lowest prevalence should be used for calculation in the formula. The formula also includes the term $(100 - p)$.
- *Absolute error (d%):* It occurs because of selecting a sample rather than examining the whole population. Sampling error

can be reduced but cannot be completely eliminated. Other terms used for this are precision or allowable error. This usually calculated as between 10 and 20% of the anticipated prevalence. As an example, if the anticipated prevalence of blindness is 9.0%, and the investigators feel that true prevalence be within 20% of the anticipated prevalence, then the value of *d* becomes 1.8% (20% of 9.0%). In case, anticipated prevalence is low (<1%), then *d* can be fixed as 0.2–0.5%.

- *Confidence interval or type-1 error rate (Z):* It is usual to work with 5% type-1 error rate, which corresponds to a Z value of 1.96. A Z of 1.96 refers to 95% probability that the true population prevalence is within "$p - d\%$ to $p + d\%$" range.
- *Design effect (Deff):* It is an adjustment made to adjust for cluster sampling methodology used in ophthalmic surveys. The design effect is high in case we have few clusters each with large participants within each cluster (cluster size) while the design effect decreases as we increase the number of clusters and decrease cluster size. Convention is to use design effect in 1.5–3.0 range. In the RAAB surveys, the design effects recommended are 1.6 for cluster size of 40, 1.7 for cluster size of 50, and 1.8 for cluster size of 60.
- *Nonresponse (NR%):* The sample size needs to be increased because despite all efforts, we will rarely have 100% participation of selected individuals in a survey. A nonresponse rate of 10% is considered acceptable and the overall sample size needs to be increased accordingly by 10%.

Example sample size calculation:
- *p%:* 7.5%
- *d%:* 0.75% (= 10% of *p*)
- Confidence interval or type-1 error rate (Zα): 1.96
- Deff: 1.8 for cluster size of 60
- NR%: 10%

$$\text{Sample size} = \frac{1.962 \times 7.5 \times (100 - 7.5)}{0.75^2}$$

$$\times 1.8 \times \frac{[(100 + 10)]}{10}$$

$$= \frac{2665.11}{0.5625} \times 1.8 \times 1.1 = 9382$$

In addition, the total population size from which the sample is to be drawn (*N*) is adjusted for by adding a finite population correction, in case the total population of district is small (convention—<100,000). It is important to note that in surveys, the type-2 error is not considered since the main purpose of survey is to estimate prevalence. However, type-2 error will come into the play, and a different formula will be used for sample size calculation, if the primary objective of the survey is to measure association between a disease and risk factor.

Sampling Methodology

The most common sampling method used in ophthalmic surveys is multistage cluster random sampling. The first stage is sampling and selection of districts in the country. Districts with larger populations have larger probability of selection, making this a *probability proportionate to size (PPS) simple random sample*. The next stage is the selection of clusters within the district. The clusters are villages and urban wards as defined by the census lists. In the National Blindness Survey, the clusters are selected from all over this district, while in the National Trachoma Prevalence Survey, one of the administrative blocks in the district was randomly selected first and then villages were selected within the block. In RAAB surveys, we take a cluster size of 60 participants per cluster, but the total number of participants aged 50 years or more may be in hundreds in each cluster. To facilitate this selection, *compact segment sampling* method is used within the cluster. Compact segment sampling involves dividing the cluster into smaller segments based on a cluster map. Each segment by itself can yield the number of participants that we need to survey. In the National Blindness Survey 2015–2018, a segment of total 400 population (all ages) will yield 60 participants aged 50 years or more, based on results of the Census 2011. Accordingly, with the help of a local volunteer, the selected cluster is divided into segments of 400 population each (six segments will be made if cluster population is 2,450), each segment is numbered on the map, and one segment is chosen randomly by draw of chits. The survey will start from any randomly selected starting household in the segment, and the team will proceed from house to house till the sample size is achieved. In case, the sample size is not achieved, then next contiguous segment is selected.

Multistage cluster random sampling method reduces the cost, but is less precise compared to the simple random sampling. To adjust for this loss of precision, we include the design effect term when calculating sample size (as described above). This method also facilitates planning for field work because a predetermined number of individuals is interviewed in each unit selected, and staff can be allocated accordingly. This method is still a probability sampling technique since the selection of districts, clusters, and segments was all done using random sampling methods. In the TRA surveys, nonprobability sampling is used wherein the district, the areas with worst hygiene and areas most likely to harbor trachoma infections are purposively selected. The results of these nonprobability TRA surveys, therefore, must never be generalized to entire districts.

Survey Duration

The cluster size if planned in a manner that 1–3 complete clusters can be covered by one team, in 1 day. In the National Blindness Survey 2015–2018, three clusters are completed per day by one team. To complete one district having 50 clusters, 9 working days are required with two teams working in parallel. Adding a period of 5 days of presurvey preparations, 1 day for local training, and 1 day for coordination with the local district administration, 3 days for travel, and 1 day of postsurvey debriefing, each district requires 20 days of work. Additionally, about 1 week is required subsequently for dual data entry and report generation. Overall, one district is realistically covered per month. In trachoma prevalence surveys, two clusters are being covered per day per team, while in the TRAs, three clusters can be covered by one team per day.

Training and Manual of Operations

A detailed manual of operations is also developed and finalized before the start of the survey. It is important that the study protocol remains constant throughout the survey and having the manual of operations ensures that if at any point of time there is a confusion about what needs to be done, the team can refer to the manual of operations and therefore be guided with the survey methodology. A copy of the manual of operations is given to the survey team for their reference, at all times.

All the staffs enrolled in the survey are trained comprehensively in the survey methodology. This includes both classroom teaching as well as a field pilot. An interobserver variation (IOV) assessment is conducted wherein the same patient is examined by two or more optometrists and two or more ophthalmologists. The findings of the teams are matched against each other and the calculation of kappa coefficient is done and recorded. A low value of kappa coefficient indicates the need for further training and discussion to bring consistency in study implementation while a high kappa value (>0.6) indicates consistency.

Survey Resources and Logistics

Managing logistics for the survey is a very important exercise. Through use of survey logistic checklists, it is ensured that all the requirements for the survey are organized well in time before the team departs for the survey district. Logistic planning also includes planning for the travel of the team from the headquarters to the survey district, identification and planning of accommodation for the team in the survey district, organizing local transport, and organizing food for the team members. If the resources are managed well, it means that the survey team can focus on the real work with minimal disturbances. Financial management is also very important since the expense of the survey can run into several lakhs of rupees.

Approval of State and District

Before starting any survey, proper approval from the State Program Officer (SPO), Chief Medical Officer (CMO), District Health Officers (DHO), and District Program Officers (DPO) is arranged to inform them about the survey activities to be conducted in their areas. The district health authorities are also requested to provide maps, list of Accredited Social Health Activist (ASHA) workers, paramedical staff, cluster details, etc. Law and order can sometimes pose problems and therefore the District Collector (DC) is always informed of the plan. The local community leaders (panchayats) are also involved in the implementation of survey. With the involvement of the district administration and health system, a detailed microplan for conduct of survey is prepared. This plan is also shared with the district health administration so that they can mobilize the health system to assist the survey team.

Survey Execution

Survey in the cluster typically consists of activities spread over 2 days—enumeration activities on day 1 and clinical evaluation and examination on day 2.

Enumeration: Two members of the survey team go to the cluster selected for the survey. Once they reach the cluster, they contend the local lusher worker and do compact segment sampling in the cluster. This involves preparing for cluster map, dividing the cluster into segments, and selection of one segment randomly by draw of chits. In the selected segment, a random starting household is identified and enumeration begins. The visited household is informed about the survey that will be done on the next day and the eligible members from the household are requested to be available on the next day for the survey team. In an enumeration sheet, the number of males and females eligible from the household are noted. Using a permanent marker or chalk, a visual marking is done near the gate of the household. The team proceeds from house to house till the required sample size is reached.

Examination: On the next day, one member from the enumeration team of the previous day brings the clinical team to the selected cluster. This person is able to guide the examination team directly to the household where the survey has to begin. In the examination team, two identified members are responsible for taking informed consent and collecting the demographic information in the study proforma. Thereafter, the study optometrists along with field supervisors conduct VA assessments. The participant is then examined by the study ophthalmologists who do lens evaluation, eye examination, and assign the cause of visual impairment or blindness. In case, the patient requires referral to a clinic or hospital, an optometrist and the local health worker accompanying the ophthalmologist counsel the participant and provide a referral card. This optometrist also is responsible for managing all the forms and keeping record of any patients that require evaluation under mydriasis. All the forms that have been filled are checked in the field at completion of a cluster to ensure completeness. After completion of one cluster, the team moves on to the next cluster. The survey investigators and the district medical officer of the CMO also visit the survey team from time to time for supervision and verification of the survey records **(Fig. 9.2.1)**.

ETHICS

The integrity, reliability, and validity of the survey rely heavily on adherence to ethical principles. All the surveys are approved by the institutional ethical board before initiation. Prior to collection of any information, a written informed consent is taken from the participant. The participant information sheet form includes all following points:
- Purpose of the survey
- Procedures involved for the participant in the survey and time involvement required
- Risks and benefits of taking part
- Costs of (or lack of costs of) taking part
- Participation is voluntary
- Participant can say no or withdraw from survey at any time without any danger or risk
- All information collected will be kept confidential to the survey team.
- Contact details of investigators.

Additionally, an aim of surveys is to provide services and all possible support to participants identified as having ocular diseases. In RAAB survey, free antibiotic and lubricating drops are provided to all the needy participants of the survey. All participants needing referral are also appropriately guided. Adequate provision of cataract surgery is made with local district authorities and NGOs. In trachoma surveys, azithromycin and epilation forceps are distributed to participants with active infection or trichiasis, respectively.

DATA ENTRY AND ANALYSIS

Data collected during the day are entered into the data entry system on the same day. The data entry system has inbuilt logical consistency checks that flags records with missing or inconsistent data. This helps in minimizing the data entry errors. Furthermore, this also identifies the records in which errors are present and these records are then shared with the survey team in the evening and the discussion takes place over minimizing them. The team is now able to ensure that the errors do not arise in the field. A second data entry is done once the survey team returns from the district to the headquarters. The first and the second data entry is compared, all nonmatched entries are then corrected by taking out the original survey records. By creating a uniform data analysis code in the statistical software, a uniform data analysis is the run on the updated dataset and the results are

SECTION 2: Basic Sciences

RAPID ASSESSMENT FOR AVOIDABLE BLINDNESS

A. GENERAL INFORMATION
Survey area: _____ ☐☐ Cluster: ☐☐☐☐ Year - month: ☐☐☐☐ - ☐☐ Individual no.: ☐☐☐
Name: _____ Sex: Male: O (1) Female: O (2) Age (years): ☐☐

Optional 1: ☐☐ Examination status:
Optional 2: ☐☐ Examined: O (1) (go to B) Refused: O (3) (go to E)
Not available: O (2) (go to E) Not able to communicate: O (4) (go to E)

Always ask: "Did you ever have any problems with your eyes?" Yes: O (1) No: O (2)
If not available - details (availability / tel number / address)

B. VISION
Uses distance glasses: No: O (1) Yes: O (2)
Uses reading glasses: No: O (1) Yes: O (2)

Presenting vision	Right eye	Left eye
Can see 6/12	O (1)	O (1)
Cannot see 6/12 but can see 6/18	O (2)	O (2)
Cannot see 6/18 but can see 6/60	O (3)	O (3)
Cannot see 6/60 but can see 3/60	O (4)	O (4)
Cannot see 3/60 but can see 1/60	O (5)	O (5)
Light perception (PL+)	O (6)	O (6)
No light perception (PL-)	O (7)	O (7)

Pinhole vision	Right eye	Left eye
Can see 6/12	O (1)	O (1)
Cannot see 6/12 but can see 6/18	O (2)	O (2)
Cannot see 6/18 but can see 6/60	O (3)	O (3)
Cannot see 6/60 but can see 3/60	O (4)	O (4)
Cannot see 3/60 but can see 1/60	O (5)	O (5)
Light perception (PL+)	O (6)	O (6)
No light perception (PL-)	O (7)	O (7)

C. LENS EXAMINATION

	Right eye	Left eye
Normal lens / minimal lens opacity:	O (1)	O (1)
Obvious lens opacity:	O (2)	O (2)
Lens absent (aphakia):	O (3)	O (3)
Pseudophakia without PCO:	O (4)	O (4)
Pseudophakia with PCO:	O (5)	O (5)
No view of lens:	O (6)	O (6)

D. MAIN CAUSE OF PRESENTING VA<6/12
(Mark only one cause for each eye)

	Right eye	Left eye	Principal cause in person
Refractive error:	O (1)	O (1)	O (1)
Aphakia, uncorrected:	O (2)	O (2)	O (2)
Cataract, untreated:	O (3)	O (3)	O (3) (F)
Cataract surg. complications:	O (4)	O (4)	O (4)
Trachoma corneal opacity:	O (5)	O (5)	O (5)
Other corneal opacity:	O (6)	O (6)	O (6)
Phthisis:	O (7)	O (7)	O (7)
Onchocerciasis:	O (8)	O (8)	O (8)
Glaucoma:	O (9)	O (9)	O (9)
Diabetic retinopathy:	O (10)	O (10)	O (10)
ARMD:	O (11)	O (11)	O (11)
Other posterior segment:	O (12)	O (12)	O (12)
All globe/CNS abnormalities:	O (13)	O (13)	O (13)
Not examined: can see 6/12	O (14)	O (14)	O (14)

E. HISTORY, IF NOT EXAMINED
(From relative or neighbour)

Believed	Right eye	Left eye
Not blind	O (1)	O (1)
Blind due to cataract	O (2)	O (2)
Blind due to other causes	O (3)	O (3)
Operated for cataract	O (4)	O (4)

F. WHY CATARACT SURGERY WAS NOT DONE
(Mark up to 2 responses, if VA<6/18, not improving with pinhole, with visually impairing lens opacity in one or both eyes)

Need not felt	O (1)
Fear of surgery or poor result	O (2)
Cannot afford operation	O (3)
Treatment denied by provider	O (4)
Unaware that treatment is possible	O (5)
No access to treatment	O (6)
Local reason (optional)	O (7)

G. DETAILS ABOUT CATARACT OPERATION

	Right eye	Left eye
Age at operation (years)	☐☐	☐☐
Place of operation		
Government hospital	O (1)	O (1)
Voluntary / charitable hospital	O (2)	O (2)
Private hospital	O (3)	O (3)
Eye camp / improvised setting	O (4)	O (4)
Traditional setting	O (5)	O (5)
Type of surgery		
Non IOL	O (1)	O (1)
IOL implant	O (2)	O (2)
Couching	O (3)	O (3)
Cost of surgery		
Totally free	O (1)	O (1)
Partially free	O (2)	O (2)
Fully paid	O (3)	O (3)
Cause of VA<6/12 after cataract surgery		
Ocular comorbidity (Selection)	O (1)	O (1)
Operative complications (Surgery)	O (2)	O (2)
Refractive error (Spectacles)	O (3)	O (3)
Longterm complications (Sequelae)	O (4)	O (4)
Does not apply - can see 6/12	O (5)	O (5)

Fig. 9.2.1: Survey form used in the National Blindness Survey 2015–2018 (sample front page).

generated. In the National Blindness Survey 2015–2018, the use of RAAB-6 software has greatly minimized the time for data analysis.

DISSEMINATION AND USE OF RESULTS

The ultimate aim of the survey is to use the results for the prevention of blindness and severe visual impairment in planning interventions. Otherwise, it becomes a redundant academic exercise. The survey should also be used to develop future programs and policies. The results of all the surveys are shared with the NPCB&VI and the concerned SPO. This helps the program managers to develop and implement various programs and interventions to address the issue of blindness and in turn this helps the nation as it strives to achieve elimination of avoidable blindness and visual impairment. Mass Drug Administration with azithromycin and implementation of safe interventions was done in Nicobar Island in 2011 with the aim to eliminate trachoma based on the results of the TRA survey done in the island in which a very high burden of active trachoma infection was observed. This led to reduction in burden of active trachoma infection to subthreshold levels in 2016, which was documented through two repeat trachoma prevalence surveys conducted in Car Nicobar.

SECTION 3: Interpretation of Images and Reports

10. Interpretation of Images

CHAPTER 10

Interpretation of Images

Pranita Sahay, Jyoti Shakrawal, Gunjan Saluja, Siddhi Goel

INTERPRETATION OF GOLDMANN VISUAL FIELDS

General Principles

Look for following while interpreting a Goldmann visual field (GVF). The report should be interpreted under following headings:
- Eye involved
- Size of stimulus used; the various size of stimulus used have been summarized in **Table 10.1**.
- The area involved general or local
- *The density of scotoma:*
  - *Absolute:* No visual sensation perceived
  - *Relative:* Depressed visual sensation perceived
- *The position of field defect*: Central, temporal, nasal, superior, and inferior
- *Shape:*
  - Sectoral (hemianopia)
  - Nonsectoral (regular or irregular)
- Differential diagnosis of conditions in which the given filed defect is found.

TABLE 10.1: Various stimuli size, diameter, and area used in Goldmann visual fields.

Size of stimulus	Diameter in mm	Area in mm²
0	0.28	1/16
I	0.56	1/4
II	1.13	1
III	2.26	4
IV	4.51	16
V	9.03	64

Specific Examples

- *Example 1* **(Fig. 10.1)**:
  - The given GVF is of the right eye and has been plotted using a stimulus size of IIIe0 and Ve0.
  - The field shows a depressed response in the inferonasal quadrant suggestive of inferior quadrantanopia.
  - Differential diagnosis of inferior quadrantanopic field defects includes:
    - Neoplasia
    - Infarction
    - Infections involving occipital lobe.
- *Example 2* **(Fig. 10.2)**:
  - The given GVF is of the right eye and has been plotted using a stimulus size of I4e0, V4e0, and I3e5.
  - The field shows a dense central scotoma.

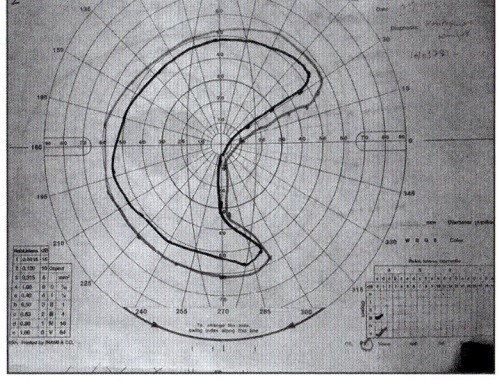

Fig. 10.1: Goldmann visual field (GVF) showing right inferior quadrantanopia.

- Differential diagnosis of this defect includes:
  - Optic neuritis
  - Hereditary optic neuropathy (bilateral central scotoma will be present)[1]
  - Toxoplasma scar
  - Neurosensory detachment (NSD) as in central serous choroidopathy
  - Macular edema
  - Macular degeneration
- *Example 3 (Figs. 10.3A and B):*
  - The given GVF shows a depressed response in the nasal quadrant of the right eye and a depressed response in the temporal quadrant of the left eye.
  - This is suggestive of right eye homonymous hemianopic field defect.
  - Differential diagnosis of these defects include:
    - Retrochiasmal lesions
    - Alzheimer's disease
    - Cortical basal ganglion degeneration
    - Mitochondrial encephalomyopathy
    - Neurosyphilis
    - Neuromyelitis optica
    - Posterior cerebral artery occlusion
    - Epilepsy
- *Example 4 (Fig. 10.4):*
  - The given GVF is of the left eye and has been plotted using a stimulus size of V4e0.
  - The field shows a dense scotoma involving the center and area surrounding it, suggestive of centrocecal scotoma.
  - Differential diagnosis of this defect includes:
    - Optic neuritis
    - Toxic optic neuropathy
    - Stargardt disease

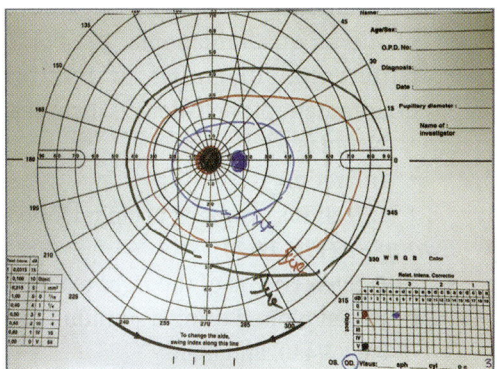

Fig. 10.2: Goldmann visual field showing right central scotoma.

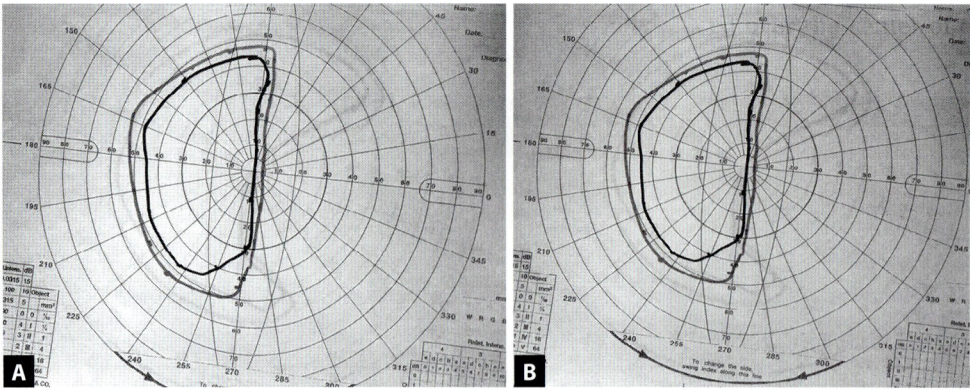

Figs. 10.3A and B: Goldmann visual field showing right homonymous hemianopia.

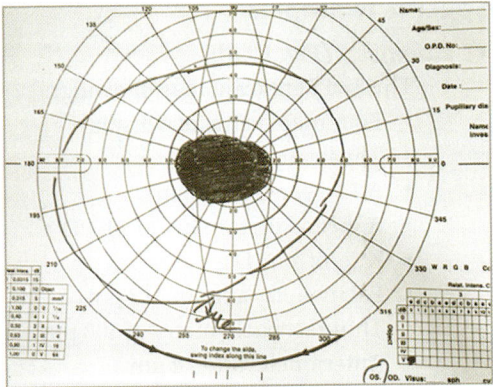

Fig. 10.4: Goldmann visual field showing left centrocecal scotoma.

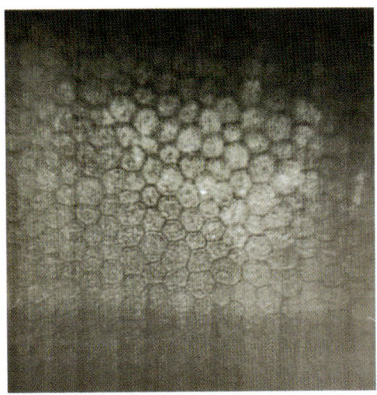

Fig. 10.5: Normal corneal endothelial cell.

INTERPRETATION OF SPECULAR MICROSCOPY

General Principles

Look for following while interpreting specular microscope images. The interpretation should be made under the following headings mentioned as follows:
- Endothelial cell shape
- Endothelial cell morphology
- Presence of cell dropout or guttae
- Differential diagnosis

Specific Examples

- *Example 1* **(Fig. 10.5)**:
  - This is specular microscope image showing:
    - Hexagonal endothelial cells
    - Cells have a bright center and dark border
    - Some variability in the cell size is visible (polymegathism)
    - No cell dropout or guttae
  - This appears to be a normal scan showing normal endothelial cells.
- *Example 2* **(Fig. 10.6)**:
  - This is a specular microscope image showing:
    - Few hexagonal endothelial cells

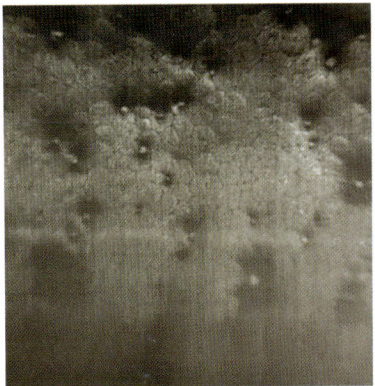

Fig. 10.6: Corneal guttae.

- Corneal guttae are present that are visible as dark areas.
- Few intervening endothelial cells between the corneal guttae have abnormal shape with missing cell boundaries.
- This image suggests the presence of corneal guttae, which can be seen in various conditions like Fuchs' endothelial corneal dystrophy, glaucoma, uveitis, and old age.
- *Example 3* **(Fig. 10.7)**: This is a specular microscope image showing:
  - Endothelial cells of variable shape (pleomorphism) and size (polymegathism)

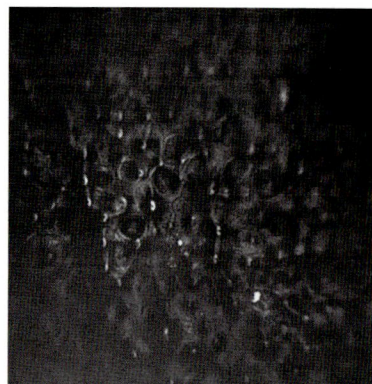

Fig. 10.7: Iridocorneal–endothelial (ICE) cells.

- The cells have a dark area with a light central spot.
- A light peripheral zone is visible with a dark border.

All the above findings suggest that this is a specular microscopy image of a case with iridocorneal endothelial syndrome. The typical appearance of this endothelial cell is called "iridocorneal–endothelial (ICE) cell".

INTERPRETATION OF PENTACAM

General Principles

Look for the following while interpreting a Pentacam map.[2] The interpretation should be made under the following headings as mentioned below. The normal values, as well as screening criteria for diagnosing keratoconus, must be remembered before going through this section (refer the chapter on Pentacam).

- Type of map
- Eye involved
- Age of patient
- K_{mean}
- K_{max}
- Pachymetry apex
- Thinnest pachymetry
- Anterior elevation
- Posterior elevation
- Differential diagnosis

Specific Examples

- *Example 1* (**Fig. 10.8**):
  - This is a Pentacam map showing:
    - Four maps refractive display
    - The left eye
    - A 12-year-old patient
    - A mean keratometry of 44.1 D
    - K_{max} of 45.3 D
    - Pachymetry apex of 512 µm
    - Thinnest pachymetry of 508 µm
    - Anterior elevation 4 µm
    - Posterior elevation 12 µm
  - This appears to be a normal scan showing with the rule corneal astigmatism.
- *Example 2* (**Figs. 10.9A and B**):
  - This is Pentacam map showing:
    - Four maps refractive display
    - Right eye
    - A 12-year-old patient
    - A mean keratometry 46.1 D
    - K_{max} of 48.2 D
    - Pachymetry apex of 511 µm
    - Thinnest pachymetry of 510 µm
    - Anterior elevation 7 µm
    - Posterior elevation 24 µm (abnormal)
  - This scan shows with the rule corneal astigmatism that appears suspicious for forme fruste keratoconus (FFKC) based on the increased posterior elevation. Hence, I would like to evaluate the Belin/Ambrósio enhanced ectasia display of this patient.
  - This is a Pentacam map showing:
    - Belin/Ambrósio enhanced ectasia display
    - The right eye
    - A 12-year-old patient
    - K_{max} of 48.2 D
    - Thinnest pachymetry of 510 µm
    - Inferotemporal displacement of the thinnest location by 0.24 mm (normal range)

CHAPTER 10: Interpretation of Images

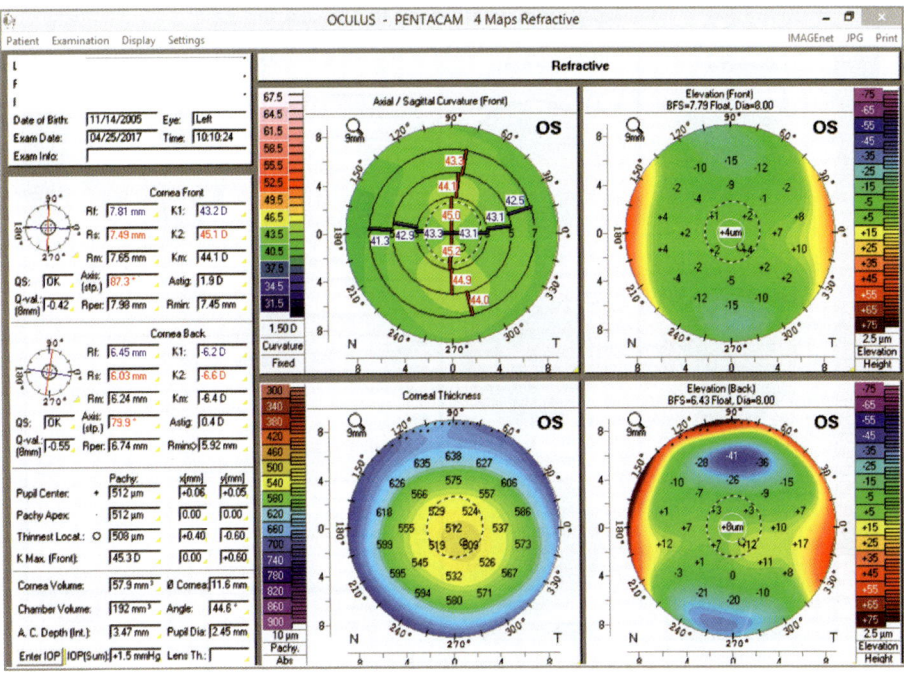

Fig. 10.8: A normal cornea.

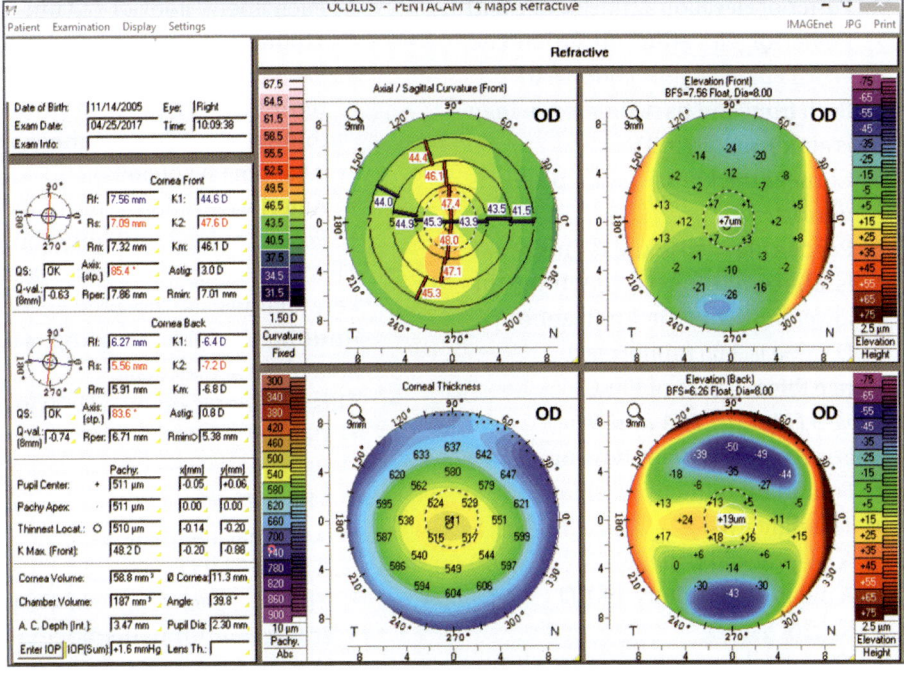

Fig. 10.9A

412 SECTION 3: Interpretation of Images and Reports

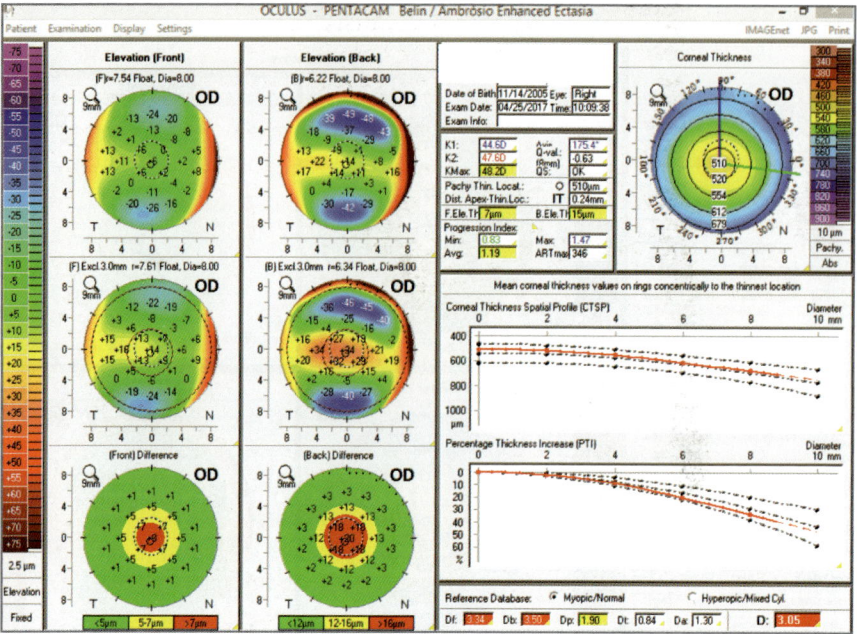

Fig. 10.9B

Figs. 10.9A and B: (A) Four maps refractive display of forme fruste keratoconus (FFKC); (B) Belin/Ambrósio enhanced ectasia display showing FFKC.

- Posterior elevation 22 μm (abnormal)
- Posterior elevation on enhanced ectasia map 34 μm (abnormal)
- Both front and back difference map is abnormal (in red).
- Corneal thickness spatial profile is normal.
- Percentage thickness increase is abnormal (curve touching the lower border in the 6 mm zone).
- D value is 3.05 (abnormal).
- Hence this is a case of FFKC.
- Example 3 **(Figs. 10.10A and B)**:
  - This is Pentacam map showing:
    - Four maps refractive display
    - The right eye
    - A 34-year-old patient
    - A mean keratometry 49.1 D
    - K_{max} of 54.9 D
    - The axial curvature map shows inferior steepening.

- Pachymetry apex of 423 μm
- Thinnest pachymetry of 410 μm
- Pachymetry map shows the inferotemporal displacement of the thinnest location on the y-axis by 0.63 mm (suspicious).
- Anterior elevation 33 μm (abnormal)
- Posterior elevation 67 μm (abnormal)
- This scan suggests that it is a case of keratoconus as the area of corneal thinning is corresponding with the area of corneal ectasia.[3]
- This is a Pentacam map showing:
  - Belin/Ambrósio enhanced ectasia display
  - The right eye
  - A 34-year-old patient
  - K_{max} of 54.9 D
  - Thinnest pachymetry of 410 μm
  - Inferotemporal displacement of the thinnest location by 0.24 mm (normal range)

CHAPTER 10: Interpretation of Images   413

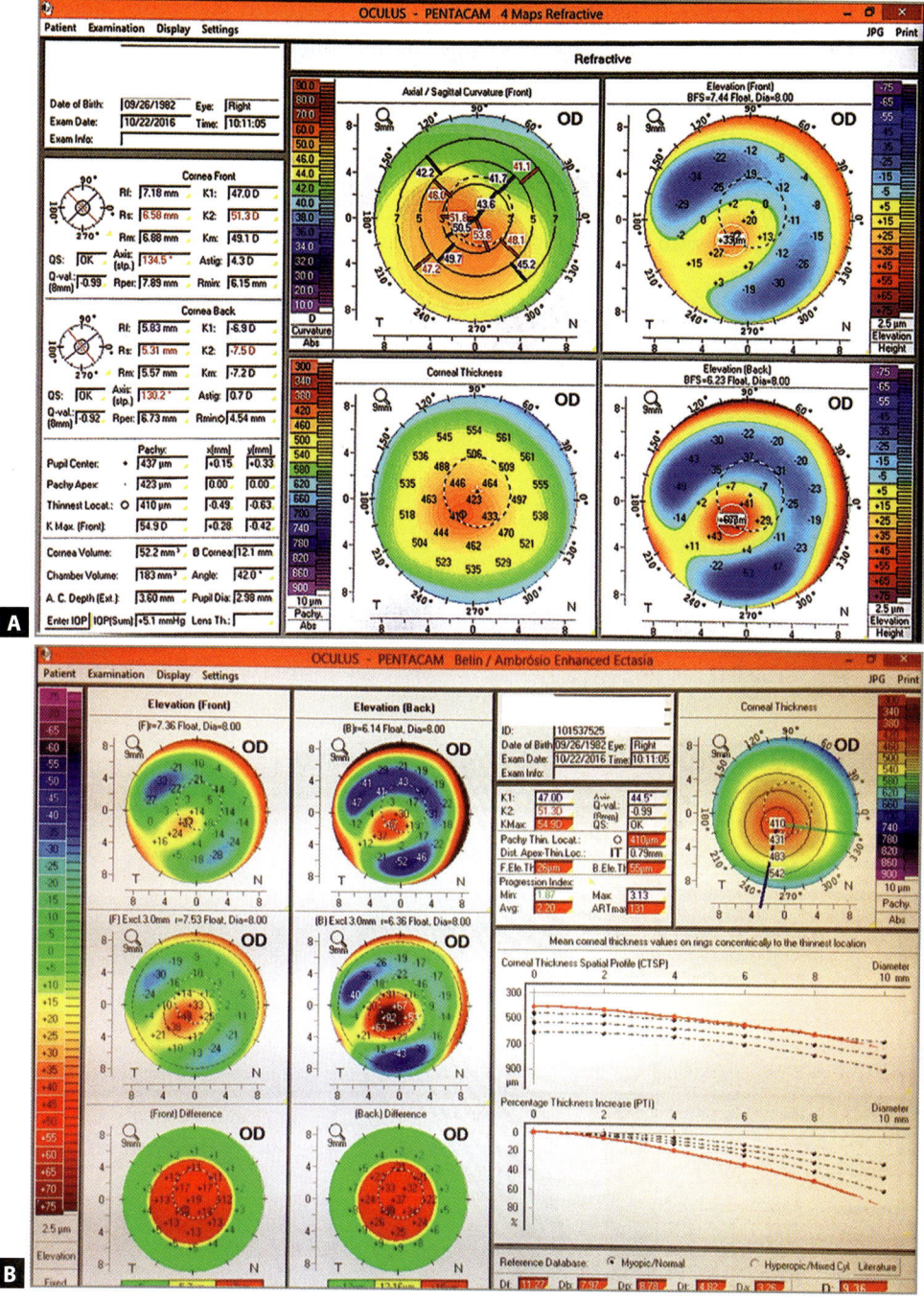

Figs. 10.10A and B: (A) Four maps refractive display; (B) Belin/Ambrósio enhanced ectasia display.

- Posterior elevation 37 µm (abnormal)
- Posterior elevation on enhanced ectasia map 82 µm (abnormal)
- Both front and back difference map is abnormal (in red).
- Corneal thickness spatial profile is abnormal (curve outside the normal range with a sudden dip at 4 mm zone).
- Percentage thickness increase is abnormal (curve outside the normal range)
- D value is 9.36 (abnormal).
- Hence this is a case of keratoconus.

■ Example 4 **(Fig. 10.11)**:
- This is a Pentacam map showing:
  - Four maps refractive display
  - The left eye
  - A 37-year-old patient
  - A mean keratometry 43.9 D
  - K_{max} of 50.6 D
- The axial curvature map shows superior flat corneal contour with an inferior band of corneal steepening in the pattern of "crab claw" or "kissing doves".
- Pachymetry apex of 495 µm
- Thinnest pachymetry of 480 µm
- Pachymetry map shows infero-temporal displacement of the thinnest location on y-axis by 1.12 mm (suspicious).
- Anterior elevation 43 µm (abnormal)
- Posterior elevation 61 µm (abnormal)
- This scan suggests a diagnosis of an ectatic corneal disorder, likely pellucid marginal corneal degeneration because the area of maximum corneal ectasia is superior to the area of corneal thinning and the typical "crab claw" appearance on the axial curvature map.

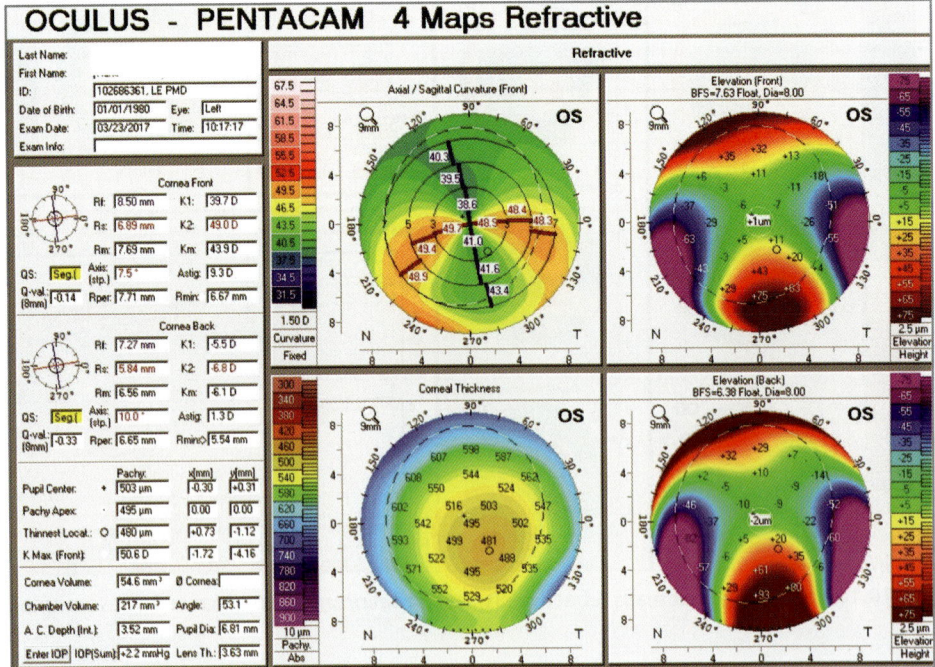

Fig. 10.11: Four maps refractive display showing pellucid marginal corneal degeneration (PMCD).

INTERPRETATION OF HUMPHREY VISUAL FIELD

Specific Examples

- *Example 1—Steps to interpret* **(Fig. 10.12A)**:
  - *Step 1:* This is a single-field analysis of right eye of a 61-year-old patient.
  - *Step 2:* By using central 30-2, Swedish interactive threshold algorithm (SITA)—fast strategy with appropriate near correction given
  - *Step 3:* The visual field is reliable.
  - *Step 4:* Total deviation probability plot shows scotoma or defect in the superior half area.
  - *Step 5:* Pattern deviation probability plot also shows a similar defect indicating localized damage, suggestive of superior arcuate going into the periphery.[4]
  - *Step 6:* Global indices are abnormal [visual field index (VFI) 71%, mean deviation (MD) –10.83 dB, and pattern standard deviation (PSD) 15.65 dB].
  - *Step 7:* Glaucoma Hemifield test is outside normal limits.[5,6]
  - *Step 8:* Anderson's criteria will be met with if these defects are reproducible on consecutive visual fields. Therefore, given visual field shows a superior arcuate scotoma breaking into the periphery, suggestive of glaucomatous damage. Clinical correlation is needed.[7]
- *Example 2* **(Fig. 10.12B)**:
  - *Step 1:* Single-field analysis of the right eye of a 56-year-old patient.
  - *Step 2:* By using central 30-2, SITA—fast strategy with appropriate near correction given
  - *Step 3:* The visual field is reliable.
  - *Step 4:* Total deviation probability plot shows scotoma or defect in nasal area inferiorly.
  - *Step 5:* Pattern deviation probability plot also shows a similar defect indicating localized damage. Global indices are abnormal (VFI 94%, MD 2.75 dB, and PSD 7.63 dB).
  - *Step 6:* Glaucoma Hemifield test is outside normal limit.
  - *Step 7:* Anderson's criteria will be met with if these defects are reproducible on consecutive visual fields. Therefore, given visual field shows an inferior nasal step, suggestive of glaucomatous damage. Clinical correlation is needed.
- *Example 3* **(Fig. 10. 12C)**:
  - *Step 1:* Single-field analysis of the right eye of a 55-year-old patient
  - *Step 2:* By using central 30-2, FASTPAC strategy with appropriate near correction
  - *Step 3:* The visual field is reliable.
  - *Step 4:* Total deviation probability plot shows superior and inferior arcuate scotoma, breaking into the periphery.
  - *Step 5:* Pattern deviation probability plot also shows a similar defect indicating localized damage.
  - *Step 6:* Global indices are abnormal (MD—26.15, PSD—7.72).
  - *Step 7:* Anderson's criteria will be met with if these defects are reproducible on consecutive visual fields. Therefore, given visual field shows a double arcuate scotoma breaking into the periphery, suggestive of advanced glaucomatous damage. Clinical correlation is needed.[8]
- *Example 4* **(Fig. 10.12D)**:
  - *Step 1:* Single field analysis of left eye of a 49-year-old patient.
  - *Step 2:* By using central 30-2, SITA—fast strategy with appropriate near correction given
  - *Step 3:* The visual field is reliable.

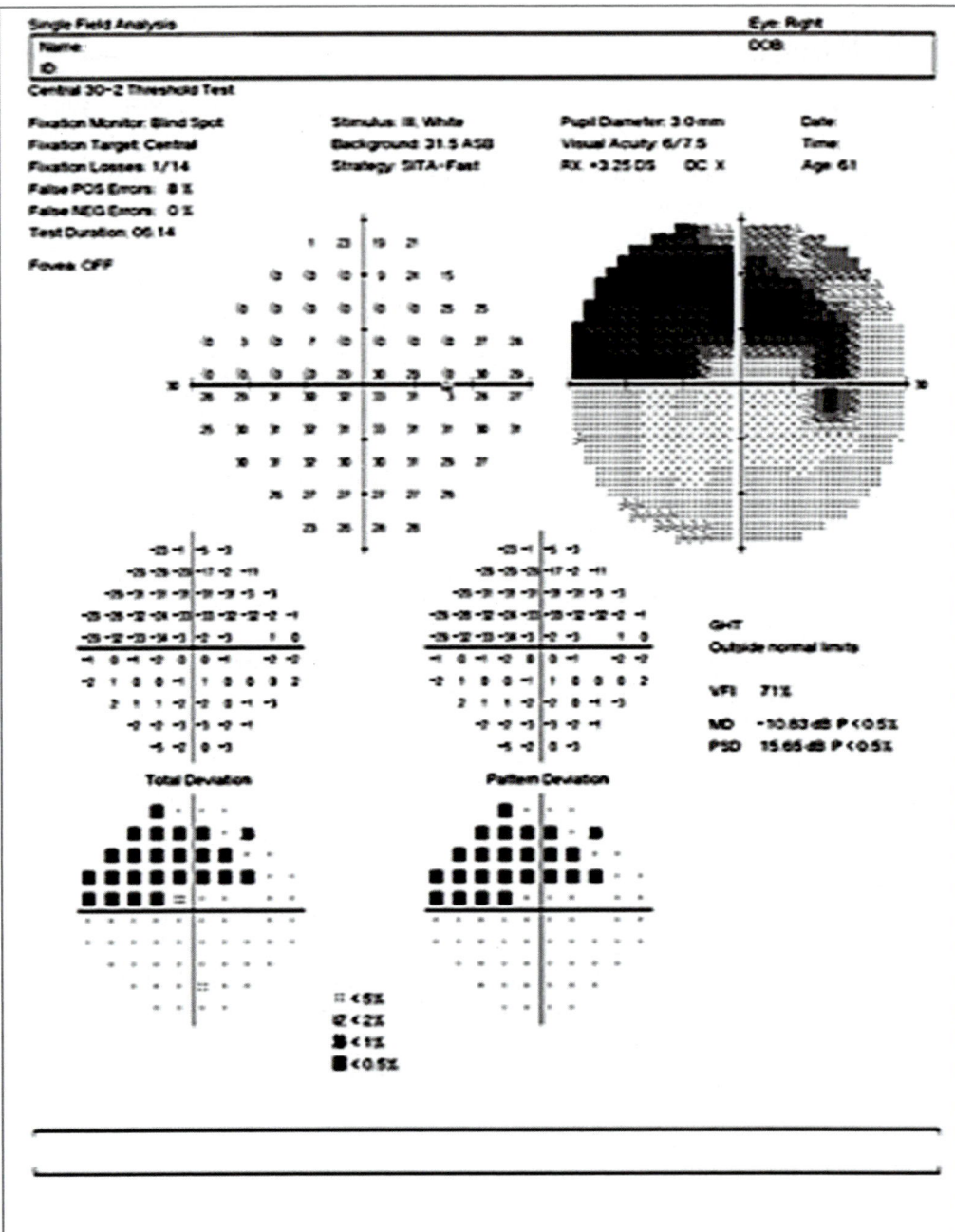

Fig. 10.12A

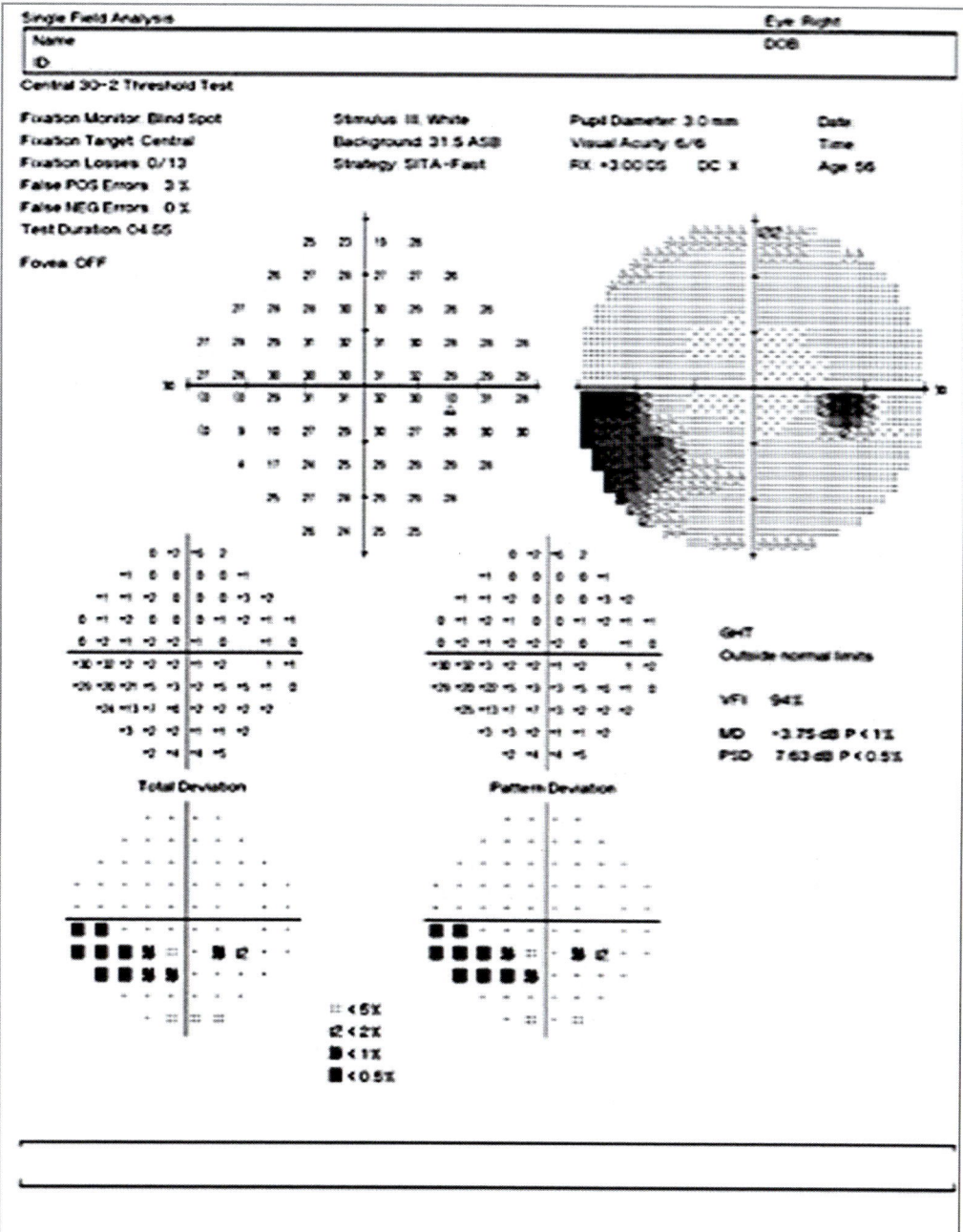

Fig. 10.12B

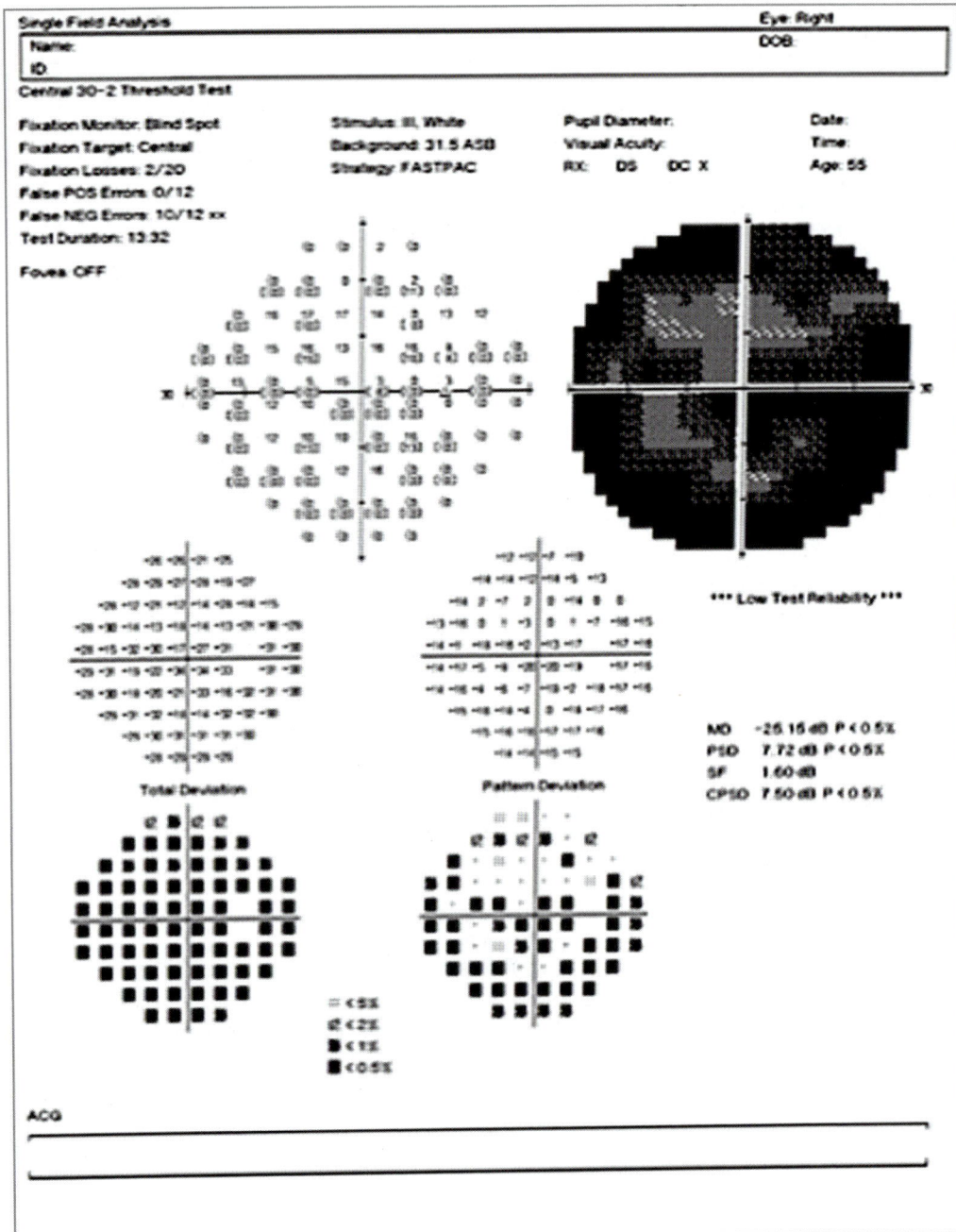

Fig. 10.12C

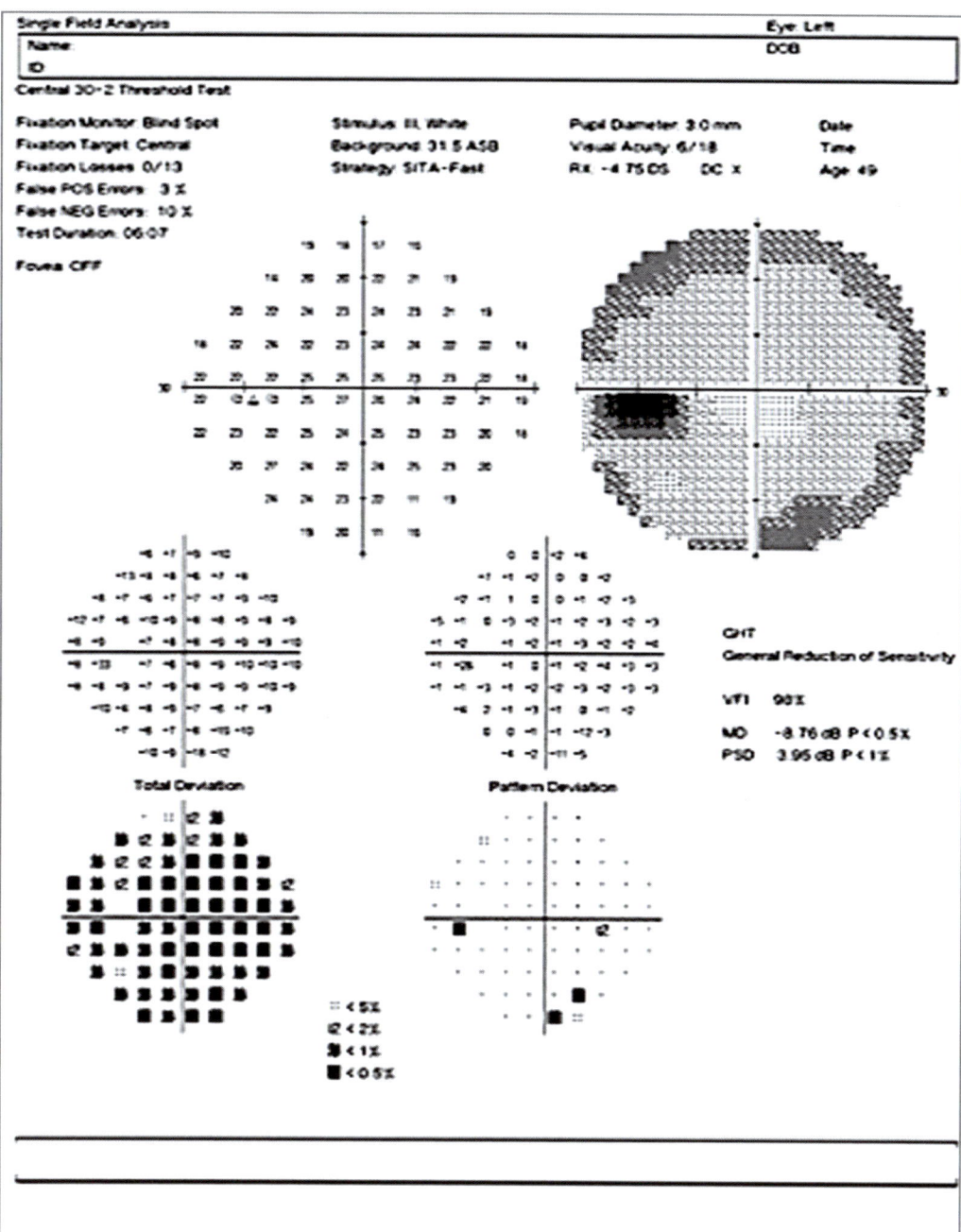

Fig. 10.12D
Figs. 10.12A to D: Humphrey visual field.

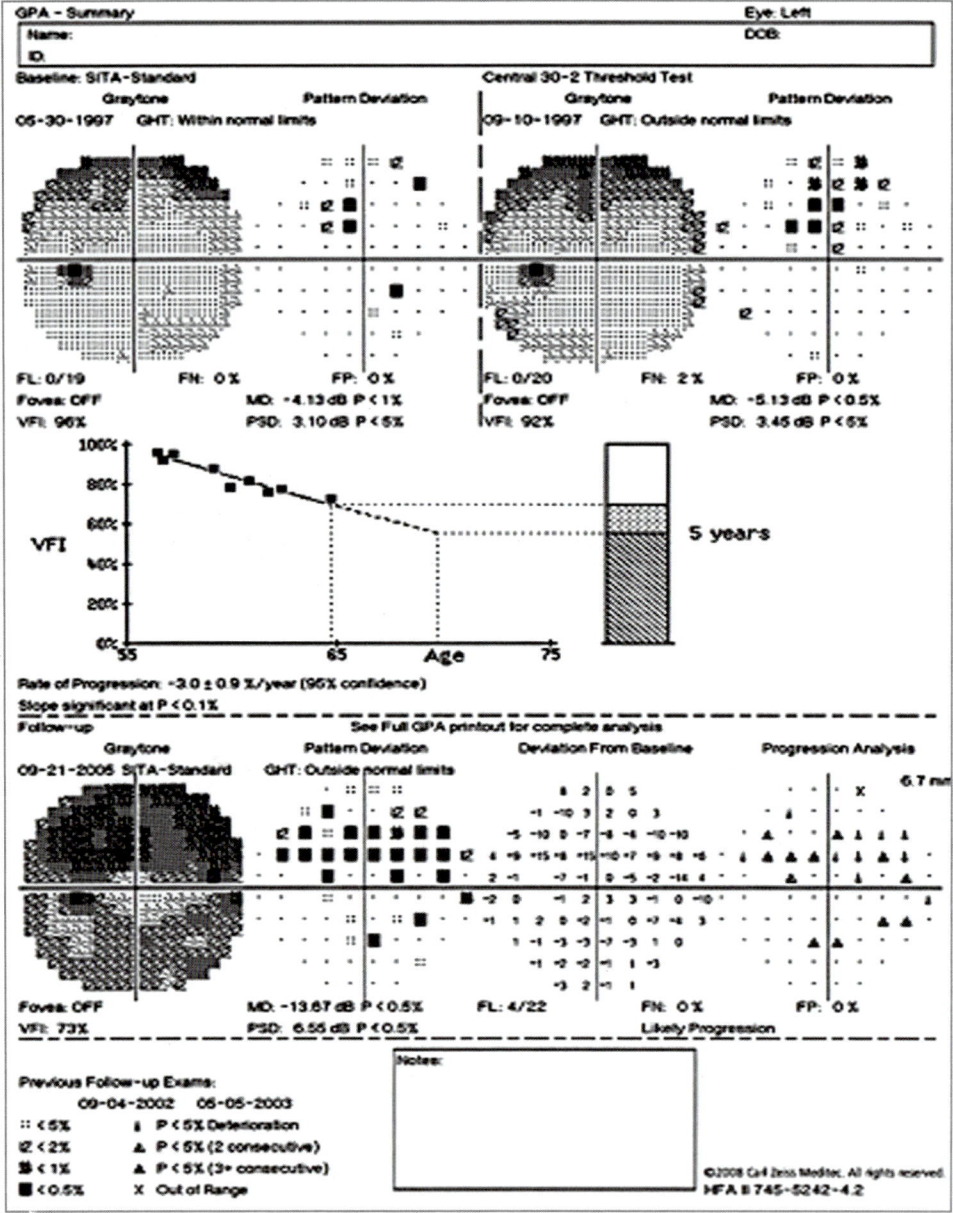

Fig. 10.13: Guided progression analysis.

- *Step 4:* Total deviation probability plot shows generalized depression, which is not present in pattern deviation probability plot, suggestive of a non-glaucomatous defect like cataract. Clinical correlation is needed.

- *Example 5* **(Fig. 10.13):**
  - *Step 1:* Guided progression analysis (GPA) report of the left eye of a patient named ....
  - *Step 2:* The upper two fields depict the baseline fields of the patient on

presentation showing VFI 96%, MD −4.13 dB, and PSD 3.10 dB.
- *Step 3:* Below that is the VFI plot with a steeper slope, showing significant progression based on VFI values. It also shows that this much amount of 3–5 years' progression is going to happen in future, if the current trend follows.
- *Step 4:* The rate of progression is −3.0 ± 0.9%/year.
- *Step 5:* Below that is the current visual field summary showing VFI 73%, MD −13.67 dB, and PSD 6.55 dB. GPA alert shows "likely progression".

INTERPRETATION OF ANTERIOR SEGMENT OPTICAL COHERENCE TOMOGRAPHY

Specific Examples

- *Example 1 (Fig. 10.14):* This is an anterior segment optical coherence tomography (ASOCT) image showing Descemet's membrane detachment with a corneal thickness of 571 µm.[9]
- *Example 2 (Fig. 10.15):* This is an ASOCT image of a case of operated endothelial keratoplasty. The total corneal thickness is 421 µm, and the thickness of donor corneal lenticule is 56 µm. The patient most likely seems to have undergone an ultrathin Descemet stripping automated endothelial keratoplasty (DSAEK) considering the graft thickness and the smooth interface.
- *Example 3 (Fig. 10.16):* This is an ASOCT image of a case of operated phakic

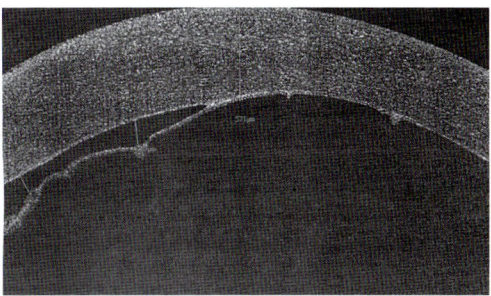

Fig. 10.14: Anterior segment optical coherence tomography (ASOCT) image showing Descemet's membrane detachment.

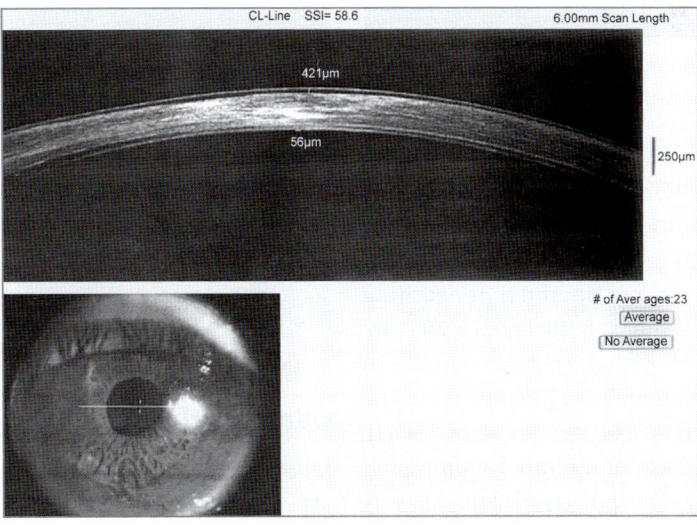

Fig. 10.15: Anterior segment optical coherence tomography image of a case of operated endothelial keratoplasty.

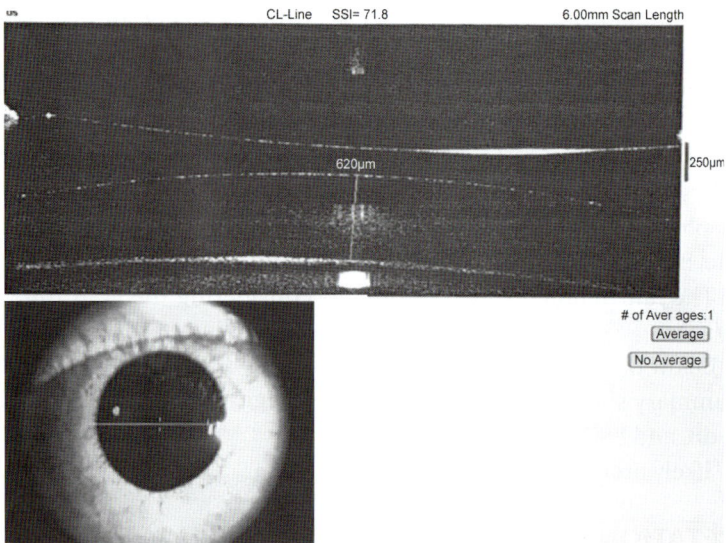

Fig. 10.16: Anterior segment optical coherence tomography image of a case of operated phakic intraocular lens.

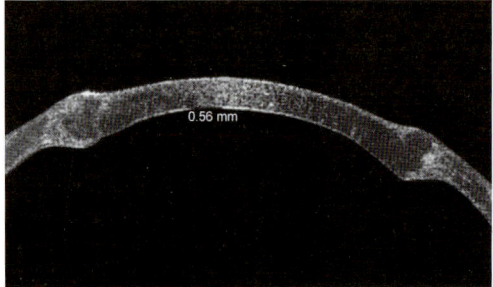

Fig. 10.17: Anterior segment optical coherence tomography image of a case of operated penetrating keratoplasty.

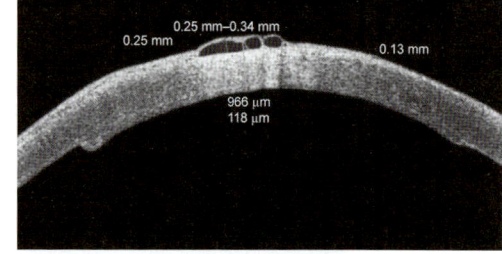

Fig. 10.18: Anterior segment optical coherence tomography image of a case of operated endothelial keratoplasty.

intraocular lens (IOL). The vault, in this case, is 620 μm.
- *Example 4 (Fig. 10.17):* This is an ASOCT image of a case of operated penetrating keratoplasty. The graft thickness is 560 μm. The image shows an irregular contour of the posterior graft–host junction.
- *Example 5 (Fig. 10.18):* This is an ASOCT image of a case of operated endothelial keratoplasty. The total corneal thickness is 966 μm, and the thickness of donor corneal lenticule is 118 μm. Corneal epithelial bullae are visible. On the basis of the presence of epithelial bullae with increased corneal thickness, this appears to be a case of failed endothelial keratoplasty.

INTERPRETATION OF RETINAL OCT

General Principles

Look for the following while interpreting an OCT image.[10] The interpretation should be made under the following headings as mentioned below. Refer to the chapter on

Optical Coherence Tomography for detailed theory on this topic (Section 4.3).

First identify the following if the scan shows these details:
- Name
- Age
- Type of OCT scan
- Date of acquisition

Then proceed with reading the OCT from the inner layers to the outer layers. Comment on the following aspects:
- Vitreous
- Vitreoretinal interface
- Retinal layers (inner to outer)
- Retinal pigmented epithelium (RPE)—Bruch's membrane complex integrity
- Choroid—thickness and pattern
- Sclera-choroidal junction

Specific Examples

- *Example 1 (Fig. 10.19) normal macular OCT scan*: This is a spectral domain macular OCT (SD-OCT) of right eye in gray scale showing the following details:
  - Vitreous is clear
  - Foveal contour is normal
  - Vitreomacular interface shows attachment of posterior hyaloid in the perifoveal region suggestive of vitreomacular adhesion.
  - Retinal layers appear normal.

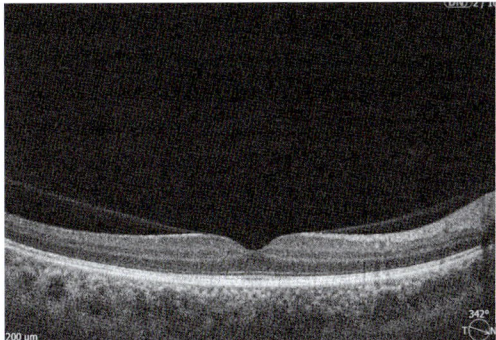

Fig. 10.19: Normal macular OCT scan.

- The retinal nerve fiber layer (RNFL) is thicker toward the right side suggesting that it is an OCT of right eye.
- The normal layers showing hyperreflectivity are:
  - RNFL
  - Internal limiting membrane
  - Inner segment–outer segment (IS-OS zone (ellipsoid zone)
  - RPE–Bruch's complex
- Choroidal vessels are visible and appear normal
- This looks like a normal macular OCT with vitreomacular adhesion.

- *Example 2 (Figs. 10.20A and B) macular edema:* This is an OCT image with a corresponding infrared retinal image showing the section through which OCT scan has been captured. This OCT scan shows the following features:
  - Vitreous is clear.
  - Foveal contour is distorted.
  - Central macular thickness (CMT) is increased to 299 microns.
  - Large cystic spaces are present predominantly in the inner retina.
  - Multiple hyperreflective spots with back-shadowing are visible in the inner nuclear and outer plexiform layer suggestive of hard exudates.
  - This looks like a macular OCT of macular edema probably diabetic macular edema.

- *Example 3 (Fig. 10.21) full-thickness macular hole:* This is a macular OCT with a corresponding infrared retinal image. The following findings are appreciated in this scan:
  - Vitreous is clear.
  - Vitreomacular interface is normal with no evidence of vitreous adhesion or traction.
  - Foveal contour is distorted.

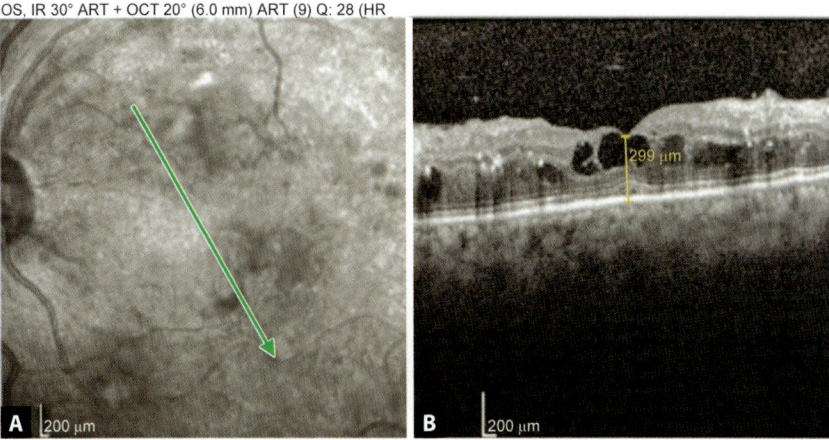

Figs. 10.20A and B: Macular edema.

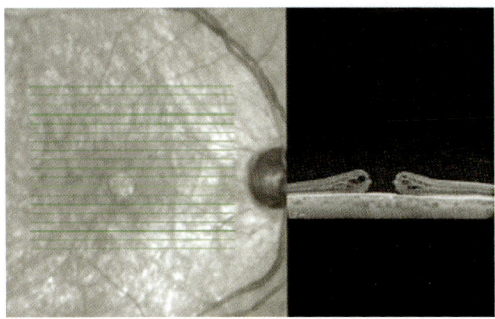

Fig. 10.21: Full-thickness macular hole.

- Full-thickness macular hole
- Intraretinal cysts are seen on both the walls.
- Height of the hole is more or less equal to base diameter.
- This is a macular OCT of a full-thickness macular hole.

▪ Example 4 **(Fig. 10.22)** choroidal neovascular membrane (CNVM): This is a macular OCT image with corresponding fundus image showing the section through which OCT scan has been captured.
 - Vitreous—clear
 - Vitreomacular interface is normal.
 - Retinal contour suggestive of staphyloma
 - CMT is increased.
 - Hyperreflective lesion is visualized arising from the choroidal tissue and is disrupting the outer retinal layers suggestive of CNVM.
 - This OCT is suggestive of CNVM probably in a myopic patient.

*Example 5 **(Fig. 10.23)** neurosensory detachment:* This is a macular OCT showing the following findings.
 ▪ Vitreous is clear.
 ▪ Vitreomacular interface is normal.
 ▪ Foveal contour appears blunted.
 ▪ Dome-shaped subfoveal serous pigment epithelial detachment (PED) of 236 micron is present.
 ▪ Shallow NSD
 ▪ CMT is 227 microns
 ▪ *This looks like an OCT of a case with central serous chorioretinopathy (CSCR).*

INTERPRETATION OF FUNDUS FLUORESCEIN ANGIOGRAPHY

General Principles

Look for the following while interpreting a fundus fluorescein angiography (FFA) image and describe under the headings as mentioned below. Refer to the chapter on FFA for detailed theory on this topic (Section 4.2).

CHAPTER 10: Interpretation of Images 425

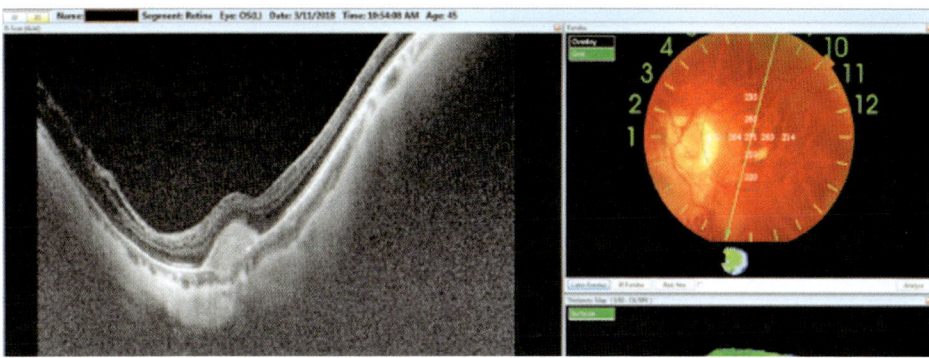

Fig. 10.22: Choroidal neovascular membrane.

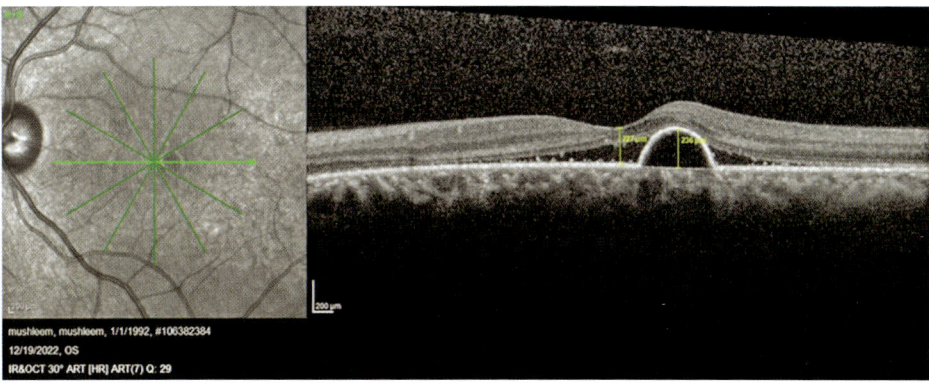

Fig. 10.23: Neurosensory detachment.

First identify the following if the scan shows these details:
- Name
- Age
- Date of acquisition

Then proceed with reading the FFA. Comment on the following aspects:
- Eye being evaluated
- Phase of scan—choroidal, arterial, arteriovenous, venous phase
- Arteries and venous caliber
- Any area of hyper-/hypofluorescence
- Change in the size and intensity of hyper-/hypofluorescence if serial scans are available
- Size of foveal avascular zone (FAZ)

Example 1 **(Fig. 10.24)** *FFA:* This is a fluorescein angiography image of right eye with the following findings:
- The FFA is captured in arteriovenous phase.
- Multiple areas of hyperfluorescence are noted.
- A smokestack pattern is visualized in the perifoveal area of hyperfluorescence.
- Multiple ink blot pattern of hyperfluorescence is noted temporal to the disc and along the superotemporal arcade.
- Clinical fundus assessment and serial FFA images can help make a complete diagnosis. However, it looks like a case of multifocal CSCR.

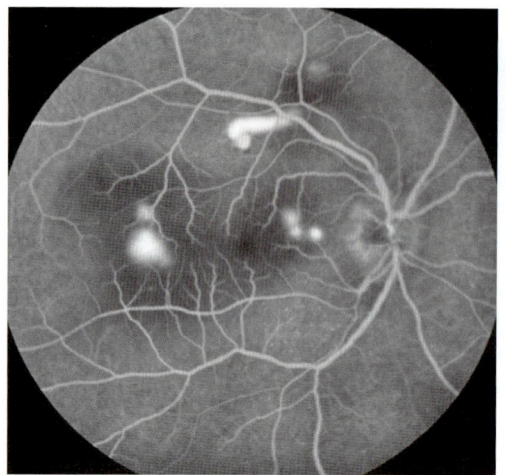

Fig. 10.24: Fundus fluorescein angiography of a case with multifocal central serous chorioretinopathy (CSCR).

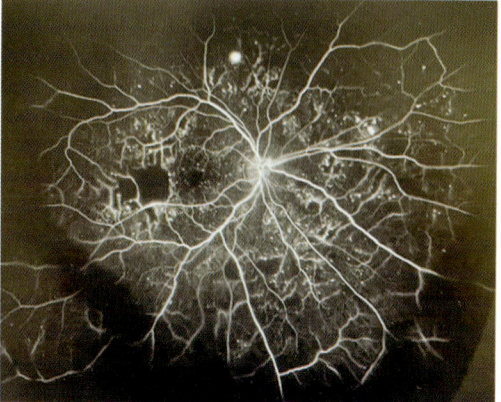

Fig. 10.25: Fundus fluorescein angiography of a case with proliferative diabetic retinopathy.

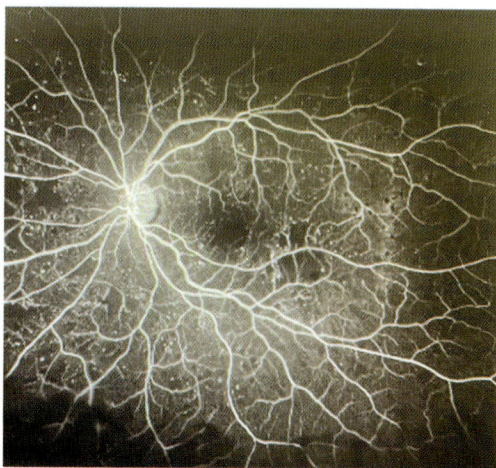

Fig. 10.26: Fundus fluorescein angiography of a case with non-proliferative diabetic retinopathy.

*Example 2 (**Fig. 10.25**) FFA:* This is a fluorescein angiography image of right eye with the following findings.
- The FFA is captured in arteriovenous phase.
- Multiple dot-like hyperfluorescence are noted likely to be microaneurysms.
- An area of diffuse hyperfluorescence is noted along the superotemporal arcade—assessment of serial scans is essential to suggest if it is neovascularization elsewhere (NVE).
- Capillary nonperfusion (CNP) areas are seen in the periphery and temporal to fovea.
- Clinical fundus assessment and serial FFA images can help make a complete diagnosis. However, it looks like a case of *proliferative diabetic retinopathy*.

*Example 3 (**Fig. 10.26**) FFA:* This is a fluorescein angiography image of left eye with the following findings.
- The FFA is captured in arteriovenous phase.
- Multiple dot-like hyperfluorescence are noted likely to be microaneurysms.
- An area of dot-like hypofluorescence is noted—can be hard exudate or hemorrhage.
- CNP areas are seen in the periphery.
- Clinical fundus assessment and serial FFA images can help make a complete diagnosis. However, it looks like a case of *nonproliferative diabetic retinopathy*.

*Example 4 (**Fig. 10.27**) FFA:* This is an FFA image of left eye with the following findings:

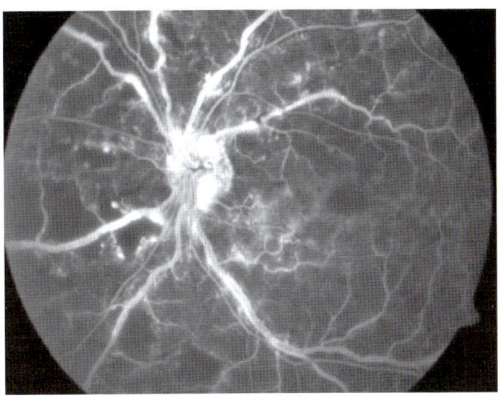

Fig. 10.27: Optical coherence tomography angiography of case showing neovascularization.

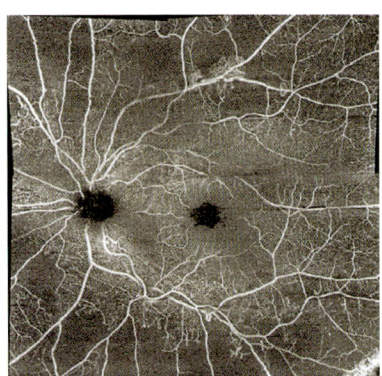

Fig. 10.29: Optical coherence tomography angiography.

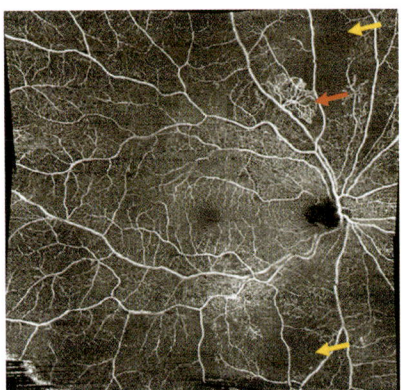

Fig. 10.28: Optical coherence tomography angiography showing vascular changes.

- The FFA is captured in arteriovenous phase.
- Dilated tortuous retinal veins are visible in all four quadrants.
- Multiple areas of CNP area visible.
- Few areas are showing dot-like hyperfluorescence suggestive of microaneurysm.
- Collateral vessels between vein and arteries are visible.
- Clinical fundus assessment and serial FFA images can help make a complete diagnosis. However, it looks like a case of *central retinal vein occlusion*.

Example 5 (**Fig. 10.28**) OCT angiography: This is an OCT—an image of right eye showing the following findings.[11,12]
- Abnormal vascular network of capillaries in the second-order vessel along the superotemporal quadrant suggestive of NVE (red arrow)
- Multiple CNP areas in the peripheral retina (yellow arrow)
- Normal FAZ[13,14]

Example 6 (**Fig. 10.29**) OCT angiography: This is an OCT—an image of left eye showing the following findings.
- Intraretinal microvascular abnormalities at the level of bifurcation of superotemporal arcade
- With venous looping in inferotemporal quadrant
- Multiple CNP areas at the mid periphery level
- Normal FAZ area[15]

REFERENCES

1. Banc A, Kedar S. Interpretation of the Visual Field in Neuro-ophthalmic Disorders. Curr Neurol Neurosci Rep. 2024;24(3):67-81.
2. Lopes BT, Ramos IC, Dawson DG, Belin MW, Ambrósio R Jr. Detection of ectatic corneal diseases based on pentacam. Z Med Phys. 2016;26(2):136-42.

3. Doctor K, Vunnava KP, Shroff R, Kaweri L, Lalgudi VG, Gupta K, et al. Simplifying and understanding various topographic indices for keratoconus using Scheimpflug based topographers. Indian J Ophthalmol. 2020;68(12):2732-43.
4. Wall M. Perimetry and visual field defects. Handb Clin Neurol. 2021;178:51-77.
5. Chen RI, Gedde SJ. Assessment of visual field progression in glaucoma. Curr Opin Ophthalmol. 2023;34(2):103-108.
6. Wu Z, Medeiros FA. Recent developments in visual field testing for glaucoma. Curr Opin Ophthalmol. 2018;29(2):141-6.
7. Upadhyaya A; Khan S; Sahay P; Goel S; Kumawat D. Delhi Journal of Ophthalmology HYPERLINK "https://ind01.safelinks.protection.outlook.com/?url=https%3A%2F%2Fjournals.lww.com%2Fdjo%2Ftoc%2F2020%2F31010&data=05%7C02%7Cpriyansh%40jaypeebrothers.com%7C4dc270319f284ed5ef0208dd09584604%7C9e7fa850fd9547b7bda2a51c357d60ae%7C0%7C0%7C638676996967084030%7CUnknown%7CTWFpbGZsb3d8eyJFbXB0eU1hcGkiOnRydWUsIlYiOiIwLjAuMDAwMCIsIlAiOiJXaW4zMiIsIkFOIjoiTWFpbCIsIldUIjoyfQ%3D%3D%7C0%7C%7C%7C&data=aWFHePNk1vDK43zdbjGMhzJJR20MSrn%2FJLx0Wpcypco%3D&reserved=0"31(1):pp. 90-5, Jul–Sep 2020.
8. McKendrick AM, Turpin A. Understanding and identifying visual field progression. Clin Exp Optom. 2024;107(2):122-9
9. Swartz T, Marten L, Wang M. Measuring the cornea: the latest developments in corneal topography. Curr Opin Ophthalmol. 2007;18(4):325-33.
10. Kanclerz P, Khoramnia R, Wang X. Current Developments in Corneal Topography and Tomography. Diagnostics (Basel). 2021;11(8):1466.
11. Sridhar U, Tripathy K. Corneal Topography. 2023 Sep 4. In: StatPearls. Treasure Island (FL): StatPearls Publishing; 2024 Jan–.
12. Rocholz R, Corvi F, Weichsel J, Schmidt S, Staurenghi G. OCT Angiography (OCTA) in Retinal Diagnostics. 2019 Aug 14. In: Bille JF (Ed). High Resolution Imaging in Microscopy and Ophthalmology: New Frontiers in Biomedical Optics. Cham (CH): Springer; 2019. Chapter 6.
13. Le PH, Kaur K, Patel BC. Optical Coherence Tomography Angiography. 2024 Oct 6. In: StatPearls. Treasure Island (FL): StatPearls Publishing; 2024 Jan–.
14. Enaholo ES, Musa MJ, Zeppieri M. Optical Coherence Tomography. 2024 Oct 6. In: StatPearls. Treasure Island (FL): StatPearls Publishing; 2024 Jan–.
15. Spaide RF, Fujimoto JG, Waheed NK, Sadda SR, Staurenghi G. Optical coherence tomography angiography. Prog Retin Eye Res. 2018;64:1-55.

Index

Page numbers followed by *f* refer to figure, *fc* refer to flowchart, and *t* refer to table

20 D lens 176*f*

A

Aberration 97
   analysis, uses of 93
   type of 98
Aberrometers 88
Abnormal corneal thickness
      distribution 80
Abscess 23*f*
Acanthamoeba 379, 381, 382
Accessory devices 63
Accredited Social Health Activist
      400
Acid mucopolysaccharides 363*f*
Acid-fast stain 377, 379
Actinic keratosis 370
Actinomyces 379
Active force generation test 355
Acute zonal occult outer
      retinopathy 210
Adaptive optical element 215
Adaptive optics 215, 216
   retinal imaging systems 216
   scanning laser ophthalmoscopy
      216
   working principle of 215*f*
Adenocarcinoma 372, 374
Adenoid cystic carcinoma 373,
      373*f*
Adnexa, infections of 375
Advanced optic nerve head
      cupping 40*f*
Aerobic bacterial cultures 381
Afterimage test 341, 343
   slides used for 341*f*
Age-related macular degeneration
      188, 203, 210, 281, 387,
      360
   dry 188, 219
   wet 190
Air-puff
   induced corneal deformation
      137
   tonometer 260
Alcian blue stain 362
Alizarin red stain 362
Allergic conjunctivitis 79
Allylamine 383

Alpha-chymotrypsin 175
Alport syndrome 94, 95*f*, 96*f*
Altered Corvis biomechanical
      index 140*f*
Alternaria species 380*f*
Alzheimer's disease 408
Amblyopia therapy 342
Ambrósio's relational thickness
      139
American optical keratometer,
      original 69
Amniotic membrane graft 105
Amplitude 205
   modulation scan 34
Amsler chart 219*t*
   interpretation 220*t*
   types of 219*t*
Amsler grid 218, 220
Anaglyph principle 344
Anderson's criteria 285, 295
Anesthetic eye drops, topical 297
Angiotensin-converting enzyme
      25
Angle alpha 342
Angle gamma 342
Angle kappa 128, 133, 342
Angle parameters 298
Angle pigmentation 250
Angular width slit 250
Anomalous retinal correspondence
      343*f*
Anophthalmic socket 51
Anterior chamber 167
   biometry 297
   depth 128*f*, 153, 157
   intraocular lens 117
   parameters 80*f*
Anterior lamellar keratoplasty 101
Anterior segment 34
   imaging 108
   optical coherence tomography
      99-101, 101*f*, 104*f*, 105,
      106, 106*f*, 108, 111*f*, 124,
      296, 300, 301, 301*t*, 421*f*,
      422*f*
      indications of 101
      interpretation of 421
      role of 108, 109, 111
      visante 100*f*, 108

   procedures 201
   surgeries 109
   trauma 105
   tumors 103
Anterior stromal scarring 59*f*
Anterior trabecular meshwork 254*f*
Antibiotics 383
Antibody 364
Antifungals 382, 383
   classification of 383*t*
Antigen 364
Antimetabolites 383
Antimicrobial sensitivity 375
Antimicrobial susceptibility testing
      381
Antivascular endothelial growth
      factor 234
Aperture type 179, 180
Apoptosis 360
Apostilbs 283*f*, 286*f*-288*f*, 290*f*-
      292*f*, 294*f*
Apparent diffusion coefficient 12
Applanation tonometry, principle
      of 263
Aqueous cells on slit lamp, clinical
      grading on 67*t*
Aqueous humor 113
Aqueous tap 361, 377
Aqueous-to-air relative intensity
      index method 67
Argon laser trabeculoplasty 246
Arruga's capsule forceps
   method 174
   tumbling technique 174
Arruga's intracapsular forceps 170,
      170*f*
Arruga's needle holder 45, 45*f*, 327,
      327*f*
Artemis digital ultrasound 126
Artemis very high-frequency
      digital ultrasound 165
Arteriovenous malformation 9
Artery forceps 45, 45*f*, 326, 327*f*,
      351, 351*f*
Artificial anterior chamber 145,
      148
A-scan 31, 34, 38, 157, 158, 162,
      162*f*, 164
   amplitude 34*t*

over IOLMaster, advantage of 166
pachymeter 123f
ultrasonography 162
Aschner phenomenon 48
Aschner-Dagnini reflex 48
Aspergillosis 359
Aspergillus 379, 382
  flavus 380f
  fumigatus 380f
  niger 380f
Aspiration cannula 169, 169f
Asteroid hyalosis 37
Astigmatic elevation map 130f
Astigmatic keratotomy 123
Astigmatism 71, 96f, 97, 259, 263
  contribution of 98f
Asymmetric bowtie 74
Atrophy 360
Autofluorescence 186
Autologous tissue 48
Automated endothelial keratoplasty 167
Automated lamellar therapeutic keratoplasty machine 149
Automated positioning system 160
Automated retinoscope 88
Avascular outer retina 232f
Avellino dystrophy 121
A-wave 205
Axial computed tomography 19f
Axial contrast computed tomography 19f, 20f, 23f, 27f, 28f
Axial keratometry map 131
Axial length 6, 157, 158
Axial noncontrast computed tomography 17f
Axial postcontrast fat suppressed T1-weighted magnetic resonance imaging 25f, 29f
Axial T1-weighted fat-suppressed postcontrast magnetic resonance imaging 16f
Axial T2-weighted fat-suppressed magnetic resonance imaging 17f
  magnetic resonance imaging 22f
Azoles 383

B

Bacilli
  gram-negative 376
  gram-positive 376
Backflush 224, 224f
Bacteria 376
  filamentous 377
  gram-negative 378
Bagolini's glasses 342, 343f
Bagolini's test 342
Balanced phaco tip, advantage of 174
Barraquer's needle holder 146f, 327, 327f
Barrett TORIC calculator 160
Barron's vacuum punch 143, 143f
Basal cell carcinoma 370, 370f
  microscopic variants of 370
Basic screening technique 33
Basophilic tumor cells, irregular islands of 370f
Bausch and Lomb keratometer 68f, 69
Beard's rule 47
Belin/Ambrósio enhanced ectasia display 77, 87
Berke's ptosis clamp 45, 45f
Berke's rule 47
Best's vitelliform macular dystrophy 200f
Best-corrected visual acuity 384, 386, 387
Best-fit
  sphere 76, 135
  concept of 129f
  TORIC ellipsoid 76
Bicanalicular stent 54
Biconvex-shaped structure 43
Bilateral extraocular muscles, bulky bellies of 26f
Bimanual vitreoretinal surgery 226
Binocular fusion 340
  slides for testing 340f
Binocular indirect ophthalmoscope 176
Binocular reading 5
Binocular single vision, grade of 339, 340f
Binocular vision 337, 341
  test for 342
Binocular visual acuity test 348
Biomechanical index 139
Biomicroscopy, technique of 58
Biopsy 377
Bjerrum's scotoma 278f
Blade breaker 145, 145f
Bleeding, causes of 49, 50
Blepharitis 376
Blepharoconjunctivitis, chronic 371

Blind
  painful eye 50
  spot 276, 277, 287f
Blindness
  burden 384
  causes of 385, 386t
  percent of 386
  prevalence of 386t
  prevention 384
  rehabilitation 384
Blood
  agar 381
  brain barrier 12
  vessels, normal 252
Blotchy pigments 253, 253f
Blumenthal's AC maintainer technique 175
Blunt-tipped forceps 351
Bodian stain 362
Bone
  lesions 15
  window 30f
Bony orbit 7
Bony orbital lesions 19
Bowman lacrimal probe 45, 46f
Branch retinal vein occlusion 233f
Branching vascular network 199
  multiple polyps with 203f
Brightbill polytef cutting block 144
Brightness modulation scan 34
Brillouin microscopy 136
Broad tangential illumination 59
Brown's syndrome 334f
Bruch's complex 193
Bruch's membrane 199
  complex 193, 423
B-scan 31, 34, 39, 228
  indications of 34
Buphthalmic eye 6
Busin glide 150f, 151
B-wave 205

C

Calibration 257
Canalicular dacryocystorhinostomy 53
Canalicular stenosis 54
Cancer-associated retinopathy 210
Cannula 221, 224
Can-opener technique 173
Capillary hemangioma 15, 18
Capillary nonperfusion 187, 190f, 233, 242f, 426
  areas 233f
  dilated veins with 191f

Capsulorhexis 173
   rescue technique 174
   run-out, causes of 173
Capsulotomy techniques 173
Cardiorespiratory arrest 183
Caroticocavernous fistula 14, 15, 26, 27*f*
Cassini 72
Castroviejo caliper 327*f*
Castroviejo corneoscleral scissors 328, 328*f*
Castroviejo marking calipers 327
Castroviejo trephine 143*f*
Cat's paw lacrimal wound retractor 46, 46*f*
Cataract 98, 153, 201, 386, 389, 394
   congenital 166
   evaluation 82
   pediatric 173
   surgery 105, 117, 166, 172, 264, 386
   surgical services, rapid assessment of 396
Cavernous carotid artery 27
Cavernous hemangioma 15, 15*f*
Cavernous malformation 15
Cavernous sinus
   enlargement of 27
   pathology 14
Cell 67
   boundaries 115
   conformation 115
   grading 67
      uveitis nomenclature classification of 67
Cellulitis 15
   orbital 14, 28, 28*f*, 50, 376
Central corneal
   thickness 122, 259
   topography 159
Central nervous system 387
Central retinal
   artery occlusion 208
   vein occlusion 191*f*, 427
Central scotoma 278*f*, 342, 408*f*
Central serous chorioretinopathy 194, 194*f*, 203, 424
   acute 194
   chronic 194
   smokestack pattern of 187*f*
Central serous
   choroidopathy 186
   retinopathy 194, 210
Central visual acuity 384
Centrocecal scotoma 279*f*, 409*f*
Cerebrospinal fluid 11, 14
   rhinorrhea 54

Cerebrovascular accident 183
Chalazion 51, 51*f*, 366
   clamp 45, 46*f*
   nonsurgical management of 51
   scoop 45, 46*f*
Charge-coupled device 88, 89*f*, 215*f*
Charles flute
   cannula 224
   needle 223*f*
Chiasmal lesion 220
Childhood blindness 388, 394
Chlamydia 382
   antigen 382
   trachomatis 382
Chloroquine 210
Chocolate agar 381
Chopper 171, 171*f*
Chopping techniques 174
Choriocapillaris 231*f*, 232*f*
Chorioretinopathy biopsies 201
Choroid sclera junction 193
Choroidal coloboma 43, 43*f*, 44*f*
Choroidal detachment 33, 35, 35*t*, 37, 37*f*, 41*f*, 299*f*
Choroidal inflammatory disease 204
Choroidal melanoma 41
Choroidal metastasis 41
Choroidal neovascular membrane 190, 190*f*, 197, 197*f*, 198*f*, 424, 425*f*
Choroidal phase 184
Choroidal tumors 204
Choroiditis, multifocal 210
Ciliary body band 252
   angle recession, abnormal widening of 252*f*
Circular optic disc 267*f*
Circumlinear vessels 272*f*
   baring of 271
Clarus 239
Classic choroidal
   neovascularization 190
Claw pattern 74
Clear corneal incision, types of 172
Clear ocular media 34
Clement Clarke's major
   synoptophore 337
Clockface arrangement 359
Closed funnel retinal detachment 36*f*
Coats' disease 42, 240
Cocci
   gram-negative 376, 378*f*
   gram-positive 378*f*

Colibri forceps 146, 146*f*, 352, 352*f*
Colibri style polack double corneal forceps 147
Colloidal iron stain 362, 363*f*
Colobomas 240
Color cup 269
Color scale, concept of 129*f*
Community-based rehabilitation 390
   matrix 392, 393*fc*
Compact segment sampling 399
Complete temporal hemianopia 291*f*
Compound nevus 366
Comprehensive biomechanical profile 141
Computed tomography 9, 14, 30, 93, 94
   acquisition of 10
   angiogram 14
   interpretation of 10
   scans 3, 26
Concave tractional retinal detachment 35
Concentric neuroretinal rim loss 268
Confocal scanning laser ophthalmoscope 183, 191, 318
   optics of 319*f*
Conjunctiva 326, 353, 360
   palpebral 372
Conjunctival
   dacryocystorhinostomy 53
Conjunctival diseases 103
Conjunctival stroma 372*f*
Conjunctival swab 377
Conjunctivitis 376
Conjunctivochalasis 103
Consecutive strabismus 354
Contact lens
   fitting 82
   sensor 262, 262*f*
   wear 119
Contact specular microscope 113
Continuous curvilinear
   capsulorhexis, concept of 173
Contour cup 269
Contrast-enhanced computed tomography imaging 10
Conventional circular cutting trephines 142
Conventional fundus cameras 242*f*

Conventional ophthalmological surveys 395
Conventional single spot systems, advantages over 212
Conventional ultrasonic pachymetry 123
Cornea 56, 59f, 72, 92, 142, 257f, 361
  anatomy of 135
  anterior segment optical coherence tomography postcorneal crosslinking of 109
  asphericity of 77
  biomechanical properties of 136
  holding flaps of 352
  Imbert-Fick's law for 257f
  irregular 71
  nonsphericity of 70
  normal anterior elevation map of 130f
  qualitative assessment of 87
  Zernike analysis of 86f
Corneal aberration 84, 91f, 96f, 97f
Corneal astigmatism 81f, 94f, 96f
Corneal biomechanics 135-137, 141
  therapeutic implications of 137
Corneal blindness 386, 387, 388, 389, 394
Corneal contact lens 246
Corneal crosslinking 125, 126, 136, 137, 140
Corneal curvature 259
Corneal decompensation 125
Corneal deformation, velocity of 138
Corneal densitometry 85
Corneal disorders 63, 64
  color coding of 63t
Corneal dystrophy classification 109
Corneal ectasia 125
Corneal edema 259, 263
Corneal endothelial punches 144
Corneal endothelium 113
Corneal guttae 120, 409f
Corneal hydrops 104f, 108, 109, 300
Corneal hysteresis 136, 261
Corneal infiltrate 110f
Corneal lens 248
Corneal marking instruments 142
Corneal opacity 101, 166, 263

Corneal optical densitometry display 82, 84f
Corneal optics, balancing of 97
Corneal pachymetry 126
  map 77f
Corneal parameters 79f
Corneal physiology 70
Corneal reflection 338
Corneal refractive surgeries 128
Corneal resistance factor 136, 261
Corneal scissors 145, 146f, 167, 167f
Corneal scraping 377
Corneal staining 65
  dyes used for 66t
Corneal stroma 113, 363f
Corneal surgery 133
Corneal thickness 104f, 126, 159
  progression analysis 77
Corneal thinning 81f
Corneal tomography 74f
Corneal topographic analysis 93
Corneal topography 72t, 80, 98f
Corneal trephines 142, 151
Corneal ulcer 67
  sequel of 111f
Corneal visualization scheimpflug technology 262, 262f
Corneal wedge 251
  formation 252f
Corner method 115
Coronal contrast-enhanced computed tomography 28f
Corvis biomechanical index 139
Corvis ST 136, 137
  clinical applications of 138
  over traditional methods, advantages of 141
  technology, principles of 137
Cottingham corneal punch 144
Cover eye 276f
Crab-claw appearance 83f
Craniopharyngiomas 11
Crescent blade 328, 328f
Crescent knife 149, 149f
Crigler's sac massage 55
Cryoextraction 174
Crystalline lens 60f, 163
Cup-disc ratio 264, 272f
Curvature map 73, 131
Curvularia species 380f
Cyclodeviation, measurement of 339
Cyst
  retinal 36f
  rupture of 365

Cystic intraorbital lesion 30f
Cysticercosis 14, 29, 366, 366f
  extraocular muscle 41, 42f
Cysticercus cellulosae 366
Cystoid 188
  changes, macular hole with 197f
  macular edema 194, 195f
Cystotome needle 169, 169f
Czapskiscope 57

D

Dacryocystectomy 54
Dacryocystorhinostomy 52, 54
  external 53
  failed 54
  intubation 54
  types of 53
Dastoor's iris repositor 169, 169f, 329, 329f
Davanger exophthalmometers 4
Deep anterior lamellar keratoplasty 102, 120, 201
  different techniques of 152
Deep retinal capillary plexus 230f, 231, 232f, 234f
Deep superior sulcus 50
Deep vascular complex 231, 232f
Deeper retinal layers 230f
Deflection length 138
Deformation amplitude 138
Dense amblyopia 341
Dense cataract 166
  measurement 159
Dense vitreous hemorrhage 166
Densely pigmented trabecular meshwork 254f
Dermoid 15
  cyst 17, 365, 365f
Descemet's membrane 150
  detachment 167, 421, 421f
  endothelial keratoplasty 120, 201
  instruments 151
  scoring 152
Descemet's stripper 15
Descemet's stripping automated endothelial keratoplasty 102, 120, 201
  busin forceps 151
  instruments 149
  scraper 150, 150f
  spatula 150
Desmarre's lamellar dissector 148
Desmoplasia 370
Deviation, angle of 338

Device 72
Diabetes 119, 120
Diabetic macular edema 188, 189*f*, 194, 196*f*, 233
Diabetic maculopathy 188
 ischemic 188
Diabetic retinopathy 186, 219, 233, 234*f*, 238, 240, 242*f*, 387, 388, 389, 394
 non-proliferative 187, 426, 426*f*
Diabetic vitrectomy surgery 227
Diamond knife 145, 145*f*
Diamond-dusted
 membrane scraper 224, 224*f*
 soft silicone tip cannula 224
Diffuse diabetic maculopathy 188
Diffuse retinal nerve fiber layer loss 270
Diffuse slit-lamp corneal image 101*f*
Diffusion-weighted images 12
Digital fundus camera 183, 183*f*
Digital subtraction angiography 27
Digitally-assisted vitreoretinal surgery 227
Diplopia 341, 342
Direct carotid-cavernous fistula 27, 27*t*
Direct focal slit illumination 58, 61
Direct goniolenses 246
Direct gonioscopy 246*f*, 248*fc*
 advantages of 248
 disadvantages of 248
Direct ophthalmoscope 178, 178*f*, 179*t*, 181, 181*t*, 182*t*, 265
 apertures of 179*f*
 head of 178*f*
Direct slit illumination 59*f*
Disc
 edema 181
 neovascularization of 187
 size 265
Distance Randot test 350
Distance stereoacuity, tests for 348
Distance visual acuity 384
Diurnal variations 70
Donor
 cornea dissection 148
 corneal tissues, evaluation of 114*f*
 dissection 149
 tissue 149
  insertion 152
Doppler ultrasound 34, 35
Double corneal forceps 147
Double-ended iris repositor 147*f*

Drugs, class of 383
Dry eye 103
 severe 360
Dual bore cannula 224
Dye 66
 extravasation of 183
Dynamic slit-lamp biomicroscopy 61, 62*f*
Dysfunctional lens index 92
Dysplasia 360
Dystrophic optic neuropathy 26
Dystrophies, hereditary 240

E

Ectasia, progression of 80
Ectatic disorders
 diagnosis of 80
 screening of 80
Elasticity 136
Electrodes 207
Electron microscopy 365
Electroretinogram 204, 207, 208, 211
 extinguishing 208*f*
 full-field 206
 leads 207*f*
 machine 204*f*
 responses, abnormal 207
 wave, normal 205*f*
Elevated bleb with microcysts 107*f*
Elevation map 76, 129
Ellipsoid 76, 193
Embryonic vascular channel 8*f*
Emission computed tomography 14
End grasping forceps 223, 223*f*
Endoilluminator 151
Endonasal dacryocystorhinostomy 53
Endophthalmitis 15, 22, 38*f*, 50, 376
 metastatic 23*f*
 ultrasonography appearance of 38
Endoscopic dacryocystorhinostomy
 advantages of 53, 54*t*
 disadvantages of 53, 54*t*
Endothelial cell
 count 116, 119
 culture 117
 density 115
 loss, bi-exponential decay model for 118
 morphology 409

Endothelial keratoplasty 102, 421*f*, 422, 422*f*
Endothelial loss 120*t*
 phases of 119*t*
Endothelium
 monitoring of 116
 research of 116
Enophthalmos 6, 50
Enucleation 48, 49, 49*t*, 50
 complications of 49
 myoconjunctival technique of 49
 scissors 45, 46*f*
 types of 49
Epidermis, basal layer of 370*f*
Epilation forceps 44, 45*f*
Epiretinal membrane 165, 197
Epithelial bullae 422
Epithelial component 373
Epithelial defect 64*f*
Epithelial cell 369
 melanoma 369*f*
Epithelium 113
Erythrocyte 372
Escherichia coli 381
Esotropia 338
Eukaryotes 376, 377
Eukaryotic cells 376
Evisceration 48, 49, 49*t*, 50
 curette 45, 46*f*
 types of 50
Exenteration 50
 types of 50*t*
Exophthalmometer 4
 types of 3, 4
Exophthalmometry 3, 4
 different types of 4
 reading 6
Exophthalmos 6
Exorbitism 6
Exotropia 338
External carotid artery 27
External limiting membrane 193, 194*f*
Extracapsular cataract extraction 120, 167
Extraconal lesions 17
Extraocular muscle 8, 25*f*, 27*f*
 cysticercosis 41
 enlargement 25
Extrusion instruments 223
Eye 203*f*, 205*f*, 206*f*, 208*f*, 331
 bank 102, 117
 cataract surgery 155*f*
 drops, topical 48
 health survey 395
  conduct of 396

internal 98f
movement, mechanical
limitation of 355
normal 251f, 342
ultrasound biomicroscopy of 301
Eyeball 360
Eyelid 360
nodule 367
Eyesuite software 295

F

Facial asymmetry 6
Familial exudative vitreoretinopathy 192, 240, 243f
Fasanella-Servat procedure 47
Fascia lata 48
Fat 11
attenuation 17f
Fat-suppressed contrast-enhanced magnetic resonance imaging 22f
Fibroblasts 370
Fibrotic sac 55
Fibrous stroma 370
Film-based fundus camera 183
Filtering bleb, evaluation of 300
Fish hook technique 175
Flat iris configuration 299f
Flieringa ring 142, 142f
use of 151
Flow cytometry 365
Fluid attenuation inversion recovery 12, 14
Fluorescein
angiogram 190f, 238
normal 185f
dye 202
intravenous injection of 184f
masking of 185
patterns, abnormal 185
pooling of 190f
staining 64f
Fontana-Masson stain 363
Food and Drug Administration 156
Forced duction test 353, 354
Forceps 147, 170
techniques 150
Foreign body forceps 223, 223f
Formalin 361
Forme fruste keratoconus 80, 82, 86, 410
refractive display of 412f

Fornices contraction 50
Four maps refractive display 413f
Fovea 343
Foveal avascular zone 184, 229, 234f
Fractal dimension 229
Frame method 115
Free-floating appearance 349
Freer periosteal elevator 45, 46f
Frequency domain optical coherence tomography 108
Frisby-Davis distance test 349
Frisby-Davis stereoacuity test 350f
Frontalis muscle 47
Fuchs endothelial corneal dystrophy 119
Full-spectrum amplitude decorrelation angiography 229
Full-thickness macular hole 423
Fundus
autofluorescence 184
camera 183, 216
fluorescein angiography 182, 191, 191f, 202t, 233, 424, 426f
advantages over 203
interpretation of 424
phases of 184
photography 215
Fungal
growth 381f
hyphae 379f
infections 367
Fungi 376
Fusarium 380f, 382
Fusional amplitudes, determination of 341

G

Gadolinium 11
Galand letterbox technique 173
Galilei 72, 86
Ganglion cell 305
analysis 312t, 316f
printout 312
complex 305
inner plexiform layer 305
layer 193, 194f, 305, 313f, 314f
Gass retinal detachment hook 225, 225f
Gaussian-shaped spectrum 159
Geuder glass injector 151f
Giemsa stain 377
Gill's lamellar dissector 149

Glass injectors 151f
Glaucoma 106, 119, 125, 137, 245, 264, 268f, 269, 272, 286, 295-297, 302, 309f, 384, 386, 388, 389, 394
congenital 125
diagnosis 280
end-stage 50
evaluation 82
Goldmann visual field of 277f, 278f
hemifield test 283f, 284, 286f-288f, 290f, 291f, 293f, 294f
malignant 301
optic disc changes of 253
probability score 323, 323f, 325f
progression 315, 317
risk assessment 140
screening 87
signs of 271f, 273
surgeries 201, 326
surgical intervention for 326
susceptibility 140
temporal raphe sign in 312f
traumatic 253
Glaucomatous optic
atrophy 273
neuropathy 266, 272
Glioma 15
Global indices 283f
Globe fixation
forceps 353, 353f
rings 142
Globe holding forceps 327, 327f
Glutaraldehyde 361
Goldmann applanation
prism 263
tonometer 256, 257, 259, 263
error in 259t
housing of 258f
parts of 257f
Goldmann lens 253f
Goldmann mires, correct alignment of 258f
Goldmann mirror 248
Goldmann perimetry 275f
Goldmann two mirror lens 247f
Goldmann visual field 274, 275, 275t, 277f, 278f, 279, 279f, 407, 407t, 408, 409f
indications of 275
interpretation of 407
normal 277
principle of 274
printout of 279
quantification of 277

Index   **435**

Goldmann-Favre syndrome 208
Goniogram 254
Goniolens
   application of 248
   obliterates cornea 246*f*
Gonioscopes 255
   sterilization of 254
Gonioscopy 64, 245, 251, 253*f*, 255
   abnormal angles on 252
   documentation of 254
   grading systems 249
   indentation 247, 248*fc*, 255
Goniosynechiae 253, 253*f*, 255
Gore-Tex strips 48
Gormaz exophthalmometers 4
Gorovoy irrigating stripper 15
Graft holder 144, 144*f*
Graft insertion 150, 151
Gram's stain 377, 378
Granit C-wave component 205
Granit P-II component 205
Granular dystrophy 101*f*, 121, 363*f*
   hyaline deposits of 60*f*
Granulomatous reaction 359
Grasping instruments 146
Green's hook 351, 351*f*
Green-light fundus
      autofluorescence 238
Grocott-Gomori methenamine 377
Ground electrodes 207
Guarded diamond knife 149
Guided progression analysis 293*f*, 315, 317*f*, 420, 420*f*
Guillotine type cutters 222
Gullstrand's illumination system 57

H

Haidinger brushes 341
Haller's layer 193
Handheld 143*f*
   keratometers 147
   slit lamp 151
Hanna trephine system 144
Haploscopic principle 330*f*, 344
Harbor trachoma infections 399
Hartmann-Shack aberrometer 88, 215
Hasner valve 52
Healed trachoma 59*f*
Healthy corneal donor tissue, specular microscopy of 118*f*
Heidelberg retina 324
   tomograph 318, 318*f*, 319*f*
      principle of 324
      printout 320*f*, 324

Heijl-Krakau method 282
Helmholtz doubling principle keratometer 69
Hemangioma 41
Hemangiopericytoma 15, 18
Hematoxylin 368*f*, 371*f*
Hemianopia 278*f*, 407
Hemispheric asymmetry 305
Hemorrhage 16*f*, 17*f*, 48, 50
   intraocular 22*f*
   intraretinal 242*f*
   scattered 191*f*
   subacute 11
   vitreous 37, 38*f*
Hemorrhagic choroidal detachment 37*f*
Hemostasis 49, 50
Hemostatic forceps 45, 45*f*, 326, 327*f*, 351
Henle's layer 193
Herbert's pits 59*f*
Hering's law 330
Herpes simplex virus 382
Hertel's exophthalmometer 3, 4, 4*f*
   advantages of 5
   disadvantages of 5
Hess chart 330, 331*f*, 332, 333*f*, 334*f*, 335
Hess screen 330, 332
Hessburg-Barron trephine 143, 143*f*
Higher-order aberrations 84
Hodapp-Parrish-Anderson classification 285, 285*t*
Hodgkin's lymphoma 25
Holocrine secretion 371
Homonymous hemianopia 408*f*
Hooks 147
Horizontal iris width 159
Horizontal specular microscope 114*f*
Horner's muscle 53
Hounsfield units 10
Hruby lens 65
Human papillomavirus 370
Humphrey field analyzer 280*f*
   examination targets 281*f*
   gaze tracker of 280*f*
Humphrey perimeter 285
Humphrey visual field 280, 282*t*, 283*f*, 286*f*-291*f*, 294*f*, 419*f*
   components of 280
   interpretation of 415
   printout 295
   strategies for 282
Hydrodelineation 173

Hydrodissection 173
Hydrogen 10
   peroxide 259
Hydroxychloroquine 210
Hyperchromatic cuboidal cells 374
Hyperechoic center suggesting scolex 30*f*
Hyperfluorescence 185, 186*f*
Hyperkeratosis 360
Hypermetropia 177
Hyperplasia 360
Hyper-reflective
   foci 196
   lesion 424
Hyper-reflectivity, causes of 194*t*
Hypertrophy 360
Hypofluorescence 185, 186*f*
Hyporeflectivity, causes of 194*t*
Hysteresis 136

I

Idiopathic blind spot enlargement, acute 210
Idiopathic orbital inflammation 15, 25, 26, 28, 28*f*
Illumination
   focal 58
   methods of 58
   modification 392
   system 57, 178
Imbert-Fick's law 256, 257*f*
   modification of 257*f*
   modified 257
Immersion scan 165, 165*f*
Immunodiagnostic methods 382
Immunohistochemical stain synaptophysin 368*f*
Immunohistochemistry 364
   antibodies 364*t*
Implant
   migration of 50
   types of 50, 51
Implantable collamer lens 106*f*
In situ hybridization 365
In vivo confocal microscopy 382
Indian Council of Medical Research 386
Indian Smith method 174
Indirect carotid-cavernous fistula 27, 27*t*
Indirect goniolenses 246, 248*t*
   features of 248
Indirect gonioscopy 248
   advantages of 248
   disadvantages of 248

Indirect illumination 60, 62
Indirect ophthalmoscope 176f, 181, 181t, 396
  parts of 176
Indocyanine green 184, 202
  administration of 202
  angiography 202, 238
  disadvantages of 203
  dye 202, 202t
  frame 203f
  phases of 202
Infections 48, 50
  adnexal 376
  chronic low-grade 359
  iatrogenic 375, 376
  nosocomial 375
  ocular 375
  parasitic 367
  postseptal 15
Inferior nasal step 286f
Inferior oblique
  strengthening procedures, types of 354
  weakening procedures, types of 353
Inferonasal quadrant 190f
Inferotemporal
  disc hemorrhage 269f
  quadrants 302
  retinal nerve fiber layer thinning 315f
Infiltrative diseases 15, 27
Inflammation 48
  intraocular 119
  optical 25
Inflammatory cells 360
Infusion cannula 222, 222f
Inherited retinal dystrophies 199
Injectable botulinum toxin 48
Inkblot pattern 186
Inner nuclear layer 193, 194f
Inner plexiform layer 193, 194f
Inner segment-outer segment junction 194f
Intensity-based techniques 228
Interdigitation zone 193
Intermediate retinal capillary plexus 231
Internal carotid artery 27
Internal eye 98f
  aberrations 97f
Internal limiting membrane 193, 194f, 308f, 311f
  forceps 223, 223f
Internal optics 91f
  balancing of 97

International Society of Clinical Electrophysiology of Vision 204, 206
International Widefield Imaging Study Group 237
Intracapsular cataract extraction 120, 167
Intraconal lesions 15
Intraconal metastasis 17
Intracorneal ring segment 84
  implantation 84, 123
Intradermal nevus 365, 366f
Intralesional steroid 51
Intramuscular metastases 27
Intraocular foreign body 29, 34, 38, 39f
Intraocular lens 92, 137, 153, 154f, 156-158, 297, 377
  dialer 171, 171f
  holding forceps 171, 171f
  master 153
    interpretation of 154
Intraocular malignancy 48
Intraocular mass 20, 21f, 22f
Intraocular metastatic lung cancer 20f
Intraocular pressure 56, 80f, 253, 256, 262
  compensation 141
  normal range of 264
  power calculation 82
Intraoperative lid height 47
Intraorbital foreign body 29
Intraorbital schwannoma 17f
Intraretinal microvascular abnormalities 187
Intubation tubes, different types of 54
IOLMaster 153f, 154f, 155, 156, 156f, 156t, 157, 157f, 157t, 158
  state advantages of 155
Iowa PK press corneal punch 145
Iridociliary sulcus, obliteration of 299f
Iridocorneal endothelial
  cells 410f
  syndrome 119, 120
Iridofundal coloboma 172
Iris 60f, 252, 352
  adhesion of 253f
  configuration 254
  cyst 299f
  insertion, site of 250f
  posterior bowing of 109f
  processes 253f, 255
  root, insertion of 250

Irisophake method 174
Irregular corneal astigmatism, detection of 132
Irregularity index 128, 133
Irrigating vectis technique 175
Irrigating wire vectis 168, 168f
Ischemia, peripheral 241
Ischemic index 241
Isopropyl alcohol 259
iTrace aberrometer 88, 88f
iTrace system 88

J

Jaeger's lid spatula 44, 45f
Jameson's hook 351, 352f
Jameson's muscle forceps 352, 352f
Javal-Schiotz keratometer 69
Josephberg-Besser scleral depressor 178f
Junctional nevus 366
Juvenile X-linked retinoschisis 240

K

Kaufmann corneal cutting block 144
Kelly's punch 328, 328f
Kelman's christmas-tree approach 173
Kelman's tip 172
Kelman-McPherson forceps 329
Keratitis 111
  infective 102, 376
Keratoacanthoma 370
Keratoconus 59f, 108, 119, 132f, 136, 139
  advanced 140f
  anterior segment optical coherence tomography classification of 108
  diagnosis of 133, 138
  early detection of 108
  eyes 102
  monitoring of 138
  Orbscan map of 132
Keratocytes 363f
Keratomes 166, 167f
Keratometer 68, 71, 147
  correct alignment in 70f
  disadvantages of 71
  incorrect alignment in 70f
  normal range of 71
  one-position 69
  parts of 69
  principle of 69, 71
  two-position 69
  types of 69

Keratometry 69, 70, 128, 159
　abnormal 79
　normal 70
　types of 71
Keratopathy 47
Keratoplasty 142
Kernel
　first-order 210
　second-order 210
Kerrison bone punch 46, 47*f*
Kinetic perimetry 274, 279
　principle of 274
King's clamp 148, 148*f*
Kissing birds 74
Kissing choroids 37*f*
Knapp procedure 354
Koeppe lens 246, 246*f*

L

Lacrimal gland 12, 19, 28*f*, 360
　lesions 19
　tumor 372
　　malignant 373
　atrophy of 360
　part of 372
　mass 15, 19*f*
Lacrimal pump 52, 53*f*
　mechanism, muscles of 53
Lacrimal sac 55
　curette 47*f*
　dimensions 52
　dissector 46, 47*f*
　parts 52
　tumor 55
Lacrimal system, infections of 376
Lagophthalmos 47
Lamellar dissection 152
Lamellar keratoplasty 148
Lamina cribrosa 368
Lamina papyracea 29*f*
Laminar dot sign 271
Lang test 348
Laser
　Doppler interferometry 123
　patterns of 213*f*
　peripheral iridotomy 264
Laser-assisted in situ
　　keratomileusis 77, 93*f*
Lateral orbital rim fractures 5
Lattice corneal dystrophy 119
Lattice dystrophy 121, 363*f*
Leber's congenital amaurosis 208
Leber's hereditary optic
　　neuropathy 191
Led bulbs 182
Lees chart 332

Lees screen 330-332
Leiberman single point cutter 144
Lens 92, 98*f*, 177
　capsule 171
　coupling fluid 113
　hook 353
　opacity classification system III
　　105
　spatula 168, 168*f*
　thickness 157, 159
　types of 248
Lens-induced secondary angle
　　closure glaucoma 111
LenStar 155, 156, 156*t*, 159, 159*f*
　over IOLMaster, advantages of
　　160
　principle of 160
Lenticonus 94
Lesions
　malignant 373
　premalignant 370
Leukoma, adherent 111*f*
Levator
　function 47
　muscle resection 47
Lid
　clamp 44, 45*f*
　contour abnormalities 47
　crease 47
　infections of 375
　lag 47
　retraction 6
　speculum 351
Lieberman gravity-action
　　punch 145
Light 392
　probe 151
Lim's forceps 326, 327*f*, 352, 352*f*
Limbal dermoid 300
Limbus 353
Linear optical coherence
　　tomography 242*f*
Lipogranulomatous inflammation,
　　chronic 366
Liquid-crystal display 350
Littmann Galilean telescope 57
Lowenstein-Jensen medium 381
Lower-order aberration 94
Low-vision 384, 389, 394
　functional 390
　magnitude of 390
　professionals 393*t*
　rehabilitation 390
　services 391
Loyez stain 362
Luedde's exophthalmometer 4,
　　5, 5*f*

Luminescence 182
Lymphangioma 16, 16*f*
Lymphocytes 359
Lymphoid hyperplasia 25
　atypical 25
Lymphoma 27
Lymphoproliferative disease 15,
　　17, 25, 27, 28

M

Mackay-Marg principle 259
Macula 35
Macular branch retinal vein
　　occlusion 191*f*
Macular corneal dystrophy 364
Macular degenerations 219
Macular dystrophy 363*f*
Macular edema 423, 424*f*
Macular hemorrhages 191*f*
Macular hole 196, 219
　full-thickness 424*f*
Macular neovascularization 234
Macular neuropathy, acute 210,
　　217
Macular optical coherence
　　tomography scan,
　　normal 423*f*
Macular telangiectasia 234
Macular thickness analysis 305
Macular threshold test 292*f*
Maddox rod test 342, 343
Maddox slides 341
Magnetic resonance 11
　angiography 27
　imaging 10, 14, 18*f*, 20*f*
　　contrast media 11
　　sequences 13
Malignant glaucoma 301
　features of 301
Manipulation gonioscopy 247,
　　248*f c*, 255
Manual optical pachymetry 123
Mass lesions 14
Massive choroidal invasion 368,
　　369*f*
Masson's trichrome stain 362, 363*f*
Mast cells 359
Maxillary sinus 30*f*
McNeill-Goldman ring 142, 142*f*
McPherson's forceps 147*f*, 170,
　　170*f*, 329*f*
Mechanical support system 57
Medial angular dermoid 17*f*
Meibomian glands 366, 371

Index

Meibomitis 376
Melanin 11, 366f
Melanocyte-associated
    retinopathy 208
Melanoma 15, 41
  cells 369f
Melles stripper 15
Membrane peeling procedures 201
Meningioma 15, 24
Metaplasia 360, 371
Metastasis 15, 20, 27, 41
Methemoglobin 11
Methenamine silver stain 372
Michelson interferometer 157, 228
Microaneurysms 187, 233f
Microangiography, optical 228
Microbiology
  methods 377
  ocular 375
  role of 375
Microincision vitrectomy
  surgery 225
  advantages of 226
  disadvantages of 226
Microkeratome 149f
Microphthalmia, bilateral 22f
Microphthalmos 48
Microscope 61, 62
Microscopy 123, 377
Microsporidia 382
Microvectis technique 175
Microvitreoretinal blade 167, 328, 328f
Midperipheral iris 299f
Minimally invasive glaucoma
  surgery 246
Mixed signal-based
  techniques 228
Mixed-cell melanoma 369f
Mobility assistive devices 392
Modern-day slit-lamp
  biomicroscopy 56
Modulation transfer function 89
Mohs' micrographic surgery 361
Molecular methods 365, 382
Monocanalicular stents 54
Monochromatic slit-light,
  ultraviolet 73
Monofilament nylon 48
Moorefield's regression analysis
  321, 322, 322f
Moria's 148f
Mosquito forceps 351
Motion artifacts 230f
Moutsouris sign 151
Mucocele 20

Mucosa-associated lymphoid
  tissue 25
Mule's evisceration spatula 45, 46f
Müller's cell membrane 205
Müller's muscle 48
  resection 47
Multifocal central serous
  chorioretinopathy 426f
Multifocal electroretinogram 209, 210
Multiple corneal foreign bodies 59f
Multiple evanescent white dot
  syndrome 210
Multiple horse shoe tears 241f
Multiple papillary infoldings 366f
Multiple stromal
  cornea opacities 101f
  fluid clefts 104f
Multispot laser 212
  neodymium-doped yttrium
    aluminum garnet 212
  system 212
Mycobacteria 379, 381
Mycotic keratitis 363f
Myocardial infarction 183
Myocysticercus 15, 30f
Myoid zone 193
Myopia 98, 99
  pathological 243
  unilateral high 6

N

Naffziger's view 6
Nagahara technique 174
Nasolacrimal duct
  obstruction, congenital 55
  system 52
Natamycin 383
National Blindness and Visual
  Impairment Survey 387t
National Blindness Survey 385, 395, 396, 402f
National Programme for Control
  of Blindness and Visual
  Impairment 394
National Trachoma Prevalence
  Survey 398
Naugle's exophthalmometer 4, 5, 5f
Nausea 183
Near stereoacuity 348
  tests for 344
Necrosis 17f
Needle-assisted technique 150
Neisseria infection 378

Neodymium-doped yttrium
  aluminum garnet laser 212
Neonatal intensive care units 388
Neoplasia 360
Neovascular age-related macular
  degeneration 234
Nerve fiber layer 193, 321
  capillary plexus 231, 232f
Nerve palsy 333f
Netherlands organization test 344, 345f
Nettleship's punctum dilator 45, 46f
Neuroblastoma, metastatic 19f
Neurofibromatosis 23, 29f
Neuromyelitis optica 24
Neuro-ophthalmology 191, 330
Neuroretinal rim 265f, 266, 267f, 268f, 270f, 273, 308f, 309f, 316f, 319f, 321
  color 266
  pallor 266
  shape 266
Neurosensory detachment 196, 408, 424, 425f
Neurosyphilis 408
Nevus
  cells 366, 366f
  benign tumors of 365
  congenital 366
NGENUITY 3D visualization
  system 227f
Nocardia 379
Nonarteritic anterior ischemic
  optic neuropathy 191, 266
Noncontact specular
  microscope 113
Noncontact tonometer 260f
Noncontact trephines 144
Nonglaucomatous optic
  atrophy 273
  neuropathy 266, 272
Non-neovascular age-related
  macular degeneration 234
Nonproliferative diabetic
  retinopathy 187, 426, 426f
  mild 187
  moderate 187
  severe 187
Nontoothed forceps 146
Normal cornea 411f
  against best-fit sphere 76f

endothelial cell 409f
endothelium, specular
    microscopy of 116f
Normative stereometric parameter 321t
Nucleus drop 43, 43f
Nutrient agar 381
Nylon 48

O

Oblique parasagittal T1-weighted fat suppressed postcontrast magnetic resonance imaging 15f
Oblique sagittal T2-weight magnetic resonance imaging 24f
Octopus perimeter 295
Ocular adnexal lymphoma 25
Ocular diseases 56
Ocular histopathology, special stains in 362t
Ocular infections 375, 376t
    barriers to 376t
Ocular pathology 360
Ocular response analyzer 123, 124, 136, 260, 260f
Ocular surface
    diseases 103
    evaluate tumors of 299
    flora, normal 375
    keratinization of 360
    squamous neoplasia 103
Oculocardiac reflex 48, 354
Oculoplasty 3, 44
Olson calibrated cornea trephine system 143
Open funnel retinal detachment 36f
Ophthalmic surveys 395
Ophthalmic ultrasound 31
Ophthalmitis, sympathetic 48
Ophthalmological surveys, uses of 395
Ophthalmology 15, 23, 365, 375, 382, 384, 395
Ophthalmoscope 176
    modifications of 181
Optic atrophy 268f
Optic cup 264, 268, 321
    changes 269
    depth 269
    shape 268
    size 268
Optic disc 265f, 268f, 272, 273, 313
    Bruch's membrane 308f
    cube 306

documentation of 272f
drusen 39, 40f
hemorrhages 264, 269
large 265f
shape 266
size 265
stereometric analysis of 321
Optic glioma 23
Optic nerve 12, 15f, 22f, 24f, 25f, 49, 361
    glioma, postcontrast magnetic resonance imaging of 24f
    head 35, 264, 267f, 272, 308f, 310f, 369f
        analysis 306, 313
        cupping, early 40f
        evaluation 264
        findings 272
        morphology, documentation of 272
        normal 265f
    infiltration 361f
    parameters 302
    pathologies 39
    sheath
        complex lesions 8, 23
        meningioma 23
Optic neuritis 14, 15, 24, 279f, 408
    bilateral 25f
Optic neuropathy 220
    glaucomatous 273t
    nonglaucomatous 273t
Optic sheath meningioma 24f
Optical biometry 159f
Optical coherence tomography 99, 103f, 105f, 106f, 108, 157, 189f, 192-194, 194f, 216, 238, 242f, 302, 310f-312f, 314f, 315, 315f, 317
    angiography 199, 227, 427f
        advantages of 231
        algorithms 228
        clinical applications of 233
        findings, interpretation of 231
        imaging artifacts 229
        limitations of 231
        ratio analysis 229
        segmentation 232f
        interpretation of 193
        intraoperative 102, 201
        normal layers in 194f
        parameters 302
        pitfalls of 313

principle of 317
recent advances in 199
types of 192, 193t
Optical low coherence interferometry 123, 124, 159
Optical principle 113, 179
Optical slit section 58
Optos 237, 239
    silverstone swept source OCT 238
Orbit
    anterior two-thirds of 35
    disorders of 3
    protocol 13
    solitary fibrous tumor of 18
Orbital bone lesions 19
Orbital capillary hemangioma 18f
Orbital flow fracture, Hess chart of 335f
Orbital imaging techniques 3, 7
Orbital plexiform neurofibroma 29f
Orbital schwannoma 17
Orbital ultrasound 8f
Orbitopathy, thyroid-associated 15, 25
Orbscan 72, 85, 86, 86t, 127, 132f, 133, 134, 134t
    early keratoconus on 134t
    pachymetry over ultrasonic pachymeter, advantages of 133
    quad map 131f
    scanning slit imaging in 127f
Orthoptic
    exercises 341
    instrument 337
Ostium, site of 53
Ota nevus 366
Outer nuclear layer 193, 194f
Outer plexiform layer 193
Outer retinal tabulation 196
Overpass phenomenon 271

P

Pachycam 123
Pachymeter probe 123f
Pachymetry 122, 134
    abnormal 80
    map 76, 131
    measurements, techniques of 123
    methods of 123
    techniques of 123, 124fc

Painful blind eye 48
Palmaris longus tendon 48
Panographic principle 344
Panophthalmitis 14, 376
Panretinal photocoagulation 240
Panstromal scar 108
Panum's area 347
Paraffin embedding 361
Parakeratosis 360
Parakeratotic cells 370
Parasites 376
Pars
    ciliaris 53
    lacrimalis 53
    plana vitrectomy 120
Partial coherence interferometry 123, 157, 158
Pascal 577 nm laser 214
Pascal dynamic contour tonometer 260
Pascal laser spots 213f
Pascal red laser 214
Paton spatula 144, 144f
Pattern deviation probability plot 284
Pattern electroretinogram, uses of 209
Pattern scanning laser trabeculoplasty 214
    gonioscopic lens 214
Pattern standard deviation 292f-294f
Paufique's knife 148, 149f
Pellicle beamsplitter 89f
Pellucid marginal corneal degeneration 74, 83f, 414f
Penetrating keratoplasty 101, 120, 422f
Penicillium species 380f
Pentacam 72, 72f, 73, 85, 86, 86t, 123, 134, 134t
    Belin 81f
    corneal rings in 85f
    indications of 79
    interpretation of 410
    nucleus staging 82
    parameters 82, 85
    topography system 85
Perfluorocarbon 165
    liquid 224
Perfusion density 229
Perimetric unit 280
Perimetry 274, 280
    types of 274

Periodic acid-Schiff stain 362, 372
Peripapillary atrophy 271, 271f, 272f
Peripapillary chorioretinal atrophy 271
Peripheral choroidal neovascularization 240
Peripheral exudative hemorrhagic chorioretinopathy 240
Peripheral iridotomy 298
Peripheral iris, configuration of 250
Peripheral retinal degeneration 242, 242f
Peripheral vessel leakage 240
Perkins applanation tonometer 259, 259f
Perl's prussian blue stain 362
Persistent fetal vasculature 38, 38f
Persistent hyperplastic primary vitreous 8, 8f
Phaco needle tip 171, 171f
Phacofracture technique 175
Phacosandwich technique 175
Phakic intraocular lens 201, 422f
Phakic lens 154
Phosphorescence 182
Photodynamic therapy 203
Photopic electroretinogram 206f
Photoreceptor
    density 217
    outer segment of 193
Phototherapeutic keratectomy 123
Phthisis bulbi 50
Pierse-Hoskins forceps 146, 146f, 353, 353f
Pigment dispersion syndrome 107, 109, 109f, 252, 254, 298, 299f
Pigmentary glaucoma 254
Pituitary adenoma 291f
Placido disc 72, 133
Plain curved scissors 352
Plain forceps 45, 45f, 326, 326f
Plain straight scissors 352
Plasma cells 359
Plastic embedding 361
Plateau iris syndrome 298, 299f
Platelet derived growth factor 212
Pleomorphic adenoma 19f, 372, 373f
Pleomorphism 115, 409
Plexiform neurofibroma 15, 28
Pneumatic cutters 222
Polack double corneal forceps 147f
Polyester mesh 48

Polyfilament 48
Polymerase chain reaction 365, 382
Polymethyl methacrylate 50
Polymorphonuclear leukocytes 359
Polypoidal choroidal neovascularization 199f
    vasculopathy 203, 203f
Polypropylene 48
Polytetrafluoroethylene 48
Positron emission tomography 14
Postenucleation socket syndrome 50
Posterior anterior lamellar therapeutic keratoplasty 101f
Posterior capsular opacification 387
Posterior corneal power 71
Posterior elevation
    abnormal 80
    map 134
Posterior polymorphous corneal dystrophy 116, 119
Posterior segment procedures 201
Posterior subcapsular cataract 156, 157
Posterior trabecular meshwork 254f
Posterior vitreous detachment 20, 35, 35t, 36, 37f, 270
Post-keratoplasty 125, 263
Post-laser peripheral iridotomy 106
Post-laser-assisted in situ keratomileusis
    ectasia 83f
    eyes 263
Post-refractive surgery biomechanics 137
Potassium hydroxide 377, 379, 379f
    wet mount 378
Power calculation formula 154f
Power map 134
Prager scleral shell 165, 165f
Pre-laser peripheral iridotomy 106
Prematurity, retinopathy of 22f, 192, 240, 388
Preseptal soft tissues 28f
Primary angle-closure
    disease 252
    glaucoma 110f
Primitive cells 376
Prism, cleaning of 259
Projection artifacts 230f

Index

Prokaryotes 376, 377
Prokaryotic cells 376
Prolene 48
Proliferative diabetic retinopathy 187, 213f, 233, 242f, 426, 426f
Proliferative vitreoretinopathy 300, 360
Proparacaine eye drops 248
Proptosis 6
    abaxial 19f, 20f
Prototype surgical lens 246
Pseudoexfoliation syndrome 58f
Pseudofluorescence 183
Pseudoplateau iris 301
Pseudoproptosis, causes of 6
Ptosis 47, 50, 278f
    amount of 47
    clamp, complications of 48
    nonsurgical management of 48
    residual 48
    surgery, complications of 47
    types of 47
Pupil
    diameter 128
    size of 207
Putterman müllerectomy 47
Pyogenic granuloma 360

Q

Quadrantanopia, inferior 407f
Qualitative keratometers 147
Quantitative analysis 115

R

RAAB-6 software 403
Radial keratotomy marker 142, 142f
Randot stereotest 346, 348f, 349f
    animals of 349f
Ray-tracing aberrometry 88
    advantages of 94
Rebound tonometer 261, 261f
Recti 354
    muscles 353
Recurrent strabismus 354
Red-green glasses 343
Red-green spectacles 345f
Refractive errors 386, 394
    rapid assessment method of 396
    uncorrected 384
Refractive surgery 71, 80, 105, 125, 137
    screening 139

Rehabilitation 389
Reichert technologies 259
Reinfection 375
Reis-Bücklers dystrophy 121
Relative afferent pupillary defect 23, 181, 273
Resorcinol phthalein sodium 183
Resuscitation, cardiopulmonary 48
Retina 176, 191f
    healthy 232f
    layer of 315f
    pediatric 240, 241
Retinal artery occlusions 233
Retinal detachment 9, 20, 20f, 35, 35f, 35t, 36f, 41, 44f, 165, 240, 241, 241f
Retinal ganglion cells, degeneration of 264
Retinal inner layers, disorganization of 196
Retinal layers 423
    splitting of 242f
Retinal nerve fiber layer 194f, 264, 269f, 270f, 272f, 304f, 306t, 307f-311f, 315f, 317f, 423
    analysis 302
    defects 270
    graph 321
    optical coherence tomography scan 315
    parameters 302
    printout 306
    thickness 303, 322
    temporal-superior-nasal-inferior-temporal graph of 305
    thinning, progressive superior 317f
Retinal optical coherence tomography, interpretation of 422
Retinal pigment epithelium 60, 184, 186f, 193, 194f, 423
    metaplasia of 360
Retinal spot diagram 89f
Retinal thickness 159
    map 195f
Retinal vascular occlusions 241
Retinal vein occlusion 192, 233
Retinoblastoma 15, 21, 22, 42f, 299, 360, 361f, 367, 368, 368f
    features of 42
    intraocular 361f

Retinopathy, melanoma-associated 210
Retinoschisis, peripheral 241, 242f
Retrobulbar fat 28f
Retrochiasmal lesions 408
Retroillumination 59, 62
Retrolaminar invasion 369f
Rhabdomyosarcoma 15, 18, 29
Rhegmatogenous retinal detachment 35
Rhinosporidiosis 371, 372f
    seeberi 371
        numerous sporangia of 372f
Rhizopus 379, 380f
Right eye 205f, 206f, 208f
    inferior retina of 213f
Riolan muscle 53
Root mean square 90
Rosenmüller valve 52
Rothman-Gilbard corneal punch 145
RPC classification 250
Ruit's technique 175
Ruler method 6

S

Sabouraud's dextrose agar 381, 381f
Sagittal curvature map 131
Sanders-Retzlaff-Kraff formula 163
Sarcoidosis 15, 25, 27, 359, 367
Sattler's layer 193
Scale readings 5
Scanning laser ophthalmoscopy 215, 216
Scanning slit
    system 127
    technology 123
Scheimpflug camera 124
Scheimpflug imaging 137
Scheimpflug principle 73f
Schepens scleral depressor 177f
Schiotz tonometer 256, 261f
Schlemm's canal 106
Schocket scleral depressor 225, 225f
Schwalbe's line 106, 251, 252, 253f
Schwannoma 15
Sclera
    choroidal junction 423
    holding flaps of 352
Scleral bands 377
Scleral dissection depth 201
Scleral flap 328
Scleral indentation 177
Scleral spur 252, 253f, 254f

Scleral tonometry 263
Scleral type lens 246, 248
Scleritis, posterior 39, 40*f*
Sclerotic scatter 59, 62, 63
Scotoma 295
  density of 407
  edges of 275
Scotopic electroretinogram 206*f*
Sebaceous cell carcinoma 371, 372*f*
Sebaceous glands 366, 371
Segmentation artifact 230
Seidel's scotoma 277*f*
Seizures 183
Selective laser trabeculoplasty 246
Self-retaining Barraquer eye speculum 351, 351*f*
Self-retaining infusion cannulas 222
Senile keratosis 370
Sepsis, active abdominal 23*f*
Serrated forceps 223, 223*f*
Shadow artifact 230, 231*f*
Shaffer's angle width determination 249*f*
Shaffer's system 249, 249*t*
Shallow retinal detachment 242*f*
Shepard percentage 349
Sherrington's law 330
Short inversion time inversion recovery 24
Sildenafil 210
Silicon
  brush tip cannula 224
  nonabsorbable sutures 48
  oil-filled eye 164
  sleeve 172
Silver methenamine stain 362, 363*f*, 364
Silver nitrate stain 377
Simcoe's cannula 169
Simcoe's irrigation 169, 169*f*
Simultaneous perception slides 339*f*, 340*f*
Single-photon
  cutting trephines 144
  emission computed tomography 14
Sinonasal masses 15
Sinskey hook 147*f*, 150, 171, 171*f*
  reverse 150, 150*f*
Skewed radial axis 75*f*, 82
Skin biopsy punches 143
Slab subtraction method 230
Sleep time intraocular pressure recording 264

Slides, types of 338
Sling surgery, materials for 48
Slit beam 61, 62
Slit scanning 127, 133
  technologies 133*t*
Slit-lamp 56, 65
  biomicroscopy 56, 61, 265
  examination 65*f*
  different filters in 66
  examination 63
    different techniques of 61*t*
    method of 61, 62
  grading of flare on 67*t*
  illumination, basic principles of 58
  optical principle of 57*f*
  parts of 56, 56*f*
Slow-flow venous malformation 15
Small incision
  cataract surgery 120, 168
  lenticule extraction 77
Smith's technique 168
Smock stack pattern 186
Snellen's E letter 96*f*
Snellen's entropion clamp 44, 45*f*
Snellen's letter 90, 92*f*
Socket contracture 50
Sodium
  fluorescein 66, 183
  hypochlorite 259
Soft calcium 11
Soft silicone tip cannula 224, 224*f*
Soft-shell technique 173
Soft-tissue
  mass 29*f*
  window 30*f*
Software system 215
Solar keratosis 370
Solid tumor 42
Spaeth grading
  angle pigmentation 251*f*
  angle width 250*f*
  peripheral iris curvature 250*f*
Spaeth system 249, 250*t*
Spatulas 147
Spectral-domain
  anterior segment optical coherence tomography 108*t*
  optical coherence tomography 192
Spectralis 239
  optical coherence tomography 316*f*
Specular endothelium 61*f*
Specular microscope 67, 112, 120, 121, 123

principle of 118
types of 113
Specular microscopy 112*f*, 116*f*, 119, 120
  interpretation of 409
Specular reflection 60, 62, 113*f*
Spheroidal degeneration, recurrence of 60*f*
Spindle-cell melanoma 369*f*
Spirochetes 377
Split-spectrum amplitude decorrelation angiography 229
Sporangia 372
Squamous cell carcinoma 370, 371*f*
Squint 330
  surgery 107, 351
  complications of 353
S-shaped iris 299*f*
S-stamp 151*f*
Standard automated perimetry 280
Staphylococcus species 378*f*
Staphyloma, posterior 39, 39*f*, 164
Staphylomatous globe 50
Stargardt's disease 199, 199*f*, 408
Static perimetry 279, 280
Steinert Descemet stripper 15
Stereo butterfly test 346
Stereo housefly card 346
Stereo tests, types of 348
Stereoacuity tests 350
Stereogram card 341
Stereopsis 340, 342, 344
  grade of 350, 350*t*
  physiologic basis of 344
  principle of tests for 344
  slides used to test 340*f*
Stevens tenotomy scissors 45, 45*f*, 352, 352*f*
Stevens-Johnson syndrome 360
Stiffness 136
  parameter 138, 139
Stimulus 207, 209
  duration of 207
  size of 407
  strength of 207
Stop-and-chop phaco 174
Strabismus 332, 354
  measurement of 338
Streptococcus pneumoniae 378
Subconjunctival ologen, bleb with 107*f*

Subepithelial corneal infiltrate 103*f*
Subfoveal choroidal thickness 196
Subluxated lens 170
Subperiosteal space 15
Subretinal injections 201
Sump syndrome 54
Superficial cells 366*f*
Superficial retinal capillary plexus 230*f*, 231, 232*f*, 234*f*
Superficial vascular
   complex 231, 232*f*
   plexus 230
Superior oblique
   palsy, Hess chart of 334*f*
   strengthening procedures, types of 354
   weakening procedures, types of 354
Superior ophthalmic vein 27*f*
Superior rectus holding forceps 326, 326*f*, 352, 352*f*
Superotemporal branch retinal vein occlusion 191*f*
Superotemporal quadrant 190*f*
Surgeries, ocular 120*t*
Surgical lens 246
Swan-Jacob lens 247*f*
Swedish interactive threshold algorithm 282, 287*f*, 291*f*, 293*f*, 294*f*, 295
Swiss cheese
   appearance 373
   pattern 373*f*
Swollen left extraocular muscles 28*f*
Synaptophore 344, 337, 337*f*, 342
   principle of 342
   slides in 338*t*

T

T sign 40*f*
Taenia solium 366
Tarsus muscle resection 47
Tear film
   assessment 109
   breakup 71
Tear meniscus 105*f*
Teflon block 144*f*
Temporal artery biopsy 361
Temporal retina 186*f*
Temporalis fascia 48
Tension glaucoma, normal 269*f*
Teratoma, benign 365
Terrien marginal degeneration 80

Therapeutic-grade corneal donor tissue, specular microscopy of 117*f*
Thickness maps 76
Thioglycollate broth 381
Thromboangiitis obliterans 26
Thrombophlebitis 183
Thyroid ophthalmopathy 14
Time-domain
   anterior segment optical coherence tomography 108*t*
   optical coherence tomography 192, 193
Tissues 14
   planes, guided identification of 201
   preparation of 361
   specimen, examination of 359
   stereotest 345
Tolosa-Hunt syndrome 28
Tonometers 263
   indentation 261
   types of 259
Tonometry 256
   types of 256, 256*fc*
Tonopen 259*f*
Tooke's knife 148, 148*f*
Toothed forceps 146, 352
Topographic analysis 89
Topographic maps 93
Topographical keratoconus classification 87
Topography
   abnormal 80
   systems 133
Toric intraocular lens 65, 94*f*
Torsion 341
Total eye aberrations 96*f*
Total higher-order aberration 91*f*
Total internal reflection 245, 245*f*
Total lower-order aberration 91*f*
Total macular thickness 305
Toxic maculopathy 219
Toxic optic neuropathy 408
Toxic retinopathy 210
Trabecular meshwork 106, 252, 253*f*
Trabecular-ciliary process distance 298
Trabeculo-iris angle 298
Trabeculotome 329, 329*f*
Trachoma 388, 389, 394
   rapid assessment 396
Tractional retinal detachment 36, 36*f*

Tram-tracking sign 24
Transcanalicular endoscopic dacryocystorhinostomy 53
Transcutaneous levator advancement 47
Transillumination 362
Transpalpebral tonometer 262
Trauma 48
   ocular 105
   orbital 30
Traumatic contusion 15
Traumatic injury, severe 50
Tripod fracture 9*f*
Tri-soft shell technique 173
Trocar 221, 221*f*
   cannula 225, 226, 226*t*
Troutman corneal punch 144
Tscherning's aberrometry 88
T-sign 39
Tuberculosis 55, 359, 367
Tumor
   benign 14, 365
   cells 368*f*, 373*f*
      cytoplasmic positivity in 368*f*
      peripheral palisading of 370*f*
   cribriform appearance of 373*f*
   intraocular 41, 41*t*, 367
   island, center of 372*f*
   malignant 14
   pigmented 365

U

Ultimate soft-shell technique 173
Ultrahigh-resolution
   anterior segment optical coherence tomography 100*f*
   optical coherence tomography 100
Ultrasonic pachymeter 122
Ultrasonic probe 162*f*
Ultrasonography 21, 31
   display 32*f*
   orientation of 32*f*
   probe 32*f*
Ultrasound 8
   biomicroscopy 9, 34, 100, 124, 296, 296*f*, 297*f*, 300, 301, 301*t*
      angle parameters measured on 298*f*
      role of 300
   high-frequency 34

Ultra-widefield
fluorescein angiography 191, 240
optical coherence tomography 199, 241
Unstable angina 183
Utrata capsulorhexis forceps 170, 170f
Uvea 176
Uveal malignant melanoma 368
Uveal melanoma 21, 21f, 48
Uveal tract, malignant melanoma of 368
Uveitis 241
chronic 359
infectious 376
pediatric 240

V

Valved small-gauge cannulas 226
van Gieson stain 363
Vannas scissors 167, 168f, 328, 328f
Vascular analysis 217
Vascular filling defects 185
Vascular lesions 14
Vascular occlusion 190
Vasovagal attacks 183
Vectographic principle 344
Vector A-scan 34
Veldman Venn technique 151
Venolymphatic malformation 15, 16, 16f
Venous phase angiogram 190f
Venous varix 15, 16
Verhoff distance 349
Vernal keratoconjunctivitis 79
Vertical axis 77
Vertical cup 269
Vessel
bayoneting of 271
diameter index 229
large 271
length density 229
Vigabatrin 210
Viscoelasticity 136
Viscoexpression 175
Vision 92f
fields of 391t
hill of 274f, 279

Vision 2020: right to sight 392
Visual acuity 385
Visual disability
certification 390
concept of 389
Visual field
frequency of 295
index 283f, 284, 286f-291f, 293f, 294f
loss 285t
grading of 285
patterns of 285
normal 274
part of 220
progression 285
testing, indications of 280
Visual function analysis summary display 92
Visual impairment
causes of 385
rapid assessment of 396
Visual rehabilitation 390, 392
Visual substitution devices 392
Visually evoked potentials 208
Vitrectomy 227
cutter 222, 222f
speed of 227
mode 222
Vitreomacular adhesion 197
Vitreomacular traction 198f
disorders 197, 219
epiretinal membrane with 198f
Vitreoretinal instruments 221
Vitreoretinal interface 423
Vitreoretinal scissors 225, 225f
Vitreoretinal status 35
Vitreoretinal surgery 225
Vitreoretinal traction 197
Vitreous 423
cutters 222
hemorrhage 37, 38f
loss 169
tap 361, 377
V-Lance blade 167
Vogt's technique 173
Vomiting 183
von Graefe's hook 353, 353f
von Graefe's knife 166, 166f

von Kossa stain 362
Voriconazole 383

W

Wavefront
analysis 89
screens 92
comparison map 93
sensor 215
verification display 89
Weakening orbicularis muscle tone 48
Well's enucleation spoon 45, 46f
Westcott conjunctival scissors 328, 328f
White-to-white diameter 153, 128, 133
Wide-field specular microscope 113
Wire speculum 326, 326f
Wire vectis 168f
method 168, 174
technique 175
World Health Organization 386
Worm's eye view 6
Worth four-dot test 343, 343f
Wound
burn 172
dehiscence 50

X

X-linked retinoschisis 208
Xylocaine 248

Y

Yoke muscle 330
Yttrium aluminum garnet capsulotomy 264

Z

Zehender exophthalmometers 4
Zeiss cirrus optical coherence tomography 304f
Zeiss four mirror lens 247f, 248
Zeiss glands 366, 371
Zernike polynomials bar graph 92
Ziehl-Neelsen stain 363, 377, 379
Zoom system 57